Management of Thyroid Nodules and Differentiated Thyroid Cancer

Sanziana A. Roman • Julie Ann Sosa
Carmen C. Solórzano
Editors

Management of Thyroid Nodules and Differentiated Thyroid Cancer

A Practical Guide

Springer

Editors
Sanziana A. Roman
Endocrine Surgery, Department of Surgery
Duke University Medical Center
Duke Cancer Institute
Durham
North Carolina
USA

Julie Ann Sosa
Department of Surgery
Duke University Medical Center
Duke Cancer Institute
Durham
North Carolina
USA

Carmen C. Solórzano
Division of Surgical Oncology and
Endocrine Surgery, Vanderbilt Endocrine
Surgery Center
Vanderbilt University Medical Center
Nashville
Tennessee
USA

ISBN 978-3-319-43616-6 ISBN 978-3-319-43618-0 (eBook)
DOI 10.1007/978-3-319-43618-0

Library of Congress Control Number: 2017931638

Printed on acid-free paper

This Springer imprint is published by Springer Nature
The registered company is Springer International Publishing AG
The registered company address is: Gewerbestrasse 11, 6330 Cham, Switzerland

Preface

Thyroid nodules are a common problem in the USA and the world. They are present in nearly 5 % of women and 1 % of men in the iodine-sufficient areas and have a much higher incidence in iodine-deficient parts of the world. With the growing use of imaging studies, such as ultrasound and computed tomography, it is estimated that more than 70 % of the adult population in the USA harbors thyroid abnormalities and nodules. While most nodules are benign, patient and physician anxiety about their presence and possible lack of familiarity with thyroid disorders can lead to either unnecessary interventions or to misdirected and inadequate treatments. Understanding the meaning of detecting such abnormalities is important for alleviating patient anxiety and undertaking the most efficient and effective diagnostic work-up and treatment.

While much has been written about thyroid nodules, we realized that a comprehensive, easy-to-follow, organized approach to understanding thyroid nodules and thyroid cancer was needed. Whether you are a primary care clinician, family practitioner, pediatrician, obstetrician/gynecologist, general endocrinologist, general surgeon, otorhinolaryngologist, nurse practitioner, physician assistant, student, trainee, or fellow, this book is designed to address numerous questions about patients with thyroid nodules and cancer. We have organized the book in specific patient presentation scenarios, ranging from small and occult thyroid nodules detected incidentally to palpable, clinical multinodular goiters, patients with benign nodules, patients with indeterminate nodules, and those with clear malignant diagnoses. It encompasses easy-to-understand diagnostic approaches, including imaging, serologic testing, and fine needle biopsies; it seeks to clarify molecular testing and to describe appropriate surgical treatment, postoperative radioactive iodine administration for differentiated thyroid cancer, and adequate thyroid hormone replacement. It describes special and often anxiety-producing patient situations such as concomitant pregnancy and thyroid nodules and cancer in children. It includes aspects of the disease which are often not discussed, such as patient quality of life after thyroid surgery and common long-term problems, and dedicates a chapter to integrative medical approaches for patients who desire such interventions.

We have brought together experts and thought leaders from the USA in the fields of thyroidology, thyroid surgery, nuclear medicine, pathology, radiology, pediatrics, and integrative medicine and have edited an up-to-date book, which we feel speaks directly to the concerns of our colleagues and our patients.

Durham, NC, USA Sanziana A. Roman, MD
Julie Ann Sosa, MD, MA
Nashville, TN, USA Carmen C. Solórzano, MD

Contents

Contributors

Erik K. Alexander, MD The Thyroid Section, Department of Medicine, Brigham & Women's Hospital and Harvard Medical School, Boston, MA, USA

Trevor E. Angell, MD The Thyroid Section, Department of Medicine, Brigham & Women's Hospital and Harvard Medical School, Boston, MA, USA

James D. Brierley, MBBS Department of Radiation Oncology, University of Toronto, Princess Margaret Cancer Centre, Toronto, ON, Canada

Denise Carneiro-Pla, MD Department of Surgery, Medical University of South Carolina, Charleston, SC, USA

M. Regina Castro, MD Division of Endocrinology, Diabetes, Metabolism, and Nutrition and Department of Internal Medicine, Mayo Clinic, Rochester, MN, USA

Joy C. Chen, MD, MS Department of Surgery, Stanford University Medical Center, Stanford, CA, USA

Kathryn E. Coan, MD Department of Surgery, Division of Surgical Oncology, Section of Endocrine Surgery, Medical College of Wisconsin, Milwaukee, WI, USA

Jennifer R. Cracchiolo, MD Department of Surgery, Head and Neck Service, Memorial Sloan Kettering Cancer Center, New York, NY, USA

Ana E. Espinosa De Ycaza, MD Endocrinology, Diabetes, Metabolism and Nutrition, Mayo Clinic, Rochester, MN, USA

Catherine A. Dinauer, MD Department of Surgery, Yale University School of Medicine, New Haven, CT, USA

Department of Pediatrics, Yale University School of Medicine, New Haven, CT, USA

Dawn M. Elfenbein, MD, MPH Department of Surgery, University of California, Irvine, Irvine, CA, USA

Nazanene H. Esfandiari, MD Internal Medicine: Metabolism, Endocrinology, & Diabetes, & Hematology/Oncology, University of Michigan, Ann Arbor, MI, USA

Paul G. Gauger, MD Division of Endocrine Surgery, Department of Surgery, University of Michigan, Ann Arbor, MI, USA

Mohiedean Ghofrani, MD Cytopathology, PeaceHealth Laboratories, Vancouver, WA, USA

Meredith E. Giuliani, MBBS, MEd Department of Radiation Oncology, University of Toronto, Princess Margaret Cancer Centre, Toronto, ON, Canada

Whitney Goldner, MD Division of Diabetes, Endocrinology and Metabolism, Department of Internal Medicine, University of Nebraska Medical Center, Omaha, NE, USA

Elizabeth Grubbs, MD Departments of Surgical Oncology, University of Texas MD Anderson Cancer Center, Houston, TX, USA

Megan R. Haymart, MD Division of Metabolism, Endocrinology, & Diabetes & Hematology/Oncology, University of Michigan Health System, Ann Arbor, MI, USA

Elizabeth H. Holt, MD, PhD Section of Endocrinology and Metabolism, Yale School of Medicine, New Haven, CT, USA

David T. Hughes, MD Division of Endocrine Surgery, Department of Surgery, University of Michigan, Ann Arbor, MI, USA

University of Michigan Hospitals and Health Centers, 2920 Taubman Center, SPC 5331, Ann Arbor, MI, USA

Electron Kebebew, MD Endocrine Oncology Branch, National Cancer Institute, National Institute of Health, Bethesda, MD, USA

Xavier Keutgen, MD Department of Surgery, Rush University Medical Center, Chicago, IL, USA

Angela M. Leung, MD, MSc Division of Endocrinology, VA Greater Los Angeles Healthcare System, UCLA David Geffen School of Medicine, Los Angeles, CA, USA

Ming Yann Lim Department of Otolaryngology, Tan Tock Seng Hospital, Singapore, Singapore

Masha Livhits, MD Endocrine Surgery, UCLA David Geffen School of Medicine, Los Angeles, CA, USA

Jonathan Mark, MD Department of Otolaryngology and Department of Internal Medicine, University of Cincinnati Medical Center, Cincinnati, OH, USA

Christopher R. McHenry, MD Case Western Reserve University School of Medicine, Department of Surgery, MetroHealth Medical Center, Cleveland, OH, USA

Naris Nilubol, MD Center for Cancer Research National Cancer Institute, Bethesda, MD, USA

Idris Tolgay Ocal, MD Pathology and Laboratory Medicine, Division of Anatomic Pathology, Department of Laboratory Medicine/Pathology, Mayo Clinic Arizona, Scottsdale, AZ, USA

Beatriz Olson, MD Endocrinology, Middlebury, CT, USA

Naykky Singh Ospina, MD Division of Endocrinology, Diabetes, Metabolism, and Nutrition and Department of Internal Medicine, Mayo Clinic, Rochester, MN, USA

Dwight H. Owen, MD Medical Oncology, Ohio State University, Columbus, OH, USA

Janice L. Pasieka, MD Department of Surgery, Sections of General Surgery and Surgical Oncology, University of Calgary, Cunning School of Medicine, Calgary, AB, Canada

Department of Surgery and Oncology, Faculty of Medicine, University of Calgary, Foothills Medical Centre, Calgary, AB, Canada

J.D. Pasternak, MD Division of General Surgery, University Health Network, Toronto, Canada

Anery Patel, MD Division of Diabetes, Endocrinology and Metabolism, Department of Internal Medicine, University of Nebraska Medical Center, Omaha, NE, USA

Snehal G. Patel, MD Department of Surgery, Division of Endocrine Surgery and Surgical Oncology, University of Pittsburgh, Pittsburgh, PA, USA

Jennifer M. Perkins, MD, MBA Division of Endocrinology, Duke University Health System, Durham, NC, USA

Scott A. Rivkees, MD Department of Pediatrics, University of Florida College of Medicine, Gainesville, FL, USA

Steven Rodgers, MD, PhD Department of Surgery, Division of Surgical Oncology, University of Miami Miller School of Medicine, Miami, FL, USA

David F. Schneider, MD, MS Section of Endocrine Surgery, Department of Surgery, University of Wisconsin, Madison, WI, USA

Ali Sepahdari, MD Radiological Sciences, Ronald Reagan UCLA Medical Center, Los Angeles, CA, USA

Manisha H. Shah, MD The Ohio State University Comprehensive Cancer Center, Arthur G. James Cancer Hospital and Richard J. Solove Research Institute, Columbus, OH, USA

Ashok R. Shaha, MD Department of Surgery, Head and Neck Service, Memorial Sloan Kettering Cancer Center, New York, NY, USA

W.T. Shen, MD Department of Surgery, Mt Zion Hospital, University of California – San Francisco, San Francisco, CA, USA

Jennifer A Sipos, MD Endocrinology and Metabolism, The Ohio State University, Columbus, OH, USA

Marius N. Stan, MD Endocrinology, Diabetes, Metabolism and Nutrition, Mayo Clinic, Rochester, MN, USA

David L. Steward, MD Department of Otolaryngology and Department of Internal Medicine, University of Cincinnati Medical Center, Cincinnati, OH, USA

Heather Stuart, MD Department of Surgery, Division of Surgical Oncology, University of Miami Miller School of Medicine, Miami, FL, USA

Department of Surgery, Sections of General Surgery and Surgical Oncology, University of Calgary, Cunning School of Medicine, Calgary, AB, Canada

Richard W. Tsang, MD Department of Radiation Oncology, University of Toronto, Princess Margaret Cancer Centre, Toronto, ON, Canada

Tracy S. Wang, MD, MPH Department of Surgery, Division of Surgical Oncology, Section of Endocrine Surgery, Medical College of Wisconsin, Milwaukee, WI, USA

Section of Endocrine Surgery, Medical College of Wisconsin, Milwaukee, WI, USA

Rebecca L. Weiss, MD Division of Endocrinology (111D), VA Greater Los Angeles Healthcare System, UCLA David Geffen School of Medicine, Los Angeles, CA, USA

James X. Wu, MD Surgery, Section of Endocrine Surgery, UCLA David Geffen School of Medicine, Los Angeles, CA, USA

Michael W. Yeh, MD Surgery, UCLA David Geffen School of Medicine, Los Angeles, CA, USA

Linwah Yip, MD Department of Surgery, Division of Endocrine Surgery and Surgical Oncology, University of Pittsburgh, Pittsburgh, PA, USA

University of Pittsburgh School of Medicine, Pittsburgh, PA, USA

Mark Zafereo, MD Departments of Head and Neck, University of Texas MD Anderson Cancer Center, Houston, TX, USA

Chapter 1
Incidence and Epidemiology

Megan R. Haymart and Nazanene H. Esfandiari

Rise in Thyroid Cancer Incidence

The incidence of thyroid cancer has tripled over the past 30 years (Fig. 1.1), with thyroid cancer now the eighth most common cancer in the United States and the fifth most common cancer in women [1–3]. Although thyroid cancers of all sizes have increased in incidence, 87 % of the rise in thyroid cancer is attributed to small papillary thyroid cancers (2 cm or smaller), which have an excellent prognosis [1]. It is estimated that in 2015, there will be 62,450 new cases of thyroid cancer but only 1,950 deaths [4]. Because of this rising incidence, thyroid cancer is projected to be the fourth most common cancer by 2030 [2, 5–9]. Not only has the incidence risen in the United States, the rise in thyroid cancer incidence has been seen across the world [10]. This rise in thyroid cancer incidence is most marked in Korea, where thyroid cancer is now the most common cancer and the incidence is close to 70/100,000 [11]. This worldwide unexplained rise in thyroid cancer incidence remains a major concern for physicians treating thyroid cancer.

The greatest rise in thyroid cancer incidence has been seen in women [12]. Women represent close to 75 % of all thyroid cancer cases and the incidence has

M.R. Haymart, MD (✉)
Division of Metabolism, Department of Internal Medicine, Endocrinology, and Diabetes and Hematology/Oncology, University of Michigan Health System, North Campus Research Complex, 2800 Plymouth Rd. Bldg. 16, Rm 408E, Ann Arbor, MI 48109, USA
e-mail: meganhay@med.umich.edu

N.H. Esfandiari, MD
Department of Internal Medicine, Metabolism, Endocrinology, and Diabetes, University of Michigan, 24, Frank Lloyd Wright Drive, Domino's Farm, Lobby C, Suite 1300, Ann Arbor, MI 48109, USA
e-mail: nazanene@med.umich.edu

S.A. Roman et al. (eds.), *Management of Thyroid Nodules and Differentiated Thyroid Cancer*, DOI 10.1007/978-3-319-43618-0_1

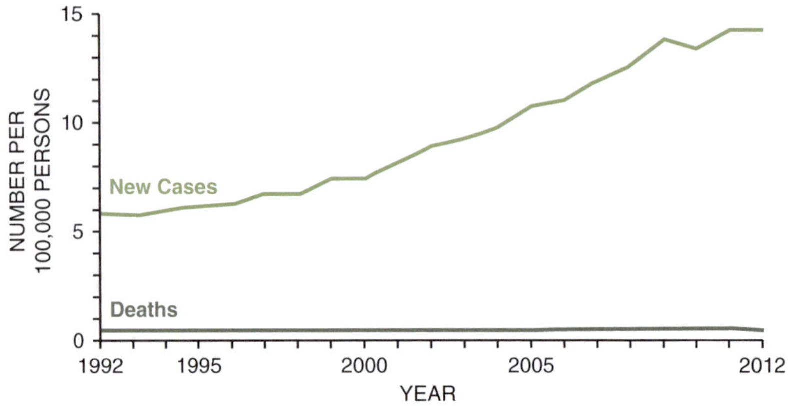

Fig. 1.1 Based on SEER data, the number of new cases of thyroid cancer was 13.5 per 100,000 men and women per year. The number of deaths was 0.5 per 100,000 men and women per year. These rates are age adjusted and based on 2008–2012 cases and deaths [5]

risen in both men and women but at a greater rate in women. From 1980 to 1983 versus 2003 to 2005, papillary thyroid cancer rates tripled among white and black females and doubled among white and black males [12]. Although two-thirds of thyroid cancers occur in patients < age 55, the fastest rise in incidence has been seen in adults over age 65 [13, 14]. Older adults have the highest incidence of thyroid cancer per 100,000, with 25.84 new cases diagnosed in patients ages 65–74 years versus 15.16 diagnosed in patients ages 20–49 [5]. Adults aged ≥65 also have the greatest growth in incidence with an annual percentage change of 8.8 % versus 6.4 % for those aged <65 years [5, 15]. The rise in incidence has been seen across race groups, but incidence rates tend to be higher among whites than blacks and among white non-Hispanics than white Hispanics and Asian Pacific Islanders [12]. Historically, thyroid cancer diagnosis has been more common in cohorts with higher socioeconomic status (SES). Based on Surveillance, Epidemiology and End Results (SEER) data from 497 counties in the United States, county papillary thyroid cancer incidence positively correlates with rates of college education, white-collar employment, and family income [15].

The Origin of Thyroid Cancer

Diagnosing thyroid cancer usually starts with identifying a thyroid nodule and/or occasionally lateral neck mass. Between 20 and 70 % of adults have thyroid nodules with older adults having a higher prevalence than younger [16, 17]. In patients with thyroid nodules, male gender, younger age, and high-risk ultrasound characteristics, such as irregular borders, solid, hypoechoic, larger size, and microcalcifications, are associated with greater likelihood of thyroid cancer [18–21].

The majority of thyroid cancers are identified with fine-needle aspiration of a thyroid nodule. Of the nodules that undergo fine needle aspiration (FNA), only 5–8 % are thyroid cancer [22–24]. Although most cancers are diagnosed by FNA, 6–21% of the thyroid operations planned for treatment of benign disease have incidental discovery of thyroid cancer postoperatively [25–27].

The most common thyroid cancer diagnosed is papillary thyroid cancer, which represents 85 % of all thyroid cancers [28]. Additional thyroid cancers include other well-differentiated cancers, such as follicular and Hürthle cell which represent approximately 10 and 3 % of thyroid cancers, respectively [28]. Medullary thyroid cancer arises from c-cells and accounts for less than 5 % of all thyroid cancers [28–30]. Anaplastic is rare and deadly and represents only 1 % of all thyroid cancers [31, 32].

Risk Factors for Thyroid Cancer

As shown in Table 1.1, there are two accepted risk factors for well-differentiated thyroid cancer: ionizing radiation and family history. Ionizing radiation is thought to cause cancer through somatic mutations and DNA strand breaks [14, 33]. When catastrophic events such as Chernobyl happen, the risk of thyroid cancer is dose and age related [34]. Children and young adults under age 20 years are most susceptible to radiation-induced thyroid cancers [14, 35, 36]. Similarly, children who underwent radiation therapy for childhood cancers, acne, treatment of enlarged thymus, etc. also have an increased risk for thyroid cancer [37]. In addition, to radiation exposure, familial nonmedullary thyroid cancer does exist. If two or more first-degree relatives have well-differentiated thyroid cancer, then it is presumed to be hereditary. However, this hereditary form of well-differentiated thyroid cancer cannot be tracked with genetic testing and is thought to represent just over 5 % of all well-differentiated thyroid cancers [38–41]. Recently, a germline variant in *HABP2* was identified in familial nonmedullary thyroid cancer [41]. Therefore, for the

Table 1.1 Accepted risk factors for thyroid cancer

Radiation
Nuclear events such as Chernobyl[a] or Fukushima[b]
Treatment of childhood cancers with ionizing (external beam) radiation Treatment of acne, thymus, etc., with ionizing (external beam) radiation Environmental exposures are currently under investigation by several researchers
Family history
RET mutations with MEN2A and MEN2B
Familial nonmedullary thyroid cancers and syndromes

[a]Chernobyl happened on April 25, 1986
[b]Meltdown of the reactor in Fukushima happened on March 11, 2011
RET RET proto-oncogene gain of function mutation is associated with the development of medullary thyroid cancer, *MEN* multiple endocrine neoplasias

majority of patients with well-differentiated thyroid cancer, there is no clear etiology of their thyroid cancer and the cancer thought to be sporadic.

In comparison, for medullary thyroid cancer, up to 1–7% of patients with apparently sporadic medullary thyroid cancer end up having germline mutations and associated syndromes MEN2A and MEN2B [42, 43]. Genetic testing can identify the RET mutation involved in development of the medullary thyroid cancer, and then subsequent testing can identify family members at risk. In addition to germline mutations, up to half of patients with sporadic medullary thyroid cancer patients have an unidentified somatic RET mutation [44].

There are no clear risk factors for anaplastic thyroid cancer. However, anaplastic thyroid cancer is thought to arise from a well-differentiated thyroid cancer, and it is more common in older adults [32]. There is an accepted "second hit" hypothesis that well-differentiated thyroid cancers typically need a second mutation, often p53, to develop anaplastic thyroid cancer [31].

Proposed Explanations for the Rise in Thyroid Cancer Incidence

Table 1.2 illustrates the two broad theories to explain the rise in thyroid cancer incidence [14]. One theory is that new or previously unidentified risk factors for thyroid cancer explain the rise in incidence. These proposed risk factors would include radiation exposure outside of known catastrophic events or treatment of childhood cancers, obesity/diabetes, autoimmune thyroid disease, and iodine deficiency or excess. Another conflicting theory is that we have detection bias or in essence overdiagnosis leading to the rise in thyroid cancer incidence. In principle, there is a large reservoir of indolent thyroid cancer, and the more we "look," the more we find. Based on this overdiagnosis theory, increased use of imaging, FNA, surgery, and

Table 1.2 Proposed explanations for the rise in thyroid cancer incidence

Novel risk factor
Background environmental radiation
Obesity/diabetes mellitus
Autoimmune thyroid disease
Iodine deficiency or excess Other environmental agents
Overdiagnosis
Greater use of neck imaging leading to more nodule detection and cancer diagnosis
More fine-needle aspirations of nodules leading to more cancer diagnosis
More surgery leading to more post op incidental cancer discovery
Greater pathologic inspection leading to more cancer diagnosis

[a]Adapted from Table 1.1. Potential Contributors to the Increasing Incidence of Thyroid Cancer in the United States, by Category [14]

pathologic inspection leads to detection of cancers that otherwise may have been unidentified. In the following section, we will explain both conflicting theories.

Explanation 1: New Risk Factor

Exposure to ionizing radiation is an accepted risk factor for well-differentiated thyroid cancer. However, typically patients aged 20 years and younger are most at risk, and in the absence of a recent catastrophic world event, such as Chernobyl or the 2011 reactor meltdown in Fukushima, Japan, this seems like an unlikely explanation for the worldwide rise in thyroid cancer incidence [14, 36]. Although some do worry that the background level of radiation exposure, especially due to increased use of CT scans, has increased and may contribute to the rise in thyroid cancer incidence, it has been estimated that pediatric CT scans account for <1% of the increased incidence of thyroid cancer [14]. Obesity and diabetes mellitus are increasingly common problems in well-developed countries. In parallel to the thyroid cancer epidemic is the obesity and diabetes epidemic [12, 45, 46]. Thus, it has been hypothesized that the thyroid cancer epidemic may be related to the rise in obesity and diabetes mellitus. A pooled analysis of five prospective studies found that obesity is an independent risk factor for thyroid cancer [47]. However, there is more conflicting data when evaluating diabetes and its relationship to thyroid cancer [48, 49]. To-date although correlations between both obesity and diabetes mellitus with thyroid cancer have been noted, causality has not been shown [47, 48].

Autoimmune thyroid disease, specifically Hashimoto's thyroiditis and Graves' disease, are common benign thyroid conditions that are similar to the thyroid cancer in the fact that they are far more common in women. There has been longstanding controversy about whether or not autoimmune thyroid disease is associated with thyroid cancer. Surgical studies have suggested a clear association, whereas studies based on FNA samples or antibodies have been less supportive [50–53]. Although thyroid cancer incidence has been rising, there is no clear data that autoimmune thyroid disease is more prevalent now than 30 years ago. Thus, this is an unlikely explanation for the recent rise in thyroid cancer incidence.

Iodine deficiency or excess is known to affect the proportions of thyroid cancer types in the world, as iodine deficiency is associated with a higher proportion of follicular thyroid cancer [54, 55]. However, the relationship between iodine levels and the recent pattern of diagnosing smaller papillary thyroid cancers is unclear [55].

Theory 2: Overdiagnosis

Suggesting that we may be tapping into a reservoir of indolent disease, the greatest rise in incidence has been in low-risk disease. Eighty-seven percent of the increase in thyroid cancer incidence is attributed to papillary thyroid cancers measuring 2 cm or smaller [1]. Since most disease detected is small, the prognosis for most patients is excellent [56]. Mortality for thyroid cancer has consistently been around 0.5 per 100,000 population [5]. Five-year disease-specific survival for localized disease is 99.8%, and for regional disease, it is 97% [2, 9]. Finally, thorough autopsy studies have revealed incidental small thyroid cancers in up to 36% of adults who die from another cause [57]. If pathologic slicing of thyroid specimens were finer, some have suggested that the actual prevalence may be as high as 100% [57]. This implies that there may be a bottomless reservoir of indolent disease. The fact that the rise in thyroid cancer incidence is primarily due to increased detection of low-risk disease and the fact that thyroid cancer is a common incidental finding on autopsy studies support the hypothesis that overdiagnosis may play an important role in the rise of thyroid cancer incidence in developed countries.

Excess thyroid imaging may be one of the reasons for the overdiagnosis of small thyroid cancers. Since at least half of all adults have thyroid nodules, increased imaging can lead to incidental nodule discovery [16, 17, 58, 59]. The rates of detection of thyroid nodules are 67% with thyroid ultrasound (US), 16% with CT and MRI, 9% with carotid duplex, and 3% with positron emission tomography (PET) or PET/CT [59–63]. Over the past 15 years, there has been a rise in the use of imaging studies that are associated with incidental thyroid nodule discovery. Based on data from a large health plan, between 1997 and 2006 use of US increased 40%, use of computed tomography (CT) doubled, and use of magnetic resonance imaging (MRI) tripled [64]. In addition to the rise in use of imaging associated with incidental cancer discovery, thyroid US is increasingly becoming an extension of the physical exam. When there is a palpable nodule, thyroid US is the preferred method of imaging [19]. Neck imaging to evaluate thyroid nodules and symptoms and neck imaging performed for other reasons have contributed to the rise in thyroid cancer incidence [65, 66].

Related to more imaging, greater use of thyroid FNA also leads to more cancer diagnosis. Use of thyroid FNAs more than doubled between 2006 and 2011 [67]. Since approximately 5–8% of thyroid nodules undergoing FNA are cancer and 20% are indeterminate, more FNAs will result in more cancer diagnoses [22–24].

More surgery may also play a role in the thyroid cancer epidemic. The number of thyroid surgeries being performed in the United States increased by 39% between 1996 and 2006 with one-third of the surgeries performed for thyroid cancer [68, 69]. Between 6 and 21% of thyroid surgeries that are planned for treatment of benign disease have an incidental discovery of thyroid cancer postoperatively [25–27]. Therefore, more thyroid surgery will result in more detection of more low-risk thyroid cancer, thus contributing to the rise in thyroid cancer incidence.

In addition to surgery, in recent years pathologic evaluation has become more detailed. Currently pathologists examine the entire thyroid and 14 versus five descriptive areas are reported [14, 70, 71]. This too could potentially contribute to the rise in thyroid cancer incidence as more small incidental cancers are detected.

Conclusion

There has been a rise in thyroid cancer incidence. Although there is an ongoing debate as to whether a new risk factor versus overdiagnosis explains the rise in incidence, most data support overdiagnosis playing a significant role in the developed countries for this finding. Regardless of etiology, this rise in thyroid cancer incidence has implications for patients, physicians, and society. As we diagnose more thyroid cancer, it becomes increasingly important to understand which patients need intensive treatment to prevent poor outcome, including death and recurrence, and which patients have low-risk disease and need minimal intervention or surveillance only.

References

1. Davies L, Welch HG. Increasing incidence of thyroid cancer in the United States, 1973–2002. JAMA. 2006;295(18):2164–7.
2. Simard EP, Ward EM, Siegel R, Jemal A. Cancers with increasing incidence trends in the United States: 1999 through 2008. CA Cancer J Clin. 2012;62(2):118–28.
3. https://www.cancer.gov/types/common-cancers National Cancer Institute. Common Cancer Types. Feb. 1, 2006.
4. American Cancer Society Cancer Facts and Figures 2015 Atlanta, Ga: American Cancer Society. Available from: http://www.cancer.org/acs/groups/content/@editorial/documents/document/acspc-044552.pdf. Cited 2015.
5. Surveillance, Epidemiology, and End Results Program (SEER). Available from: www.seer.cancer.gov. Cited 2015.
6. National Cancer Institute at the National Institutes of Health; Common Cancer Types. Available from: http://www.cancer.gov/cancertopics/types/commoncancers. Cited 2015.
7. Rahib L, Smith BD, Aizenberg R, Rosenzweig AB, Fleshman JM, Matrisian LM. Projecting cancer incidence and deaths to 2030: the unexpected burden of thyroid, liver, and pancreas cancers in the United States. Cancer Res. 2014;74(11):2913–21.
8. Esserman LJ, Thompson Jr IM, Reid B. Overdiagnosis and overtreatment in cancer: an opportunity for improvement. JAMA. 2013;310(8):797–8.
9. Siegel R, Naishadham D, Jemal A. Cancer statistics, 2012. CA Cancer J Clin. 2012; 62(1):10–29.
10. Brito JP, Morris JC, Montori VM. Thyroid cancer: zealous imaging has increased detection and treatment of low risk tumours. BMJ. 2013;347:f4706.
11. Ahn HS, Kim HJ, Welch HG. Korea's thyroid-cancer "epidemic"--screening and overdiagnosis. N Engl J Med. 2014;371(19):1765–7.
12. Enewold L, Zhu K, Ron E, Marrogi AJ, Stojadinovic A, Peoples GE, et al. Rising thyroid cancer incidence in the United States by demographic and tumor characteristics, 1980–2005. Cancer Epidemiol Biomarkers Prev. 2009;18(3):784–91.
13. The American Cancer Society. Available from: www.cancer.org. Cited 2015.
14. Davies L, Morris L, Haymart M, Chen A, Goldenberg D, Morris J, et al. AACE Endocrine Surgery Scientific Committee Disease Review Statement: on the Increasing Incidence of Thyroid Cancer. Endocr Pract. 2015;21(6):686–96.
15. Morris LG, Sikora AG, Tosteson TD, Davies L. The increasing incidence of thyroid cancer: the influence of access to care. Thyroid. 2013;23(7):885–91.

16. Tan GH, Gharib H. Thyroid incidentalomas: management approaches to nonpalpable nodules discovered incidentally on thyroid imaging. Ann Intern Med. 1997;126(3):226–31.
17. Rojeski MT, Gharib H. Nodular thyroid disease. Evaluation and management. N Engl J Med. 1985;313(7):428–36.
18. Smith-Bindman R, Lebda P, Feldstein VA, Sellami D, Goldstein RB, Brasic N, et al. Risk of thyroid cancer based on thyroid ultrasound imaging characteristics: results of a population-based study. JAMA Intern Med. 2013;173(19):1788–96.
19. Cooper DS, Doherty GM, Haugen BR, Kloos RT, Lee SL, Mandel SJ, et al. Revised American Thyroid Association management guidelines for patients with thyroid nodules and differentiated thyroid cancer. Thyroid. 2009;19(11):1167–214.
20. Fish SA, Langer JE, Mandel SJ. Sonographic imaging of thyroid nodules and cervical lymph nodes. Endocrinol Metab Clin North Am. 2008;37(2):401–17, ix.
21. Haugen BR, Alexander EK, Bible KC, Doherty GM, Mandel SJ, Nikiforov YE, et al. 2015 American Thyroid Association Management Guidelines for Adult Patients with Thyroid Nodules and Differentiated Thyroid Cancer: The American Thyroid Association Guidelines Task Force on Thyroid Nodules and Differentiated Thyroid Cancer. Thyroid. 2016;26(1):1–133.
22. Alexander EK, Kennedy GC, Baloch ZW, Cibas ES, Chudova D, Diggans J, et al. Preoperative diagnosis of benign thyroid nodules with indeterminate cytology. N Engl J Med. 2012;367(8):705–15.
23. Yassa L, Cibas ES, Benson CB, Frates MC, Doubilet PM, Gawande AA, et al. Long-term assessment of a multidisciplinary approach to thyroid nodule diagnostic evaluation. Cancer. 2007;111(6):508–16.
24. Gharib H, Papini E, Paschke R, Duick DS, Valcavi R, Hegedus L, et al. American Association of Clinical Endocrinologists, Associazione Medici Endocrinologi, and European Thyroid Association medical guidelines for clinical practice for the diagnosis and management of thyroid nodules: Executive Summary of recommendations. J Endocrinol Invest. 2010;33(5):287–91.
25. Deveci MS, Deveci G, LiVolsi VA, Gupta PK, Baloch ZW. Concordance between thyroid nodule sizes measured by ultrasound and gross pathology examination: effect on patient management. Diagn Cytopathol. 2007;35(9):579–83.
26. Haymart MR, Cayo M, Chen H. Papillary thyroid microcarcinomas: big decisions for a small tumor. Ann Surg Oncol. 2009;16(11):3132–9.
27. Ito Y, Higashiyama T, Takamura Y, Miya A, Kobayashi K, Matsuzuka F, et al. Prognosis of patients with benign thyroid diseases accompanied by incidental papillary carcinoma undetectable on preoperative imaging tests. World J Surg. 2007;31(8):1672–6.
28. Hundahl SA, Fleming ID, Fremgen AM, Menck HR. A National Cancer Data Base report on 53,856 cases of thyroid carcinoma treated in the U.S., 1985–1995. Cancer. 1998;83(12):2638–48.
29. Saad MF, Ordonez NG, Rashid RK, Guido JJ, Hill Jr CS, Hickey RC, et al. Medullary carcinoma of the thyroid. A study of the clinical features and prognostic factors in 161 patients. Medicine. 1984;63(6):319–42.
30. Giuffrida D, Gharib H. Current diagnosis and management of medullary thyroid carcinoma. Ann Oncol Off J Eur Soc Med Oncol/ESMO. 1998;9(7):695–701.
31. Smallridge RC, Marlow LA, Copland JA. Anaplastic thyroid cancer: molecular pathogenesis and emerging therapies. Endocr Relat Cancer. 2009;16(1):17–44.
32. Nagaiah G, Hossain A, Mooney CJ, Parmentier J, Remick SC. Anaplastic thyroid cancer: a review of epidemiology, pathogenesis, and treatment. J oncol. 2011;2011:542358.
33. Nikiforova MN, Stringer JR, Blough R, Medvedovic M, Fagin JA, Nikiforov YE. Proximity of chromosomal loci that participate in radiation-induced rearrangements in human cells. Science. 2000;290(5489):138–41.
34. Zablotska LB, Nadyrov EA, Rozhko AV, Gong Z, Polyanskaya ON, McConnell RJ, et al. Analysis of thyroid malignant pathologic findings identified during 3 rounds of screening (1997–2008) of a cohort of children and adolescents from belarus exposed to radioiodines after the Chernobyl accident. Cancer. 2015;121(3):457–66.

35. Schonfeld SJ, Lee C, Berrington de Gonzalez A. Medical exposure to radiation and thyroid cancer. Clin Oncol. 2011;23(4):244–50.
36. Furukawa K, Preston D, Funamoto S, Yonehara S, Ito M, Tokuoka S, et al. Long-term trend of thyroid cancer risk among Japanese atomic-bomb survivors: 60 years after exposure. Int J Cancer. 2013;132(5):1222–6.
37. de Vathaire F, Haddy N, Allodji R, Hawkins M, Guibout C, El-Fayech C, et al. Thyroid radiation dose and other risk factors of thyroid carcinoma following childhood cancer. J Clin Endocrinol Metab. 2015;100:4282–90. jc20151690.
38. Fallah M, Pukkala E, Tryggvadottir L, Olsen JH, Tretli S, Sundquist K, et al. Risk of thyroid cancer in first-degree relatives of patients with non-medullary thyroid cancer by histology type and age at diagnosis: a joint study from five Nordic countries. J Med Genet. 2013;50(6):373–82.
39. Sippel RS, Caron NR, Clark OH. An evidence-based approach to familial nonmedullary thyroid cancer: screening, clinical management, and follow-up. World J Surg. 2007;31(5):924–33.
40. Nose V. Familial non-medullary thyroid carcinoma: an update. Endocr Pathol. 2008;19(4):226–40.
41. Gara SK, Jia L, Merino MJ, Agarwal SK, Zhang L, Cam M, et al. Germline HABP2 mutation causing familial nonmedullary thyroid cancer. N Engl J Med. 2015;373(5):448–55.
42. Eng C, Mulligan LM, Smith DP, Healey CS, Frilling A, Raue F, et al. Low frequency of germline mutations in the RET proto-oncogene in patients with apparently sporadic medullary thyroid carcinoma. Clin Endocrinol (Oxf). 1995;43(1):123–7.
43. Elisei R, Romei C, Cosci B, Agate L, Bottici V, Molinaro E, et al. RET genetic screening in patients with medullary thyroid cancer and their relatives: experience with 807 individuals at one center. J Clin Endocrinol Metab. 2007;92(12):4725–9.
44. Elisei R, Cosci B, Romei C, Bottici V, Renzini G, Molinaro E, et al. Prognostic significance of somatic RET oncogene mutations in sporadic medullary thyroid cancer: a 10-year follow-up study. J Clin Endocrinol Metab. 2008;93(3):682–7.
45. Flegal KM, Carroll MD, Kuczmarski RJ, Johnson CL. Overweight and obesity in the United States: prevalence and trends, 1960–1994. Int J obes Relat Metab Disord J Int Assoc Study Obes. 1998;22(1):39–47.
46. Menke A, Casagrande S, Geiss L, Cowie CC. Prevalence of and trends in diabetes among adults in the United States, 1988–2012. JAMA. 2015;314(10):1021–9.
47. Kitahara CM, Platz EA, Freeman LE, Hsing AW, Linet MS, Park Y, et al. Obesity and thyroid cancer risk among U.S. men and women: a pooled analysis of five prospective studies. Cancer Epidemiol Biomarkers Prev. 2011;20(3):464–72.
48. Aschebrook-Kilfoy B, Sabra MM, Brenner A, Moore SC, Ron E, Schatzkin A, et al. Diabetes and thyroid cancer risk in the National Institutes of Health-AARP Diet and Health Study. Thyroid. 2011;21(9):957–63.
49. Kitahara CM, Platz EA, Beane Freeman LE, Black A, Hsing AW, Linet MS, et al. Physical activity, diabetes, and thyroid cancer risk: a pooled analysis of five prospective studies. Cancer Causes Control. 2012;23(3):463–71.
50. Ye ZQ, Gu DN, Hu HY, Zhou YL, Hu XQ, Zhang XH. Hashimoto's thyroiditis, microcalcification and raised thyrotropin levels within normal range are associated with thyroid cancer. World J Surg Oncol. 2013;11:56.
51. Repplinger D, Bargren A, Zhang YW, Adler JT, Haymart M, Chen H. Is Hashimoto's thyroiditis a risk factor for papillary thyroid cancer? J Surg Res. 2008;150(1):49–52.
52. Fiore E, Rago T, Scutari M, Ugolini C, Proietti A, Di Coscio G, et al. Papillary thyroid cancer, although strongly associated with lymphocytic infiltration on histology, is only weakly predicted by serum thyroid auto-antibodies in patients with nodular thyroid diseases. J Endocrinol Invest. 2009;32(4):344–51.
53. Anil C, Goksel S, Gursoy A. Hashimoto's thyroiditis is not associated with increased risk of thyroid cancer in patients with thyroid nodules: a single-center prospective study. Thyroid. 2010;20(6):601–6.

54. Lawal O, Agbakwuru A, Olayinka OS, Adelusola K. Thyroid malignancy in endemic nodular goitres: prevalence, pattern and treatment. Eur J Surg Oncol Journal Eur Soc Surg Oncol Br Assoc Surg Oncol. 2001;27(2):157–61.
55. Feldt-Rasmussen U. Iodine and cancer. Thyroid. 2001;11(5):483–6.
56. Ho AS, Davies L, Nixon IJ, Palmer FL, Wang LY, Patel SG, et al. Increasing diagnosis of subclinical thyroid cancers leads to spurious improvements in survival rates. Cancer. 2015;121(11):1793–9.
57. Harach HR, Franssila KO, Wasenius VM. Occult papillary carcinoma of the thyroid. A "normal" finding in Finland. A systematic autopsy study. Cancer. 1985;56(3):531–8.
58. Davies L, Ouellette M, Hunter M, Welch HG. The increasing incidence of small thyroid cancers: where are the cases coming from? Laryngoscope. 2010;120(12):2446–51.
59. Ezzat S, Sarti DA, Cain DR, Braunstein GD. Thyroid incidentalomas. Prevalence by palpation and ultrasonography. Arch Intern Med. 1994;154(16):1838–40.
60. Jin J, McHenry CR. Thyroid incidentaloma. Best Pract Res Clin Endocrinol Metab. 2012;26(1):83–96.
61. Steele SR, Martin MJ, Mullenix PS, Azarow KS, Andersen CA. The significance of incidental thyroid abnormalities identified during carotid duplex ultrasonography. Arch Surg. 2005;140(10):981–5.
62. Cohen MS, Arslan N, Dehdashti F, Doherty GM, Lairmore TC, Brunt LM, et al. Risk of malignancy in thyroid incidentalomas identified by fluorodeoxyglucose-positron emission tomography. Surgery. 2001;130(6):941–6.
63. Youserm DM, Huang T, Loevner LA, Langlotz CP. Clinical and economic impact of incidental thyroid lesions found with CT and MR. AJNR Am J Neuroradiol. 1997;18(8):1423–8.
64. Smith-Bindman R, Miglioretti DL, Larson EB. Rising use of diagnostic medical imaging in a large integrated health system. Health Aff (Millwood). 2008;27(6):1491–502.
65. Brito JP, Al Nofal A, Montori VM, Hay ID, Morris JC. The impact of subclinical disease and mechanism of detection on the rise in thyroid cancer incidence: a population-based study in Olmsted County, Minnesota During 1935 Through 2012. Thyroid. 2015;25(9):999–1007.
66. Van den Bruel A, Francart J, Dubois C, Adam M, Vlayen J, De Schutter H, et al. Regional variation in thyroid cancer incidence in belgium is associated with variation in thyroid imaging and thyroid disease management. J Clin Endocrinol Metab. 2013;98(10):4063–71.
67. Sosa JA, Hanna JW, Robinson KA, Lanman RB. Increases in thyroid nodule fine-needle aspirations, operations, and diagnoses of thyroid cancer in the United States. Surgery. 2013;154(6):1420–6.
68. Sun GH, DeMonner S, Davis MM. Epidemiological and economic trends in inpatient and outpatient thyroidectomy in the United States, 1996–2006. Thyroid. 2013;23(6):727–33.
69. Loyo M, Tufano RP, Gourin CG. National trends in thyroid surgery and the effect of volume on short-term outcomes. Laryngoscope. 2013;123(8):2056–63.
70. Verkooijen HM, Fioretta G, Pache JC, Franceschi S, Raymond L, Schubert H, et al. Diagnostic changes as a reason for the increase in papillary thyroid cancer incidence in Geneva, Switzerland. Cancer Causes Control. 2003;14(1):13–7.
71. Ghossein R, Asa SL, Barnes L, Chan J, Harrison JB, Heffess CS, et al. College of American Pathologists, Northfield, IL. Protocol for the Examination of Specimens From Patients With Carcinomas of the Thyroid Gland. Based on AJCC/UICC TNM. 7th ed. 2011.

Part I
The Thyroid Nodule

Chapter 2
The Clinically Detected and Palpable Thyroid Nodule

Whitney Goldner and Anery Patel

Abbreviations

ATC	Anaplastic thyroid cancer
FAP	Familial adenomatous polyposis
FTC	Follicular thyroid cancer
FMTC	Familial medullary thyroid cancer
MEN	Multiple endocrine neoplasia
MTC	Medullary thyroid cancer
PTC	Papillary thyroid cancer

Introduction

Thyroid nodules are common, but they are not always easy to detect clinically or by physical exam. Historically, nodules were discovered only if they had a visible or palpable neck mass. Additionally, nodules were suspected if a patient had compressive symptoms in the anterior neck or symptoms of hormone deficiency or excess. Before the advent and routine use of imaging, thyroid nodules were estimated to occur in approximately 5–10 % of people, when discovered by palpation alone [1–3]. Even in the most experienced hands, physicians may fail to detect smaller nodules (less than 1 cm) [4]. Large anterior thyroid nodules can be palpable and easy to visualize, but smaller or posterior nodules frequently are not palpable, but may be associated with compressive symptoms [5, 6]. Variations in individual

W. Goldner, MD (✉) • A. Patel, MD
Division of Diabetes, Endocrinology and Metabolism, Department of Internal Medicine, University of Nebraska Medical Center,
984120 Nebraska Medical Center, Omaha, NE 68198-4120, USA
e-mail: wgoldner@unmc.edu; anery.patel@unmc.edu

S.A. Roman et al. (eds.), *Management of Thyroid Nodules and Differentiated Thyroid Cancer*, DOI 10.1007/978-3-319-43618-0_2

anatomy of the neck can also make the thyroid exam difficult and thyroid nodules even less likely to be palpable. In kyphotic persons, or those with shorter necks, the thyroid may be situated more inferiorly either near the sternal notch or substernal, making it difficult to palpate [7].

As ultrasound and cross-sectional imaging of the neck with computed tomography (CT) or magnetic resonance imaging (MRI) became available, many non-palpable thyroid nodules have been incidentally detected. The prevalence of thyroid nodules is now estimated to be 20–60 %, depending on age, gender, and geographic location [1, 3, 6, 8]. This is consistent with previous observations in autopsy studies reporting the prevalence of thyroid nodules as high as 50 % [4, 9].

Even though many nodules are asymptomatic and incidentally noted, there is a subset of nodules that are identified because of presenting symptoms or based on physical examination. Physical assessment is a valuable first step in evaluating neck masses for patients with symptoms suggestive of a thyroid nodule and thyroid hormone deficiency or excess or for those who are at high risk for nodules or thyroid cancer based on personal or family history.

Thyroid cancer is now the eighth most common cancer in the United States and the fifth most common cancer in women, with its incidence rising approximately 5 % per year over the last 10 years [10] (see Chap. 1). When looking at the total number of thyroid nodules, it is estimated that approximately 5–10 % of all thyroid nodules are malignant [11, 12], and similar rates of thyroid cancer have been reported in patients who have solitary or multiple thyroid nodules [13]. However, it is now recognized that the overall risk of malignancy in an individual nodule is dependent on age, gender, radiation exposure, family history, and imaging characteristics of the nodule, as well as history and physical examination characteristics [14]. Nodules occurring at extremes of age, particularly in men, are more likely to be malignant [1]. Symptoms, such as rapid growth, hoarseness, fixation to surrounding tissues, and the development of cervical lymphadenopathy make the risk of malignancy in thyroid nodules higher [14]. Thyroid nodules and some thyroid cancers are also more commonly associated with specific hereditary genetic syndromes (Table 2.1). A good physical examination may not only identify a thyroid abnormality or lymphadenopathy but also can identify other physical findings that may be associated with genetic syndromes or medical conditions that have increased risk for thyroid nodules or cancer.

Symptoms

Most patients with thyroid nodules have no hyper- or hypothyroid symptoms. They are often asymptomatic; a minority of nodules can be detected by physical examination, and more are detected incidentally with imaging. If the nodules are palpable, patients can present with a slowly enlarging mass in the neck. The most common symptoms associated with thyroid nodules are those due to pressure on or invasion of adjacent structures and can include dysphagia, globus sensation, compressive/constrictive feeling in the neck, hoarseness or change in speech quality, difficulty

Table 2.1 Hereditary thyroid cancer syndromes

Syndrome	Rate of thyroid cancer	Associated conditions	Pattern of inheritance and mutations
Gardner's syndrome (FAP)	2–12 % with PTC [15] with mean age at diagnosis of 28 years	Gastrointestinal polyps Osteomas Epidermoid cysts Desmoid tumors [16]	Autosomal dominant tumor suppressor APC gene
Cowden's syndrome (PTEN hamartoma syndrome)	Two-thirds with thyroid pathology including multinodular goiter, follicular adenomas, FTC, and PTC [17]	Multiple hamartomas Breast cancer Endometrial cancer	Autosomal dominant tumor suppressor PTEN gene
Carney complex	15 % of patients with PTC and FTC [18]	Adrenal and pituitary gland pathology Myxomas of the soft tissue, heart, skin, and brain Schwannomas Testicular tumors Lentigines	Autosomal dominant PRKA1α gene
Werner syndrome	18 % of patients with thyroid malignancy including PTC, FTC, ATC [19]	Soft tissue sarcomas Melanomas Osteosarcomas	Autosomal recessive WRN gene
Familial Non-medullary Thyroid cancer	3.2–9.4 % of all thyroid cancer cases [20]	Differentiated thyroid cancer of follicular origin in two or more first-degree relatives [21]	Not identified
MEN 2, FMTC	25 % cases of MTC [22, 23]	MEN 2A – pheochromocytoma, hyperparathyroidism MEN 2B – pheochromocytoma, mucosal neuromas, ganglioneuromatosis of GI tract, megacolon	Autosomal dominant RET proto-oncogene

breathing, and cosmetic concerns. Occasionally, they can also cause anterior neck pain with radiation to the ears [7]. There can be pain in the thyroid itself when there has been acute hemorrhage into the nodule and there is associated inflammation or rapid growth [24]. In extremely large goiters, patients can have a Pemberton's sign, which is facial flushing upon elevation of the arms above the head, due to partial obstruction of the superior vena cava [7]. If a nodule is visible and palpable, it is possible to deduce how quickly the nodule has grown and if symptoms have been stable or changing. Patients who present with symptoms of tracheal or esophageal compression, vocal cord paralysis, or persistent hoarseness may be more likely to harbor malignancy [14].

If nodules are functioning, they can be associated with symptoms of hyperthyroidism. Autonomously hyperfunctional thyroid nodules can be either solitary or multiple and can lead to thyrotoxicosis. If a thyroid nodule is noted in a patient with symptoms of tachycardia, anxiety, tremor, heat intolerance, weight loss, and frequent bowel movements, this is suggestive of a toxic thyroid nodule. However, Graves' disease can also present with hyperthyroid symptoms [25] along with a diffusely enlarged thyroid, or asymmetric enlargement, which can simulate a nodule. Additional clinical characteristics that can be associated with Graves' disease, that are not seen with a toxic nodule, include the presence of ophthalmopathy and dermopathy. Patients with ophthalmopathy, or thyroid eye disease, can have periorbital edema, proptosis, exophthalmos, lid lag, stare, and conjunctival injection [26]. Dermopathy can present as non-pitting edema, usually of the lower extremities in the pretibial area. If a patient presents with thyroid dysfunction associated with ophthalmopathy, the pretibial area should be carefully examined for subtle signs of dermopathy, such as localized thickening of the skin with reddish discoloration [27].

A slowly growing, diffusely enlarged thyroid or thyroid nodule associated with typical symptoms [28] such as dry skin, cold sensitivity, fatigue, muscle cramps, voice changes, and constipation could suggest hypothyroidism.

Family History and Cancer Syndromes

Several familial syndromes are associated with increased risk of thyroid cancer. These include Gardner's syndrome, PTEN hamartoma syndrome (Cowden's syndrome), Carney complex, Werner syndrome, familial non-medullary thyroid carcinoma, multiple endocrine neoplasia type 2 (MEN 2), and familial medullary thyroid carcinoma (FMTC) [15–23, 29] (Table 2.1).

Hirschsprung disease and McCune-Albright, Peutz-Jeghers, Pendred, and ataxia-telangiectasia syndromes also have been reported to be associated with thyroid cancer, but the links are less established [29]. If family history is significant for any of these syndromes, it is important to not only evaluate for thyroid nodules but also for the non-thyroid manifestations of these syndromes (Table 2.1).

Radiation Exposure

Studies have shown that children exposed to ≥1 Gy of ionizing radiation are at higher risk of development of thyroid nodules at a rate of 2 % annually [30], and these nodules have a higher risk of malignancy, estimated at 20–50 % [31]. This risk can persist for over 50 years [31]. Additionally, a history of external radiation exposure in low or medium doses (40–50 Gy) given to patients with lymphoma or head and neck cancer, particularly in childhood, is a highly concerning risk factor for both benign and malignant nodules [32].

Iodine Exposure

The risk of thyroid disease from iodine exposure is U-shaped which shows potential harm for the patients from both iodine deficiency and iodine excess [33]. Iodine deficiency and excess can both cause thyroid dysfunction; iodine deficiency has also been associated with a diffusely enlarged thyroid and goiter [34] and can trigger formation of nodules. The possible mechanism is due to chronic stimulation by TSH and the effects of increased reactive oxygen species in the iodine-deficient thyroid [35].

Physical Examination

Knowing how to perform a good physical examination of the thyroid and neck is essential. First, it is important to know the anatomy of the neck, which will help the examiner identify essential landmarks (Fig. 2.1). The thyroid is made up of a right and left thyroid lobe and the connection in the middle is the isthmus. Some people may have a pyramidal lobe, which extends superiorly from the isthmus

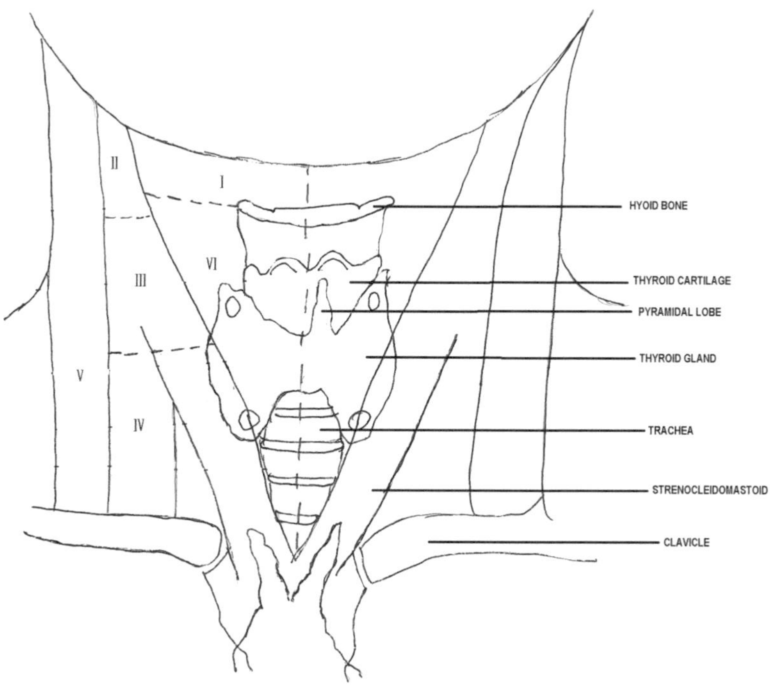

Fig. 2.1 Neck anatomy including cervical lymph node levels

(usually on the left), just lateral to the midline [7]. Each lobe is approximately 2–4 cm in size and the right lobe can be slightly larger than the left. When palpating the thyroid gland, one should first palpate the cricoid cartilage. The isthmus is usually situated caudal to it; hence, identifying the cricoid cartilage first will indicate where the isthmus should be [7]. Once the isthmus is located, then the right and left lobes can be identified and palpated medial to the sternocleidomastoid muscles. Examination should include both inspection and palpation of the neck in good light with the patient sitting upright with their neck straight or slightly extended [36]. In this position, goiters and many nodules can be visible when swallowing. For some patients, it may be necessary to provide a cup of water to facilitate swallowing [36].

The neck and thyroid can be examined using two different methods. The first is with the examiner sitting or standing behind the patient and using both hands to come around anteriorly to palpate the thyroid gland (Fig. 2.2). Both lobes and the isthmus are palpated simultaneously with the pads of the second, third, and fourth fingers. The second method is for the examiner to stand to the side of a seated patient and examine the thyroid and neck with one hand, using the pads of the thumb for one lobe and the pads of the second, third, and fourth fingers for the opposite lobe (Fig. 2.3). The isthmus can be palpated in the same fashion. After palpation of the thyroid, examination of the neck lymph nodes, level 1–6 (Fig. 2.1), should be performed, and this is usually done with the examiner either behind the patient or facing the patient and using both hands to palpate both sides of the lateral neck.

It is helpful to develop a stepwise approach to the thyroid and neck examination and important to document specific characteristics of the examination. These characteristics include overall size of the thyroid gland in vertical and horizontal dimensions, consistency of the thyroid gland, the presence of masses or nodules including their size and characteristics (firm, soft, woody, or hard), adherence to adjacent

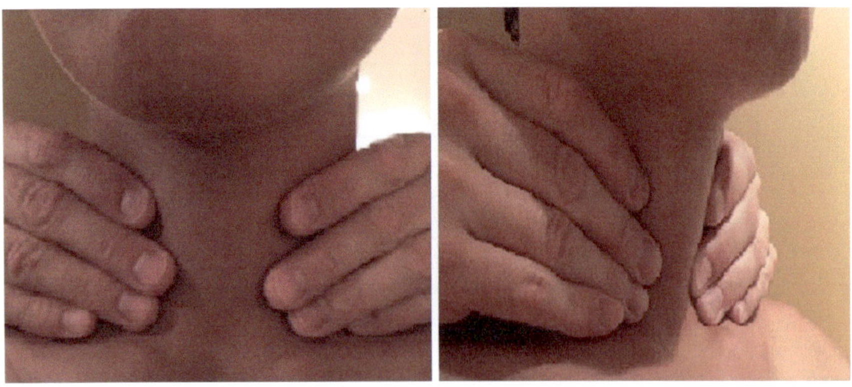

Fig. 2.2 Examination of the thyroid gland using the two hand method

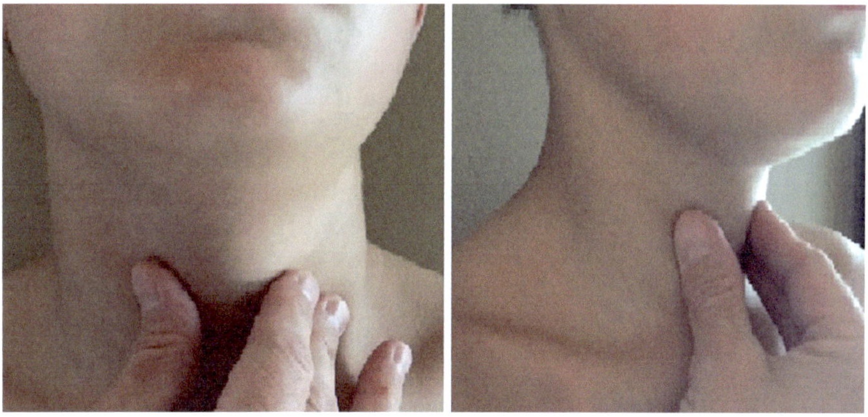

Fig. 2.3 Examination of the thyroid gland using the one hand method

structures, rise with swallowing, and tenderness. It is also important to examine the cervical lymph nodes and identify any enlarged lymph nodes in the neck and their locations (levels 1–6). Examination of the thyroid while swallowing may enable palpation of the inferior aspect of the gland or nodule and identification of nodules or an enlarged gland that may be situated behind the clavicles or sternum. It will also help to determine if the mass is fixed to adjacent structures or freely movable with deglutition.

The trachea should also be palpated by placing the thumb and index finger on either side of the trachea and follow the path up to the suprasternal notch as a large thyroid lobe or a nodule can cause lateral deviation of the trachea and inspiratory stridor [7].

Differential Diagnosis

Even though many palpable masses of the anterior neck are thyroid nodules, it is important to note that not all neck masses are thyroid nodules. The differential diagnosis for palpable neck masses includes but is not limited to thyroid nodules, enlarged lymph nodes, thyroglossal duct cysts, dermoid cysts, branchial cleft cysts, a diffusely enlarged thyroid gland (goiter), prominent sternocleidomastoid muscles or cervical musculature, cervical neck lipoma, contralateral hypertrophy due to agenesis or previous removal of one thyroid lobe, and lymphoma. The location of the mass and associated symptoms will aid in the differentiation of these etiologies. Lymphoma can be associated with night sweats, weight loss, and diffuse cervical lymphadenopathy. Muscular prominence can be associated with lateral neck pain over the sternocleidomastoid muscles, rather than pain in the thyroid gland itself. Additionally, symptoms suggestive of hyperthyroidism or hypothyroidism can be nonspecific and do not always present classically.

The Next Step

If there is a clinical suspicion of a thyroid nodule, the next step in evaluation is to obtain a thyroid ultrasound and serum TSH. The thyroid ultrasound can provide valuable clinical information about the size and imaging characteristics of the thyroid gland itself, any thyroid nodules, lymph nodes, or other masses in the neck. If the patient is found to have a low serum TSH, then additional workup for thyrotoxicosis will need to be performed (see Chap. 9). If the serum TSH is normal or elevated, and thyroid ultrasound confirms a thyroid nodule, then fine-needle aspiration biopsy (FNA) should be considered, depending on clinical and imaging characteristics. If the TSH is high, then further evaluation for hypothyroidism will also need to be performed.

Conclusion

Physical examination and palpation of the neck and thyroid is important in the evaluation of neck masses or suspected thyroid nodules. It is important in screening of high-risk populations, as well as in the evaluation of suspicious symptoms. It is not to be used as the sole evaluation, but it is a very useful initial tool in the overall workup of a suspected thyroid nodule.

References

1. Mazzaferri EL. Management of a solitary thyroid nodule. N Engl J Med. 1993;328(8):553–9.
2. Rojeski MT, Gharib H. Nodular thyroid disease. Evaluation and management. N Engl J Med. 1985;313(7):428–36.
3. Stanicic J, Prpic M, Jukic T, Boric M, Kusic Z. Thyroid nodularity–true epidemic or improved diagnostics. Acta Clin Croat. 2009;48(4):413–8.
4. Tan GH, Gharib H. Thyroid incidentalomas: management approaches to nonpalpable nodules discovered incidentally on thyroid imaging. Ann Intern Med. 1997;126(3):226–31.
5. Wiest PW, Hartshorne MF, Inskip PD, Crooks LA, Vela BS, Telepak RJ, et al. Thyroid palpation versus high-resolution thyroid ultrasonography in the detection of nodules. J Ultrasound Med Off J Am Inst Ultrasound Med. 1998;17(8):487–96.
6. Brander A, Viikinkoski P, Tuuhea J, Voutilainen L, Kivisaari L. Clinical versus ultrasound examination of the thyroid gland in common clinical practice. J Clin Ultrasound. 1992;20(1):37–42.
7. Daniels GH. Physical examination of the thyroid gland. In: Braverman LE, Utiger RD, editors. Werner & Ingbar's the thyroid: a fundamental and clinical text. 8th ed. Philadelphia: Lipincott Williams & Wilkins; 2000. p. 462–6.
8. Brander AE, Viikinkoski VP, Nickels JI, Kivisaari LM. Importance of thyroid abnormalities detected at US screening: a 5-year follow-up. Radiology. 2000;215(3):801–6.
9. Burguera B, Gharib H. Thyroid incidentalomas. Prevalence, diagnosis, significance, and management. Endocrinol Metab Clin North Am. 2000;29(1):187–203.

10. Pellegriti G, Frasca F, Regalbuto C, Squatrito S, Vigneri R. Worldwide increasing incidence of thyroid cancer: update on epidemiology and risk factors. J Cancer Epidemiol. 2013;2013:965212.
11. Gharib H, Papini E, Valcavi R, Baskin HJ, Crescenzi A, Dottorini ME, et al. American Association of Clinical Endocrinologists and Associazione Medici Endocrinologi medical guidelines for clinical practice for the diagnosis and management of thyroid nodules. Endocr Pract Off J Am Coll of Endocrinol Am Ass Clin Endocrinol. 2006;12(1):63–102.
12. Morris LG, Sikora AG, Tosteson TD, Davies L. The increasing incidence of thyroid cancer: the influence of access to care. Thyroid Off J AmThyroid Ass. 2013;23(7):885–91.
13. Belfiore A, La Rosa GL, La Porta GA, Giuffrida D, Milazzo G, Lupo L, et al. Cancer risk in patients with cold thyroid nodules: relevance of iodine intake, sex, age, and multinodularity. Am J Med. 1992;93(4):363–9.
14. Cooper DS, Doherty GM, Haugen BR, Kloos RT, Lee SL, Mandel SJ, et al. Revised American Thyroid Association management guidelines for patients with thyroid nodules and differentiated thyroid cancer. Thyroid Off J AmThyroid Ass. 2009;19(11):1167–214.
15. Feng X, Milas M, O'Malley M, LaGuardia L, Berber E, Jin J, et al. Characteristics of benign and malignant thyroid disease in familial adenomatous polyposis patients and recommendations for disease surveillance. Thyroid Off J AmThyroid Ass. 2015;25(3):325–32.
16. Jarrar AM, Milas M, Mitchell J, Laguardia L, O'Malley M, Berber E, et al. Screening for thyroid cancer in patients with familial adenomatous polyposis. Ann Surg. 2011; 253(3):515–21.
17. Mazeh H, Sippel RS. Familial nonmedullary thyroid carcinoma. Thyroid Off J AmThyroid Ass. 2013;23(9):1049–56.
18. Stratakis CA, Courcoutsakis NA, Abati A, Filie A, Doppman JL, Carney JA, et al. Thyroid gland abnormalities in patients with the syndrome of spotty skin pigmentation, myxomas, endocrine overactivity, and schwannomas (Carney complex). J Clin Endocrinol Metab. 1997;82(7):2037–43.
19. Ishikawa Y, Sugano H, Matsumoto T, Furuichi Y, Miller RW, Goto M. Unusual features of thyroid carcinomas in Japanese patients with Werner syndrome and possible genotype-phenotype relations to cell type and race. Cancer. 1999;85(6):1345–52.
20. Ron E, Kleinerman RA, LiVolsi VA, Fraumeni Jr JF. Familial nonmedullary thyroid cancer. Oncology. 1991;48(4):309–11.
21. Sippel RS, Caron NR, Clark OH. An evidence-based approach to familial nonmedullary thyroid cancer: screening, clinical management, and follow-up. World J Surg. 2007; 31(5):924–33.
22. Rowland KJ, Moley JF. Hereditary thyroid cancer syndromes and genetic testing. J Surg Oncol. 2015;111(1):51–60.
23. Wells Jr SA, Asa SL, Dralle H, Elisei R, Evans DB, Gagel RF, et al. Revised American Thyroid Association guidelines for the management of medullary thyroid carcinoma. Thyroid Off J AmThyroid Ass. 2015;25(6):567–610.
24. Davies L, Randolph G. Evidence-based evaluation of the thyroid nodule. Otolaryngol Clin North Am. 2014;47(4):461–74.
25. Bahn Chair RS, Burch HB, Cooper DS, Garber JR, Greenlee MC, Klein I, et al. Hyperthyroidism and other causes of thyrotoxicosis: management guidelines of the American Thyroid Association and American Association of Clinical Endocrinologists. Thyroid Off J AmThyroid Ass. 2011;21(6):593–646.
26. Dolman PJ. Evaluating Graves' orbitopathy. Best Pract Res Clin Endocrinol Metab. 2012;26(3):229–48.
27. Fatourechi V. Thyroid dermopathy and acropachy. Best Pract Res Clin Endocrinol Metab. 2012;26(4):553–65.
28. Garber JR, Cobin RH, Gharib H, Hennessey JV, Klein I, Mechanick JI, et al. Clinical practice guidelines for hypothyroidism in adults: cosponsored by the American Association of Clinical Endocrinologists and the American Thyroid Association. Thyroid Off J AmThyroid Ass. 2012;22(12):1200–35.

29. Nose V. Thyroid cancer of follicular cell origin in inherited tumor syndromes. Adv Anat Pathol. 2010;17(6):428–36.
30. DeGroot LJ. Clinical review 2: diagnostic approach and management of patients exposed to irradiation to the thyroid. J Clin Endocrinol Metab. 1989;69(5):925–8.
31. Furukawa K, Preston D, Funamoto S, Yonehara S, Ito M, Tokuoka S, et al. Long-term trend of thyroid cancer risk among Japanese atomic-bomb survivors: 60 years after exposure. Int J Cancer. 2013;132(5):1222–6.
32. Fogelfeld L, Wiviott MB, Shore-Freedman E, Blend M, Bekerman C, Pinsky S, et al. Recurrence of thyroid nodules after surgical removal in patients irradiated in childhood for benign conditions. N Engl J Med. 1989;320(13):835–40.
33. Laurberg P, Bulow Pedersen I, Knudsen N, Ovesen L, Andersen S. Environmental iodine intake affects the type of nonmalignant thyroid disease. Thyroid Off J AmThyroid Ass. 2001;11(5):457–69.
34. Braverman LE. Iodine and the thyroid: 33 years of study. Thyroid Off J AmThyroid Ass. 1994;4(3):351–6.
35. Zimmermann MB, Galetti V. Iodine intake as a risk factor for thyroid cancer: a comprehensive review of animal and human studies. Thyroid Res. 2015;8:8.
36. Salvatore D, Davies TF, Schlumberger M-J, Hay ID, Larsen PR. Thyroid physiology and diagnostic evaluation of patients with thyroid disoders. In: Williams textbook of endocrinology. 12th ed. Philadelphia: Saunders Elsevier; 2011. p. 327–61.

Chapter 3
Ultrasound of the Thyroid and Soft Tissues of the Neck

Jennifer A Sipos

Introduction

Thyroid nodules are a common entity and have an increasing frequency with age; they may be seen in up to 50 % of individuals over the age of 70 [1]. Fortunately, the majority of nodules are benign. Though the exact prevalence of malignancy in all nodules is not exactly known, it is estimated that 7–14 % of thyroid nodules are cancerous [2, 3]. The risk of malignancy is inversely related to patient age; there is a 2.2 % decrease per year in the relative risk of malignancy in a given nodule between the ages of 20 and 60 years, with stabilization thereafter [4]. Given the high prevalence of nodularity and the relative paucity of malignancy, it is the sometimes-daunting task of the clinician to discern which nodules require further evaluation.

Ultrasonography is highly sensitive and specific for visualizing structures in the neck. Simple to perform in the outpatient setting, it is an inexpensive imaging modality that does not expose the patient to ionizing radiation. Current machines are portable and affordable while still offering a high-resolution image that allows visualization of very small nodules and accurate identification of critical nodule characteristics such as microcalcifications and extrathyroidal extension. An ultrasound exam in the office provides real-time feedback regarding the presence or absence of thyroid nodules; palpation is neither a sensitive nor accurate means of identifying thyroid nodules. One study found that palpation missed 55 % of nodules measuring up to 2 cm [5]. Another study noted that 16 % of patients referred for evaluation of a palpable nodule had no corresponding nodule on US [6]. Accordingly, US of the neck is the initial recommended test for evaluation of a patient suspected of having a thyroid nodule [7].

J.A. Sipos, MD
Endocrinology and Metabolism, The Ohio State University, Columbus, OH 43210, USA
e-mail: Jennifer.Sipos@osumc.edu

S.A. Roman et al. (eds.), *Management of Thyroid Nodules and Differentiated Thyroid Cancer*, DOI 10.1007/978-3-319-43618-0_3

Thyroid Scintigraphy

While ultrasonography is the recommended initial imaging modality in the assessment of thyroid nodules, some patients may require additional studies for further characterization of the nature of the lesion. Thyroid scintigraphy offers insight into the functionality of a thyroid nodule. Taking advantage of the process of organification of iodine to make thyroid hormone, scintigraphy utilizes radiotracers that similarly can pass through the sodium-iodine symporter (NIS) on the surface of the follicular cell. The most commonly used compounds are iodine isotopes: iodine-123 (^{123}I) sodium iodide, iodine-131 (^{131}I), or iodine-124 (^{124}I). Iodine-123 is the ideal imaging tracer because it has a low radiation burden compared to ^{131}I yet still offers excellent thyroid imaging. A promising new isotope, ^{124}I, emits positrons and is being examined for its utility in conjunction with PET scanning [8]. It is currently only available for investigational purposes, however. Additionally, ^{99m} Tc-pertechnetate is frequently used in thyroid scintigraphy. Though it is not a metabolic substrate, ^{99m}Tc-pertechnetate can pass through NIS and offers the added benefit of complete washout from thyroid cells within 30 min [9]. Pregnancy and breastfeeding are absolute contraindications for scintigraphy as the radiotracer can impact fetal and infant thyroid function.

Thyroid scans with the various isotopes are acquired by gamma-camera on a parallel-hole collimator. Additionally, tracer uptake can be quantified in an uptake study (6- or 24-h uptake test), though interference by dietary intake of iodine and certain medications can create significant competitive interference, falsely altering the results of the exam. For the purposes of evaluating a patient with a nodule, a qualitative thyroid map or scan is typically sufficient. A "hot" or "toxic" nodule readily incorporates the nuclear tracer into the nodule for production of excess thyroid hormone, whereas a "cold" or "nonfunctioning" nodule does not actively take up the isotope. Nodules that exhibit comparable tracer uptake to the surrounding normal thyroid tissue are termed "warm" or isofunctioning. Hot or toxic nodules are only rarely malignant and therefore typically can forgo further diagnostic evaluation [7]. On the other hand, nodules that are "cold" or "warm" by scintigraphy may harbor malignancy and therefore may require further evaluation by FNA. It is important to note, however, that most cold/warm nodules are ultimately benign.

Thyroid scintigraphy is moderately sensitive for detecting functioning nodules; depending on the isotope used, it ranges between 83 and 91 % [10]. The specificity of a radioiodine scan is very low, however, because superimposed normal thyroid tissue or cystic lesions may alter the uptake of the isotopes. Scintigraphy, therefore, should be limited to those patients in whom a high clinical suspicion exists for a functioning nodule, namely, those with a low serum TSH [7] (see Fig. 3.1).

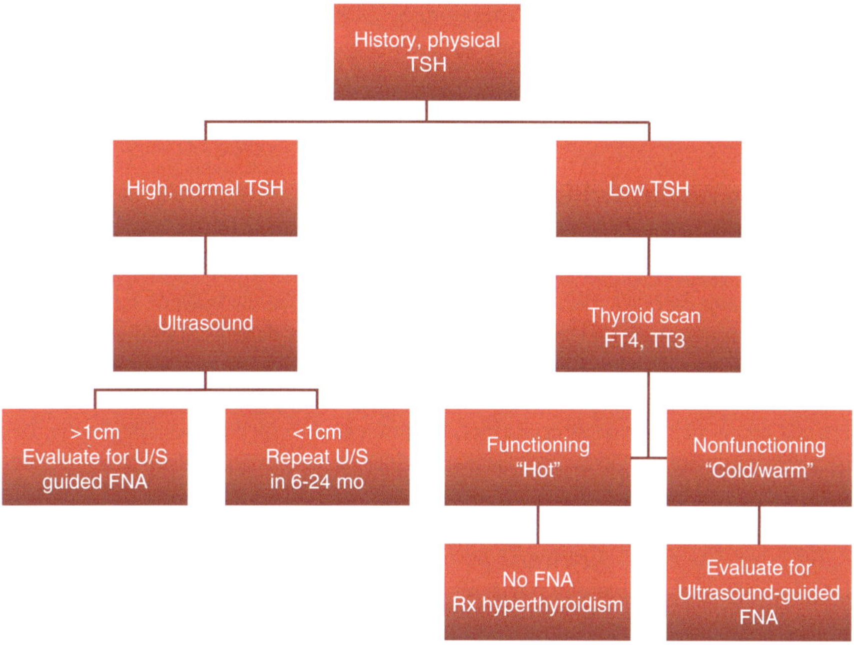

Fig. 3.1 The diagnostic algorithm for a thyroid nodule

Initial Approach to the Patient Suspected of Having a Nodule

The discovery of a thyroid nodule over 1 cm should prompt measurement of the serum TSH [7]. In a patient with a high or normal TSH, the likelihood of identifying a hyperfunctioning nodule is very low. The great majority of nodules in such patients will be either cold or warm on scanning; further evaluation of the need for FNA will be based solely on the sonographic features. As such, in patients with a normal or high TSH, scintigraphy is unnecessary (see Fig. 3.1) [7]. Conversely, a patient with a low TSH and one or more nodules requires scintigraphy to determine if the nodule(s) is(are) toxic and may be observed, or if further interrogation by fine needle aspiration is required in the event of a warm or cold nodule [7]. Consideration to scintigraphy may also be given in a patient with a cytologic diagnosis of follicular neoplasm, particularly if the serum TSH is in the low-normal range [11]. Molecular testing of such indeterminate nodules has largely replaced this approach in clinical practice, however [12].

Most benign and nearly all malignant nodules concentrate radioiodine less avidly than the surrounding normal thyroid tissue. Approximately 5 % of thyroid cancers, however, will concentrate pertechnetate but not radioiodine [13]. Such nodules may appear warm or hot on pertechnetate scans [14]. Consequently, it is recommended that patients with functioning nodules on ^{99m}Tc-pertechnetate scans should undergo confirmatory imaging with radioiodine to determine their functional status [15].

Clinician-Performed Ultrasonography

Ultrasonography is rapidly gaining popularity among non-radiologists for use in the clinical setting. In point of fact, use of ultrasonography at the bedside has become a mandatory component of training for some surgery residencies and all endocrinology fellowships. The high prevalence of thyroid nodules, particularly the nonpalpable variety, necessitates a simple stratification tool to distinguish the benign lesions from those requiring further evaluation. As such, ultrasonography has become an extension of the physical examination in the evaluation of the patient with a thyroid nodule. Indeed, a properly trained clinician can provide a similarly informative exam as that of a radiologist [16].

The benefits of an ultrasound performed by a non-radiologist are manifold. Long-recognized as a more powerful tool when simultaneously performed and interpreted by the same individual, US exams increasingly are being done instead by technologists with subsequent interpretation of the images by a radiologist. Subtle findings on US such as comet-tail signs or microcalcifications easily can be missed when only static images are reviewed. Real-time sonography, in contrast, reveals a wealth of information about the subtle morphologic characteristics of a lesion and the background thyroid parenchyma. Further, the ability to visualize a structure in multiple planes offers a unique radiologic opportunity to create a three-dimensional image, providing important details regarding geographic relationships with nearby anatomic structures. These clues can provide additional context regarding the risk of malignancy or benignity for any given nodule.

From the patient's perspective, clinician-performed exams may be preferable; the endocrinologist or surgeon can provide immediate feedback to the patient regarding the exam findings, rather than waiting for the radiologist's report. These results can then prompt an immediate action, such as an FNA or counseling regarding the need for surgery, in the case of a suspicious nodule or lymph node. In fact, a study of 223 patients referred to a multidisciplinary thyroid nodule clinic revealed that the use of ultrasonography in the clinic altered the management in 63 % of patients [6].

For patients with a diagnosis of thyroid cancer, performing the appropriate initial surgery is a critical determinant of outcome, to minimize the risk of residual disease [7]. Thyroid cancer has a high predilection for metastatic spread to the locoregional lymph nodes; macroscopic nodal disease may be seen in up to 50 % of patients [17–19]. Preoperative US of the neck for identification of suspicious cervical lymph nodes is strongly recommended for all patients undergoing thyroidectomy for a malignant or suspicious cytologic diagnosis [7]. An appropriate initial surgery reduces the morbidity associated with multiple operations, which are often required when the diagnosis of nodal metastases is made after the thyroidectomy [20]. Additionally, the identification of nodal metastases alters the staging and, ultimately, may result in a modification of the treatment strategy [19]. When performed by a radiologist, the presence (or absence) of nodal metastases often is not assessed on preoperative ultrasound, unless specifically requested by the ordering physician. Indeed, one study found that the preoperative US performed in a radiology center missed 88 and 93 % of patients with suspicious central and lateral lymph nodes requiring FNA compared to the findings of an US exam by a surgeon [21]. Moreover, the findings on clinician-performed exam changed the surgical approach in 45 % of patients compared to the initial assessment based on the radiologic diagnoses [21].

Performance of the Ultrasound Exam

Although sonography is a relatively simple procedure to perform, there are a few essential components of the exam that should be reviewed. It is critical to place the patient in the supine position with the neck hyperextended. Such positioning allows structures in the inferior neck and superior mediastinum to be more readily visualized. Attempts to identify the inferior parathyroid glands, a substernal goiter, or mediastinal lymph nodes may be unsuccessful if this important detail is overlooked. Occasionally, it may be necessary to place a pillow or towel roll between the patient's shoulders to achieve greater extension of the neck.

The optimal method for performance of the sonographic exam has not been defined; it is of utmost importance though to cover all areas of the neck. Additionally, the inspection should include both the transverse and longitudinal (sagittal) views. When evaluating a patient with a thyroid nodule, assessment of the lymph nodes, particularly in the lateral neck, provides important clues regarding the malignancy risk. Identification of a suspicious lymph node increases the likelihood of cancer and may warrant FNA of the node in lieu of the thyroid [7] (see Fig. 3.2 normal neck anatomy).

Sonographic Risk Stratification

Ultrasonography is a highly sensitive tool for the identification of thyroid nodules; screening for such lesions identifies nodules in up to 40 % of patients [22], with increasing incidence with advanced age [1]. The high prevalence of nodules and the relative infrequency of malignancy mandate a method of stratification, as there are insufficient resources to perform an FNA of every thyroid lesion identified. Various individual sonographic features have a high specificity for identification of malignancy [23]; the absence of one of these features, however, does not rule out the possibility of a cancerous nodule.

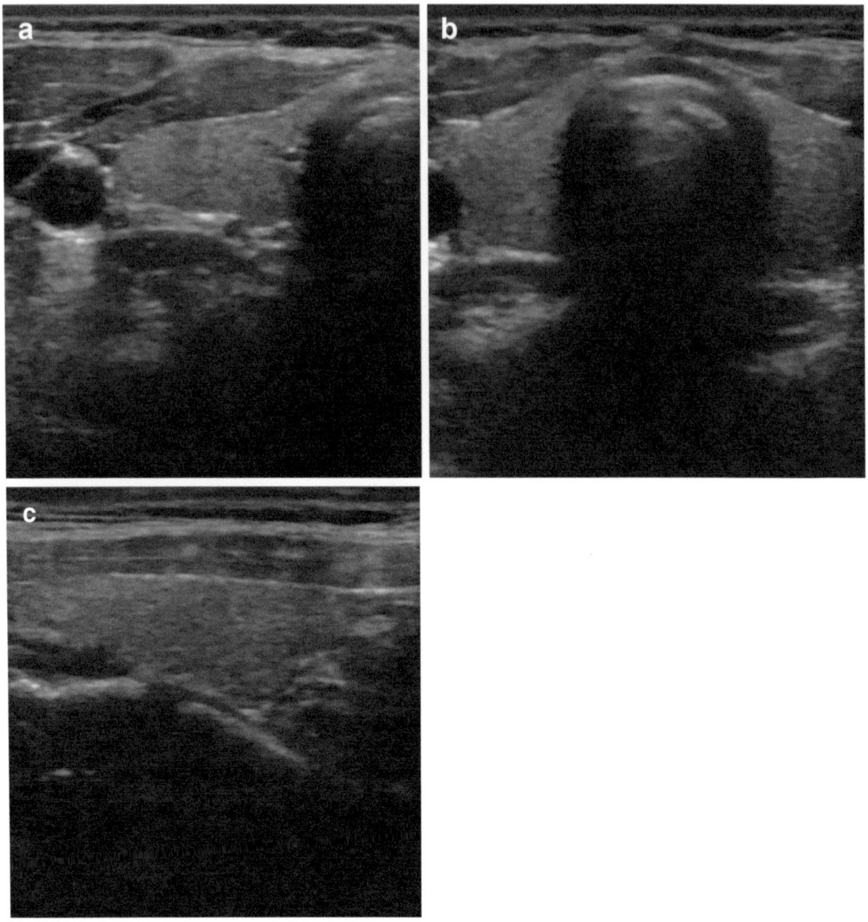

Fig. 3.2 (**a**) Transverse view of a normal right lobe of the thyroid. (**b**) Transverse view normal isthmus and left lobe. (**c**) Longitudinal view normal thyroid

Nodule Size, Composition, and Number

Nodule size does not correlate with malignancy risk, though nearly all consensus guidelines stratify nodules for FNA based on their largest dimension. This size threshold is a necessity, however, as it is increasingly recognized that microcarcinomas are highly prevalent and represent an indolent, clinically inconsequential tumor in the vast majority of cases [24]. The various size thresholds for FNA (see Table 3.1) have been chosen because clinically significant tumors may exist in nodules above this limit [7]. Smaller nodules, even when harboring suspicious US features, may be followed with serial US exams for growth; such a change could potentially indicate a more aggressive lesion which would then warrant interrogation with FNA.

Table 3.1 Summary of 2015 American Thyroid Association recommendations for fine needle aspiration biopsy of thyroid nodules

Nodule features on ultrasound	Recommended FNA based on nodule size
High and intermediate suspicion for malignancy	≥1 cm
Low suspicion for malignancy	≥1.5 cm
Very low suspicion for malignancy (completely cystic/simple cyst)	≥2 cm vs. observation without FNA is also an option
Benign features (cystic)	No FNA unless symptomatic or cosmetic reasons

Nodule composition is important to note on US exam. The greater the cystic content of a nodule, the lower the likelihood of malignancy [25]. Although rare, a simple cyst (no solid component) has virtually no risk of malignancy and can forgo FNA entirely [7, 25].

Echogenicity

Thyroid parenchyma has a medium gray echotexture compared to the surrounding structures in the neck. A lesion that is of the same echogenicity as normal thyroid tissue is termed isoechoic. Those nodules which have a brighter appearance than that of the normal thyroid are labeled hyperechoic. Nodules that are either iso- or hyperechoic have a lower likelihood of malignancy. Most nodules are hypoechoic or darker than the normal thyroid parenchyma. Hypoechogenicity of a nodule is associated with a higher risk of malignancy. Indeed, most malignant nodules are hypoechoic; the majority of hypoechoic nodules, however, are not cancerous. A nodule with an echotexture that is darker than the surrounding strap muscles is termed markedly hypoechoic. Such a finding has a very high specificity for malignancy [23]. A nodule that is completely black is designated anechoic; these lesions are typically simple cysts (see Fig. 3.3).

Nodule Shape

The natural growth plane of a benign nodule is horizontal in a supine patient (or the nodule width). Growth opposite of this plane is suggestive of an aggressive lesion (see Fig. 3.4). Nodule height that is greater than the nodule width has been reported to have a specificity of 91 % for identification of malignancy, though the sensitivity for this feature is significantly lower [26].

Nodule margins are an important feature to assess for malignancy risk. The interface between the thyroid nodule and the surrounding normal parenchyma may be well demarcated (Fig. 3.4a) or poorly defined. It is important to note that

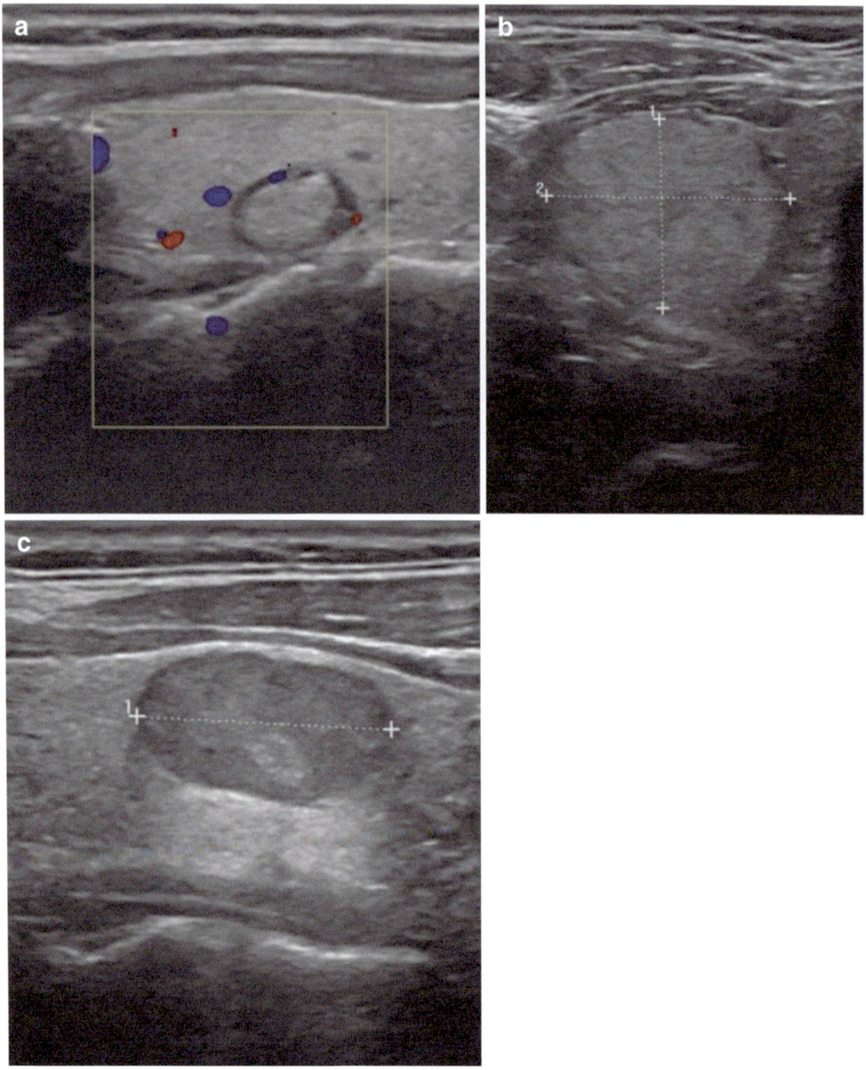

Fig. 3.3 (**a**) Isoechoic nodule. (**b**) Hyperechoic nodule. (**c**) Hypoechoic nodule. (**d**) Markedly hypoechoic nodule with lobulated borders. (**e**) Anechoic nodule (simple cyst)

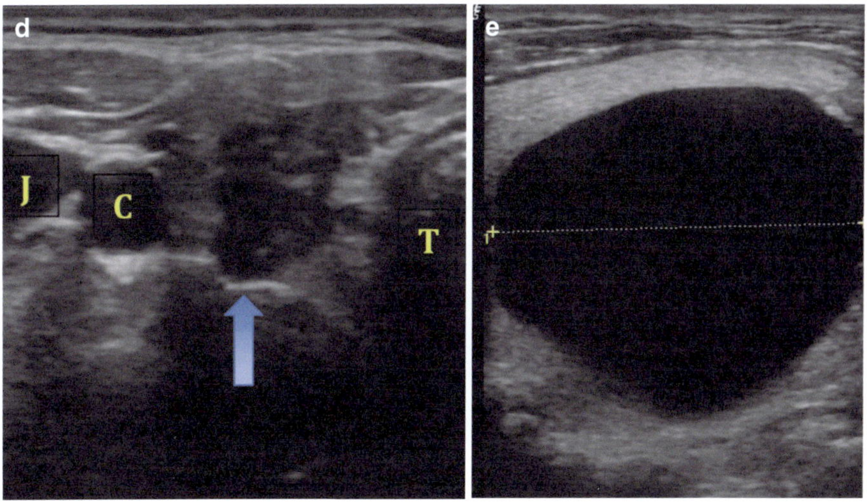

Fig. 3.3 (continued)

a poorly defined margin does not necessarily translate to increased risk of malignancy and is not the same as an irregular margin. Isoechoic or mildly hypoechoic nodules are more likely to have a poorly defined border and carry a low risk of malignancy (Fig. 3.3b). In contrast, nodules that have a microlobulated, spiculated, or infiltrative margin have a high malignancy risk [26] (see Fig. 3.5).

Calcifications

Calcifications are identified on sonography as bright echogenic foci (hyperlucencies). Typically divided into one of three categories, microcalcifications, macrocalcifications (or coarse calcifications), and eggshell (linear), the risk of malignancy varies with each type (see Fig. 3.6a). Microcalcifications are associated with the highest risk of malignancy, though the presence of any of the three increases the risk in any given nodule.

Microcalcifications are defined as punctate hyperlucencies (1 mm or less in size) and lack signal dropout posteriorly (see Fig. 3.6a). Macrocalcifications, in contrast, are greater than 1 mm in dimension and are associated with signal dropout posteriorly. The loss of signal results from the failure of the US wave to penetrate the calcification; consequently, the entire sound wave is sent back to the probe (see Fig. 3.6b). Such coarse calcifications within a nodule are not uniformly associated with malignancy [27]. The coexistence of coarse calcifications

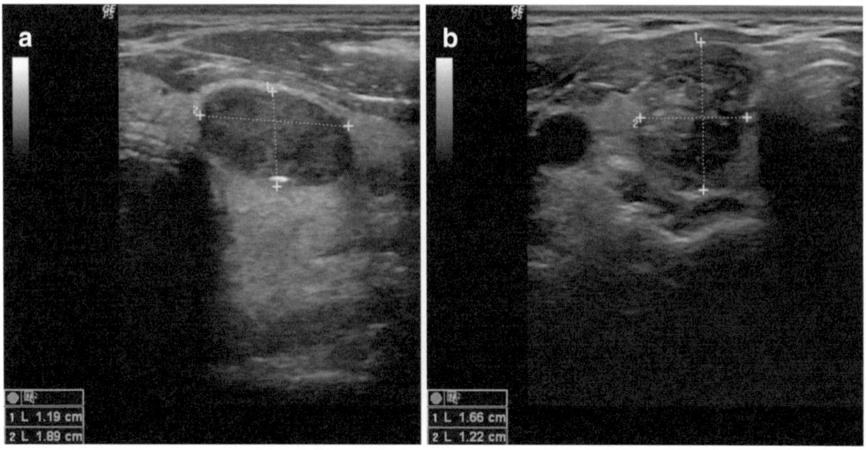

Fig. 3.4 (**a**) Nodule width greater than height. (**b**) Nodule height greater than width

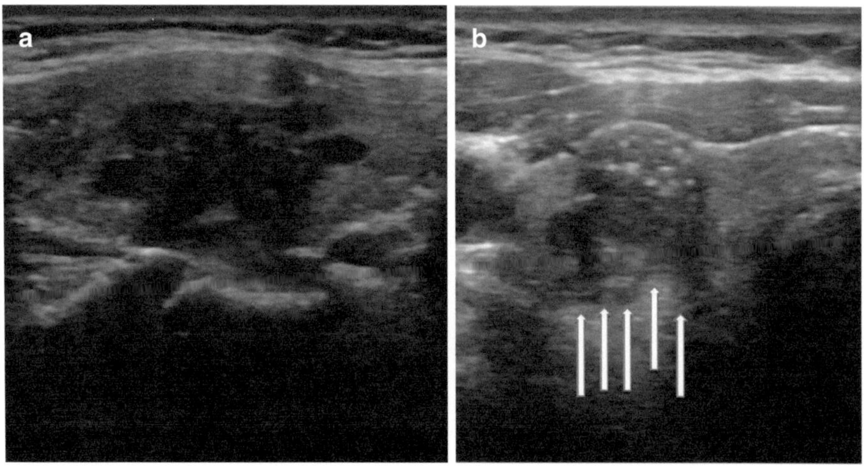

Fig. 3.5 (**a**) Microlobulated margin. (**b**) Infiltrative margin

and microcalcifications within a single nodule confers the same risk as microcalcifications alone [28, 29]. Eggshell calcifications may be described as intact or interrupted. The interrupted variety is associated with a greater malignancy risk [30, 31].

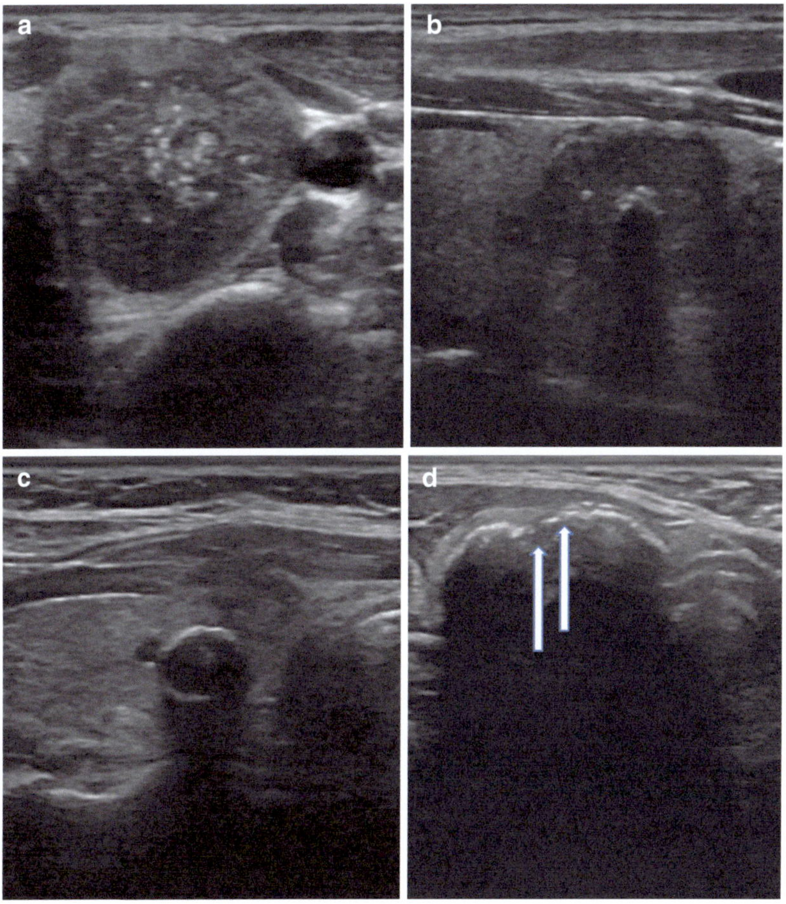

Fig. 3.6 (**a**) Microcalcifications. (**b**) Coarse calcification. (**c**) Continuous eggshell calcification. (**d**) Interrupted eggshell calcification

Vascularity

Early studies have suggested that the pattern of blood flow within a nodule can be used as an additional tool to identify suspicious nodules [29, 32, 33]. More recent reviews of the topic have shown that intranodular vascularity is not associated with malignancy risk on multivariate logistic regression analysis [34].

Benign US Findings

Not all US features are associated with malignancy; various findings on sonography may be strongly associated with benignity. Among the more common reassuring findings are spongiform nodules. These nodules have a "honeycomb" appearance and are composed of multiple tiny cystic structures divided by thin septations involving more than 50 % of the nodule (see Fig. 3.7a).

Colloid, a normal component of the thyroid follicle and the locale for the formation of thyroid hormone, may be identified on sonography. Insipissated colloid may be seen as a comet-tail sign (ring-down artifact or cat's eye). The energy of the ultrasound wave as it strikes the colloid crystals creates a vibration which influences their return to the transducer after the initial reflected signal. The result is a hyperlucency with a posterior tail or stepladder artifact (see Fig. 3.7b). The comet-tail sign, when found within a cystic area, is a reassuring finding most commonly associated with colloid nodules and resolving hematomas. Although rare, it may be seen in PTC, but is typically found within a solid component of the lesion [35].

Pattern Recognition

Quantification of the risk of malignancy in a given nodule based on its individual ultrasound features can be challenging, even in the hands of an experienced sonographer. Indeed, the identification of a single US parameter cannot satisfactorily identify the entire subset of patients who require FNA, as the requisite sensitivity and specificity cannot be achieved with any one sonographic feature. Additionally,

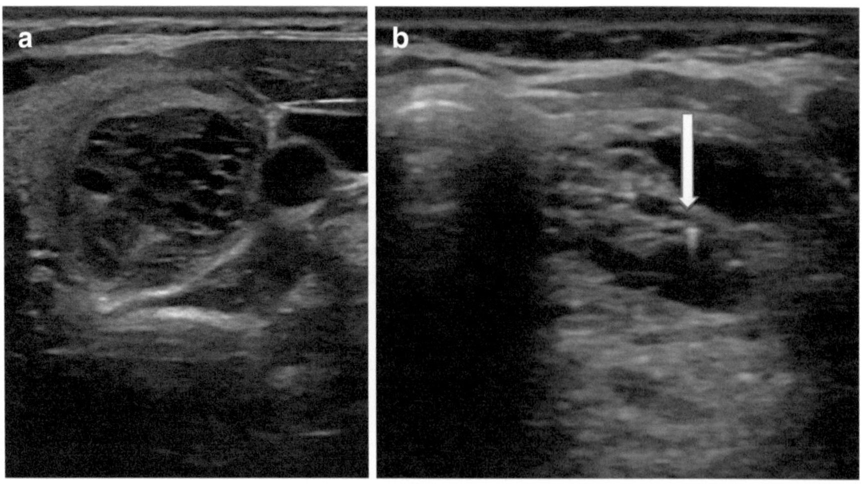

Fig. 3.7 (**a**) Spongiform nodule. (**b**) Comet-tail sign

the interobserver variability of individual US characteristics is unacceptably low. Instead, the majority of thyroid nodules should be classified into one of several US patterns; such a classification system has been reported to have a high interobserver correlation [36, 37]. Borrowing terminology from breast cancer imaging, various authors have proposed a thyroid imaging reporting and data system (TIRADS) for categorization of thyroid nodules based on their sonographic appearance [36, 38]. Additionally, the American Thyroid Association has created a system of pattern recognition for stratification of thyroid nodules into various risk categories [7]. This system assigns a risk of malignancy and provides a recommendation regarding the size threshold for FNA and is explained below (See Table 3.1 and Chap. 4, "Thyroid Nodule Biopsy").

High Suspicion Nodules

A solid hypoechoic nodule or a cystic nodule with a solid component that is hypoechoic and has at least one of the following features, irregular margins (infiltrative or microlobulated), microcalcifications, taller-than-wide shape, interrupted rim calcifications, or evidence of extrathyroidal extension, is considered to be high risk nodules [7]. This group of lesions has been found to carry an estimated risk of malignancy of 70–90 % [7]. As such, it is recommended that nodules in this category should undergo FNA when they are 1 cm or larger [7].

Intermediate Suspicion Nodules

Hypoechoic solid nodules with smooth margins and lacking microcalcifications, extrathyroidal extension, or taller-than-wide shape are of intermediate suspicion [7]. This sonographic pattern has the highest sensitivity for identification of PTC at 60–80 % but carries a lower specificity than in the high risk group [7]. For this reason, it is also recommended that these nodules are considered for FNA at the 1 cm threshold [7].

Low Suspicion Nodules

Hyperechoic or isoechoic solid nodules or partially cystic nodules with an eccentric solid component have a lower suspicion for malignancy, 5–10 % [7]. Nodules in this category do not have any high risk features, including microcalcifications, extrathyroidal extension, or taller-than-wide shape. The threshold for FNA for these low risk nodules is 1.5 cm or larger [7].

Very Low Suspicion Nodules

Nodules that are partially cystic (and lacking all of the features in the above categories) or spongiform have a very low likelihood of malignancy (<3 %) [7]. Such nodules may be observed or considered for FNA if larger than 2 cm [7].

Benign Nodules

Simple cysts (lacking any solid component) are very unlikely to be malignant and do not require FNA for diagnostic purposes [7]. Occasionally, patients may request FNA for relief of compressive symptoms with drainage of the cystic contents. In such cases, a small amount of the aspirate should also be sent for cytologic analysis.

Indications for FNA of Smaller Nodules

It is recommended that all patients undergoing sonographic evaluation for suspected thyroid nodules should also have an examination of the anterior neck for the presence of nodal metastases [7]. The identification of a suspicious lymph node should prompt an FNA for cytologic analysis and measurement of thyroglobulin in the needle washout [7]. If the suspected primary site of malignancy is a subcentimeter thyroid nodule, consideration may be given to aspiration of this lesion [7].

Additionally, patients with a high risk for thyroid cancer may warrant FNA of subcentimeter nodules [7]. Such high risk patients include those with a strong family history of thyroid cancer or those with a history of childhood radiation to the head/neck. Additional concerning clinical features include voice change, pain, cough, immobility with swallowing, or associated lymphadenopathy [7, 39]. Though not rigorously studied, the likelihood malignancy in the presence of any one of these features was over 70 % according to one study [39].

Lymph Node Evaluation

Because of the high frequency of nodal metastases in thyroid cancer and the impact that sonographically suspicious nodes have on prognosis and management, it is important to examine all patients with a nodule for the presence of suspicious lymph nodes in the anterior neck [7]. The sensitivity and specificity of US for detecting nodal metastases is variably reported in the literature; experience of the sonographer and study design can significantly impact the rates of detection. One important limitation of US, certain areas of the neck may not be adequately interrogated sonographically, including behind the trachea or in the superior mediastinum. Computed tomography

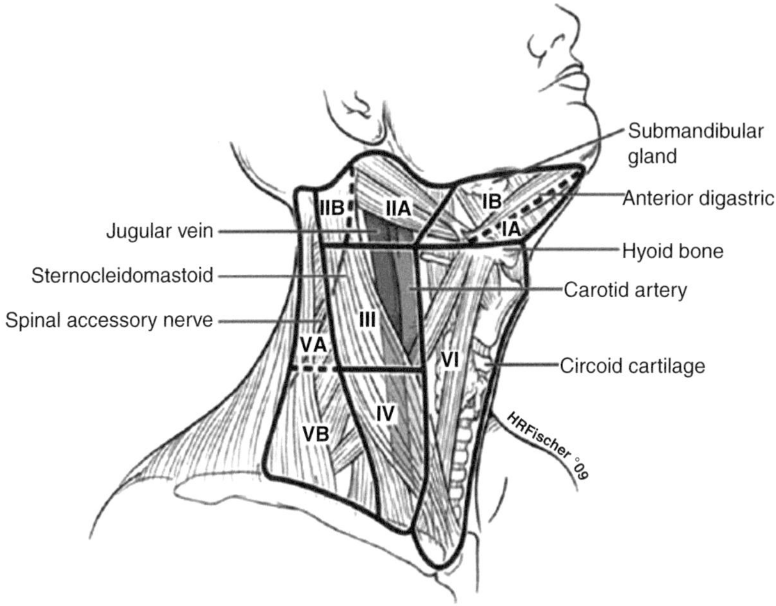

Fig. 3.8 Lymph node compartments of the neck

or magnetic resonance imaging of the neck may be required to allow better visualization in select individuals, particularly those with bulky or extensive nodal involvement [7]. A further limitation of US is that the central neck nodes are often difficult to visualize prior to thyroidectomy [40]. In contrast, inspection of the lateral neck compartments is more sensitive for identification of suspicious adenopathy [41].

Once a suspicious node is detected and cytologically confirmed, communication of the involved nodal compartments to the surgeon (if the surgeon is not performing the US exam) is of paramount importance. The most widely accepted system for reporting nodal locations is the surgical lymph node compartments (see Fig. 3.8) [7]. Compartment-directed removal of the sonographically suspicious nodes and any other lymphatic structures seen intraoperatively is the recommended surgical approach to nodal disease [7].

Benign Lymph Node Sonographic Appearance

Though many benign lymph nodes are not visible on US, those that are enlarged and reactive may be more readily appreciated [42]. The classic appearance of a benign node is a fusiform (oval)-shaped hypoechoic structure with a hyperechoic stripe (hilum) in the center [43] (see Fig. 3.9). The hilar stripe represents the entry of vasculature and lymphatic outflow from the node [43]. The vascularity in a benign lymph node should superimpose on the area of the hilar stripe [44] (see Fig. 3.9).

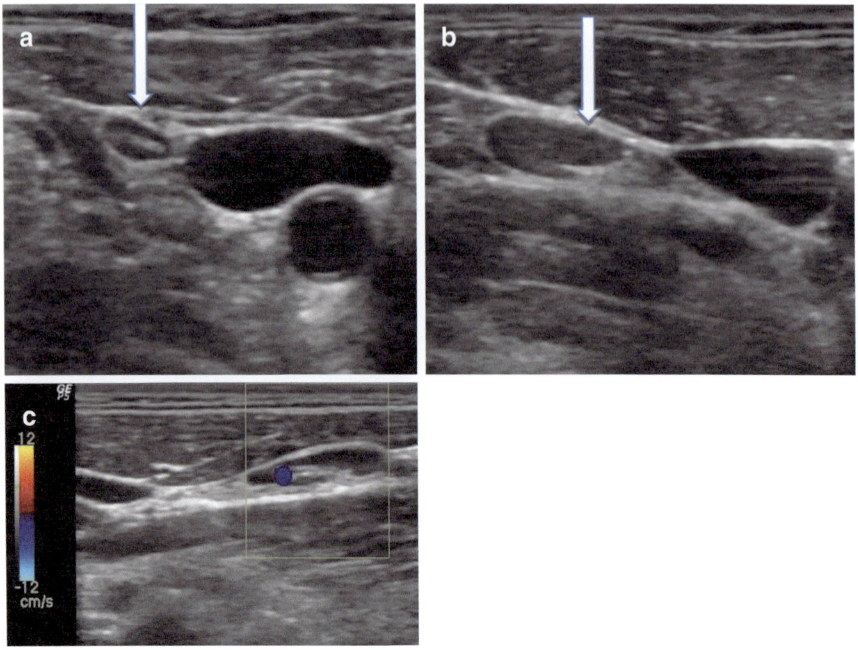

Fig. 3.9 (**a**) Benign lymph node with prominent hilar stripe. (**b**) Benign, reactive lymph node with hilar stripe. (**c**) Doppler flow within a benign lymph node

Malignant Lymph Node Sonographic Appearance

Neoplastic infiltration typically begins at the outer cortex of the node; disappearance of the hilum may be the earliest indication of a malignant transformation [43]. Though the absence of a hilum is commonly seen in malignant lymph nodes, it is not a specific indicator; the hilar stripe is not always visible in benign nodes [45]. A more suspicious finding may be seen as the node converts from oval to a rounded appearance with progression of the peripheral infiltration [42, 45]. An objective means to assess the "roundness" of a node is the Solbiati Index—the long-to-short axis ratio [43]. A ratio of greater than 2.0 is consistent with an elongated or benign node (Fig. 3.10a); a ratio less than 2.0 indicates a more rounded node, suspicious for malignancy (Fig. 3.10b) [43].

Echogenicity of a node may be a marker of a malignant transformation. Benign nodes are typically hypoechoic (darker than the thyroid tissue or the same echogenicity as the surrounding muscles) [46]; a malignant lesion may be hyperechoic

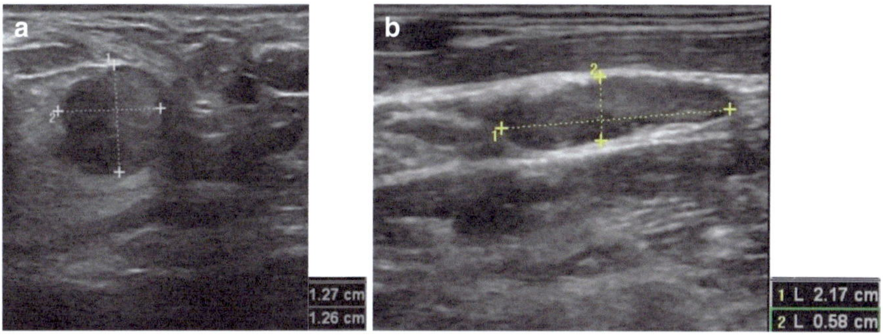

Fig. 3.10 (**a**) Rounded node. Solbiati Index is 1.0. (**b**) Fusiform node. Solbiati Index is 3.75 (2.17/0.58)

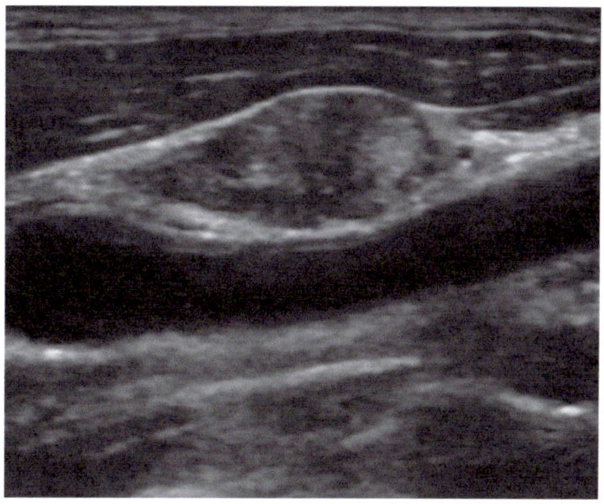

Fig. 3.11 Heterogeneous malignant node

or isoechoic [47]. Heterogeneity of a node may be seen if there are areas of cystic degeneration or foci of malignant infiltration (see Fig. 3.11) [47].

Cystic degeneration within a lymph node is a common finding in young adults and children with metastatic thyroid cancer; these tumors may undergo liquefaction necrosis as they outgrow their blood supply [48]. Cystic change may also be seen in well-differentiated tumors that retain the ability to produce colloid [48]. Identification of a cystic lymph node in the neck should prompt high clinical suspicion for a malignancy, the mean specificity of this finding in a thyroid cancer patient is over 95 % [23] (see Fig. 3.12).

Calcifications within a lymph node are also highly specific for malignancy, reaching nearly 100 % (see Fig. 3.13) [40, 45]. In patients with PTC, the punctate calcifications often represent psammoma bodies [40, 45]. Though less commonly seen, calcifications may occur in metastatic nodes of patients with MTC [49]. These

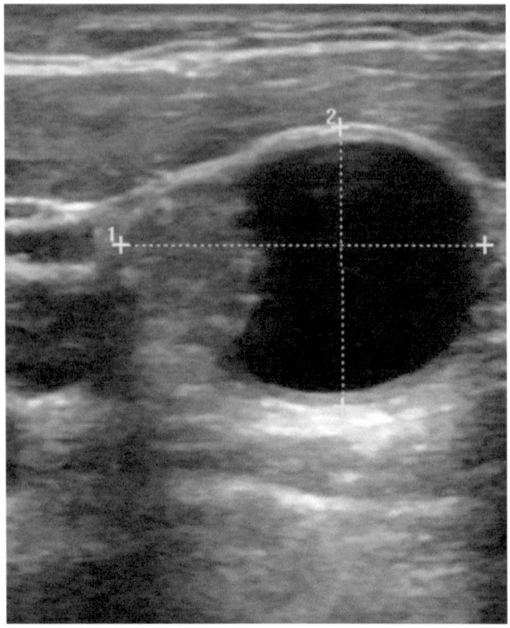

Fig. 3.12 Partially cystic malignant lymph node

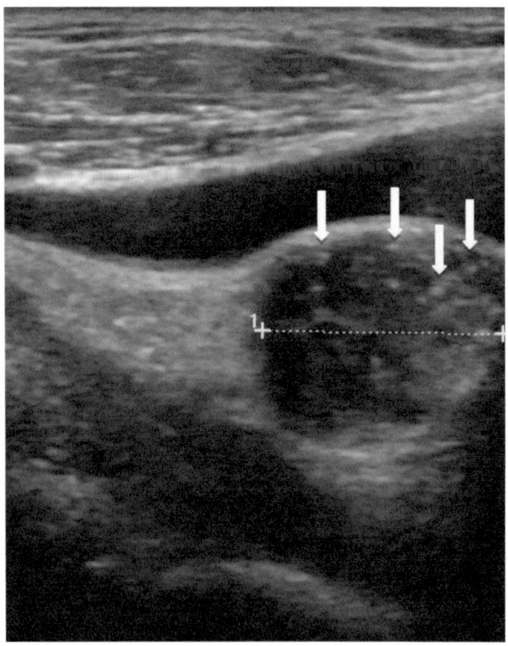

Fig. 3.13 Microcalcifications in a malignant node

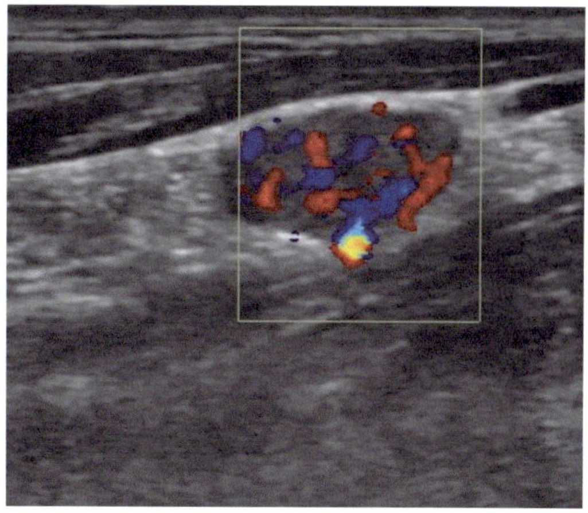

Fig. 3.14 Chaotic Doppler flow in a malignant node

calcifications are more likely to be coarse (>1 cm with posterior signal dropout) and are thought to the result of calcium deposits surrounded by amyloid [49].

Doppler flow can help assess the presence of malignancy within a lymph node. The normal flow within the hilum is disrupted as the malignant cells infiltrate the node; neovascularization creates chaotic flow throughout the node and into the periphery (see Fig. 3.14) [44]. It is important to recognize, however, that the Doppler settings may require adjustment to be able to detect the blood flow in these small vessels. The settings should include high sensitivity on the power Doppler with a low wall filter and a low pulse repetition frequency [44].

Other Sonographic Findings in the Neck

It is important to have a firm understanding of neck anatomy when performing ultrasonography. Various embryonic remnants and other nonmalignant pathologic processes may be mistaken for malignancy. The thyroglossal duct may be seen as a cystic structure anterior to the trachea, typically between the hyoid bone and the thyroid bed (see Fig. 3.15). The thyroglossal duct can be visualized as a distinct mass or it may be attached to the thyroid [50]. Additionally, the thymus may be visible in the superior mediastinum, particularly in children and young adults; less commonly, it may be seen in the lateral neck (cervical thymus) [51]. The characteristic appearance of the thymus is a lacelike mass with fibrous septations and internal hyperlucencies (see Fig. 3.16) [51]. A pharyngoesophageal diverticulum may be confused for a metastatic central neck node with internal calcifications. These lesions are typically located in the thyroid bed and may be visibly contiguous with the esophagus in the sagittal view; mobility with swallowing may be another clue to the diagnosis [52]. A parathyroid adenoma may be mistaken for a

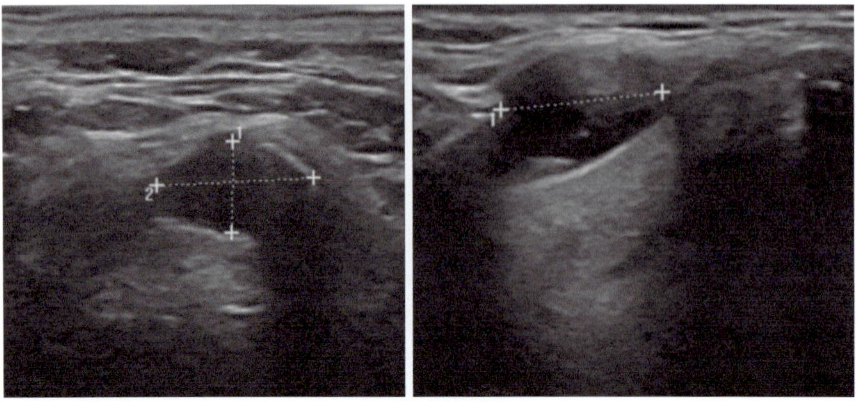

Fig. 3.15 Transverse and sagittal views of thyroglossal cyst

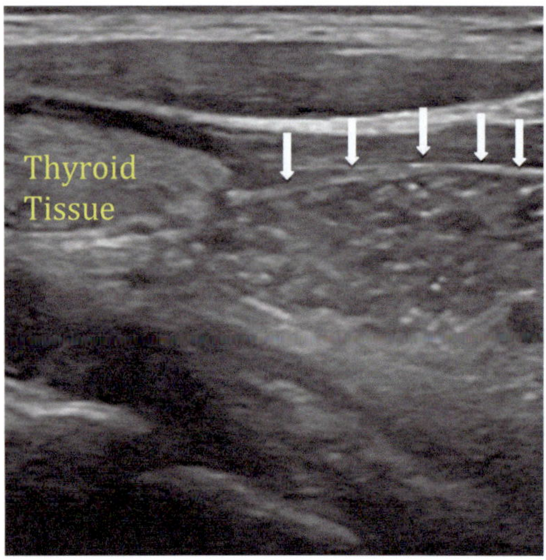

Fig. 3.16 Sagittal view of the thymus inferior to the lower pole of the thyroid

posterior thyroid nodule or a suspicious central neck node. Typically located in the region of the midpole below the inferior pole of the thyroid, these uniformly hypoechoic densities are oval with well-defined margins (see Fig. 3.17) [53]. The Doppler flow is typically concentrated on one end of the lesion—polar feeding

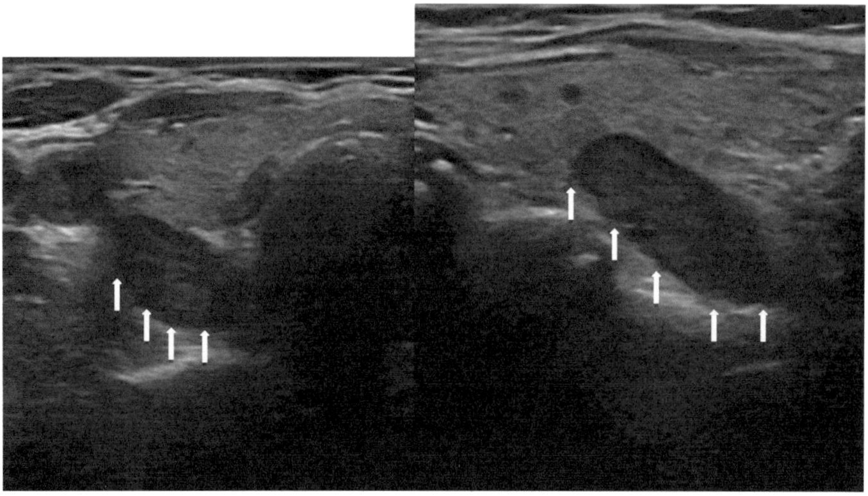

Fig. 3.17 Transverse and sagittal views of a parathyroid adenoma

vessel [53]. Alternatively, the Doppler flow may also be distributed throughout the mass [53].

References

1. Mazzaferri EL. Management of a solitary thyroid nodule. N Engl J Med. 1993;328(8):553–9.
2. Yang J, et al. Fine-needle aspiration of thyroid nodules: a study of 4703 patients with histologic and clinical correlations. Cancer. 2007;111(5):306–15.
3. Yassa L, et al. Long-term assessment of a multidisciplinary approach to thyroid nodule diagnostic evaluation. Cancer. 2007;111(6):508–16.
4. Kwong N, et al. The Influence of patient age on thyroid nodule formation, multinodularity, and thyroid cancer risk. J Clin Endocrinol Metab. 2015;100(12):4434–40.
5. Brander A, et al. Clinical versus ultrasound examination of the thyroid gland in common clinical practice. J Clin Ultrasound. 1992;20(1):37–42.
6. Marqusee E, et al. Usefulness of ultrasonography in the management of nodular thyroid disease. Ann Intern Med. 2000;133(9):696–700.
7. Haugen BR, et al. 2015 American Thyroid Association Management guidelines for adult patients with thyroid nodules and differentiated thyroid cancer: The American Thyroid association guidelines task force on thyroid nodules and differentiated thyroid cancer. Thyroid. 2016;26(1):1–133.
8. Van Nostrand D, et al. (124)I positron emission tomography versus (131)I planar imaging in the identification of residual thyroid tissue and/or metastasis in patients who have well-differentiated thyroid cancer. Thyroid. 2010;20(8):879–83.
9. Wong KT, et al. Current role of radionuclide imaging in differentiated thyroid cancer. Cancer Imaging. 2008;8:159–62.
10. Bahn RS, Castro MR. Approach to the patient with nontoxic multinodular goiter. J Clin Endocrinol Metab. 2011;96(5):1202–12.

11. Cooper DS, American Thyroid Association Guidelines Taskforce on Thyroid, N, et al. Revised American Thyroid Association management guidelines for patients with thyroid nodules and differentiated thyroid cancer. Thyroid. 2009;19(11):1167–214.
12. Alexander EK, et al. Preoperative diagnosis of benign thyroid nodules with indeterminate cytology. N Engl J Med. 2012;367(8):705–15.
13. Reschini E, et al. The trapping-only nodules of the thyroid gland: prevalence study. Thyroid. 2006;16(8):757–62.
14. Arnold JE, Pinsky S. Comparison of 99mTc and 123I for thyroid imaging. J Nucl Med. 1976;17(4):261–7.
15. Shambaugh 3rd GE, et al. Disparate thyroid imaging. Combined studies with sodium pertechnetate Tc 99m and radioactive iodine. JAMA. 1974;228(7):866–9.
16. Hamer PW, Aspinall SR, Malycha PL. Clinician-performed ultrasound in assessing potentially malignant thyroid nodules. ANZ J Surg. 2014;84(5):376–9.
17. Mazzaferri EL, Jhiang SM. Long-term impact of initial surgical and medical therapy on papillary and follicular thyroid cancer. Am J Med. 1994;97(5):418–28.
18. Grant CS, et al. Risks and adequacy of an optimized surgical approach to the primary surgical management of papillary thyroid carcinoma treated during 1999–2006. World J Surg. 2010;34(6):1239–46.
19. Bardet S, et al. Macroscopic lymph-node involvement and neck dissection predict lymph-node recurrence in papillary thyroid carcinoma. Eur J Endocrinol. 2008;158(4):551–60.
20. Urken ML, et al. Management of recurrent and persistent metastatic lymph nodes in well-differentiated thyroid cancer: a multifactorial decision-making guide for the thyroid cancer care collaborative. Head Neck. 2015;37(4):605–14.
21. Carneiro-Pla D, Amin S. Comparison between preconsultation ultrasonography and office surgeon-performed ultrasound in patients with thyroid cancer. World J Surg. 2014;38(3):622–7.
22. Sharen G, et al. Retrospective epidemiological study of thyroid nodules by ultrasound in asymptomatic subjects. Chin Med J (Engl). 2014;127(9):1661–5.
23. Sipos JA. Advances in ultrasound for the diagnosis and management of thyroid cancer. Thyroid. 2009;19(12):1363–72.
24. Davies L, Welch HG. Increasing incidence of thyroid cancer in the United States, 1973–2002. JAMA. 2006;295(18):2164–7.
25. Frates MC, et al. Prevalence and distribution of carcinoma in patients with solitary and multiple thyroid nodules on sonography. J Clin Endocrinol Metab. 2006;91(9):3411–7.
26. Moon WJ, et al. Benign and malignant thyroid nodules: US differentiation–multicenter retrospective study. Radiology. 2008;247(3):762–70.
27. Moon HJ, et al. Diagnostic performance of gray-scale US and elastography in solid thyroid nodules. Radiology. 2012;262(3):1002–13.
28. Kwak JY, et al. Thyroid imaging reporting and data system for US features of nodules: a step in establishing better stratification of cancer risk. Radiology. 2011;260(3):892–9.
29. Papini E, et al. Risk of malignancy in nonpalpable thyroid nodules: predictive value of ultrasound and color-Doppler features. J Clin Endocrinol Metab. 2002;87(5):1941–6.
30. Kim DS, et al. Sonographic features of follicular variant papillary thyroid carcinomas in comparison with conventional papillary thyroid carcinomas. J Ultrasound Med. 2009;28(12):1685–92.
31. Park YJ, et al. Thyroid nodules with macrocalcification: sonographic findings predictive of malignancy. Yonsei Med J. 2014;55(2):339–44.
32. Cappelli C, et al. The predictive value of ultrasound findings in the management of thyroid nodules. QJM. 2007;100(1):29–35.
33. Cerbone G, et al. Power Doppler improves the diagnostic accuracy of color Doppler ultrasonography in cold thyroid nodules: follow-up results. Horm Res. 1999;52(1):19–24.
34. Moon HJ, et al. Can vascularity at power Doppler US help predict thyroid malignancy? Radiology. 2010;255(1):260–9.
35. Malhi H, et al. Echogenic foci in thyroid nodules: significance of posterior acoustic artifacts. AJR Am J Roentgenol. 2014;203(6):1310–6.

36. Russ G, et al. Prospective evaluation of thyroid imaging reporting and data system on 4550 nodules with and without elastography. Eur J Endocrinol. 2013;168(5):649–55.
37. Cheng SP, et al. Characterization of thyroid nodules using the proposed thyroid imaging reporting and data system (TI-RADS). Head Neck. 2013;35(4):541–7.
38. Park JY, et al. A proposal for a thyroid imaging reporting and data system for ultrasound features of thyroid carcinoma. Thyroid. 2009;19(11):1257–64.
39. Hamming JF, et al. The value of fine-needle aspiration biopsy in patients with nodular thyroid disease divided into groups of suspicion of malignant neoplasms on clinical grounds. Arch Intern Med. 1990;150(1):113–6.
40. Park JS, et al. Performance of preoperative sonographic staging of papillary thyroid carcinoma based on the sixth edition of the AJCC/UICC TNM classification system. AJR Am J Roentgenol. 2009;192(1):66–72.
41. Ahn JE, et al. Diagnostic accuracy of CT and ultrasonography for evaluating metastatic cervical lymph nodes in patients with thyroid cancer. World J Surg. 2008;32(7):1552–8.
42. Kuna SK, et al. Ultrasonographic differentiation of benign from malignant neck lymphadenopathy in thyroid cancer. J Ultrasound Med. 2006;25(12):1531–7; quiz 1538–40.
43. Solbiati L, et al. Ultrasound of thyroid, parathyroid glands and neck lymph nodes. Eur Radiol. 2001;11(12):2411–24.
44. Ahuja AT, et al. Power Doppler sonography of metastatic nodes from papillary carcinoma of the thyroid. Clin Radiol. 2001;56(4):284–8.
45. Leboulleux S, et al. Ultrasound criteria of malignancy for cervical lymph nodes in patients followed up for differentiated thyroid cancer. J Clin Endocrinol Metab. 2007;92(9): 3590–4.
46. Ying M, Ahuja A. Sonography of neck lymph nodes. Part I: normal lymph nodes. Clin Radiol. 2003;58(5):351–8.
47. Ahuja A, Ying M. Sonography of neck lymph nodes. Part II: abnormal lymph nodes. Clin Radiol. 2003;58(5):359–66.
48. Wunderbaldinger P, et al. Cystic lymph node metastases in papillary thyroid carcinoma. AJR Am J Roentgenol. 2002;178(3):693–7.
49. Gorman B, et al. Medullary thyroid carcinoma: role of high-resolution US. Radiology. 1987;162(1 Pt 1):147–50.
50. Hong HS, et al. Ultrasonography of various thyroid diseases in children and adolescents: a pictorial essay. Korean J Radiol. 2015;16(2):419–29.
51. Sakai F, et al. Ultrasonography of thymoma with pathologic correlation. Acta Radiol. 1994;35(1):25–9.
52. Kwak JY, Kim EK. Sonographic findings of Zenker diverticula. J Ultrasound Med. 2006;25(5):639–42.
53. Kobaly K, Mandel SJ, Langer JE. Clinical review: Thyroid cancer mimics on surveillance neck sonography. J Clin Endocrinol Metab. 2015;100(2):371–5.

Chapter 4
Thyroid Nodule Biopsy

Denise Carneiro-Pla

Background

Thyroid nodule biopsy has been the most effective tool of thyroid nodule evaluation in patients who are eu- or hypothyroid since it gained popularity in the 1980s in the USA [1–4]. FNA was vastly used in Scandinavia for many years before initial reports in the early 1970s were published [5–10]. Using the clinical information, ultrasound characteristics, and cytology [see chapter 5], the clinician can decide which nodules can be followed safely over time as opposed to nodules requiring surgical excision to confirm or rule out malignancy.

Usually, thyroid gland biopsy is performed using fine-needle aspiration (FNA). This method allows collection of enough cells to evaluate nuclear features without causing significant bleeding. Although core biopsy of the thyroid can be done, it is usually not recommended because of the risk of significant hematoma. The information gained from a core biopsy is not superior to that gained from a FNA, except for the rare cases of thyroid lymphoma. However, patients with lymphoma will often undergo an open incisional biopsy as a substitute for a core biopsy [11].

Ultrasound-guided FNA biopsy has proven to be more accurate when compared to FNA guided by palpation alone and has higher adequacy rates [12–15]. When performed under US guidance, the ultrasonographer can direct the biopsy needle to the more suspicious areas within the nodule containing micro- or macrocalcifications, hypervascular regions, or more solid portions while avoiding cystic collections or central necrotic areas, which can decrease the yield of FNA.

D. Carneiro-Pla, MD, FACS
Oncologic and Endocrine Surgery Division at the Department of Surgery,
Medical University of South Carolina, 114 Doughty Street, Charleston, SC 29425, USA
e-mail: carneiro@musc.edu

S.A. Roman et al. (eds.), *Management of Thyroid Nodules and Differentiated Thyroid Cancer*, DOI 10.1007/978-3-319-43618-0_4

Indications

The American Thyroid Association provides guidelines to assist the clinician in choosing which thyroid nodules require FNA (Table 4.1) [16]. These guidelines are more conservative than the previous recommendations. As a generalized summary, hypoechoic solid nodules or a solid hypoechoic component of a partially cystic nodule ≥1 cm with one of these high suspicion features – irregular margins (infiltrative, microlobulated), microcalcifications, taller-than-wide shape on a transverse image on US, rim calcifications with small extrusive soft tissue component, and evidence of extrathyroidal invasion – should be biopsied. Nodules with intermediate suspicion features such as hypoechoic solid nodule with smooth margins without microcalcifications, extrathyroidal extension, or taller-than-wide shape should be biopsied when ≥1 cm. Nodules with low suspicion features, which are isoechoic or hyperechoic solid nodules, or partially cystic lesions with eccentric solid areas, without microcalcification, irregular margin or extrathyroidal invasion, or taller-than-wide shape should be biopsied when are larger than 1.5 cm. However, nodules with very low suspicion patterns for malignancy (spongiform or partially cystic nodules without any of the sonographic features described in low, intermediate, or high suspicion patterns) can be biopsied only when they reach 2 cm in size or can be observed without FNA with periodic US. Purely cystic lesions should be only aspirated if symptomatic or for cosmetic reasons, and no longer need to be evaluated for recurrence because of the low possibility of malignancy on the cystic wall on those patients.

In the author's opinion, smaller nodules with suspicious features should be biopsied if the diagnosis of malignancy would lead to surgical intervention, especially nodules close to the thyroid capsule, isthmus, or in the upper thyroid pole next to the cricothyroid muscle, which are known for metastasizing early on. The current guidelines do not strongly indicate more aggressive FNA biopsy of these small lesions in patients at a higher risk for thyroid cancer such as in patients with history of thyroid cancer in one or more first-degree relatives, exposure to ionizing radiation in childhood or adolescence, personal history of thyroid cancer, PET-positive nodules, multiple endocrine neoplasia 2/familial medullary thyroid cancer history, RET proto-oncogene mutation, or calcitonin >100 pg/mL. Again, in the author's opinion, these patients can be considered for biopsy earlier if the clinician would treat surgically if a small lesion was found to be positive on FNA.

Table 4.1 Summary of the 2015 American Thyroid Association recommendations for fine-needle aspiration biopsy of thyroid nodules

Nodule features on ultrasound	Recommended FNA based on nodule size
High and intermediate suspicion for malignancy	≥1 cm
Low suspicion for malignancy	≥1.5 cm
Very low suspicion for malignancy	≥2 cm vs observation without FNA is also an option
Benign features (cystic)	No FNA unless symptomatic or cosmetic reasons

The American Association of Clinical Endocrinologists, Associazione Medici Endocrinologi, and European Thyroid Association Medical Guidelines for diagnosis and management of thyroid nodules suggest that solid and hypoechoic thyroid nodules should be biopsied when larger than 1 cm or at any size if the patient presents with any risk factor for thyroid cancer as described above [17].

Materials for Thyroid Nodule Fine-Needle Aspiration Biopsy

The ultrasonographer will require the following materials for fine-needle aspiration: a 10-cc syringe, a 25- or 27-gauge sterile needle usually 1–1.5 inches in length depending on the patient's body habitus and location of the thyroid nodule, alcohol pads, gauze to wipe the excess gel, sterile probe cover, gloves, and lidocaine without epinephrine for local analgesia. Some clinicians prefer using a biopsy gun for ease of aspiration (Fig. 4.1). Larger bore needles should be avoided to prevent bleeding from the site of the biopsy and to avoid aspirating excess blood with the sample. For specimen processing, glass slides and 95 % ethanol solution for fixation along with ThinPrep or Hanks solution to wash the needle content are required (Fig. 4.2). For the clinicians who also assess the sample adequacy, a microscope with a set of Diff-Quik stains for slide preparation is necessary.

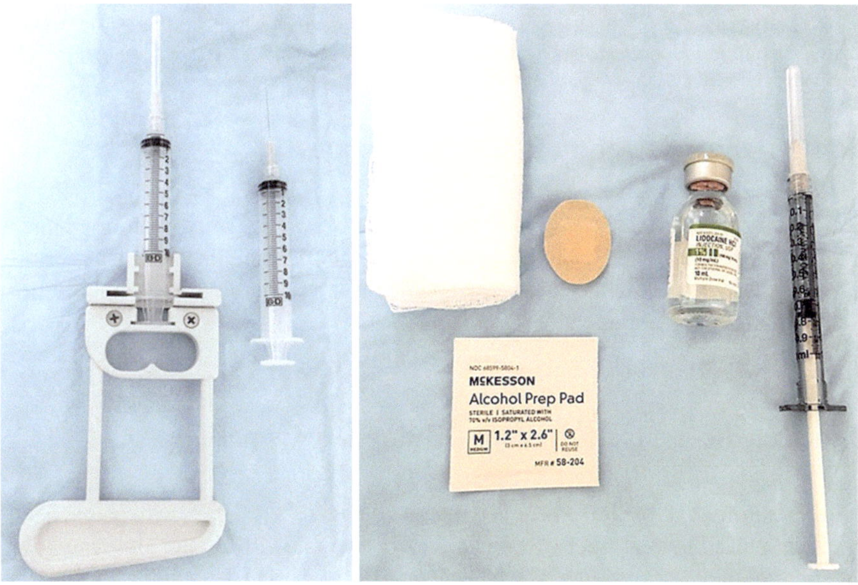

Fig. 4.1 Material for fine-needle aspiration biopsy of the thyroid gland. Picture from *left* to *right*: biopsy gun, 10-cc syringe with 27-gauge needle, gauze, alcohol pad, Band-Aid, lidocaine without epinephrine, and tuberculin syringe for local anesthesia injection

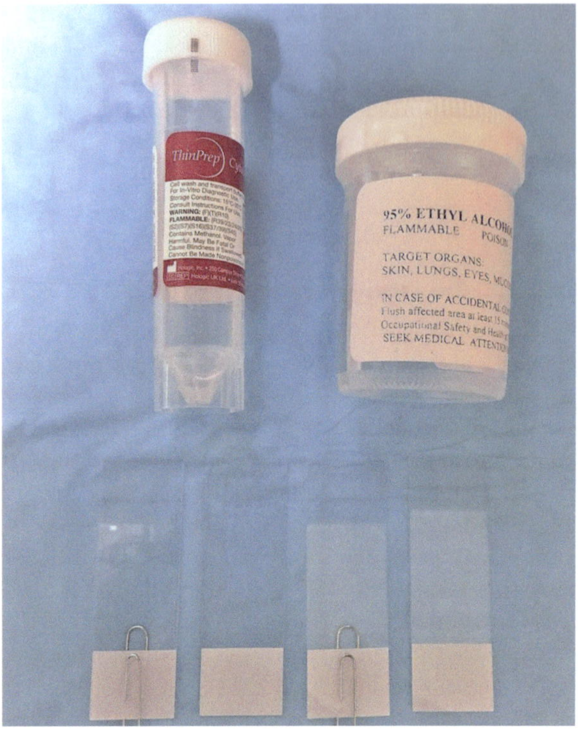

Fig. 4.2 Material for specimen preparation following fine-needle aspiration biopsy of thyroid nodule picture from *top* to *bottom*: ThinPrep solution, 95 % ethanol for fixation, and glass slides with paper clips placed on every other slide

Fine-Needle Aspiration Biopsy Techniques

Fine-needle aspiration of the thyroid has a higher sensitivity when performed under ultrasound guidance [12–15]. However, because an ultrasound system is not available in every office, palpable thyroid nodules can still be biopsied without ultrasound guidance if absolutely necessary.

Fine-Needle Aspiration Biopsy Guided by Palpation

During this procedure, the patient is lying down with cervical hyperextension, using a pillow placed behind the patient's shoulders (Fig. 4.3), while the clinician holds the thyroid nodule between his or her fingers (Fig. 4.4). The person performing the fine-needle aspiration will be standing on the opposite side of the lesion, so the needle is introduced from the neck midline in an effort to avoid going through large

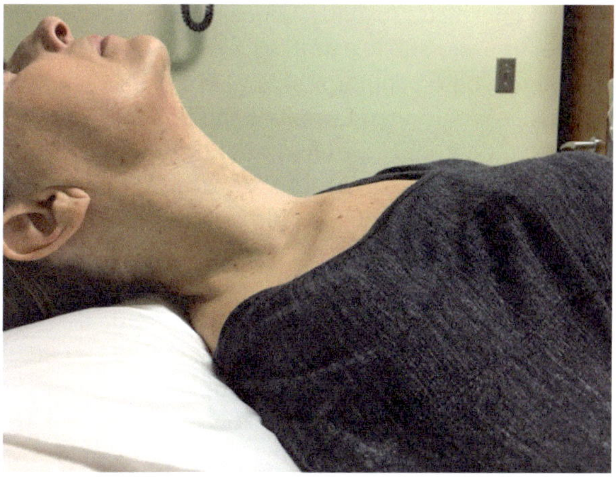

Fig. 4.3 Patient positioning for thyroid nodule biopsy with cervical hyperextension

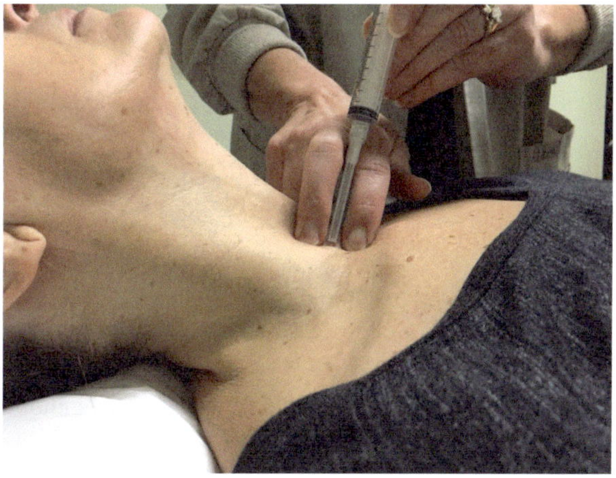

Fig. 4.4 Demonstration of fine-needle aspiration of a thyroid nodule guided by palpation

muscles and blood vessels. The patient is asked not to swallow or speak during the procedure to preclude movement of the thyroid. As mentioned above, one of the disadvantages of this technique is the imprecise needle placement due to lack of direct nodule visualization during the procedure.

Fine-Needle Aspiration Biopsy Guided by Ultrasonography

There are two main methods of aspiration of thyroid nodules under US guidance: transverse and longitudinal approaches.

With the transverse approach, the US probe is placed anterior to the nodule in question which should be positioned in the middle of the screen. A small button of local anesthetic (usually lidocaine without epinephrine) is injected in the subcutaneous area. The use of local anesthesia is optional, since the pain of injection is at times more uncomfortable than the fine needle puncture itself. The ultrasonographer would then introduce the fine needle exactly in next to the middle of the probe transversely, which should coincide with the middle of the screen where the nodule is located (Fig. 4.5). With this technique, the entire length of the needle cannot be visualized. The ultrasonographer should look for the subtle appearance of the needle on the screen at the time it enters the lesion in question. At this point, the needle is moved in and out with short and quick movements, back and forth inside of the nodule which can be done while aspirating the nodule or not. When the sample is collected, the aspiration should be released and the needle should be removed smoothly. This movement is the key for FNA of the thyroid and this repetitive motion should occur for approximately 10 seconds during each pass. The fine needle will collect the tissue in the bore by capillary action even if no active aspiration is applied, which is an important technique to decrease the blood in the aspirate, especially in hypervascular lesion biopsies. For most thyroid FNA guided by US, an adequate specimen is obtained with three passes. The advantage of the transverse technique is that it requires slightly less precision in the placement of the needle when compared to the longitudinal method; however, it can also be less accurate because the exact location of the tip of the needle is unknown unless the ultrasonographer can identify the needle tip appearing and disappearing from the screen while inside of the thyroid lesion with these short movements in and out of the imaged nodule.

On the longitudinal approach, the probe is placed 90 degrees with the skin and the needle is introduced next to the middle of the probe at its narrow edge (Fig. 4.6). The needle will only be seen while directly under the probe, which is usually marked with a line; therefore, it is paramount that the probe is 90 degrees to the skin before the needle is introduced. As the ultrasonographer chooses the probe placement, it is important to make sure the thyroid nodule is close to the place where the needle will be entering the skin to make sure the lesion can be reached with a 1–1.5-inch needle. With this technique, the length of the needle is seen in its entirety with its tip visualized at all times; consequently, the sampled area can be specifically chosen (Fig. 4.7). The advantage of this technique is precision of sampling. A disadvantage of this method is that it requires more training and skill since it is more difficult to keep the needle under visualization exactly under the center of the narrow portion of the probe.

Following the aspiration of the nodule, light local pressure should be applied to stop superficial bleeding in the event it occurs. Scanning of the thyroid after the last pass should be done to make sure there is no evidence of active or significant bleeding. This usually manifests by rapid enlargement of the nodule, thyroid capsule or surrounding planes and pain. If there is a hematoma, it should be followed with US for a short period of time for stability. Even without the occurrence of a hematoma, it is normal for the patient to feel some discomfort when talking and swallowing; therefore, patients should be educated before and after the procedure.

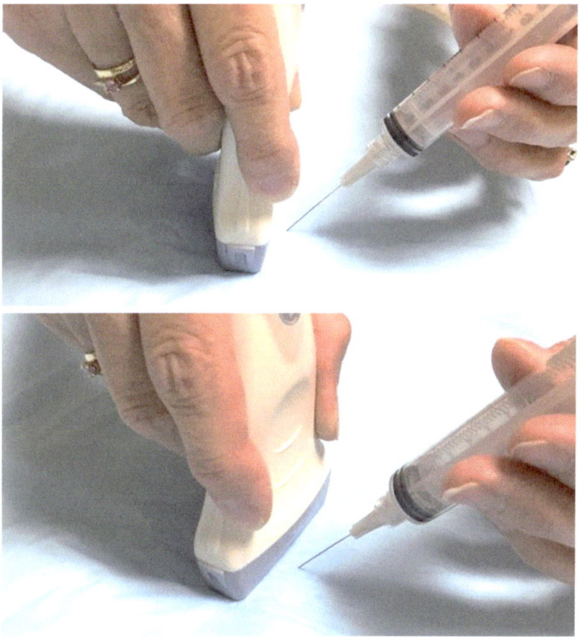

Fig. 4.5 Transverse technique for ultrasound guided fine-needle aspiration biopsy of a thyroid nodule

Specimen Processing

When a sample is collected using any of the above described techniques, the clinician should promptly prepare the slides to prevent air-dried specimens, which will jeopardize the quality of the results. The content aspirated and present inside of the needle should be quickly sprayed on the top of a slide and smeared, as shown in Fig. 4.8a–c. The needle should be disconnected from the syringe to aspirate a few cc of air so there is enough pressure to spray the specimen onto the slide. If the needle is not detached from the syringe, and air is aspirated, the specimen will be dislodged and trapped into the syringe, and it will be difficult to transfer it onto the slide. Air should not be aspirated without first disconnecting the needle. The patient's name and medical record number should be written on each slide, and every other slide should have a paper clip on its tip to prevent "sticking" of the slides and therefore damage to the sample (Fig. 4.2). Following the smearing of the specimen, the slides should be quickly placed in ethanol for fixation for subsequent Papanicolaou staining. The content on the tip of the needle and inside of the syringe should be washed out with ThinPrep or Hanks solution, which later will be spun at the cytopathology lab to collect additional cells (Fig. 4.9). Occasionally, the sample is trapped in the hub of the needle, and it is not easily removed. In that case, a useful technique is to place the needle into a rubber top (from a blood collection tube without the vacuum) and "flick" the needle hub against the slide. This will release the material onto the slide (Fig. 4.10).

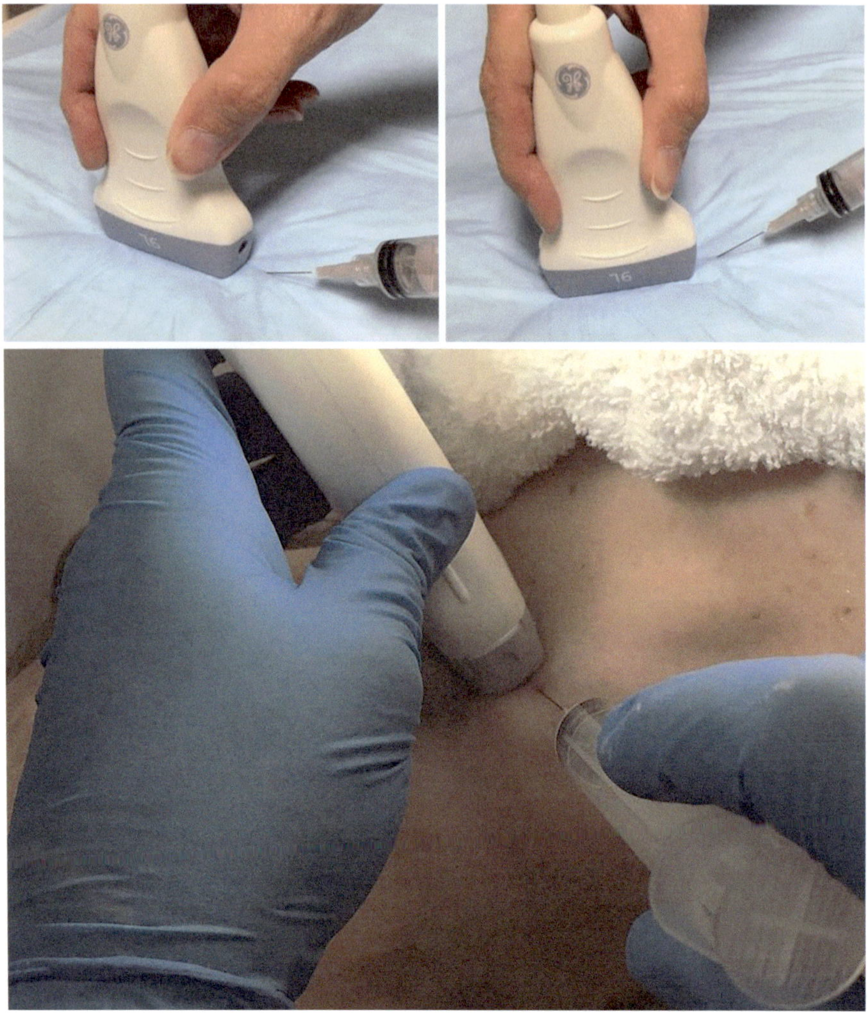

Fig. 4.6 Longitudinal technique for ultrasound guided fine-needle aspiration of a thyroid

When sample adequacy is evaluated immediately after its collection, the slides are air-dried for Diff-Quik staining. At least five to six groups of follicular cells, each containing ten cells, should be present in at least two slides for the sample to be considered adequate.

Complications

The two most common complications of FNA of the thyroid are hematoma and vasovagal response to the procedure.

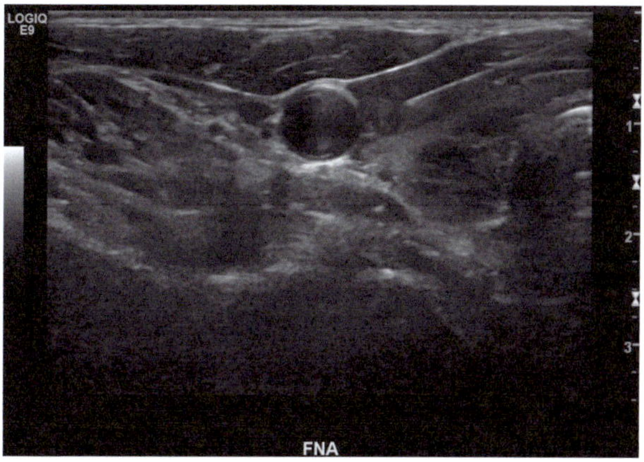

Fig. 4.7 Ultrasound image of longitudinal technique of fine-needle aspiration of right thyroid nodule

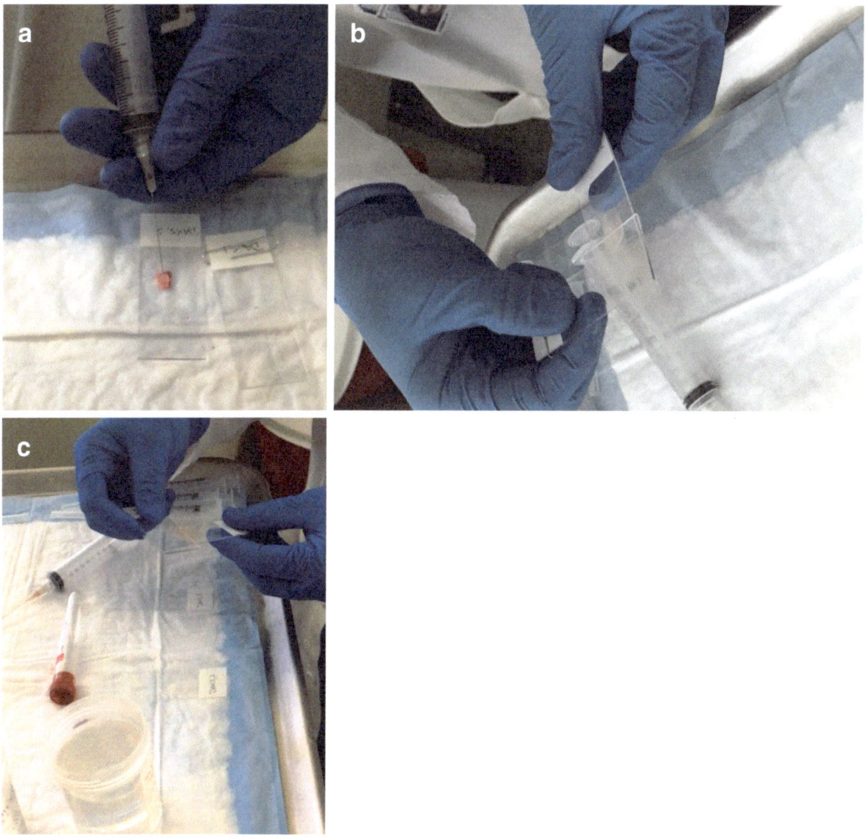

Fig. 4.8 **(a–c)**. Smearing of fine needle aspirate on glass slide. Demonstration of air aspiration before smear

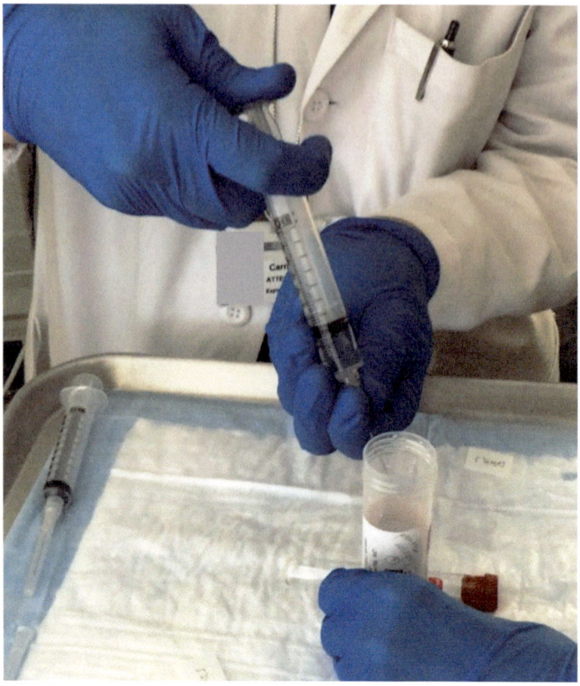

Fig. 4.9 Specimen preparation of fine-needle aspiration biopsy of a thyroid nodule with washout of the needle content on ThinPrep or Hanks solution

Several measures can be taken to prevent a hematoma: stopping anticoagulants before FNA, avoid large vessels in the path of the needle, use fine needles with gauges 25 or higher, avoid excess suction on the FNA, and avoid core biopsies. Bleeding will usually occur when the solid portion of a complex cyst is subjected to biopsy. Bleeding is usually self-contained; however, it can be large enough to cause obstructive symptoms. It can be painful and cause significant compression for a few days to weeks. The effect of bleeding from an FNA can be seen months after FNA, and presents as loss of planes and inflammatory changes during thyroidectomy.

A few patients will have vasovagal symptoms during FNA. The patient should be lying down for the procedure, which will help. Usually, patients become bradycardic, hypotensive, diaphoretic and nauseated. If this occurs, the procedure should be stopped, and supportive measures such as oxygen, vital signs monitoring, Trendelenburg positioning or elevated lower extremities with a pillow under the knees, and a cold compress to the forehead for comfort are usually all that is necessary. Physicians should be prepared for the rare circumstance when CPR may be needed.

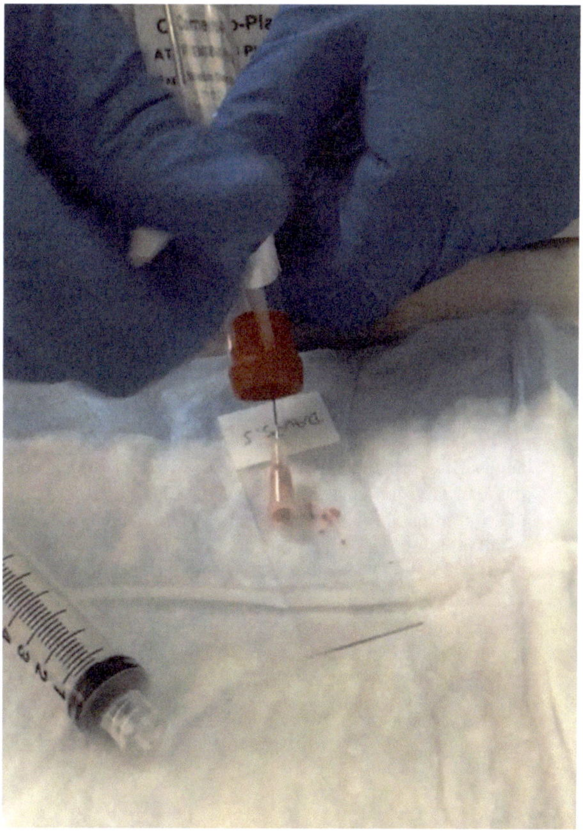

Fig. 4.10 Technique to remove specimen trapped in the hub of the needle

References

1. Miller JM, Hamburger JI, Kini S. Diagnosis of thyroid nodules. Use of fine-needle aspiration and needle biopsy. JAMA. 1979;241(5):481–4.
2. Kini SR, Miller JM, Hamburger JI, Smith MJ. Cytopathology of papillary carcinoma of the thyroid by fine needle aspiration. Acta Cytol. 1980;24(6):511–21.
3. Gharib H, Goellner JR. Diagnosis of amyloidosis by fine-needle aspiration biopsy of the thyroid. N Engl J Med. 1981;305(10):586.
4. Miller TR, Abele JS, Greenspan FS. Fine-needle aspiration biopsy in the management of thyroid nodules. West J Med. 1981;134(3):198–205.
5. Nilsson G. Marginal vacuoles in fine needle aspiration biopsy smears of toxic goiters. Acta Pathol Microbiol Scand A. 1972;80(3):289–93.
6. Nilsson G. Lymphoid infiltration in toxic goitres studied with fine needle aspiration biopsy. Acta Endocrinol (Copenh). 1972;71(3):480–90.
7. Crockford PM, Bain GO. Fine-needle aspiration biopsy of the thyroid. Can Med Assoc J. 1974;110(9):1029–32.
8. Droese M, Kempken K. Fine-needle aspiration biopsy in the diagnosis of thyroid diseases (author's transl). Med Klin. 1976;71(6):229–34.

9. Bodo M, Dobrossy L, Sinkovics I, Tarjan G, Daubner K. Fine-needle biopsy of thyroid gland. J Surg Oncol. 1979;12(4):288–97.
10. Fox CH. Innovation in medical diagnosis–the Scandinavian curiosity. Lancet. 1979;1(8131): 1387–8.
11. Stein SA, Wartofsky L. Primary thyroid lymphoma: a clinical review. J Clin Endocrinol Metab. 2013;98(8):3131–8.
12. Mittendorf EA, Tamarkin SW, McHenry CR. The results of ultrasound-guided fine-needle aspiration biopsy for evaluation of nodular thyroid disease. Surgery. 2002;132(4):648–53; discussion 53–4.
13. Cesur M, Corapcioglu D, Bulut S, Gursoy A, Yilmaz AE, Erdogan N, et al. Comparison of palpation-guided fine-needle aspiration biopsy to ultrasound-guided fine-needle aspiration biopsy in the evaluation of thyroid nodules. Thyroid. 2006;16(6):555–61.
14. Izquierdo R, Arekat MR, Knudson PE, Kartun KF, Khurana K, Kort K, et al. Comparison of palpation-guided versus ultrasound-guided fine-needle aspiration biopsies of thyroid nodules in an outpatient endocrinology practice. Endocr Pract. 2006;12(6):609–14.
15. Can AS. Cost-effectiveness comparison between palpation- and ultrasound-guided thyroid fine-needle aspiration biopsies. BMC Endocr Disord. 2009;9:14.
16. Haugen BR, Alexander EK, Bible KC, Doherty GM, Mandel SJ, Nikiforov YE, et al. 2015 American Thyroid Association Management guidelines for adult patients with thyroid nodules and differentiated thyroid cancer: the American Thyroid Association guidelines task force on thyroid nodules and differentiated thyroid cancer. Thyroid. 2016;26(1):1–133.
17. Gharib H, Papini E, Paschke R, Duick DS, Valcavi R, Hegedus L, et al. American Association of Clinical Endocrinologists, Associazione Medici Endocrinologi, and European Thyroid Association medical guidelines for clinical practice for the diagnosis and management of thyroid nodules. J Endocrinol Invest. 2010;33(5 Suppl):1–50.

Chapter 5
The Bethesda System for Reporting Thyroid Cytopathology (BSRTC)

Idris Tolgay Ocal and Mohiedean Ghofrani

Thyroid Fine Needle Aspiration: The Bethesda System for Reporting Thyroid Cytopathology (BSRTC)

Fine needle aspiration (FNA) has been reported as "the most accurate and cost-effective method for evaluating thyroid nodules" by the 2015 American Thyroid Association (ATA) Management Guidelines for Adult Patients with Thyroid Nodules and Differentiated Thyroid Cancer [1]. FNA is a safe and simple procedure and can be performed by palpation in an outpatient office or under image guidance (see Chap. 4). While ultrasound guidance (USG) is not a requirement for FNA of palpable thyroid nodules, more and more thyroid FNAs have been performed by USG. There is also accumulating evidence that USG improves diagnostic accuracy and reduces nondiagnostic rates [2–4]. Ultrasound has also been suggested to be complementary in managing thyroid nodules that were found to be suspicious for malignancy by cytology, with lower risk of malignancy observed for those thyroid nodules showing benign ultrasonographic findings [5–7].

Sensitivity and specificity of thyroid FNA have been measured in the last few decades, and it has been proven as a highly sensitive tool for evaluation of thyroid nodules [8–15]. It has also been established that the sensitivity and specificity of thyroid FNA is greatest for both benign and malignant diagnoses, while in the indeterminate categories, the surgical correlates lack accuracy. To further complicate this issue, there is no shortage of terminology among cytopathologists for reporting this group of FNAs.

I.T. Ocal, MD (✉)
Pathology and Laboratory Medicine, Division of Anatomic Pathology, Department of Laboratory Medicine/Pathology, Mayo Clinic Arizona, 13400 East Shea Boulevard, Scottsdale, AZ 85259, USA
e-mail: ocal.tolgay@mayo.edu

M. Ghofrani, MD
Cytopathology, PeaceHealth Laboratories, Vancouver, WA, USA

S.A. Roman et al. (eds.), *Management of Thyroid Nodules and Differentiated Thyroid Cancer*, DOI 10.1007/978-3-319-43618-0_5

In clinical practice, for diagnoses other than benign and malignant, terminology such as "atypical," "indeterminate," "suspicious," "cannot rule out," and similar wording is prone to cause significant confusion, not only for the clinicians, but also among the expert cytopathologists reviewing the same specimen. Obviously, this is not a mere academic reason to seek a unifying terminology but is an important clinical, patient care concern. Thyroid FNA diagnoses must be communicated with the clinical team appropriately to assure the best clinical management decisions. Both the surgeon and the patient must be aware of the significance of the FNA diagnosis to ensure evidence-based decision-making.

To standardize the terminology for thyroid FNA reporting and to provide better communication among physicians, the National Cancer Institute (NCI) hosted the multidisciplinary "Thyroid Fine Needle Aspiration State of the Science" conference in Bethesda, Maryland, on October 22–23, 2007, with 154 registrants including pathologists, surgeons, endocrinologists, and radiologists. The meeting was organized by Andrea Abati, M.D.

The outcome of this conference was detailed in an atlas in 2010 [16]. According to the Bethesda system, a six-tiered reporting system is suggested that included three atypical/indeterminate categories as outlined below.

1. Nondiagnostic or unsatisfactory
2. Benign
3. Atypia of undetermined significance or follicular lesion of undetermined significance (AUS/FLUS)
4. Follicular neoplasm/suspicious for follicular neoplasm (including oncocytic lesions)
5. Suspicious for malignancy
6. Malignant

In the years following the publication of this reporting system, multiple studies confirmed the utility of the Bethesda terminology [17–21]. Few institutional modifications and suggestions were also reported [22–28]. However, currently, this system seems to be the most widely accepted terminology for reporting thyroid cytology in the literature. It is important, however, to note that institutional variations depending on patient populations and interobserver variability among cytopathologists are well established [29–32]. Therefore, it is highly recommended that each practice collect their own data with case distributions and malignancy risks. We will look into the categories in detail and point out possible areas of weakness, particularly in the "indeterminate" categories, with clinical implications and malignancy risks for each category.

Components of Thyroid Fine Needle Aspiration

Follicular Cells The main cellular components of thyroid FNA are the follicular cells (see Fig. 5.1), the primary functional cells of thyroid parenchyma, responsible for production of thyroid hormones. Cells are arranged in three-dimensional groups

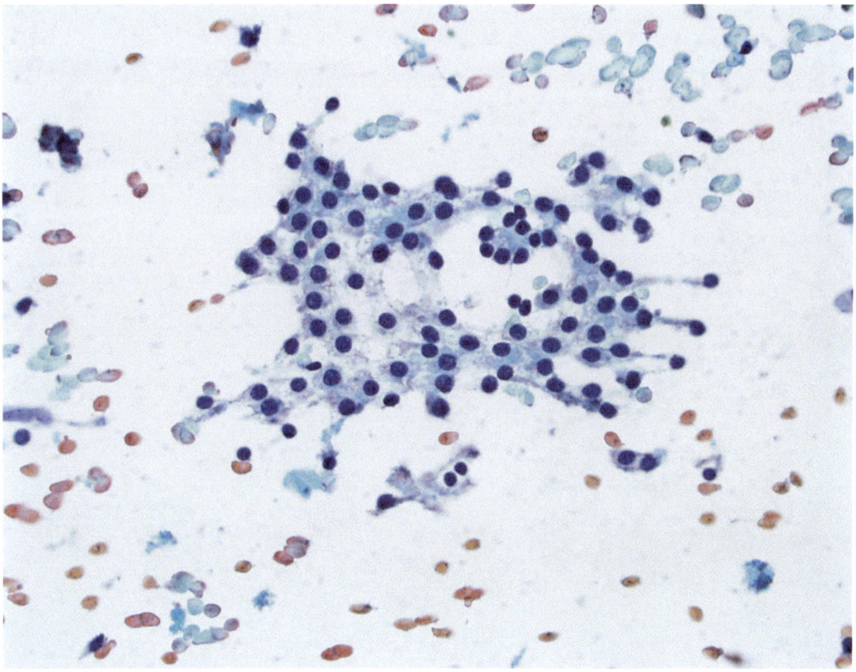

Fig. 5.1 Follicular cells. Bland follicular cells with round-to-oval nuclei, smooth nuclear contours; cytoplasm is fine and friable

of variable sizes with colloid in the central lumen storing thyroglobulin. On FNA specimens, cells may be seen individually or forming intact follicles on smeared slides. C-cells, responsible for calcitonin production, are not identified in thyroid FNAs unless they form a neoplastic mass.

Oncocytic (Hürthle) Cells These are large, epithelial cells with abundant, granular cytoplasm, engorged with mitochondria (see Fig. 5.2). Although the term oncocyte (meaning "swollen cell") may be more appropriate, Hürthle cell terminology has been entrenched in medical practice and is used commonly. While similar morphologic changes can also be seen in thyroid C-cells, the term Hürthle cell implies a follicular cell origin.

Colloid Colloid is the storage form of thyroglobulin that is packed inside follicles in the thyroid. It is a homogeneous, viscous material with characteristic smearing pattern on FNA slides. Pathologists who perform thyroid FNAs can easily identify colloid grossly by the smearing characteristics and shiny, smooth, and homogeneous, honey-like features on glass slides before fixation.

Inflammatory Cells Both acute and chronic inflammatory cells can be seen in thyroid FNAs and may be secondary to infectious and autoimmune inflammatory processes and neoplasias of the hematolymphoid system.

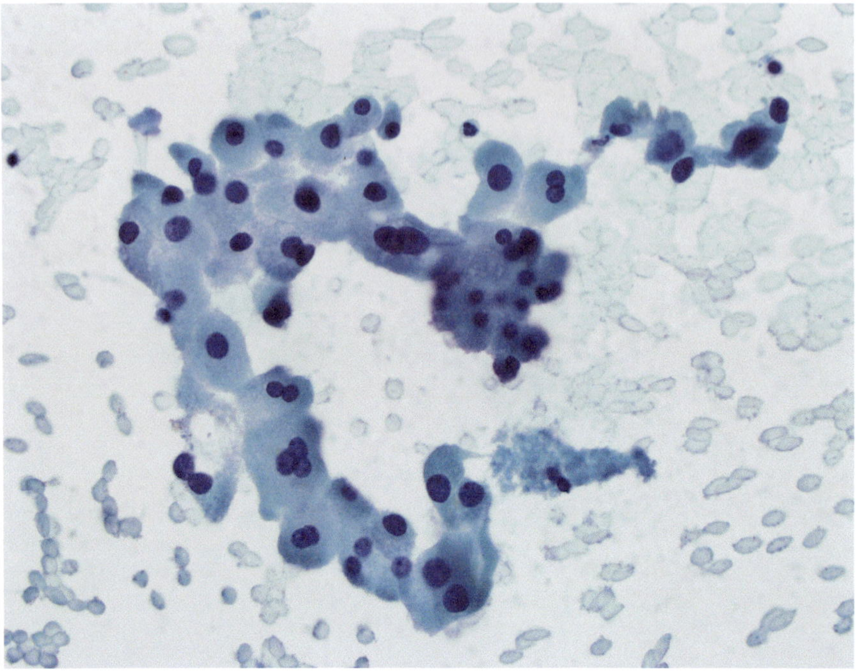

Fig. 5.2 Hürthle cells. Group of cells with abundant, granular cytoplasm and single or multiple, round-to-oval, smooth nuclei. There may be prominent nucleoli

Macrophages Macrophages serve as scavenger cells in tissue. In the thyroid, they may be seen in association with thyroid cysts, where they are characterized by their vacuolated ("foamy") cytoplasm with or without pigment (mostly hemosiderin) (see Fig. 5.3).

Stromal and Vascular Components Depending on the underlying pathologic processes, vascular, stromal, neural, or skeletal muscle fragments may be present in thyroid FNA specimens.

Diagnostic Categories

Nondiagnostic or Unsatisfactory

The main reason for specifying adequacy of thyroid FNA specimens is to avoid false-negative diagnoses. To reduce the risk of false negatives, the cytopathologist should be able to identify the tissue appropriately. This, however, involves multiple parameters including the operator, slide preparation, proper fixation and staining, and also the inherent characteristics of the nodule itself, such as solid vs. cystic components, hemorrhage into the lesion, degenerative or necrotic changes

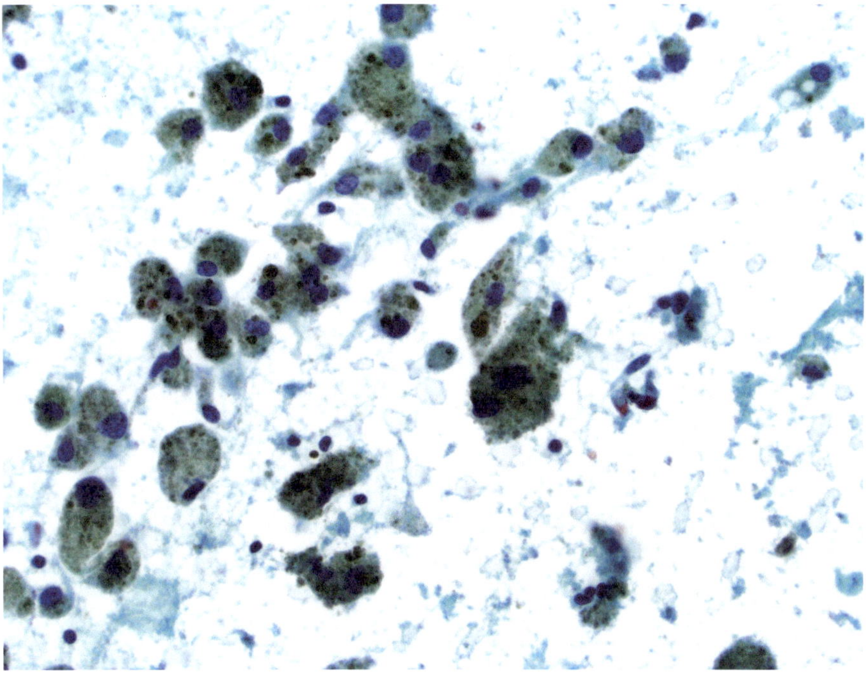

Fig. 5.3 Cyst contents with abundant pigment-laden histiocytes

and amount of sclerosis, calcification, or ossification involving the nodule. Therefore, there is no single criterion for the adequacy of thyroid FNAs. It should also be noted that the adequacy discussion applies to specimens that would otherwise be reported as benign; in other words, if a specimen is considered for any diagnosis other than benign, it should not be reported as nondiagnostic or unsatisfactory, but instead findings should be communicated in an appropriate manner in the pathology report. In this context, the value of detailed verbal or written communication cannot be overemphasized. While in certain practices, a terminology of nondiagnostic implies the features and findings are not "diagnostic for a specific entity," and the term unsatisfactory is used when there is insufficient material for proper evaluation; the two forms a single diagnostic category in the Bethesda system.

One of the earlier reports on quantitative criteria for adequacy was from Dr. Goellner at Mayo Clinic giving actual numbers of follicular cells necessary for adequacy [33]. While "adequacy" reflects much more than the number of follicular cells on glass slides, this proposal by Goellner has remained useful for reporting thyroid cytology for decades and was also included in the Bethesda terminology. For this purpose, six groups of well-visualized cells, each with ten follicular cells, should be considered an "adequate" specimen for evaluation of thyroid nodules in the appropriate setting. This means that the cytologic specimen should be sufficient to identify the "lesion," with clinical and preferably radiologic correlates.

The exceptions to the quantitative requirements for adequacy are those that would identify the lesion in the thyroid as anything other than benign or otherwise guide the clinical or surgical management of the patient. Examples include colloid nodules or inflammatory processes where the follicular cell component may not be well represented or not present at all in the aspirate smears.

Cyst contents without sufficient follicular epithelial cells are considered nondiagnostic. The main concern for these cases is a cystic papillary thyroid carcinoma. In such instances, the aspirates are reported as nondiagnostic with a statement that the FNA shows "cyst contents only." Still, such smears have a very low risk of malignancy particularly for nodules smaller than 4 cm in size and those that shrink after the FNA procedure [34].

Similarly, obscuring blood, preservation and/or fixation artifacts, and staining problems can render the specimen nondiagnostic even if the cellularity is quantitatively "sufficient."

While there are wide variations in the literature for the nondiagnostic category, overall it averages around 10 % [14, 15, 35–40]. In a meta-analysis including a large series in the post-Bethesda era, Bongiovanni reported an average nondiagnostic rate of 13 %, ranging from 1.8 to 23.6 %, in over 25 thousand FNAs [20].

The risk of malignancy for nondiagnostic specimens is difficult to assess in small series without sufficient follow-up, because the majority of these cases do not lead to surgical intervention. The studies that report a malignancy risk for this group with surgical follow-up overestimate the malignancy risk because of selection bias, i.e., the patients with surgical follow-up usually have additional indications for excision, such as increasing size, clinical symptoms, or abnormal or suspicious findings on imaging that skew the risk stratification for these patients. Overall, the malignancy risk with nondiagnostic specimens is actually very low. While it ranges from 0.6 to 39 % in different series, depending on how the data is collected, the malignancy risk is especially low for nodules without suspicious radiologic findings and smaller lesions [15, 35–37, 39, 41, 42]. In a study including 393 cases with an original nondiagnostic FNA but with adequate cytologic, surgical, or ultrasound follow-up, only 2.3 % were associated with malignancy [41]. In this series, the risk increased significantly with each 1 cm increase in any dimension of the nodule [41].

The overall inadequacy rate may decrease with ultrasound guidance [2, 3]. On-site evaluation of thyroid FNAs, with or without USG, may also prove helpful in further reducing the nondiagnostic rate of thyroid FNAs [38, 43, 44]. However, it should be emphasized that more important than any USG or aspiration technique is the experience and competency of the operator performing the procedure and also the cytologist evaluating the specimen [45]. The Bethesda system recommendation for nondiagnostic aspirates is a repeat FNA but "no sooner than 3 months later," preferably with ultrasound guidance and rapid, on-site adequacy evaluation. While ultrasound guidance is likely to reduce the nondiagnostic rate, similar to on-site evaluation, there is no convincing data in the literature that requires a specific time interval for a repeat aspirate. Actually, recent studies that looked into this recommendation did not find any basis for a 3-month period in their series [46, 47]. Furthermore, no contraindication is proven for immediate repeat aspirate, either. On the other hand, it seems reasonable to allow the tissue repair to prevent overinterpretation of reparative/reactive changes as an atypical or neoplastic process particularly by an inexperienced cytopathologist. However, additional factors, including patient compliance, clinical and ultrasonographic findings, and operator experience should all be considered in deciding the most appropriate follow-up. This is particularly evidenced by studies that showed clinical and radiologic follow-up was as acceptable as a repeat aspirate for initially nondiagnostic thyroid FNAs, particularly in the absence of suspicious radiologic findings [41, 48, 49].

Benign

While FNA diagnosis of thyroid nodules can be utilized for confirmation of malignancy or determination of the extent of surgery, the primary purpose of a thyroid FNA is to document that the nodule is benign and no surgical excision is necessary. As the overwhelming majority of thyroid nodules are benign, in most practices, at least 60 % of thyroid FNAs are reported as such [9, 11, 14, 15, 33]. Therefore, thyroid FNA has been an extremely useful tool in prevention of many unnecessary thyroidectomies. When a benign diagnosis is rendered on cytology, the nodule can safely be followed clinically and radiologically, and no further immediate diagnostic studies are indicated [50].

The benign diagnosis includes multiple entities, including benign follicular nodule, colloid nodule, and inflammatory conditions.

Benign follicular nodule is the most common diagnosis for thyroid FNAs. As the name implies, this group consists of follicular-patterned lesions, which encompasses a large and diverse group of lesions including the broad term of "follicular hyperplastic nodules" and also some "follicular adenomas." Follicular hyperplastic nodules include multinodular or uninodular goiters, dominant hyperplastic nodules, nodules in the background of Graves' disease, and colloid nodules (see below). Generally, differentiation of these entities on cytology has little or no clinical significance, as their clinical management will be the same, or in the case of Graves' disease, the diagnosis is usually established on clinical grounds.

The main cytologic characteristic of a benign follicular nodule is presence of colloid and a mixture of bland follicular cells, commonly including Hürthle cells. Therefore, proper identification of colloid on cytologic material is very important. It is common for colloid to "wash off" with fixation. Therefore, it is best seen on stained air-dried smears as dark blue-magenta-colored material. Colloid may be thick, dark, and cracked, or it may be "watery" as clouds of bluish tinge on smears (see Fig. 5.4). To an untrained eye, it may be difficult to differentiate colloid from serum.

When specimens show abundant colloid, even in the absence of follicular cells, those cases are reported as "benign" or "colloid nodule" as the malignancy risk for such lesions is considered to be extremely low [51]. However, in practice, this is a relatively rare occurrence. These can be considered as one end of the spectrum of "macrofollicular lesions." The term colloid nodule should be reserved for those lesions that are clearly dominated by definite colloid on smears. Additionally, the

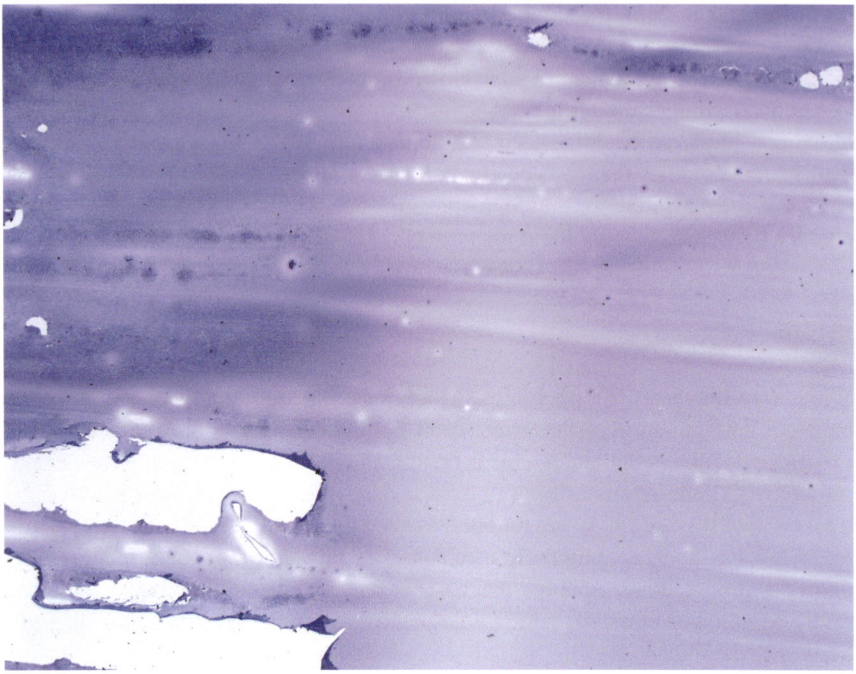

Fig. 5.4 Colloid. Homogeneous, viscous, gel-like material that forms smooth smears on glass slides. It may crack or fold on the edges

cytologic findings should be supported by the imaging characteristics of the nodule sampled. A specimen with abundant colloid should not be reported as benign or adequate if the ultrasonographic features are consistent with a solid lesion.

In addition to colloid, follicular epithelial cells are commonly seen in smears from benign follicular nodules (see Fig. 5.5). They may be seen as sheets or follicles of various sizes. It is important to note that a minor component of microfollicles can be seen in benign follicular nodules, and presence of microfollicles in such a background should not be interpreted as atypical or follicular neoplasm. Follicles show a range of sizes and three-dimensional intact follicles can be seen. As the size of the follicles decrease, it is more likely to see colloid in the center of the follicles. Depending on the aspiration technique and the size of the needle, occasional thick tissue fragments may be seen; however, in a fine needle aspiration specimen, three-dimensional groups of follicles (instead of occasional individual follicles) should not be seen. Cellularity may be low to moderate and occasionally marked; however, there is a mixture of follicular architecture, ranging from small to large macrofollicles, flat sheets, and occasional microfollicles.

It is at this point pertinent to mention what constitutes a microfollicle. So far, the best definition of a microfollicle is by Renshaw as "less than 15 cells, arranged in a circle that is at least two-thirds complete, and flat." Microfollicles can also be seen as small, compact, three-dimensional "spheres" with colloid in the center.

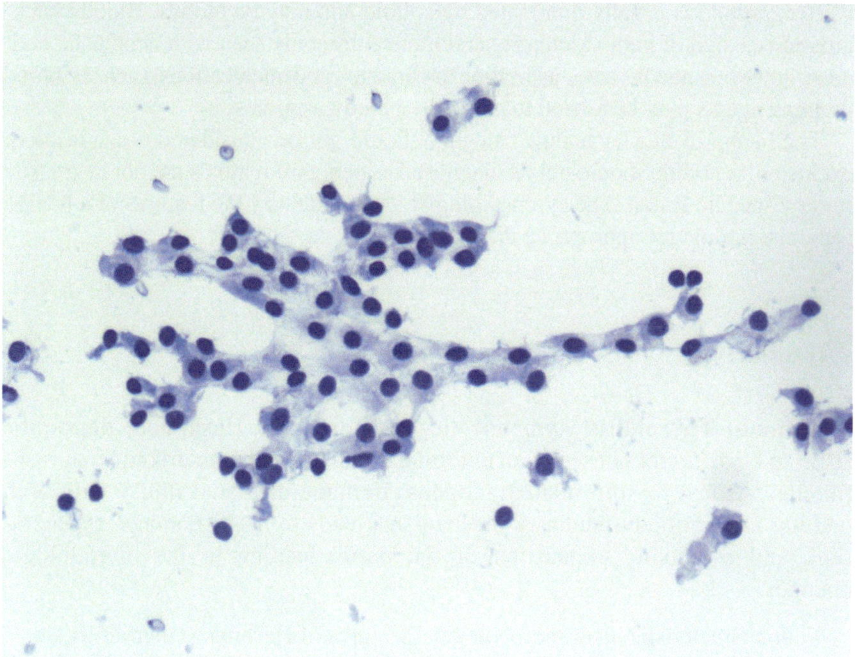

Fig. 5.5 Benign follicular nodule. Bland follicular epithelial cells without nuclear atypia

Follicular epithelial cells are bland, with moderate to abundant cytoplasm. Cytoplasm may be smooth or granular depending on the amount of cytoplasmic organelles and the metabolic activity of the cells. During the aspiration and smearing of the specimen, the cytoplasm may be ripped off, and scattered naked nuclei may be present in the background. Nuclei of normal follicular cells have a very slight variation in size, shape, and chromatin pattern. They are round to oval, monotonous cells with smooth, homogeneous chromatin. The nuclear membrane is usually very smooth and regular, without indentations, grooves, or intranuclear inclusions. Occasionally, one or two small, inconspicuous nucleoli may be seen but without angulations.

Hürthle cells or oncocytes are commonly seen as a part of benign follicular nodules. While Hürthle cell terminology for oncocytic lesions of the thyroid is a misnomer as Hürthle cells are actually the C-cells of dogs [52], it has been well established in the literature and clinical practice to use the name Hürthle for oncocytic cells in this location. Hürthle cells have abundant cytoplasm filled with mitochondria, which gives a homogeneously granular appearance to these cells. Nuclei are round to oval, moderately enlarged, and usually with a single prominent nucleolus. Hürthle cells may also show marked nuclear enlargement, membrane irregularities, and hyperchromasia, which should not be interpreted as atypia or malignancy. It should be noted that there may be "early Hürthle cells" with features intermediate between bland follicular epithelial cells and Hürthle cells.

Background is usually dominated by colloid and may be bloody. Bloody background is a sign of high vascularity and more commonly seen with neoplastic nodules; however, needle size, aspiration technique, and medications such as blood thinning agents may be related to markedly bloody aspirates.

The benign follicular nodule category should not be considered a diagnosis of exclusion. A nodule should not be diagnosed as benign if features are not diagnostic for any specific lesion. The cytopathologist should identify the features of a benign follicular nodule for appropriate diagnosis.

Thyroiditis

Hashimoto Thyroiditis Lymphocytic thyroiditis and Hashimoto thyroiditis seem to be different phases of an autoimmune disease characterized by autoantibodies against thyroid-related antigens. Immune-mediated injury with both cellular and antibody-mediated mechanisms leads to tissue damage, regeneration, and eventually exhaustion of the tissue leading to the morphologic changes.

Four characteristic histo-morphological features of Hashimoto thyroiditis are:

1. Lymphocytic infiltration with germinal centers
2. Hürthle cell metaplasia
3. Follicular atrophy (microfollicles)
4. Fibrous bands of scarring (fibrous variant)

However, Hashimoto thyroiditis is not a single pathologic entity, and there is a wide variation of morphologic features differing in severity and predominant morphologic feature on histology (see Fig. 5.6). Similarly, features of Hashimoto thyroiditis on cytology show marked variations. The major cytologic features of Hashimoto thyroiditis (see Fig. 5.7) are:

1. Presence of a mixed population of lymphoid cells including small, mature lymphocytes, reactive lymphocytes, and occasional plasma cells. Germinal centers may be identified on cytologic smears.
2. Sheets and scattered Hürthle cells with granular cytoplasm, enlarged nuclei, and prominent nucleoli usually predominate the follicular epithelial component on cytology.
3. Presence of microfollicles is not a sign of follicular neoplasia and should not be over-interpreted in these cases.
4. Stromal fragments with capillaries are also seen associated with Hashimoto thyroiditis.

Commonly, the lymphocytic cells seem to intermingle with the epithelial clusters; however, the only finding of Hashimoto thyroiditis may be a slight but definite chronic inflammatory infiltrate in the background of a cellular thyroid aspirate with a mixed Hürthle cell population.

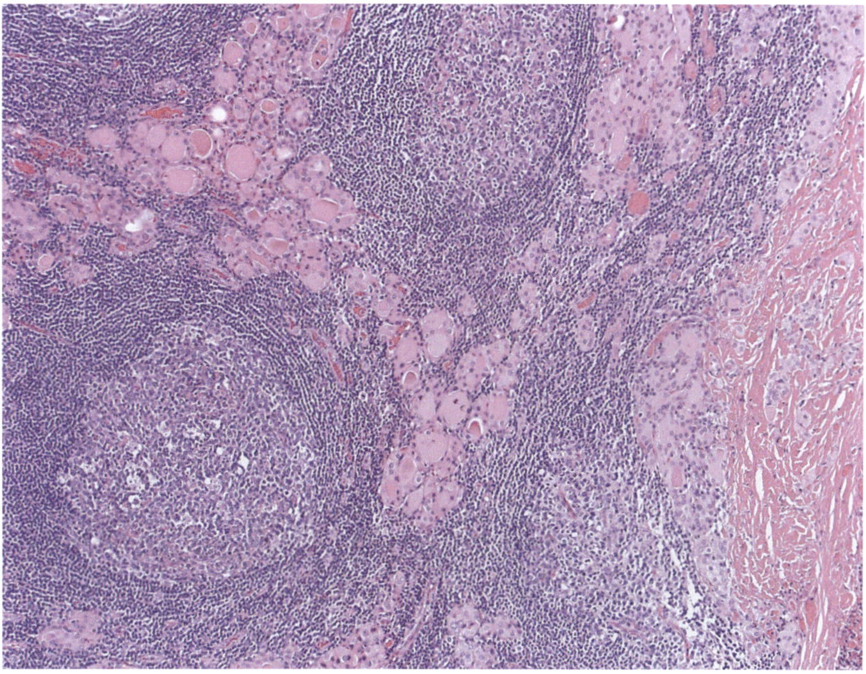

Fig. 5.6 Hashimoto thyroiditis. Histologic section shows thyroid parenchyma infiltrated by abundant lymphoid cells with germinal centers. Follicular epithelial component shows atrophy and prominent Hürthle cell changes

No minimum cytologic requirements are established for diagnosis of Hashimoto thyroiditis on cytology. Some require identification of all four components, including capillaries in smears, while others may report presence of a lymphoid infiltrate as evidence of lymphocytic (Hashimoto) thyroiditis.

Granulomatous Thyroiditis This is an idiopathic disease, usually seen in middle-aged women with painful thyroiditis, often with fever. It is usually bilateral; however, it may be asymmetrical and rarely aspirated. Diagnosis of granulomatous thyroiditis may be possible on aspiration cytology; however, the cellularity varies depending on the activity of the inflammation. The findings are those of a granulomatous inflammation with foreign body type, multinucleated giant cells, the most characteristic finding of this disease (see Fig. 5.8); however, it should be emphasized that multinucleated giant cells can commonly be seen in a variety of thyroid aspirates with and without malignancy, and mere presence of multinucleated cells should not be interpreted as granulomatous thyroiditis. Epithelioid histiocytes and well-formed granulomas may be seen on cytology, some surrounding colloid. Follicular epithelial cells may be abundant in the background, including Hürthle cells. Colloid may be minimal.

Acute Thyroiditis Acute thyroiditis has a typical clinical presentation and usually is not subjected to FNA, unless a drainage and microbiology culture are planned.

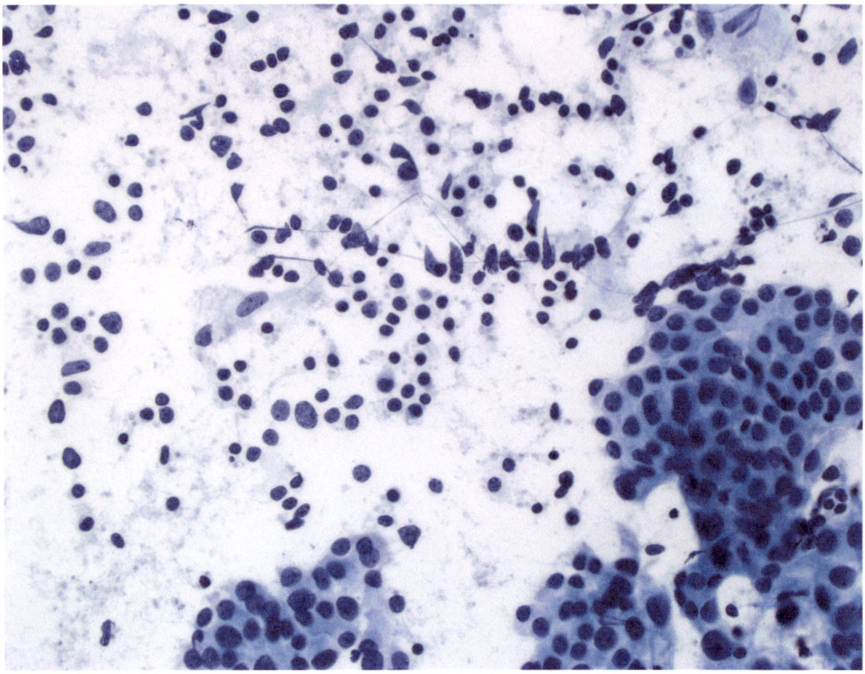

Fig. 5.7 Hashimoto thyroiditis. Most characteristic features of Hashimoto thyroiditis are cellular smears with variable amount of lymphocytic infiltrate and Hürthle cells

FNA material shows abundant acute inflammation and background debris (see Fig. 5.9). Follicular epithelial cells may be a minor component in the background if identified at all. Epithelial cells usually show reactive atypia, which should not be interpreted as neoplastic.

Graves' Disease Graves' disease is an autoimmune thyroiditis, more commonly seen in middle-aged women as diffuse hyperplasia of the thyroid. The patients are usually diagnosed clinically with hyperthyroidism. The disease usually involves the thyroid in a diffuse fashion and is not aspirated. Occasionally, asymmetrical involvement and nodules may be seen on imaging or palpation that may be followed with FNA.

The cytologic features of Graves' disease are not specific and clinical correlation is very helpful. Overall, findings are similar to other benign follicular nodules; however the cellularity may be marked and raise concern for follicular neoplasia. Smears are cellular with mixed follicular cells showing micro- and macrofollicles, a very helpful feature in differentiating these lesions from follicular neoplasms, particularly for those cases where the background colloid is minimal. Occasional papillary hyperplastic groups may be seen, but clinical history and absence of nuclear atypia should steer the cytologist from over-interpreting these as papillary carcinoma.

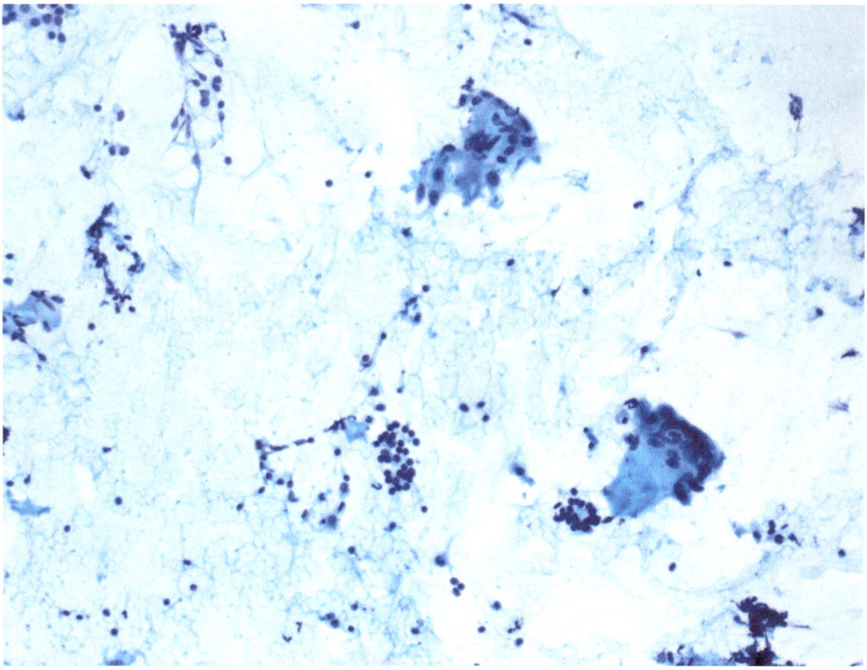

Fig. 5.8 Subacute thyroiditis. Bland follicular cells, lymphocytes, and multinucleated giant cells are seen

A mixed lymphoid background with or without Hürthle cells may be present; however, it is usually much less pronounced than Hashimoto thyroiditis.

Riedel Thyroiditis This is a very rare form of thyroiditis characterized by marked fibrosis extending outside the thyroid parenchyma, raising concern for malignancy. Cytologically, specimens are usually not cellular and may show mixed chronic inflammation with relative lack of follicular cells and colloid. In this clinical setting, the most important finding is the absence of a cytologically diagnostic malignancy, such as anaplastic carcinoma or sarcoma.

Atypia of Undetermined Significance or Follicular Lesion of Undetermined Significance (AUS/FLUS)

This is the most controversial category in the Bethesda system; however, it serves a specific purpose in reporting and management of thyroid nodules with certain morphologic features. It should be noted that this category does not pertain to a single type of lesion or pathologic correlate but should rather be considered to be any type of lesion identified on cytology with a malignancy risk higher than benign but lower

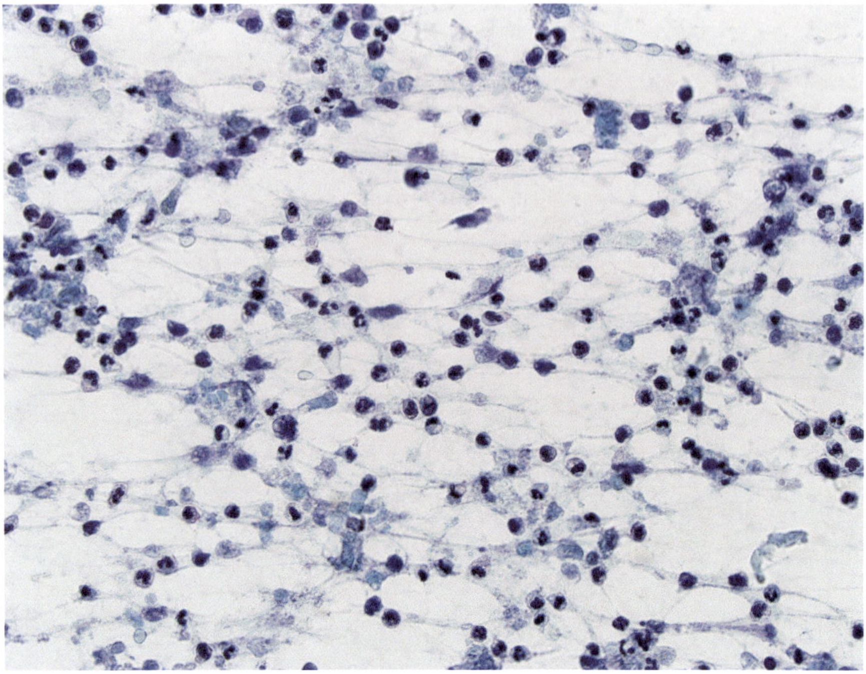

Fig. 5.9 Acute thyroiditis. Acute inflammatory infiltrate. Follicular cells may not be identified in smears

than follicular neoplasia/suspicious for follicular neoplasia or suspicious for malignancy, i.e., in the range of 5–15 % [16]. This is the range that is considered by some to be not high enough for immediate surgical intervention but too high for routine follow-up. The definition of AUS/FLUS is broad and covers multiple scenarios. The most common scenarios described in the Bethesda system involve those lesions where there is a small but definitive concern for a follicular neoplasm, Hürthle cell neoplasm, or malignancy (papillary thyroid carcinoma); however, atypia involving lymphoid or other cells types including medullary carcinoma can also be in this category. The lesion may not be well represented on the aspirate slides due to various reasons such as low cellularity, obscuring hemorrhage, and preservation/staining artifacts, or the clinical background may only partially explain the atypia seen in the specimen, such as Hashimoto thyroiditis, history of radiation exposure, or drugs such as carbimazole.

In the Bethesda system, specific situations are listed with a final "not otherwise categorized." To prevent overutilization of this category as a "wastebasket" diagnosis, a recommendation was made to limit this category in the range of 7 % of all thyroid FNAs. As expected, the reproducibility of this category is far from perfect [32] and the terminology is used differently in many practices [23, 53]. Additionally, the recommended malignancy risks for this group showed marked variability in the literature, usually exceeding the expected range of 5–15 % [27, 54–61].

Since BSRTC became more widely accepted and used, the risk stratification of the atypical category showed significant variations not only among institutions but also how it is reported. While the Bethesda system does not recommend subdividing the AUS/FLUS category, many suggested that the atypical category should be reported in subgroups with descriptive qualifiers as they represent different risks of malignancy. Considering the recent reported findings in the current literature, this category can, at least theoretically, be divided into the following subgroups [27, 54–62]:

1. AUS with nuclear atypia, concerning for papillary thyroid carcinoma (PTC); however, findings are not sufficient for a diagnosis of "suspicious for malignancy" or "malignancy." These mostly include atypia in a limited number of cells. There is a significant body of literature showing that this group has the highest risk of malignancy, ranging from 28 to 56 %.

   These cases show focal nuclear enlargement and nuclear membrane irregularities including grooves and homogenous pale chromatin in an otherwise benign FNA (see Fig. 5.10). It should be noted that, in many series, it may be appropriate to place these cases into the "suspicious for malignancy" category instead of AUS. It is of great importance for the cytopathologist to interpret

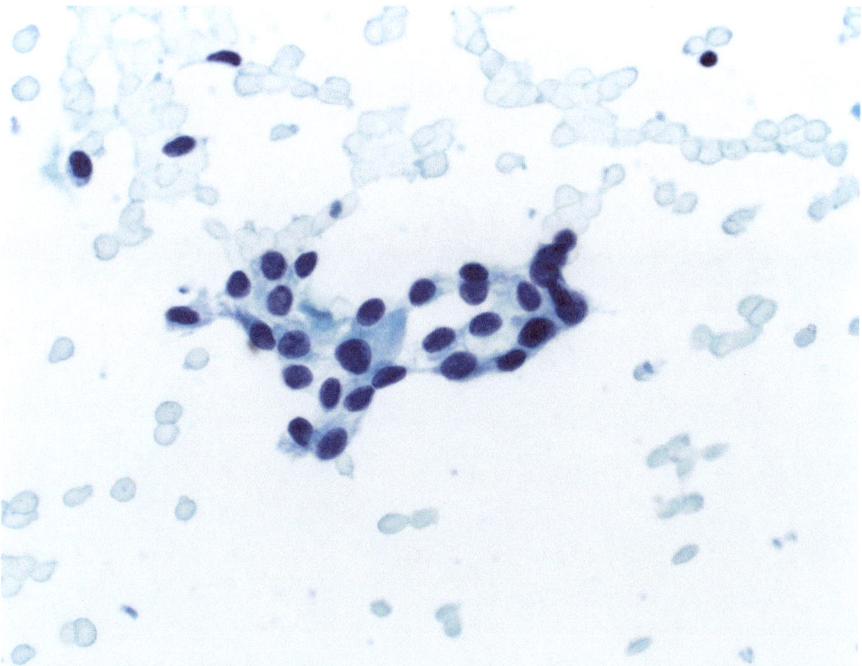

Fig. 5.10 Atypical of undetermined significance. Small, cohesive epithelial cells with finely granular chromatin and nuclear grooves. Nuclei are somewhat more elongated than round. No Hürthle cell morphology is evident. In isolation, this epithelial group raises concern; however, it is not sufficient for the cytologic diagnosis of suspicious for PTC or malignancy

cytologic atypia and features of PTC appropriately. Only those cases that the nuclear features cannot be explained by reactive changes in the background of Hashimoto thyroiditis, history of radiation, medications, identifiable cyst-lining cells, etc., should be reported as atypical. Similarly, if there is a pattern of atypical features or a separately identifiable population of cells with atypical features raising concern for PTC, those should be reported as "suspicious for malignancy." In many institutions, any intranuclear cytoplasmic invaginations (INCI) seen in follicular epithelial cells on a well-fixed, appropriately stained slide are reported as at least suspicious for malignancy, not AUS. For these reasons, the reader should become familiar with the diagnostic features of PTC described in the sections below.

AUS with prominent microfollicles in a sparsely cellular specimen or in the background of a mixed pattern where findings are not supportive of a diagnosis of follicular neoplasm (see Fig. 5.11). Overall, the risk of malignancy in this category is relatively low, on average 5–25 %, depending on how the data is obtained. In our experience, the risk is closer to the lower end of the spectrum.

2. *AUS with predominance of Hürthle cells* in a sparsely cellular specimen or in the background of Hashimoto thyroiditis or multinodular goiter. This category seems to be more heterogeneous and complex; however, it seems to have a very low risk of malignancy, less than 10 % in most series.

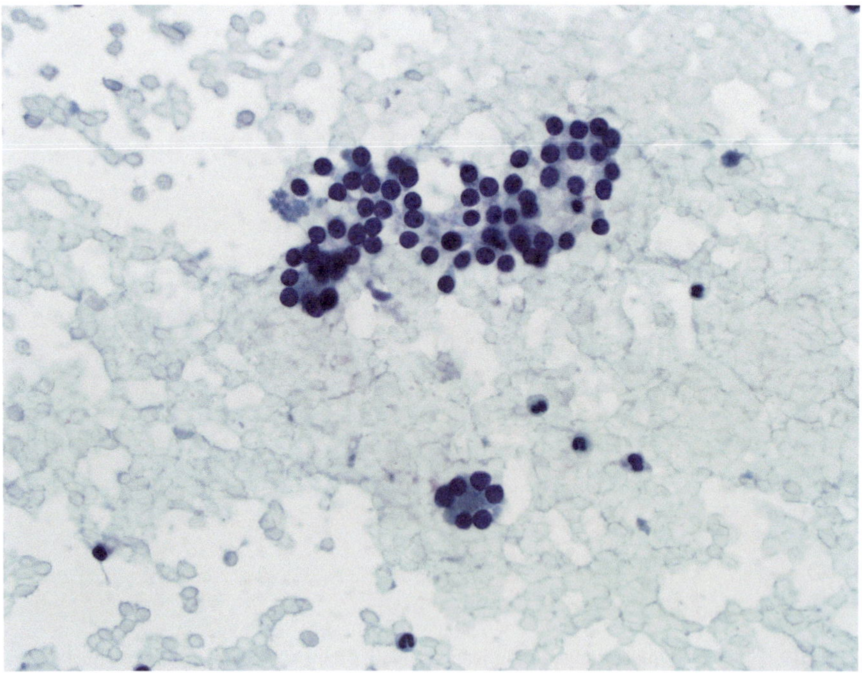

Fig. 5.11 Microfollicles. Bland follicular cells forming flat or three-dimensional groups with 15 cells or less

Some authors further characterize Hürthle cells as those with dysplasia and those without dysplasia; however the reproducibility of this practice is not well established, mostly because Hürthle cells associated with benign proliferations commonly show nuclear enlargement, chromatin clumping, hyperchromasia, nuclear membrane irregularities, and degenerative changes with or without high nuclear-to-cytoplasmic (N/C) ratios. However, if there is a monotonous population of Hürthle cells, particularly without background benign features or Hashimoto thyroiditis, it is still appropriate to report these cases AUS/FLUS.

3. *AUS, not otherwise specified* (*NOS*), involving other cellular components, including lymphoid cells in Hashimoto thyroiditis or atypia that cannot be characterized due to specimen processing and staining problems. History of radiation exposure including radioactive iodine and other drugs may also show nuclear atypia, which may be diagnosed as AUS/FLUS. Cytologic changes seen in cyst-lining cells can also be in this group. Obviously, this is a mixed group with overall risk of malignancy averaging 8–36 %.

   It is important to clearly communicate the cytologic findings in the pathology report. If the clinical team is not aware of the significance of the findings and relative risks that are associated with individual diagnoses, it is best to include a comment about clinical significance in reporting individual cases. This is best accomplished by obtaining institutional data as there is significant variation in risk of malignancy in different practice settings [55, 63].

   In most practices, the next step after a diagnosis of AUS/FLUS is repeat aspiration. Similar to the discussion for nondiagnostic aspirates, an appropriate interval of 3 months has been suggested, but there is no evidence to support this interval. In over half of AUS/FLUS cases, a repeat FNA will be diagnostic, most often with a benign diagnosis [37, 64–66], thus significantly reducing unnecessary thyroid surgery.

   It should also be noted that the malignancy risk associated with only surgically excised cases show an erroneously elevated malignancy risk for this category, as those cases may have additional clinical or imaging findings suspicious for malignancy.

Follicular Neoplasm/Suspicious for Follicular Neoplasm (Including Oncocytic Lesions)

Follicular-patterned lesions form the largest and most heterogeneous group in the thyroid ranging from benign, non-neoplastic follicular hyperplasias to follicle-forming infiltrating carcinomas. These lesions share common morphologic features on cytology, and FNA is not a reliable tool for differentiating these lesions on cytologic grounds. Diagnosis of malignancy relies on histologic evidence of an infiltrative lesion, which cannot be assessed on aspiration specimens. Therefore, a follicular neoplasia (FN) diagnosis on cytology covers the main differential of cellular hyperplastic nodules, follicular adenomas, follicular carcinomas, and follicular variant of papillary thyroid carcinoma (FVPTC). A recently updated terminology for some of the lesions that used to be included in the category of encapsulated follicular variant of papillary carcinoma, i.e., "noninvasive follicular thyroid neoplasm with papillary-like nuclear features" (NIFTP), should also be included in this differential (see discussion below) [67]. In a recent study, 56 % of these benign lesions that were surgically removed had a preoperative cytologic diagnosis of follicular neoplasm [68]. In addition, some rare tumors, such as medullary carcinomas, poorly differentiated thyroid carcinomas, parathyroid proliferations, and some metastatic carcinomas, may also be reported as FN [69].

In the Bethesda system, the FN category is considered to carry a malignancy risk of 15–30 %. Considering the heterogeneous nature of this category, it is possible to divide this group into subgroups with separate morphologic characteristics and corresponding malignancy risks.

1. *Bland hypercellular follicular lesions*: Benign follicular hyperplasia is the most common histologic lesion in the thyroid, and FNA can easily classify these lesions as benign with high sensitivity and specificity. However, those lesions with marked cellularity, overcrowding, and abundant microfollicles with scant background colloid enter the spectrum of FN (see Fig. 5.12). Even in histologic sections, definitive diagnosis depends on complete evaluation of the entire capsule of the lesion, which is not possible on cytology. Therefore, the spectrum

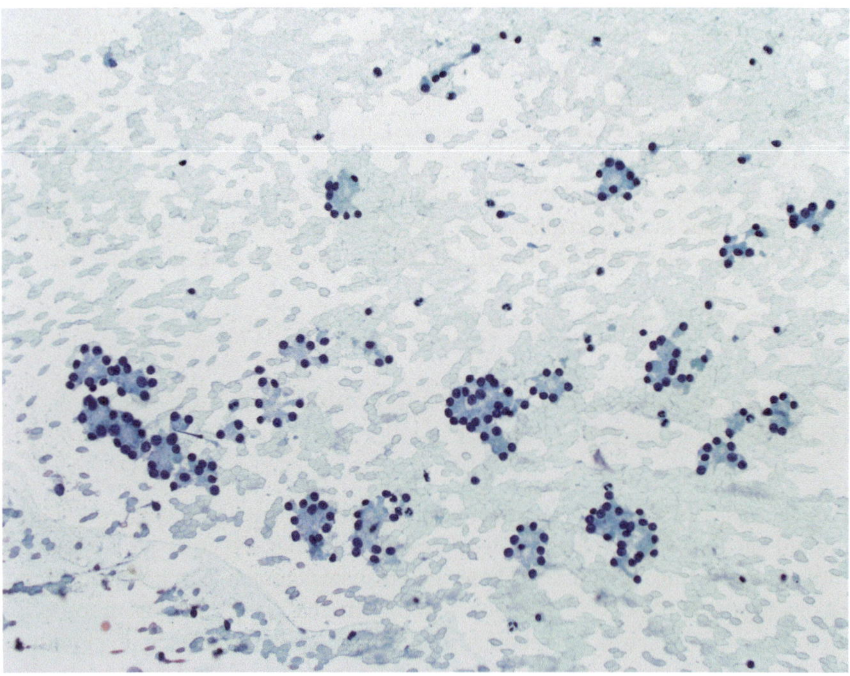

Fig. 5.12 Bland hypercellular follicular lesions. Bland follicular epithelial cells with abundant microfollicles in the background of scant to absent colloid. No nuclear atypia is present

of lesions in this group includes cellular hyperplastic nodules on one end and invasive follicular carcinomas on the other. Increased nuclear-to-cytoplasmic (N/C) ratios, marked cellularity, dyscohesion, and three-dimensional clusters have been suggested as possible signs of "malignancy" in this group; however, these have not been proven to be reproducible in larger studies [70, 71].

The border between the Bethesda system categories of AUS/FLUS and FN is not well defined; however, increased cellularity with microfollicles and "uniformity" of both cells and architecture are reliable signs of neoplasia. Characteristically, there are more cells than colloid in FN.

Overall risk of malignancy in this group of FN shows a wide range in different clinical practices, depending on the terminology used, but seems to be in the range of 25–30 % [14, 15, 42, 65, 72–75].

2. *Microfollicular lesions with nuclear atypia*: Cases that show nuclear features of PTC should not be diagnosed as FN, and those with concern for the possibility of PTC should be reported as suspicious for malignancy. However, it has been well documented that characteristic nuclear features of PTC may not be obvious, particularly in follicular variant of PTC (FVPTC) [76–81]. Therefore, these lesions are commonly diagnosed with other follicular-patterned lesions in the FN category.

   For FNAs with a prominent follicular pattern and only rare nuclear membrane irregularities, the most appropriate diagnosis may still be FN; however, we believe that if the pathologist considers PTC in the differential diagnosis of an otherwise classic FN pattern, it should be noted in the cytology report. This has been supported by the fact that the majority of malignancies associated with FN diagnoses are PTC, particularly FVPTC [14, 15, 65, 72, 74, 75, 82]. It is important to note that cases where the pathologist renders an FN diagnosis with a possibility of PTC have a significantly higher risk of malignancy on excision [78, 83], usually intermediate between the FN and suspicious categories, commonly greater than 50 %. Any atypical nuclear features, particularly nuclear enlargement, grooves, and syncytial clusters, are highly significant and, due to their associated increased risk of malignancy, should be reported (see Fig. 5.13).
3. *Hürthle cell neoplasias*: Hürthle cells are morphologically distinct follicular cells with abundant, granular cytoplasm with enlarged, round-to-oval nuclei and prominent nucleoli. Cytoplasmic granularity is the result of abundant mitochondria, which also show irregular morphologic features [84].

   Hürthle cells are modified follicular cells, and, morphologically, similar features may be seen in different tumors in the thyroid and also in other organs (oncocytic neoplasms of the salivary gland, kidney, esophagus, etc.). Therefore, it is unlikely that these are a specific or separate type of cells but instead an end point in cellular differentiation. Abundant granular cytoplasm with large, round-to-oval nuclei and conspicuous nucleoli can also be seen in some cases of papillary thyroid carcinoma (PTC) and medullary thyroid carcinoma (MTC); however, those should not be diagnosed as Hürthle cell neoplasia but PTC and MTC, respectively. As with any other PTC, the diagnosis of Hürthle cell variant is made on the nuclear features. While some nuclear enlargement and nuclear membrane

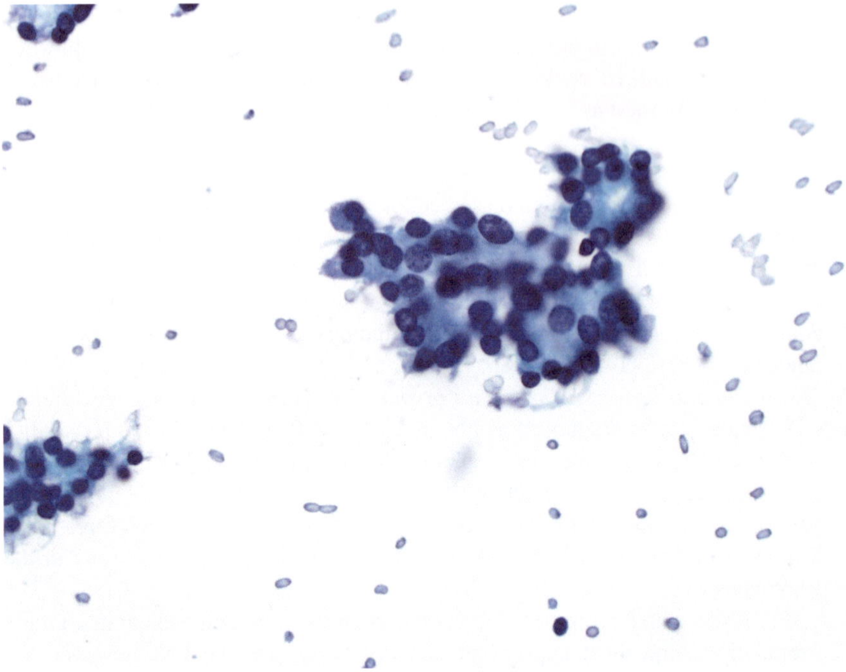

Fig. 5.13 Microfollicular lesions with nuclear atypia. Cohesive clusters forming microfollicles; however, anisonucleosis and areas of chromatin clumping and clearing are evident

irregularities may be seen in Hürthle cell lesions, finely granular chromatin and intranuclear pseudoinclusions are not features of Hürthle cells and should raise concern for PTC. Although not truly a Hürthle cell lesion, occasional MTCs with abundant granular cytoplasm may have overlapping morphologic features. Typical neurosecretory granules of MTC stain red in Romanowsky stains, in contrast to the blue staining granularity of Hürthle cells [16, 85].

Follicular neoplasm, Hürthle cell type (FNHCT), is the terminology suggested by the Bethesda system where the risk of malignancy for this diagnosis was reported to be the same as other follicular neoplasias, i.e., 15–30 %. The diagnostic features of the FNHCT are the same as FN of non-Hürthle cell type. Specimens show abundant cellularity with a dominant monotonous population of Hürthle-type cells with little or no colloid in the background (see Fig. 5.14). Most Hürthle cell lesions show little or no cohesive characteristics, and large three-dimensional clusters are only rarely seen in Hürthle cell tumors. When present, they are highly suggestive of FNHCT. It should also be noted that Hürthle cells are common components of benign follicular nodules and Hashimoto thyroiditis. Therefore, the mere presence of an abundant Hürthle cell component is not an atypical finding in the background of such benign lesions. Hürthle cells should be considered atypical or neoplastic when the cytologic specimen is dominated by a monotonous Hürthle cell component. Some cytologic features have also been suggested

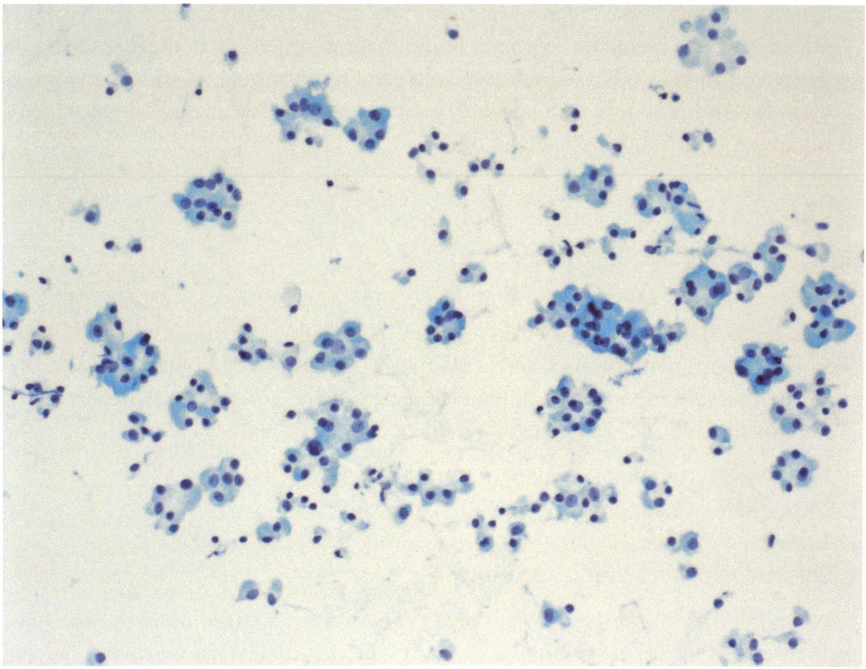

Fig. 5.14 Hürthle cell neoplasm. Monotonous population of abundant Hürthle cells with no colloid in the background. Surgical excision of this lesion showed a Hürthle cell carcinoma with angioinvasion

to identify malignancy in oncocytic lesions, such as small cell or large cell dysplasia, dyscohesion, scant colloid, and syncytia formation; however, these features are more significant for the diagnosis of Hürthle cell tumors than diagnosis of Hürthle cell carcinoma on cytologic grounds [86].

BSRTC places these lesions in the same risk category with other FNs. We believe Hürthle cell neoplasia is an uncommon diagnosis and should be reserved for those with an abundant, monotonous population of Hürthle cells with dyscohesion, minimal to absent of colloid, and lack of features of chronic thyroiditis. When these criteria are applied, the risk of malignancy is probably close to the non-Hürthle cell FN. However, depending on how strictly the criteria are applied, the risk of malignancy may be significantly lower, due to the fact that Hürthle cells are very commonly seen in nonneoplastic thyroid nodules.

4. *Follicular neoplasias, not otherwise specified*:

As with other classification schemes, not all cases can be categorized into certain groups, and there will be cases with morphologic features not specific enough for any further classification. In our experience, some medullary carcinomas, parathyroid lesions, poorly differentiated carcinomas, and some metastatic lesions may show features of FN. Chronic thyroiditis should be briefly mentioned in this section as aspirates may show features resembling FN. If clinical history of thyroiditis is present or any of the morphologic features of thyroiditis are identified, including chronic inflammation (other than those present in peripheral blood), admixed Hürthle cells, and transgressing vessels, a cytologic diagnosis of FN should be made with extreme caution, if ever, as the overwhelming majority of such cases are benign [87].

Suspicious for Malignancy

This is not a specific category with defined morphologic features but instead an intermediate group of lesions where a diagnosis of malignancy is suspected but cannot be definitively established. In the Bethesda system, certain scenarios are listed as patterns that fall into this category [16]:

1. Patchy malignant nuclear changes in a benign background
2. Incomplete nuclear changes of malignancy
3. Features of malignancy in a sample with very low cellularity
4. Nuclear atypia in a cystic background

Although these descriptions may give the cytologist an idea about the morphologic features that are commonly associated with this diagnosis, we do not believe that it is possible to group and categorize all cases that are suspicious for malignancy. Additionally, there is no convincing evidence that categorizing different suspicious patterns has any clinical significance or specific malignancy risks. Instead, it should be considered as when the diagnosis of malignancy, mostly PTC, cannot be established with certainty (see Fig. 5.15). It should be noted that this is an intermediate category without set morphologic borders, similar to the atypical group, and the definition and practical applications will be quite subjective and operator dependent. It is recommended that individual practices collect their own data to document the risk of malignancy associated with this diagnosis in their practice.

This category comprises about 1.3–9 % of all thyroid FNAs and, as expected, shows variations in different patient populations and cytology practices [14, 15, 37, 42]. It is important to note that, particularly in the older literature, the suspicious and follicular neoplasia categories may have been reported together [9, 33, 88].

The malignancy risk for this category is also variable and operator/population dependent. In the Bethesda system, the malignancy risk for this category is suggested to be in the range of 60–75 %, which seems to be in line with the majority of reported series. In Bongiovanni's meta-analysis of multiple series with a combined case number of over 25,000, the average malignancy risk was 75 % [20]. More recently, however, the Endocrine Pathology Society has introduced the term "noninvasive follicular thyroid neoplasm with papillary-like nuclear features" (NIFTP) for a subset of thyroid tumors that were previously called malignant [67]. In a small series published by Maletta [68], 27 % of cases of NIFTP were preoperatively interpreted as suspicious for malignancy. As this is a new terminology that classifies cases that were previously called malignant as benign, the long-term impact of this change on malignancy risk is yet to be determined in larger series.

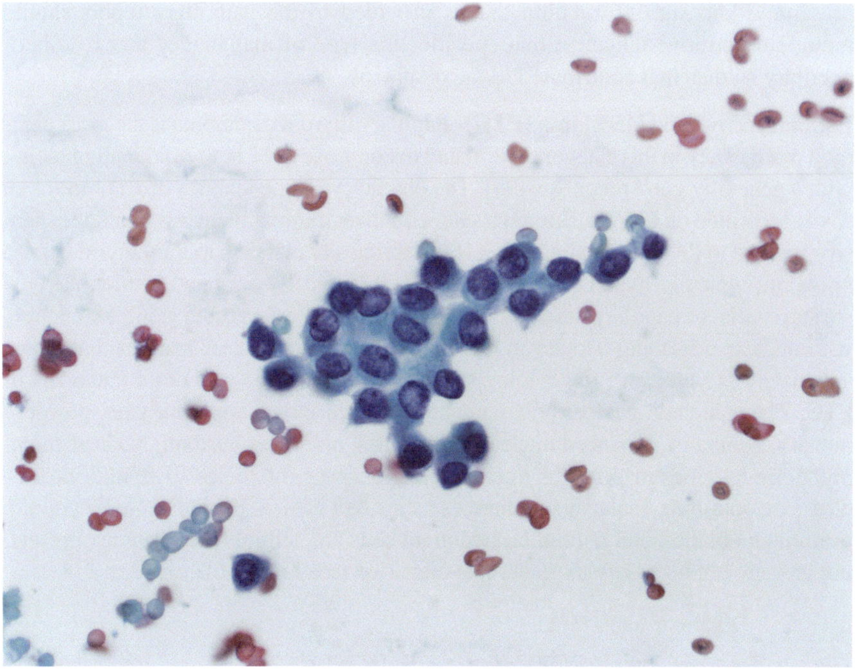

Fig. 5.15 Suspicious for papillary thyroid carcinoma. Small cohesive epithelial group with nuclear membrane irregularities that, in isolation, may not be sufficient for diagnosis of papillary thyroid carcinoma. Surgical excision of this lesion showed papillary carcinoma

The majority of malignancies in the suspicious category are PTC, as expected. Therefore, most centers follow-up with a lobectomy for these cases, usually with intraoperative frozen section evaluation. We believe that these cases should be the primary indication for frozen section evaluation of thyroid nodules. However, it has been also suggested that a total thyroidectomy would be a more cost-effective approach for these patients [89]. The 2015 ATA guidelines strongly recommend surgical management similar to that of malignant cytology depending on clinical and imaging features and patient preference.

For the majority of cases, the suspicion is for PTC; however, depending on the morphologic features, other tumors such as medullary carcinoma, lymphoma, or metastatic lesions can be reported in this group. Literature on these non-PTC cases is limited and likely to show a malignancy risk close to or above the risk for "suspicious for PTC."

Malignant

In approximately 4–8 % of thyroid FNAs, a definitive diagnosis of malignancy can be rendered [14]. These are cases where the diagnostic morphologic, immunophenotypic, or molecular features for a specific thyroid malignancy are adequately present. Additional information that is provided in the pathology report should include descriptive language that specifies the type of malignancy and results of ancillary studies that contributed to the diagnosis.

Papillary Thyroid Carcinoma (PTC) Papillary thyroid carcinoma is the most common malignancy in this category, estimated to comprise 80 % of thyroid malignancies, with a generally good prognosis [90]. The classic cytologic features of PTC are often easily identified on FNA, making it a safe, effective, minimally invasive, and inexpensive method to diagnose malignancy [16]. Aspirates of classic papillary thyroid carcinoma are typically hypercellular, with the cells typically arranged in monolayered sheets, swirls, or papillary structures. These papillary clusters often exhibit branching with nuclear palisading. However, it is the characteristic nuclear features that, when adequately present, give the cytologist the most assurance to render a diagnosis of PTC. These include nuclear enlargement and often elongation with pale, powdery nuclear chromatin, enhanced nuclear membranes, and micronucleoli. Nuclear membrane irregularities manifest as linear nuclear grooves (more sensitive) and intranuclear cytoplasmic inclusions (more specific). Thick ("bubble gum") colloid, psammoma bodies, and multinucleated giant cells are helpful features when present, but they are not necessary to render this diagnosis (see Fig. 5.16).

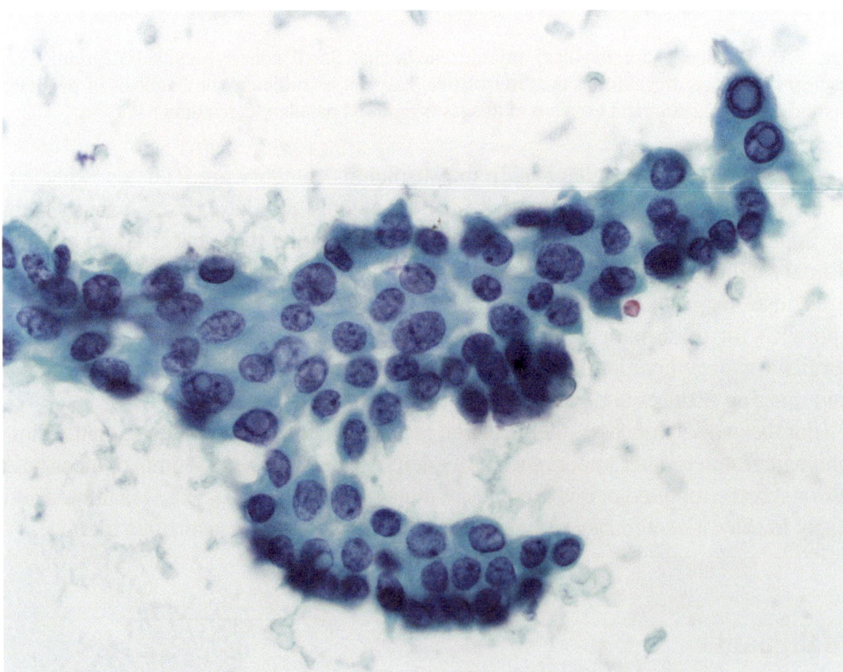

Fig. 5.16 Papillary thyroid carcinoma: Cohesive cluster of epithelial cells with anisocytosis, nuclear membrane irregularities including prominent intranuclear pseudoinclusions, more specific feature of this diagnosis

Although a few immunochemical markers have been suggested as helpful in establishing a diagnosis of PTC, most cases can be confidently diagnosed based on the cytomorphologic features alone. However, many cytologic variants of PTC have been described, including but not limited to follicular (predominantly microfollicles) [91], macrofollicular (>50 % macrofollicular architecture) [92], cystic (hypervacuolated tumor cells and macrophages) [93], oncocytic (granular cytoplasm) [94], Warthin-like (oncocytic tumor cells in a lymphoplasmacytic background) [95], tall cell (an aggressive PTC with elongated tumor cells that are three times higher than wide) [96], and columnar cell (also aggressive with stratified, elongated nuclei) [97] variants. The classic cytologic features of PTC may be more subtle in these variants, which may hinder a definitive diagnosis and relegate the case to the previously mentioned indeterminate categories [98].

A subgroup of encapsulated follicular variant of PTC has been identified to behave in a benign fashion. This subgroup is characterized by the absence of capsular or vascular invasion (i.e., noninvasive), lack of psammoma bodies, mitotic activity less than 3 per 10 high-power fields, no tumor necrosis, and none of the cytomorphologic characteristics of other PTC variants (such as tall cell, solid, etc.). A new terminology, namely, "noninvasive follicular thyroid neoplasm with papillary-like nuclear features" (NIFTP) has been proposed for these tumors by the Endocrine Pathology Society to avoid the term "carcinoma" [67]. However, it should be kept in mind that these lesions may show diagnostic features of PTC on preoperative cytologic evaluation. In a series of 96 histologically proven NIFTP cases, 2 had been called malignant on cytology [68].

Medullary Thyroid Carcinoma (MTC) Medullary thyroid carcinoma is an aggressive differentiated cancer arising from parafollicular C-cells, accounting for approximately 5 % of all thyroid malignancies [99]. Most cases are sporadic, which typically present as a solitary thyroid nodule in adulthood, while the less common hereditary forms associated with multiple endocrine neoplasia 2 (MEN2) are usually identified as multifocal disease at an earlier age [90]. On FNA cytology, MTC is characterized by cellular smears composed of plasmacytoid, spindled, and/or epithelioid/Hürthloid cells [16]. The cells are typically dyscohesive and show variation in nuclear size and shape, with frequent binucleation and multinucleation. Given the neuroendocrine nature of parafollicular C-cells that give rise to MTC, nuclear chromatin has a granular ("salt-and-pepper") appearance, and nucleoli are inconspicuous (see Fig. 5.17). Cytoplasmic secretory granules may also be seen. The presence of intranuclear cytoplasmic inclusions and extracellular amyloid (which often appears like thick "bubble gum" colloid) may cause confusion with PTC. In contrast to colloid, amyloid does not exhibit typical cracking artifact, and if Congo red stain is performed on the cytologic preparation, it should exhibit characteristic apple-green refringence on polarizing microscopy.

Rare cytologic variants of MTC have been described, including the small cell, giant cell, clear cell, squamoid, melanotic, and mucinous variants [100]. Architecturally, besides the dispersed cell pattern, other rare presentations include rosette forming, follicular, papillary, and trabecular patterns. These different variants

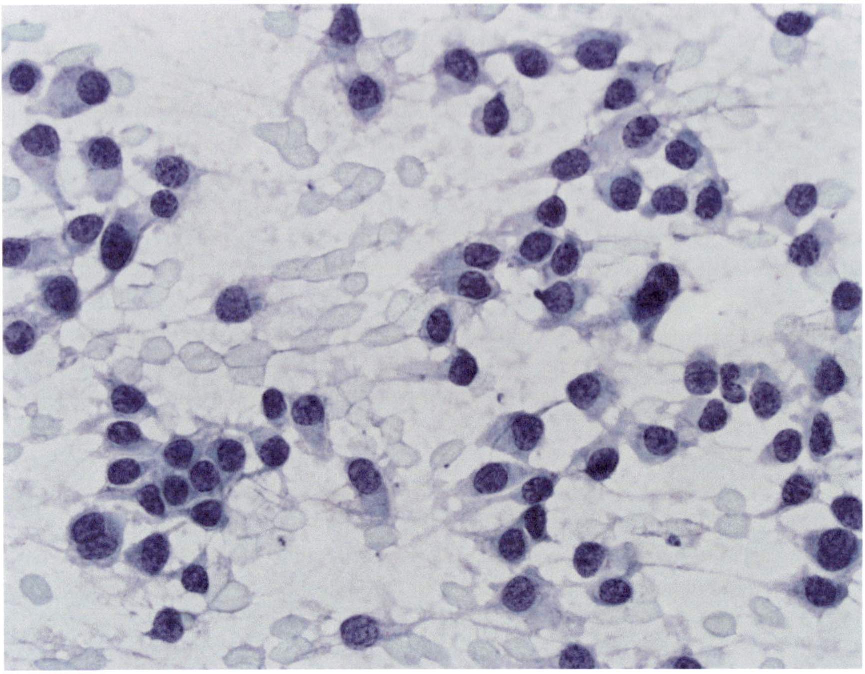

Fig. 5.17 Medullary thyroid carcinoma: Cellular specimen with scattered dyscohesive cells, some with binucleation. Characteristic "salt-and-pepper" granularity of the chromatin is a feature of neuroendocrine differentiation

may pose a challenge in the diagnosis of MTC. Fortunately, immunochemistry for calcitonin can help establish a diagnosis of MTC in its classic and variant forms, with sensitivity ranging from about 75 % in sporadic cases to 100 % in hereditary cases. Calcitonin immunostain is also relatively specific for MTC, although nonspecific staining may be seen in oncocytic neoplasms. Immunostains for carcinoembryonic antigen (CEA) and chromogranin A may also provide additional confirmatory evidence for a diagnosis of MTC. The sensitivity of CEA stain is comparable to calcitonin, but it is less specific, as it is elevated in a variety of benign and malignant conditions [101]. Since MTC is not a follicular cell-derived malignancy, negative thyroglobulin stain can serve as a pertinent negative in the FNA workup of suspected MTC. If cytologic material is not sufficient for confirmatory immunostains, measurement of serum calcitonin and CEA may be recommended [102].

Poorly Differentiated Thyroid Carcinoma (PDTC) Poorly differentiated thyroid carcinoma is a moderately aggressive thyroid malignancy that shows only limited cytologic features of follicular differentiation. In original descriptions of this tumor, the cells were noted to form large round to oval groups or "insulae" [103]. However, both insular and non-insular (trabecular and solid) histologic patterns of PDTC are currently recognized [90], with FNA smears showing variable proportions of cells in cohesive groups or presenting as single dyscohesive cells [16]. Cytologically, these tumors are characterized by a high cell/colloid ratio. PDTC nuclei are small with only mild to at most moderate atypia, but the abundance of mitotic figures and necrosis are clues to the more aggressive nature of this tumor. PDTC may present as a focal finding in an otherwise well-differentiated (papillary, follicular, or Hürthle cell) carcinoma, or its cytologic features may overlap with other tumors (especially follicular neoplasms and medullary thyroid carcinoma), which may lead to its misclassification [104].

Undifferentiated (Anaplastic) Thyroid Carcinoma (UTC) Undifferentiated (anaplastic) thyroid carcinoma is the most aggressive of thyroid malignancies with the poorest survival compared to well-differentiated and poorly differentiated thyroid carcinomas [90]. They mostly occur in the elderly. By definition, these tumors show no specific thyroid differentiation. Well-prepared FNA smears are highly cellular (unless there is marked fibrosis), with giant cells, spindle cells, and squamoid cells exhibiting marked pleomorphism including single or multiple bizarre nuclei [16]. There is coarse chromatin clumping with one or more prominent nucleoli. Mitotic figures (including atypical forms) and necrosis are often prominent; excessive necrosis may diminish the number of diagnostic cells. Osteoclast-like giant cells may be present. Due to invasion of adjacent structures, extrathyroidal elements such as skeletal muscle may be seen in the FNA sample. Since by definition UTC shows no specific thyroid differentiation, TTF-1 and thyroglobulin immunochemistry are usually negative [105]. The most reliable immunostain for UTC is pankeratin but even that stain is negative in up to half of cases. This misleading staining pattern may raise the possibility of sarcoma, but it should be noted that primary sarcomas of the thyroid are extremely rare.

Squamous Cell Carcinoma (SQC) Squamous cell carcinoma of the thyroid is a rare but also highly aggressive thyroid malignancy. Cytologically, it is exclusively composed of large pleomorphic epithelial cells with keratinization, usually associated with necrosis [90]. Cytologically and immunophenotypically, SQC of the thyroid is identical to SQC of other sites, thus correlation with clinical and imaging findings is necessary to rule out metastasis. SQC may be confused with UTC exhibiting abundant squamoid cells, but this distinction is not clinically significant as the management for both malignancies is similar [106].

Primary Lymphoma Primary lymphoma is a relatively uncommon thyroid malignancy, comprising approximately 5 % of thyroid tumors and extranodal lymphomas [90]. Preexisting Hashimoto thyroiditis is a risk factor for developing primary thyroid lymphoma, the vast majority of which are of B-cell type and are thought to arise from mucosa-associated lymphoid tissue (MALT) [107]. Hodgkin lymphoma and plasma cell neoplasms of the thyroid are rare, often representing direct extension from a nearby lymph node or thymic mass and MALT-type lymphoma with prominent plasmacytic differentiation, respectively. The FNA cytomorphology will depend on the specific type of lymphoma [16]. Large cell lymphoma typically presents as a dense, dyscohesive population of large atypical lymphocytes, similar to large cell lymphoma of other sites. Cytoplasmic fragments (lymphoglandular bodies) are commonly seen. Extranodal marginal zone B-cell lymphoma, on the other hand, is characterized by a mixed lymphoplasmacytic population, which may be difficult to distinguish from thyroiditis [108]. Therefore, if appropriate cytologic material is available, ancillary studies such as flow cytometry, immunochemistry, or molecular testing are usually necessary to arrive at a definitive diagnosis [109].

Secondary Tumors Secondary tumors of the thyroid may be the result of hematolymphoid spread of distant malignancies [110] or direct extension from adjacent organs such as the pharynx, larynx, trachea, esophagus, cervical lymph nodes, cervical soft tissue, and mediastinum [111]. Although in clinical series metastases to the thyroid are less common and usually present as solitary masses, in autopsy series up to 25 % of patients with disseminated malignancy are found to have thyroid involvement, typically in the form of multiple variably sized nodules. The most common primary malignancies include kidney, breast, lung, uterus, stomach, colorectal, melanoma, and leukemia/lymphoma [112, 113]. Rare cases of metastatic nasopharyngeal carcinoma [114], choriocarcinoma [115], and sarcoma [116] have also been reported in the thyroid. FNA diagnosis of secondary thyroid malignancy is often aided by immunochemistry and clinical history of a known extrathyroidal tumor, although occasionally the thyroid tumor may be the first manifestation of disease [117].

The positive predictive value of malignancy in a thyroid FNA is over 97 % [42]. Surgical management of a malignant diagnosis is generally thyroidectomy, except for certain diagnoses including metastasis, lymphoma, and undifferentiated carcinoma, which should be determined based on the individual features of the case.

References

1. Haugen BR, Alexander EK, Bible KC, Doherty GM, Mandel SJ, Nikiforov YE, et al. 2015 American Thyroid Association Management Guidelines for adult patients with thyroid nodules and differentiated thyroid cancer: The American Thyroid Association Guidelines Task Force on thyroid nodules and differentiated thyroid cancer. Thyroid. 2016;26:1–133.
2. Cesur M, Corapcioglu D, Bulut S, Gursoy A, Yilmaz AE, Erdogan N, et al. Comparison of palpation-guided fine-needle aspiration biopsy to ultrasound-guided fine-needle aspiration biopsy in the evaluation of thyroid nodules. Thyroid. 2006;16:555–61.
3. Danese D, Sciacchitano S, Farsetti A, Andreoli M, Pontecorvi A. Diagnostic accuracy of conventional versus sonography-guided fine-needle aspiration biopsy of thyroid nodules. Thyroid. 1998;8:15–21.
4. Deandrea M, Mormile A, Veglio M, Motta M, Pellerito R, Gallone G, et al. Fine-needle aspiration biopsy of the thyroid: comparison between thyroid palpation and ultrasonography. Endocr Pract. 2002;8:282–6.
5. Chung YS, Yoo C, Jung JH, Choi HJ, Suh YJ. Review of atypical cytology of thyroid nodule according to the Bethesda system and its beneficial effect in the surgical treatment of papillary carcinoma. J Korean Surg Soc. 2011;81:75–84.

6. Kwak JY, Kim EK, Kim MJ, Hong SW, Choi SH, Son EJ, et al. The role of ultrasound in thyroid nodules with a cytology reading of "suspicious for papillary thyroid carcinoma". Thyroid. 2008;18:517–22.
7. Lee MJ, Hong SW, Chung WY, Kwak JY, Kim MJ, Kim EK. Cytological results of ultrasound-guided fine-needle aspiration cytology for thyroid nodules: emphasis on correlation with sonographic findings. Yonsei Med J. 2011;52:838–44.
8. Jo VY, Renshaw AA, Krane JF. Relative sensitivity of thyroid fine-needle aspiration by tumor type and size. Diagn Cytopathol. 2013;41:871–5.
9. Gharib H, Goellner JR. Fine-needle aspiration biopsy of the thyroid: an appraisal. Ann Intern Med. 1993;118:282–9.
10. Amrikachi M, Ramzy I, Rubenfeld S, Wheeler TM. Accuracy of fine-needle aspiration of thyroid. Arch Pathol Lab Med. 2001;125:484–8.
11. Cramer H. Fine-needle aspiration cytology of the thyroid: an appraisal. Cancer. 2000;90:325–9.
12. Ravetto C, Colombo L, Dottorini ME. Usefulness of fine-needle aspiration in the diagnosis of thyroid carcinoma: a retrospective study in 37,895 patients. Cancer. 2000;90:357–63.
13. Wu HH, Jones JN, Osman J. Fine-needle aspiration cytology of the thyroid: ten years experience in a community teaching hospital. Diagn Cytopathol. 2006;34:93–6.
14. Yang J, Schnadig V, Logrono R, Wasserman PG. Fine-needle aspiration of thyroid nodules: a study of 4703 patients with histologic and clinical correlations. Cancer. 2007;111:306–15.
15. Yassa L, Cibas ES, Benson CB, Frates MC, Doubilet PM, Gawande AA, et al. Long-term assessment of a multidisciplinary approach to thyroid nodule diagnostic evaluation. Cancer. 2007;111:508–16.
16. Ali SZ, Cibas ES, SpringerLink (Online service). The Bethesda system for reporting thyroid cytopathology definitions, criteria and explanatory notes. Boston, MA: Springer Science+Business Media, LLC, 2010:1 online resource.
17. Rabaglia JL, Kabbani W, Wallace L, Holt S, Watumull L, Pruitt J, et al. Effect of the Bethesda system for reporting thyroid cytopathology on thyroidectomy rates and malignancy risk in cytologically indeterminate lesions. Surgery. 2010;148:1267–72; discussion 72–3.
18. Crowe A, Linder A, Hameed O, Salih C, Roberson J, Gidley J, et al. The impact of implementation of the Bethesda system for reporting thyroid cytopathology on the quality of reporting, "risk" of malignancy, surgical rate, and rate of frozen sections requested for thyroid lesions. Cancer Cytopathol. 2011;119:315–21.
19. Ohori NP, Schoedel KE. Variability in the atypia of undetermined significance/follicular lesion of undetermined significance diagnosis in the Bethesda system for reporting thyroid cytopathology: sources and recommendations. Acta Cytol. 2011;55:492–8.
20. Bongiovanni M, Spitale A, Faquin WC, Mazzucchelli L, Baloch ZW. The Bethesda system for reporting thyroid cytopathology: a meta-analysis. Acta Cytol. 2012;56:333–9.
21. Mehra P, Verma AK. Thyroid cytopathology reporting by the bethesda system: a two-year prospective study in an academic institution. Patholog Res Int. 2015;2015:240505.
22. Singh RS, Wang HH. Eliminating the "atypia of undetermined significance/follicular lesion of undetermined significance" category from the Bethesda system for reporting thyroid cytopathology. Am J Clin Pathol. 2011;136:896–902.
23. Krane JF, Vanderlaan PA, Faquin WC, Renshaw AA. The atypia of undetermined significance/follicular lesion of undetermined significance:malignant ratio: a proposed performance measure for reporting in the Bethesda system for thyroid cytopathology. Cancer Cytopathol. 2012;120:111–6.
24. Ustun H, Astarci HM, Altunkaya C, Yilmaz S, Barin A, Ekici S, et al. Fine-needle aspiration of follicular patterned lesions of the thyroid: diagnosis, management, and follow-up according to thyroid Bethesda system. Acta Cytol. 2012;56:361–9.
25. Walts AE, Bose S, Fan X, Frishberg D, Scharre K, de Peralta-Venturina M, et al. A simplified Bethesda system for reporting thyroid cytopathology using only four categories improves intra- and inter-observer diagnostic agreement and provides non-overlapping estimates of malignancy risks. Diagn Cytopathol. 2012;40 Suppl 1:E62–8.

26. Baloch ZW, Mandel SJ, LiVolsi VA. Are we ready to modify the Bethesda thyroid fine-needle aspiration classification scheme? Cancer Cytopathol. 2013;121:171–4.
27. Onder S, Firat P, Ates D. The Bethesda system for reporting thyroid cytopathology: an institutional experience of the outcome of indeterminate categories. Cytopathology. 2014;25:177–84.
28. Ustun B, Chhieng D, Van Dyke A, Carling T, Holt E, Udelsman R, et al. Risk stratification in follicular neoplasm: a cytological assessment using the modified Bethesda classification. Cancer Cytopathol. 2014;122:536–45.
29. Broome JT, Solorzano CC. The impact of atypia/follicular lesion of undetermined significance on the rate of malignancy in thyroid fine-needle aspiration: evaluation of the Bethesda system for reporting thyroid cytopathology. Surgery. 2011;150:1234–41.
30. Kiernan CM, Broome JT, Solorzano CC. The Bethesda system for reporting thyroid cytopathology: a single-center experience over 5 years. Ann Surg Oncol. 2014;21:3522–7.
31. Park JH, Yoon SO, Son EJ, Kim HM, Nahm JH, Hong S. Incidence and malignancy rates of diagnoses in the bethesda system for reporting thyroid aspiration cytology: an institutional experience. Korean J Pathology. 2014;48:133–9.
32. Unpublished data on "Intereobserver variability in interpretation of thyroid fine needle aspiration biopsies using the Bethesda system for reporting of thyroid cytology- A focus on atypical cells of undetermined significance/follicular lesion of undetermined significance" from the CAP Cytopathology Committee members; Vijayalakshmi Padmanabhan MBBS, MD, MPH, Carrie Marshall MD, Guliz A Barkan MD, Mohiedean Ghofrani MD, Idris Tolgay Ocal, M.D., Charles Sturgis, Rhona Souers, Daniel F.I. Kurtycz, MD.
33. Goellner JR, Gharib H, Grant CS, Johnson DA. Fine needle aspiration cytology of the thyroid, 1980 to 1986. Acta Cytol. 1987;31:587–90.
34. Choi KU, Kim JY, Park DY, Lee CH, Sol MY, Han KT, et al. Recommendations for the management of cystic thyroid nodules. ANZ J Surg. 2005;75:537–41.
35. Deniwar A, Hambleton C, Thethi T, Moroz K, Kandil E. Examining the Bethesda criteria risk stratification of thyroid nodules. Pathol Res Pract. 2015;211:345–8.
36. Marchevsky AM, Walts AE, Bose S, Gupta R, Fan X, Frishberg D, et al. Evidence-based evaluation of the risks of malignancy predicted by thyroid fine-needle aspiration biopsies. Diagn Cytopathol. 2010;38:252–9.
37. Theoharis CG, Schofield KM, Hammers L, Udelsman R, Chhieng DC. The Bethesda thyroid fine-needle aspiration classification system: year 1 at an academic institution. Thyroid. 2009;19:1215–23.
38. Wu HH, Rose C, Elsheikh TM. The Bethesda system for reporting thyroid cytopathology: an experience of 1,382 cases in a community practice setting with the implication for risk of neoplasm and risk of malignancy. Diagn Cytopathol. 2012;40:399–403.
39. Al Maqbali T, Tedla M, Weickert MO, Mehanna H. Malignancy risk analysis in patients with inadequate fine needle aspiration cytology (FNAC) of the thyroid. PLoS One. 2012;7, e49078.
40. Gharib H, Goellner JR, Johnson DA. Fine-needle aspiration cytology of the thyroid. A 12-year experience with 11,000 biopsies. Clin Lab Med. 1993;13:699–709.
41. Anderson TJ, Atalay MK, Grand DJ, Baird GL, Cronan JJ, Beland MD. Management of nodules with initially nondiagnostic results of thyroid fine-needle aspiration: can we avoid repeat biopsy? Radiology. 2014;272:777–84.
42. Jo VY, Stelow EB, Dustin SM, Hanley KZ. Malignancy risk for fine-needle aspiration of thyroid lesions according to the Bethesda system for reporting thyroid cytopathology. Am J Clin Pathol. 2010;134:450–6.
43. Cerit M, Yucel C, Gocun PU, Poyraz A, Cerit ET, Taneri F. Ultrasound-guided thyroid nodule fine-needle biopsies – comparison of sample adequacy with different sampling techniques, different needle sizes, and with/without onsite cytological analysis. Endokrynol Pol. 2015;66:295–300.
44. Ghofrani M, Beckman D, Rimm DL. The value of onsite adequacy assessment of thyroid fine-needle aspirations is a function of operator experience. Cancer. 2006;108:110–3.

45. de Meer SG, Schreinemakers JM, Zelissen PM, Stapper G, Sie-Go DM, Rinkes IH, et al. Fine-needle aspiration of thyroid tumors: identifying factors associated with adequacy rate in a large academic center in the Netherlands. Diagn Cytopathol. 2012;40 Suppl 1:E21–6.
46. Singh RS, Wang HH. Timing of repeat thyroid fine-needle aspiration in the management of thyroid nodules. Acta Cytol. 2011;55:544–8.
47. Lubitz CC, Nagarkatti SS, Faquin WC, Samir AE, Hassan MC, Barbesino G, et al. Diagnostic yield of nondiagnostic thyroid nodules is not altered by timing of repeat biopsy. Thyroid. 2012;22:590–4.
48. Chung J, Youk JH, Kim JA, Kwak JY, Kim EK, Ryu YH, et al. Initially non-diagnostic ultrasound-guided fine needle aspiration cytology of thyroid nodules: value and management. Acta Radiol. 2012;53:168–73.
49. Yoon JH, Moon HJ, Kim EK, Kwak JY. Inadequate cytology in thyroid nodules: should we repeat aspiration or follow-up? Ann Surg Oncol. 2011;18:1282–9.
50. Haugen B. American Thyroid Association Management Guidelines for adult patients with thyroid nodules and differentiated thyroid cancer. Thyroid. 2015;26(1):1–133.
51. Baloch ZW, LiVolsi VA, Asa SL, Rosai J, Merino MJ, Randolph G, et al. Diagnostic terminology and morphologic criteria for cytologic diagnosis of thyroid lesions: a synopsis of the National Cancer Institute Thyroid Fine-Needle Aspiration State of the Science Conference. Diagn Cytopathol. 2008;36:425–37.
52. Rosai J, Carcangiu ML, DeLellis RA, American Registry of Pathology, Universities Associated for Research and Education in Pathology, Center for Medical Education Technologies (Rockville Md.). Tumors of the thyroid gland. Atlas of tumor pathology Third series,. Washington, D.C.: Published by the Armed Forces Institute of Pathology, under the auspices of Universities Associated for Research and Education in Pathology,, 1994:1 computer laser optical disc.
53. Bongiovanni M, Krane JF, Cibas ES, Faquin WC. The atypical thyroid fine-needle aspiration: past, present, and future. Cancer Cytopathol. 2012;120:73–86.
54. Chen JC, Pace SC, Khiyami A, McHenry CR. Should atypia of undetermined significance be subclassified to better estimate risk of thyroid cancer? Am J Surg. 2014;207:331–6; discussion 5–6.
55. Ho AS, Sarti EE, Jain KS, Wang H, Nixon IJ, Shaha AR, et al. Malignancy rate in thyroid nodules classified as Bethesda category III (AUS/FLUS). Thyroid. 2014;24:832–9.
56. Horne MJ, Chhieng DC, Theoharis C, Schofield K, Kowalski D, Prasad ML, et al. Thyroid follicular lesion of undetermined significance: evaluation of the risk of malignancy using the two-tier sub-classification. Diagn Cytopathol. 2012;40:410–5.
57. Hyeon J, Ahn S, Shin JH, Oh YL. The prediction of malignant risk in the category "atypia of undetermined significance/follicular lesion of undetermined significance" of the Bethesda system for reporting thyroid cytopathology using subcategorization and BRAF mutation results. Cancer Cytopathol. 2014;122:368–76.
58. Olson MT, Clark DP, Erozan YS, Ali SZ. Spectrum of risk of malignancy in subcategories of 'atypia of undetermined significance'. Acta Cytol. 2011;55:518–25.
59. Park HJ, Moon JH, Yom CK, Kim KH, Choi JY, Choi SI, et al. Thyroid "atypia of undetermined significance" with nuclear atypia has high rates of malignancy and BRAF mutation. Cancer Cytopathol. 2014;122:512–20.
60. Renshaw AA. Does a repeated benign aspirate change the risk of malignancy after an initial atypical thyroid fine-needle aspiration? Am J Clin Pathol. 2010;134:788–92.
61. Wu HH, Inman A, Cramer HM. Subclassification of "atypia of undetermined significance" in thyroid fine-needle aspirates. Diagn Cytopathol. 2014;42:23–9.
62. Gocun PU, Karakus E, Bulutay P, Akturk M, Akin M, Poyraz A. What is the malignancy risk for atypia of undetermined significance? three years' experience at a university hospital in Turkey. Cancer Cytopathol. 2014;122:604–10.
63. Iskandar ME, Bonomo G, Avadhani V, Persky M, Lucido D, Wang B, et al. Evidence for overestimation of the prevalence of malignancy in indeterminate thyroid nodules classified as Bethesda category III. Surgery. 2015;157:510–7.

64. Wong LQ, LiVolsi VA, Baloch ZW. Diagnosis of atypia/follicular lesion of undetermined significance: an institutional experience. Cytojournal. 2014;11:23.
65. Faquin WC, Baloch ZW. Fine-needle aspiration of follicular patterned lesions of the thyroid: diagnosis, management, and follow-up according to National Cancer Institute (NCI) recommendations. Diagn Cytopathol. 2010;38:731–9.
66. Baloch Z, LiVolsi VA, Jain P, Jain R, Aljada I, Mandel S, et al. Role of repeat fine-needle aspiration biopsy (FNAB) in the management of thyroid nodules. Diagn Cytopathol. 2003;29:203–6.
67. Nikiforov YE, Seethala RR, Tallini G, et al. Nomenclature revision for encapsulated follicular variant of papillary thyroid carcinoma: a paradigm shift to reduce overtreatment of indolent tumors. JAMA Oncol. 2016.
68. Maletta F, Massa F, Torregrossa L, et al. Cytological features of "non-invasive follicular thyroid neoplasm with papillary-like nuclear features" and their correlation with tumor histology. Hum Pathol. 2016.
69. Ocal IT, Ghofrani M. Follicular neoplasias of thyroid, fine-needle aspiration cytology. Pathology Case Reviews. 2015;20:115–20.
70. Deshpande V, Kapila K, Sai KS, Verma K. Follicular neoplasms of the thyroid. Decision tree approach using morphologic and morphometric parameters. Acta Cytol. 1997;41:369–76.
71. Lubitz CC, Faquin WC, Yang J, Mekel M, Gaz RD, Parangi S, et al. Clinical and cytological features predictive of malignancy in thyroid follicular neoplasms. Thyroid. 2010;20:25–31.
72. Baloch ZW, Fleisher S, LiVolsi VA, Gupta PK. Diagnosis of "follicular neoplasm": a gray zone in thyroid fine-needle aspiration cytology. Diagn Cytopathol. 2002;26:41–4.
73. Goldstein RE, Netterville JL, Burkey B, Johnson JE. Implications of follicular neoplasms, atypia, and lesions suspicious for malignancy diagnosed by fine-needle aspiration of thyroid nodules. Ann Surg. 2002;235:656–62; discussion 62–4.
74. Lee SH, Baek JS, Lee JY, Lim JA, Cho SY, Lee TH, et al. Predictive factors of malignancy in thyroid nodules with a cytological diagnosis of follicular neoplasm. Endocr Pathol. 2013;24:177–83.
75. Williams BA, Bullock MJ, Trites JR, Taylor SM, Hart RD. Rates of thyroid malignancy by FNA diagnostic category. J Otolaryngology – Head & Neck Surgery = Le Journal d'oto-rhino-laryngologie et de chirurgie cervico-faciale. 2013;42:61.
76. Baloch ZW, Gupta PK, Yu GH, Sack MJ, LiVolsi VA. Follicular variant of papillary carcinoma. Cytologic and histologic correlation. Am J Clin Pathol. 1999;111:216–22.
77. Manimaran D, Karthikeyan TM, Khan DM, Raman RT. Follicular variant of papillary thyroid carcinoma: cytological indicators of diagnostic value. J Clinical and Diagnostic Research JCDR. 2014;8:46–8.
78. Logani S, Gupta PK, LiVolsi VA, Mandel S, Baloch ZW. Thyroid nodules with FNA cytology suspicious for follicular variant of papillary thyroid carcinoma: follow-up and management. Diagn Cytopathol. 2000;23:380–5.
79. Powari M, Dey P, Saikia UN. Fine needle aspiration cytology of follicular variant of papillary carcinoma of thyroid. Cytopathology. 2003;14:212–5.
80. Shih SR, Shun CT, Su DH, Hsiao YL, Chang TC. Follicular variant of papillary thyroid carcinoma: diagnostic limitations of fine needle aspiration cytology. Acta Cytol. 2005;49:383–6.
81. Ustun B, Chhieng D, Prasad ML, Holt E, Hammers L, Carling T, et al. Follicular Variant of Papillary Thyroid Carcinoma: Accuracy of FNA Diagnosis and Implications for Patient Management. Endocr Pathol. 2014;25(3):257–64.
82. Pu RT, Yang J, Wasserman PG, Bhuiya T, Griffith KA, Michael CW. Does Hurthle cell lesion/neoplasm predict malignancy more than follicular lesion/neoplasm on thyroid fine-needle aspiration? Diagn Cytopathol. 2006;34:330–4.
83. Deveci MS, Deveci G, LiVolsi VA, Baloch ZW. Fine-needle aspiration of follicular lesions of the thyroid. Diagnosis and follow-Up Cytojournal. 2006;3:9.

84. Nesland JM, Sobrinho-Simoes MA, Holm R, Sambade MC, Johannessen JV. Hurthle-cell lesions of the thyroid: a combined study using transmission electron microscopy, scanning electron microscopy, and immunocytochemistry. Ultrastruct Pathol. 1985;8:269–90.
85. Kini SR, Miller JM, Hamburger JI, Smith MJ. Cytopathologic features of medullary carcinoma of the thyroid. Arch Pathol Lab Med. 1984;108:156–9.
86. Renshaw AA. Hurthle cell carcinoma is a better gold standard than Hurthle cell neoplasm for fine-needle aspiration of the thyroid: defining more consistent and specific cytologic criteria. Cancer. 2002;96:261–6.
87. Carson HJ, Castelli MJ, Gattuso P. Incidence of neoplasia in Hashimoto's thyroiditis: a fine-needle aspiration study. Diagn Cytopathol. 1996;14:38–42.
88. Cersosimo E, Gharib H, Suman VJ, Goellner JR. "Suspicious" thyroid cytologic findings: outcome in patients without immediate surgical treatment. Mayo Clin Proc. 1993;68:343–8.
89. Leiker AJ, Yen TW, Cheung K, Evans DB, Wang TS. Cost analysis of thyroid lobectomy and intraoperative frozen section versus total thyroidectomy in patients with a cytologic diagnosis of "suspicious for papillary thyroid cancer". Surgery. 2013;154:1307–13; discussion 13–4.
90. DeLellis RA. Pathology and genetics of tumours of endocrine organs. Lyon: IARC Press; 2004.
91. Fulciniti F, Benincasa G, Vetrani A, Palombini L. Follicular variant of papillary carcinoma: cytologic findings on FNAB samples-experience with 16 cases. Diagn Cytopathol. 2001;25:86–93.
92. Fadda G, Fiorino MC, Mule A, LiVolsi VA. Macrofollicular encapsulated variant of papillary thyroid carcinoma as a potential pitfall in histologic and cytologic diagnosis. A report of three cases. Acta Cytol. 2002;46:555–9.
93. Goellner JR, Johnson DA. Cytology of cystic papillary carcinoma of the thyroid. Acta Cytol. 1982;26:797–808.
94. Moreira AL, Waisman J, Cangiarella JF. Aspiration cytology of the oncocytic variant of papillary adenocarcinoma of the thyroid gland. Acta Cytol. 2004;48:137–41.
95. Baloch ZW, LiVolsi VA. Warthin-like papillary carcinoma of the thyroid. Arch Pathol Lab Med. 2000;124:1192–5.
96. Ghossein R, Livolsi VA. Papillary thyroid carcinoma tall cell variant. Thyroid. 2008;18:1179–81.
97. Jayaram G. Cytology of columnar-cell variant of papillary thyroid carcinoma. Diagn Cytopathol. 2000;22:227–9.
98. Mesonero CE, Jugle JE, Wilbur DC, Nayar R. Fine-needle aspiration of the macrofollicular and microfollicular subtypes of the follicular variant of papillary carcinoma of the thyroid. Cancer. 1998;84:235–44.
99. Ghofrani M, Ocal IT. Medullary thyroid carcinoma: a brief review of pathogenesis, diagnosis, and treatment. Pathology Case Reviews. 2015;20:204–9.
100. Pusztaszeri MP, Bongiovanni M, Faquin WC. Update on the cytologic and molecular features of medullary thyroid carcinoma. Adv Anat Pathol. 2014;21:26–35.
101. Akbulut S, Sogutcu N. A high level of carcinoembryonic antigen as initial manifestation of medullary thyroid carcinoma in a patient with subclinical hyperthyroidism. Int Surg. 2011;96:254–9.
102. Filie AC, Asa SL, Geisinger KR, Logani S, Merino M, Nikiforov YE, et al. Utilization of ancillary studies in thyroid fine needle aspirates: a synopsis of the National Cancer Institute Thyroid Fine Needle Aspiration State of the Science Conference. Diagn Cytopathol. 2008;36:438–41.
103. Carcangiu ML, Zampi G, Rosai J. Poorly differentiated ("insular") thyroid carcinoma. A reinterpretation of Langhans' "wuchernde Struma". Am J Surg Pathol. 1984;8:655–68.
104. Ghofrani M, Sosa JA, Ocal IT, Angeletti C. Fine needle aspiration of poorly differentiated oxyphilic (Hurthle cell) thyroid carcinoma: a case report. Acta Cytol. 2006;50:560–2.

105. Miettinen M, Franssila KO. Variable expression of keratins and nearly uniform lack of thyroid transcription factor 1 in thyroid anaplastic carcinoma. Hum Pathol. 2000;31:1139–45.
106. Bolfi F, Domingues MA, Sobrinho-Simoes M, Soares P, Celestino R, Castilho EC, et al. Primary squamous cell carcinoma of the thyroid diagnosed as anaplastic carcinoma: failure in fine-needle aspiration cytology?. Case Rep Pathol. 2014;2014:301780.
107. Pedersen RK, Pedersen NT. Primary non-Hodgkin's lymphoma of the thyroid gland: a population based study. Histopathology. 1996;28:25–32.
108. Lerma E, Arguelles R, Rigla M, Otal C, Cubero JM, Bague S, et al. Comparative findings of lymphocytic thyroiditis and thyroid lymphoma. Acta Cytol. 2003;47:575–80.
109. Boonyaarunnate T, Olson MT, Ali SZ. Impact of flow cytometry in thyroid cytopathology. Acta Cytol. 2013;57:562–6.
110. Chung AY, Tran TB, Brumund KT, Weisman RA, Bouvet M. Metastases to the thyroid: a review of the literature from the last decade. Thyroid. 2012;22:258–68.
111. Nakhjavani M, Gharib H, Goellner JR, Heerden JA. Direct extension of malignant lesions to the thyroid gland from adjacent organs: report of 17 cases. Endocr Pract. 1999;5:69–71.
112. HooKim K, Gaitor J, Lin O, Reid MD. Secondary tumors involving the thyroid gland: a multi-institutional analysis of 28 cases diagnosed on fine-needle aspiration. Diagn Cytopathol. 2015;43:904–11.
113. Nakhjavani MK, Gharib H, Goellner JR, van Heerden JA. Metastasis to the thyroid gland. A report of 43 cases. Cancer. 1997;79:574–8.
114. Chiumento C, Fiorentino A, Castaldo G, Fusco V. A case of thyroid metastasis of nasopharyngeal cancer. Tumori. 2011;97:24e-6e.
115. Lam KY, Lo CY. Metastatic tumors of the thyroid gland: a study of 79 cases in Chinese patients. Arch Pathol Lab Med. 1998;122:37–41.
116. Darouassi Y, Touati MM, Chihani M, Nadour K, Boussouga M, Ammar H, et al. Chondrosarcoma metastasis in the thyroid gland: a case report. J Med Case Rep. 2014;8:157.
117. Heffess CS, Wenig BM, Thompson LD. Metastatic renal cell carcinoma to the thyroid gland: a clinicopathologic study of 36 cases. Cancer. 2002;95:1869–78.

Chapter 6
Cross-Sectional Imaging for the Evaluation of Thyroid Nodules and Cancer

James X. Wu, Masha Livhits, Ali Sepahdari, and Michael W. Yeh

Introduction

Cross-sectional imaging is routinely used for most solid tumors in all phases of therapy: as part of the initial workup, preoperative planning, disease monitoring, and surveillance. Thyroid nodules and suspected thyroid cancers differ from other solid organ malignancies in several key aspects that diminish the utility and need for cross-sectional imaging: (1) The superficial anatomic location allows for comprehensive imaging with neck ultrasound alone in most cases, (2) detection of distant disease in patients with thyroid cancer is accomplished with radioiodine scanning following total thyroidectomy, and (3) the presence of distant metastases preoperatively does not alter initial management, which consists of total thyroidectomy in almost all cases. Furthermore, neck ultrasound can be done in the outpatient setting by the endocrinologist or endocrine surgeon, has lower cost compared to

J.X. Wu, MD (✉) • M. Livhits, MD • M.W. Yeh, MD
Endocrine Surgery, UCLA David Geffen School of Medicine, Los Angeles, CA, USA
e-mail: JamesWu@mednet.ucla.edu; mlivhits@mednet.ucla.edu; myeh@mednet.ucla.edu

A. Sepahdari, MD
Radiological Sciences, UCLA David Geffen School of Medicine, Los Angeles, CA, USA
e-mail: asepahdari@mednet.ucla.edu

S.A. Roman et al. (eds.), *Management of Thyroid Nodules and Differentiated Thyroid Cancer*, DOI 10.1007/978-3-319-43618-0_6

cross-sectional imaging, and does not involve radiation or intravenous contrast. This chapter reviews the circumstances when supplemental cross-sectional imaging is useful and also how to manage thyroid lesions found incidentally on cross-sectional imaging.

Initial Evaluation of Thyroid Nodules

In patients with palpable thyroid disease, the American Thyroid Association (ATA) 2015 guidelines for the management of thyroid nodules and thyroid cancer recommend routine initial diagnostic thyroid ultrasound [1, 2]. All subsequent workup depends on ultrasound findings. If neck ultrasound is negative, no further imaging is required. Suspicious findings on ultrasound may prompt serum TSH testing, fine needle aspiration biopsy, and/or radioiodine scanning to evaluate for lesion for the risk of malignancy. Cross-sectional imaging does not further inform the indication for these tests and procedures. Moreover, cross-sectional imaging should not be substituted for neck ultrasound unless there is an absence of ultrasound expertise. In clinical scenarios where ultrasound expertise is lacking, patients should be referred to higher volume centers for management of their thyroid disease when feasible.

Incidentally Detected Thyroid Nodules

With the rising utilization of CT, MRI, and PET scanning, an increasing number of thyroid nodules are discovered incidentally. Incidental thyroid lesions are detected in up to 16 % of CT and MRI scans and 2 % of PET scans [3–5]. Cross-sectional imaging alone is currently not sufficient for thyroid lesions. Neck ultrasound is still indicated. Cross-sectional imaging alone underestimates multi-nodularity when compared to neck ultrasound [6]. Consequently, the official recommendation by the ATA is to obtain thyroid ultrasound for all thyroid nodules incidentally detected on cross-sectional imaging [1, 2]. In addition, obtaining a fine needle aspiration biopsy (FNAB) at the time of ultrasound should be strongly considered because the rate of malignancy in incidentally discovered thyroid nodules is significant; the malignancy rate in thyroid nodules detected on neck CT and MRI ranges from 4 to 11 %, and the malignancy rate among hypermetabolic lesions seen on PET/CT can be as high as 42 % [6–8]. Of note, diffuse thyroidal uptake seen on PET scanning likely represents an inflammatory thyroiditis rather than a thyroid nodule; a thyroid ultrasound is still indicated to survey for thyroid nodules.

Indeterminate Thyroid Nodules

A significant number of thyroid nodules are cytologically indeterminate (Bethesda categories 3 and 4). Surgical excision has generally been recommended for indeterminate thyroid nodules despite the fact that the prevalence of malignancy is relatively low, ranging from 5 to 30 % [9]. Recently, molecular testing has gained considerable attention as a means of risk stratifying indeterminate thyroid nodules. That said, considerable interest remains in using PET for the same purpose. A meta-analysis by Wang et al. in 2013 determined that PET imaging could predict benign versus malignant disease in indeterminate thyroid nodules with a high negative predictive value and moderate positive predictive value [10]. However, due to limited and conflicting evidence, the ATA guidelines do not recommend routine PET imaging for thyroid nodules with indeterminate cytology [2].

Initial Preoperative Evaluation for Thyroid Cancer

For patients with suspected or biopsy-proven thyroid cancer undergoing preoperative evaluation, the 2015 ATA guidelines on imaging for thyroid cancer do not recommend routine cross-sectional imaging prior to initial surgery [11]. Neck ultrasound can provide sufficient information about the primary lesions and regional lymph nodes for preoperative planning in the vast majority of cases. Unlike most other solid tumors, staging and screening for distant metastases is performed postoperatively using serum thyroglobulin and/or functional radioiodine imaging instead of preoperative cross-sectional imaging [1]. This is because the detection of distant metastases prior to initial surgery does not obviate the need for total thyroidectomy. Even patients with metastatic disease need total thyroidectomy to properly receive radioactive iodine therapy, and thyroidectomy also allows disease monitoring using serum thyroglobulin. The minority of patients that may benefit from supplemental cross-sectional imaging are patients with clinical or sonographic evidence of locally advanced disease. Specific considerations and indications for each cross-sectional imaging modality (CT, MRI, PET) are described below.

Computed Tomography

Supplemental CT scanning in addition to ultrasound should be considered when there is an advanced primary tumor, bulky lymphadenopathy, or signs and symptoms of local invasion. The specific indications for preoperative CT scanning for

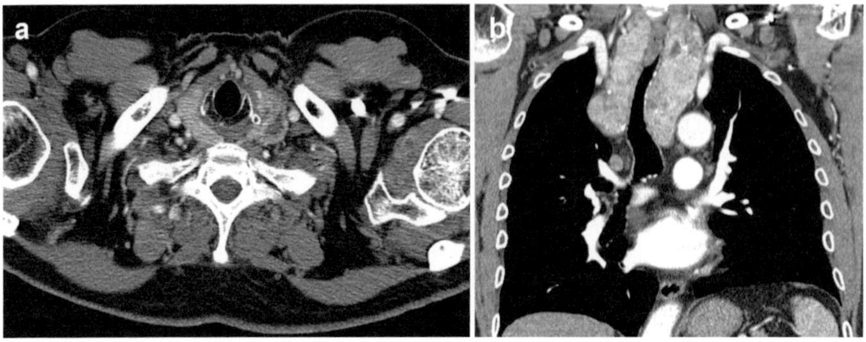

Fig. 6.1 Axial (**a**) and coronal (**b**) images from CT chest with intravenous contrast demonstrating a multi-nodular goiter with an enlarged thyroid gland, thyroid nodules with calcifications, and extension into the mediastinum

initial surgery for thyroid surgery are listed in Box 6.1. Sonographically, extrathyroidal extension and invasion of local structures will appear as a blurry or indistinct border (see Fig. 6.1). Locoregionally advanced disease is present in approximately 10–15 % patients with well-differentiated thyroid cancer [12, 13]. However, at our academic practice, only 5 % or less of patients with thyroid cancer require supplemental cross-sectional imaging in addition to neck ultrasound.

Box 6.1. Indications for Preoperative CT for Initial Surgery for Thyroid Cancer

- Clinical evidence of local invasion:
  - Hoarseness, voice changes
  - Stridor
  - Dysphagia
  - Fixed mass on exam
- Sonographic evidence of invasion of aerodigestive or vascular structures
- Large primary tumor and/or mediastinal extension
- Extensive nodal extension into:
  - Mediastinum
  - Deep structures of neck
- Lack of thyroid ultrasound capability/expertise

CT scanning allows better visualization of structures in the deep/posterior neck and mediastinum, i.e., those areas that lie at the limits of the acoustic window accessible by ultrasound. When extracapsular extension is suspected, CT scanning is reported to be 29–78 % sensitive and 91–99 % specific for invasion of the trachea, esophagus, carotid artery, internal jugular vein, or recurrent laryngeal nerve [14]. Additionally, CT scanning carries the advantages of being widely available, reproducible, and user independent.

Assessment of the primary tumor and lymph nodes should include scanning from the skull base to the mediastinum. Intravenous contrast is needed to facilitate visual differentiation of tissues and should be used in all cases unless specifically contraindicated by allergy or renal insufficiency.

Iodinated contrast interferes with the uptake of radioactive iodine, an important component of thyroid cancer treatment. Thus, postoperative radioactive iodine ablation should be delayed for at least one month after the administration of iodinated contrast [15]. Because of this interaction, it is important to only obtain CT scanning when indicated. Finally, if CT scanning is performed, the decision to do so should be communicated clearly between surgeon and endocrinologist.

Magnetic Resonance Imaging

MRI is principally used for patients with an indication for cross-sectional imaging that have a contraindication for CT scanning, typically patients who have a known allergy to iodinated CT contrast. Since the gadolinium contrast used with MRI scanning does not interact with radioactive iodine, MRI may also be considered in patients with a strong, urgent indication for radioactive iodine therapy. The drawbacks to MRI include long image acquisition times, which can lead to motion artifact or feelings of claustrophobia, and increased risk of nephrogenic systemic fibrosis in patients with renal failure [16].

MRI images with and without contrast should be obtained. Thyroglobulin produced in lymph node metastases is hyperintense on T1-weighted scans (see Fig. 6.2). Papillary thyroid cancer typically has lower mean T2 signal intensity ratio (SIR) and apparent diffusion coefficient (ADC) than benign nodules; using T2 SIR and ADC combined, MRI has 93 % sensitivity and 93 % specificity for discrimination between PTC and benign nodules [17].

When dynamic contrast MRI was compared to US-guided FNAB in the evaluation of multinodular goiter for underlying thyroid cancer in 26 consecutive patients, Tunca et al. reported 100 % sensitivity and 100 % NPV compared to 71.4 % and 91.7 % sensitivity and NPV, respectively, for US-FNAB [18].

Positron Emission Tomography

The images generated by PET are low resolution and not suitable for operative planning. Similar to other solid organ malignancies, the primary use of PET scans is to evaluate for the presence of distant metastases (see Fig. 6.3). However, for the initial

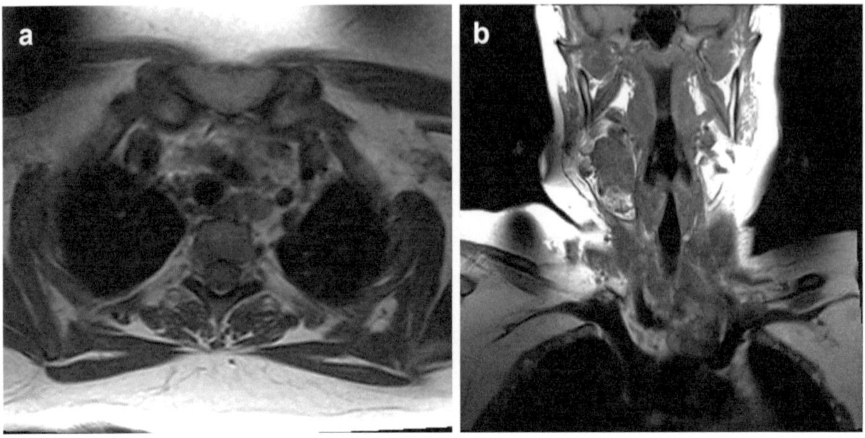

Fig. 6.2 T1 weighted axial (**a**) and coronal (**b**) images of MRI demonstrating paratracheal and neck lymphadenopathy in a patient with recurrent papillary thyroid carcinoma after total thyroidectomy

evaluation of thyroid cancer, this is achieved postoperatively with radioactive iodine scanning. Moreover, given their relatively low metabolic activity, most primary thyroid tumors and up to 70 % of metastases are non-FDG avid [19–22]. Thus, there is no role for PET or combined PET/CT scans for the initial evaluation of thyroid cancer.

Surveillance for Persistent or Recurrent Thyroid Cancer

Following surgery for thyroid cancer, patients should be assessed for persistent or recurrent disease using serum thyroglobulin (either on thyroid hormone therapy or after stimulation with recombinant human TSH) in combination with a neck ultrasound at 6–12 months postoperatively. The presence of disease as indicated by serum thyroglobulin or neck ultrasound may prompt further imaging. In patients who have undergone less than a total thyroidectomy or did not undergo radioiodine ablation, the absolute value of thyroglobulin is less meaningful, but an elevation in serum thyroglobulin from baseline should raise suspicion.

Conceptually, persistent/recurrent thyroid cancer can be classified as being either cervical or extracervical, with the former usually being managed surgically and the latter often being managed nonsurgically. The degree of thyroglobulin elevation provides some guide as to the anatomic location of persistent/recurrent disease, with the most common presentation being a small-volume locoregional lymph node recurrence associated with a thyroglobulin level in the single digits [23]. For such cases, ultrasound imaging alone is adequate. Patients with suspected extracervical disease may be evaluated with (1) diagnostic whole body scanning with radioactive iodine, (2) thin-cut non-contrast chest CT, or (3) 18 F-FDG PET scanning.

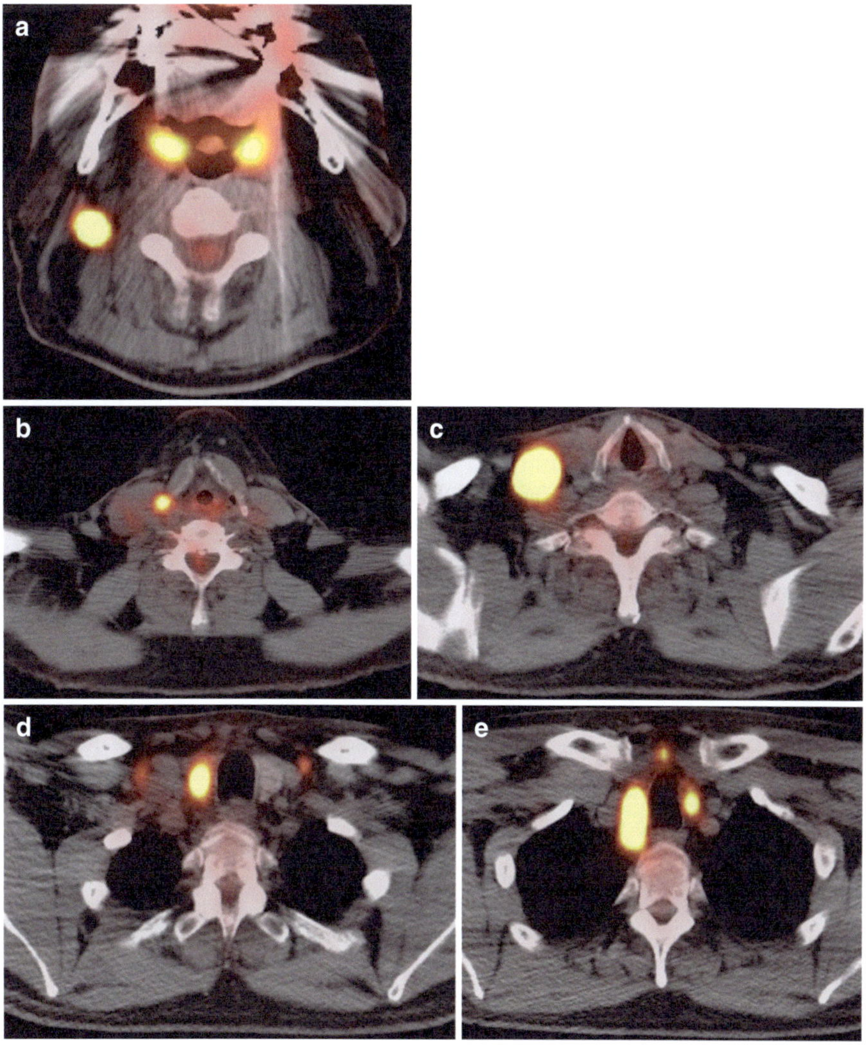

Fig. 6.3 Axial images from an 18-FDG PET/CT demonstrating (**a**, **b**, **c**) hypermetabolic lymphadenopathy in left neck levels II–V and a (**d**, **e**) hypermetabolic right thyroid nodule in patient diagnosed with metastatic papillary thyroid carcinoma

18 F-FDG PET scanning is most strongly indicated in the patient with suspected extracervical disease and negative radioactive iodine imaging [24–27]. The 2015 ATA guidelines recommend PET scanning in patients with negative RAI imaging and thyroglobulin greater than 10 ng/ml [2]. As some high-grade tumors dedifferentiate, they may lose their affinity for iodine and simultaneously become more hypermetabolic on PET scan [28]. The sensitivity and specificity of PET/CT in I^{131}-negative patients with suspicion of persistent or recurrent disease has been reported at 81 and 89 % [29]. The sensitivity of PET/CT may be improved with TSH stimulation [30].

Similar to the indications for chest CT in the initial evaluation for thyroid nodules and thyroid cancer, CT should be considered when there is extensive bulky lymphadenopathy and/or signs and symptoms of local invasion of aerodigestive structures. Additionally, chest CT should be obtained in patients with negative US and high serum thyroglobulin (>10 ng/ml) or rising serum thyroglobulin. While MRI can be considered as an alternative imaging modality for the neck, it is not as sensitive for pulmonary nodules as chest CT.

Conclusion

Cross-sectional imaging is uncommonly indicated in the evaluation of thyroid nodules and thyroid cancer. Supplemental cross-sectional imaging should only be performed in addition to neck ultrasound when there is evidence of extensive disease or invasion of aerodigestive structures. For thyroid cancer surveillance after initial surgery, cross-sectional imaging should be used to evaluate patients with negative neck ultrasound but high or rising levels of thyroglobulin.

References

1. Cooper DS, Doherty GM, Haugen BR, Hauger BR, Kloos RT, Lee SL, et al. Revised American Thyroid Association management guidelines for patients with thyroid nodules and differentiated thyroid cancer. Thyroid. 2009;19(11):1167–214.
2. Haugen BR, Alexander EK, Bible KC, Doherty G, Mandel SJ, Nikiforov YE, et al. 2015 American Thyroid Association Management Guidelines for adult patients with thyroid nodules and differentiated thyroid cancer. Thyroid. 2016;26(1):1–133.
3. Yoon DY, Chang SK, Choi CS, Yun EJ, Seo YL, Nam ES, et al. The prevalence and significance of incidental thyroid nodules identified on computed tomography. J Comput Assist Tomogr. 2008;32(5):810–5.
4. Cohen MS, Arslan N, Dehdashti F, Doherty GM, Lairmore TC, Brunt LM, et al. Risk of malignancy in thyroid incidentalomas identified by fluorodeoxyglucose-positron emission tomography. Surgery. 2001;130(6):941–6.
5. Youserm D, Huang T, Loevner LA, Langlotz CP. Clinical and economic impact of incidental thyroid lesions found with CT and MR. Am J Neuroradiol. 1997;18(8):1423–8.
6. Shetty SK, Maher MM, Hahn PF, Halpern EF, Aquino SL. Significance of incidental thyroid lesions detected on CT: correlation among CT, sonography, and pathology. Am J Roentgenol. 2006;187(5):1349–56.
7. Are C, Hsu JF, Schoder H, Shah JP, Larson SM, Shaha AR. FDG-PET detected thyroid incidentalomas: need for further investigation? Ann Surg Oncol. 2007;14(1):239–47.
8. Jin J, Wilhelm SM, McHenry CR. Incidental thyroid nodule: patterns of diagnosis and rate of malignancy. Am J Surg. 2009;197(3):320–4.
9. Cibas ES, Ali SZ. The Bethesda system for reporting thyroid cytopathology. Am J Clin Pathol. 2009;132(5):658–65.
10. Wang N, Zhai H, Lu Y. Is fluorine-18 fluorodeoxyglucose positron emission tomography useful for the thyroid nodules with indeterminate fine needle aspiration biopsy? A meta-analysis of the literature. J Otolaryngol Head Neck Surg. 2013;42:38.

11. Yeh MW, Bauer AJ, Bernet VA, Ferris RL, Loevner LA, Mandel SJ, et al. American Thyroid Association Statement on preoperative imaging for thyroid cancer surgery. Thyroid. 2015;25(1):3–14.
12. Andersen PE, Kinsella J, Loree TR, Shaha AR, Shah JP. Differentiated carcinoma of the thyroid with extrathyroidal extension. Am J Surg. 1995;170(5):467–70.
13. McCaffrey TV, Bergstralh EJ, Hay ID. Locally invasive papillary thyroid carcinoma: 1940–1990. Head Neck. 1994;16(2):165–72.
14. Seo YL, Yoon DY, Lim KJ, Cha JH, Yun EJ, Choi CS, et al. Locally advanced thyroid cancer: can CT help in prediction of extrathyroidal invasion to adjacent structures? AJR Am J Roentgenol. 2010;195(3):W240–4.
15. Padovani RP, Kasamatsu TS, Nakabashi CC, Camacho CP, Andreoni DM, Malouf EZ, et al. One month is sufficient for urinary iodine to return to its baseline value after the use of water-soluble iodinated contrast agents in post-thyroidectomy patients requiring radioiodine therapy. Thyroid. 2012;22(9):926–30.
16. Yang L, Krefting I, Gorovets A, Marzella L, Kaiser J, Boucher R, et al. Nephrogenic systemic fibrosis and class labeling of gadolinium-based contrast agents by the Food and Drug Administration. Radiology. 2012;265(1):248–53.
17. Noda Y, Kanematsu M, Goshima S, Kondo H, Watanabe H, Kawada H, et al. MRI of the thyroid for differential diagnosis of benign thyroid nodules and papillary carcinomas. Am J Roentgenol. 2015;204(3):W332–5.
18. Tunca F, Giles Y, Salmaslioglu A, Poyanli A, Yilmazbayhan D, Terzioglu T, et al. The preoperative exclusion of thyroid carcinoma in multinodular goiter: dynamic contrast-enhanced magnetic resonance imaging versus ultrasonography-guided fine-needle aspiration biopsy. Surgery. 2007;142(6):992–1002; discussion e1–2.
19. Feine U, Lietzenmayer R, Hanke JP, Held J, Wohrle H, Muller-Schauenburg W. Fluorine-18-FDG and iodine-131-iodide uptake in thyroid cancer. J Nucl Med. 1996;37(9):1468–72.
20. Oh JR, Byun BH, Hong SP, Chong A, Kim J, Yoo SW, et al. Comparison of (1)(3)(1)I whole-body imaging, (1)(3)(1)I SPECT/CT, and (1)(8)F-FDG PET/CT in the detection of metastatic thyroid cancer. Eur J Nucl Med Mol Imaging. 2011;38(8):1459–68.
21. Nakajo M, Nakajo M, Jinguji M, Tani A, Kajiya Y, Tanabe H, et al. Diagnosis of metastases from postoperative differentiated thyroid cancer: comparison between FDG and FLT PET/CT studies. Radiology. 2013;267(3):891–901.
22. Jeong HS, Baek CH, Son YI, Choi JY, Kim HJ, Ko YH, et al. Integrated 18F-FDG PET/CT for the initial evaluation of cervical node level of patients with papillary thyroid carcinoma: comparison with ultrasound and contrast-enhanced CT. Clin Endocrinol (Oxf). 2006;65(3):402–7.
23. Robbins RJ, Srivastava S, Shaha A, Ghossein R, Larson SM, Fleisher M, et al. Factors influencing the basal and recombinant human thyrotropin-stimulated serum thyroglobulin in patients with metastatic thyroid carcinoma. J Clin Endocrinol Metab. 2004;89(12):6010–6.
24. Grünwald F, Kälicke T, Feine U, Lietzenmayer R, Scheidhauer K, Dietlein M, et al. Fluorine-18 fluorodeoxyglucose positron emission tomography in thyroid cancer: results of a multicentre study. Eur J Nucl Med. 1999;26(12):1547–52.
25. Schlüter B, Bohuslavizki KH, Beyer W, Plotkin M, Buchert R, Clausen M. Impact of FDG PET on patients with differentiated thyroid cancer who present with elevated thyroglobulin and negative 131I scan. J Nucl Med. 2001;42(1):71–6.
26. Wang W, Macapinlac H, Larson SM, Yeh SD, Akhurst T, Finn RD, et al. [18F]-2-fluoro-2-deoxy-D-glucose positron emission tomography localizes residual thyroid cancer in patients with negative diagnostic (131)I whole body scans and elevated serum thyroglobulin levels. J Clin Endocrinol Metab. 1999;84(7):2291–302.
27. Mosci C, Iagaru A. PET/CT imaging of thyroid cancer. Clin Nucl Med. 2011;36(12):e180–5.
28. Robbins RJ, Wan Q, Grewal RK, Reibke R, Gonen M, Strauss HW, et al. Real-time prognosis for metastatic thyroid carcinoma based on 2-[18F]fluoro-2-deoxy-D-glucose-positron emission tomography scanning. J Clin Endocrinol Metab. 2006;91(2):498–505.

29. Razfar A, Branstetter BF, Christopoulos A, Lebeau SO, Hodak SP, Heron DE, et al. Clinical usefulness of positron emission tomography-computed tomography in recurrent thyroid carcinoma. Arch Otolaryngol Head Neck Surg. 2010;136(2):120–5.
30. Leboulleux S, Schroeder PR, Busaidy NL, Auperin A, Corone C, Jacene HA, et al. Assessment of the incremental value of recombinant thyrotropin stimulation before 2-[18F]-Fluoro-2-deoxy-D-glucose positron emission tomography/computed tomography imaging to localize residual differentiated thyroid cancer. J Clin Endocrinol Metab. 2009;94(4):1310–6.

Chapter 7
Surveillance of Benign Thyroid Nodules

Elizabeth H. Holt

Introduction

This chapter will address current controversial issues in the management of cytologically benign thyroid nodules. Optimal follow-up of benign thyroid nodules is an area of debate. It is well known that a subset of cytologically benign thyroid nodules grow over time; however, growth often can be perceived as a sign of concern. Identification of growing nodules for rebiopsy is an area of interest. Fine needle aspiration (FNA) of thyroid nodules is associated with an error rate of approximately 5 %. Whether rebiopsy of cytologically benign thyroid nodules will improve the accuracy of the diagnosis is controversial. Management of large thyroid nodules greater than 3–4 cm in size is an area of ongoing debate. Some investigators find these nodules to be more likely to yield false-negative results on FNA and more likely to be malignant; as a result, these nodules are often removed surgically. The use of molecular diagnostics to improve the accuracy of FNA biopsy results and avoid unnecessary surgery for cytologically indeterminate nodules is a growing area in thyroid cancer research. Molecular tests may be of value as well for cytologically benign nodules, in some cases.

E.H. Holt, MD, PhD
Section of Endocrinology and Metabolism, Yale School of Medicine, New Haven, CT, USA
e-mail: elizabeth.holt@yale.edu

S.A. Roman et al. (eds.), *Management of Thyroid Nodules and Differentiated Thyroid Cancer*, DOI 10.1007/978-3-319-43618-0_7

Long-Term Monitoring of Benign Thyroid Nodules

Monitoring of cytologically benign thyroid nodules by ultrasound surveillance is a common practice and one recommended by the American Thyroid Association (ATA) [1]. The goal of surveillance is to detect increase in size of the nodule or a change in the nodule's ultrasound appearance that renders it more suspicious. Nodules that grow or become more suspicious in appearance are recommended for rebiopsy (below).

How much growth should be considered significant was evaluated by Brauer et al. [2], who investigated the variability of thyroid nodule measurement by ultrasound by different radiologists. They found an interobserver variability of 48 % at measuring nodule volume. They concluded that a change in nodule volume of 49 % or more is needed to be considered a significant sign of shrinkage or growth.

Durante et al. [3] followed 992 Italian patients over 5 years with ultrasound. They defined nodule growth as an increase of 20 % in 2 dimensions with a minimum of 2 mm increase. With those criteria, 11.1 % of nodules grew during the study period. Nodule growth was associated with multiple nodules, larger-sized nodules, and male sex. They concluded that most nodules do not grow over time. Papini et al. [4] studied a small group of 41 patients prospectively over 5 years and found that, on average, nodules grew in volume from 1.46 ± 0.77 to 2.12 ± 1.46 ml. Overall, 56 % of nodules grew during the observation period. Erdogan et al. [5] followed 531 nodules in 420 patients for a mean time of 39.7 ± 29.8 months in a moderately iodine-deficient area. They found 1/3 of thyroid nodules grew during the time of the study, while 1/3 remained stable in size and 1/3 decreased in size.

Overall, then there appears to be controversy regarding the percentage of nodules that grow while under surveillance. Differences in results may come from differences in the definition of growth, interobserver variability in measurement, and different patient populations. The majority of nodules that grow are benign. As noted in the current ATA guidelines [1], there are no long-term surveillance studies for thyroid nodules beyond 5 years, so there is little to guide how long to monitor thyroid nodules after a benign cytologic diagnosis beyond 5 years.

Value of Repeat FNA in Monitoring Thyroid Nodules

It is estimated that biopsy of thyroid nodules has on average a 4–5 % false-negative rate [6, 7]. Several investigators have addressed the question of whether reaspiration of nodules is of value in improving the false-negative rate. Many of these studies are limited by lack of information about why a given nodule was selected for rebiopsy. In addition, many of the studies include nodules biopsied without ultrasound guidance.

Amrikachi et al. [6] found a rate of only 0.8 % malignancy on repeat FNA of previously cytologically benign thyroid nodules, suggesting that repeat biopsy may not be necessary. Dwarakanathan et al. [8] studied repeat FNA and its effect on diagnosis. They found that repeat FNA confirmed a benign diagnosis in 93 % of patients. Of those where a benign diagnosis was not confirmed, 30 % had malignancy on final pathology. They concluded that repeat FNA was valuable in improving diagnostic accuracy. Flanagan et al. [9] found that repeat FNA for benign nodules yielded 1/70 with malignancy on cytopathology. An additional 17 were indeterminate, of which 7 were malignant on final histopathology. Overall they found that the initial FNA was 81.7 % sensitive for malignancy, and with a second FNA, the sensitivity rose to 90.4 %. False-negative rates went down from 17.1 to 11.4 % with a second biopsy. This study does not indicate if the biopsies were done under ultrasound guidance or not, nor does it explain how nodules were selected for rebiopsy. Similarly, Furlan et al. [10] found that rebiopsy increased accuracy by 22.6 %, sensitivity by 13.8 %, and specificity by 6.2 %. The investigators did not indicate if ultrasound guidance was used for these biopsies. Illouz et al. [11] performed 895 biopsies on 298 nodules followed over a mean of 5 years. These nodules were performed without ultrasound guidance. Thirty-five nodules later had malignant or suspicious results. Ultrasound characteristics did not identify the patients at risk for malignant or suspicious results. They concluded that up to 3 FNA biopsies should be performed to ensure malignancy is not missed. Nou et al. [12] followed 1369 patients with 2010 cytologically benign nodules over an average of 8.5 years. FNA was performed under ultrasound guidance. During that time 45 patients had repeat thyroid biopsy due to nodule growth, of which 18 false-negative thyroid malignancies were identified and removed. Most of these patients waited 2–4 years for malignancy to be diagnosed, and none had advanced disease developed during that time. The investigators concluded that a repeat biopsy 2–4 year after an initial benign result would safely identify nodules whose initial biopsy was false negative. Oertel et al. [13] conducted a retrospective review of all patients who underwent FNA biopsy at Washington Hospital Center 1998–2006. They found that benign FNA lead to benign surgical pathology in 90 % of patients. If the nodule was benign on repeat aspiration, the odds of finding benign surgical pathology increased to 98 %. In this study, the majority of the FNAs were palpation guided. How nodules were selected for repeat FNA was not described. They concluded that repeat FNA should be performed for benign nodules one year after benign FNA. Orlandi et al. [14] performed FNA biopsy on their patients on an annual basis. Over time they found that 97.7 % remained benign, but 0.98 % became suspicious and 1.3 % had papillary thyroid carcinoma as the diagnosis, ultimately. Of those that were later found to be suspicious or malignant, 25 % were diagnosed on the second biopsy and 75 % on the third biopsy. The authors concluded that three biopsies for a nodule are appropriate to ensure malignancy is not missed. Of note, they did not indicate whether ultrasound guidance was used for their biopsies. Rosario et al. [15] repeated FNA biopsy after 12–18 months if nodules showed significant growth (>50 % increase in volume) or if the nodules developed suspicious ultrasound characteristics. In their cohort, 11.4 % of the nodules demonstrated suspicious ultrasound characteristics, of which 17.6 % had malignancy on repeat FNA. Also in their cohort, 9.6 % of the nodules showed growth, of which 1.3 % had malignancy on repeat FNA.

In comparison, Erdogan et al. [16] studied 457 reaspirations of benign thyroid nodules. They found the initial diagnosis did not change in 98.6 % of cases. Their reaspirations yielded 0.7 % papillary thyroid cancer and 3.5 % suspicious for thyroid cancer. While they acknowledged that reaspiration of a suspicious appearing nodule may be of value, they did not recommend routine reaspiration of cytologically benign thyroid nodules.

Growth of nodules has been a reason for rebiopsy. This was evaluated by Alexander et al. [17] who followed 268 patients with benign biopsies over time ranging from 1 month to 5 years. They found 89 % of nodules grew more than 15 % in volume over the study period. Rebiopsy was performed on 74 of 330 nodules with an average increase in volume of 69 %. Only one of 74 nodules rebiopsied was malignant. They concluded that most nodules grow over time and that this growth is not necessarily a sign of malignancy.

In conclusion, there is some evidence that routine repeat FNA biopsy of cytologically benign nodules may increase the likelihood of discovering a malignancy. Some of the studies supporting this statement included biopsies performed by palpation rather than by ultrasound guidance, thus likely reducing their diagnostic accuracy. The applicability of those studies to current-day practice of performing biopsy under ultrasound guidance is unknown. Whether repeat FNA biopsy of all cytologically benign thyroid nodules is cost-effective has not been studied.

The current ATA guidelines note that high-suspicion ultrasound appearance rather than growth of the nodule is a better predictor of malignancy. Therefore, the recommendation is that for cytologically benign nodules with suspicious ultrasound appearance, a repeat ultrasound and biopsy be performed within 12 months. For nodules with low to intermediate suspicious ultrasound pattern and benign cytopathology, the ATA recommends repeat ultrasound at 1–2 years. If there is evidence on ultrasound of growth (as defined as 20 % increase in at least two nodule dimensions with minimal increase of 2 mm or a greater than 50 % increase in volume) or development of new suspicious ultrasound characteristics, biopsy could be repeated, or surveillance carried on. They recommend that for nodules with very low suspicion pattern, such as spongiform nodules, the utility of follow-up ultrasound for growth is limited, and repeat ultrasound can be done at ≥24 months [1].

The Large (≥4 cm) Nodule with Benign FNA

As noted above, it is estimated that biopsy of thyroid nodules has on average a 4–5 % false-negative rate [6, 7] overall, but that error rate may not apply to all nodules. There is concern that larger thyroid nodules (typically defined as those nodules measuring greater than or equal to 4 cm) are more likely to yield false-negative results on fine needle aspiration (FNA) and/or that these nodules are more likely to be malignant than their smaller counterparts. These questions have been examined by numerous investigators, with conflicting results.

Several studies showed no relationship between nodule size and risk of false-negative cytology. Albuja-Cruz et al. [18] studied 1068 consecutive patients with FNA and surgery at a single tertiary care center. Of those, 212 had nodules greater than or equal to 4 cm. Biopsy was performed under ultrasound guidance in 98 % of cases. They found no decrease in reliability of FNA based on nodule size and concluded that large nodule size should not be an independent criterion for surgery. In a study from the Mayo Clinic, Porterfield et al. [19] did a retrospective study of 4 years of data and 742 thyroid nodules ≥3 cm with benign cytology on ultrasound-guided needle biopsy. Of these patients, 145 went to surgery and only one proved to be a false negative (0.7 %). They concluded that size ≥3 cm should not be an independent indication for surgery. Bohacek et al. [20] studied patients with 1000 ultrasound-guided thyroid biopsies, of which 67 % were benign, and of those benign nodules, 26 % went to surgery due to compressive symptoms or other worrisome features. They found no association between size of cytologically benign nodules and risk of malignancy at histopathology. Kamran et al. [21] conducted a retrospective cohort analysis of 7348 nodules evaluated by ultrasound-guided biopsy between 1995 and 2009 at an academic medical center. Of those nodules with benign FNA, 1502 were removed due to clinical concern. Overall, 1.1 % of these cytologically benign nodules proved to be malignant on final pathology. No correlation between nodule size and risk of false-negative FNA was found. Kuru et al. [22] studied 213 patients with nodules ≥3 cm who all had thyroidectomy based on nodule size and regardless of ultrasound-guided FNA biopsy results. They found a false-negative rate for FNA biopsy in nodules ≥4 cm of 4.3 %, but this was not statistically significantly different from the false-negative rate for smaller nodules in their cohort. Mehanna et al. [23] evaluated 262 cases who underwent ultrasound-guided FNA and had a thyroidectomy. Of that group, there were 55 nodules ≥3 cm with benign cytopathology, of which a 10.9 % false-negative rate for biopsies was found on final histology. This false-negative rate did not differ significantly from the false-negative rate for nodules measuring <3 cm. Raj et al. [24] studied a group of 223 patients with nodules ≥4 cm who were evaluated preoperatively by ultrasound-guided FNA, and all had thyroidectomy due to concerns about nodule size. There was no smaller size nodule comparison group. They found only one missed malignancy from 118 patients with benign cytology. They concluded that FNA biopsy can be used with confidence to exclude malignancy even in large thyroid nodules. Rosario et al. [25] studied 151 patients with thyroid nodules ≥4 cm who had thyroidectomy regardless of their cytology result. It is unclear from their methods whether biopsy was performed under ultrasound guidance. They found the negative predictive value of benign cytology for nodules ≥4 cm was 96.4 %. Their conclusion was that the false-negative rate for cytology in thyroid nodules ≥4 cm does not justify routine resection of thyroid nodules in this size range. Shrestha et al. [26] studied 540 patients with 695 nodules of varying sizes who had a thyroidectomy. They found no significant difference in the rates of false-negative biopsies in larger (≥4 cm) thyroid nodules. They concluded that large nodule size should not be an indication for thyroidectomy. Yoon et al. [27] studied 206 patients with thyroid nodules measuring ≥3 cm with a variety of ultrasound-guided biopsy results, who went to thyroidectomy. Of those patients, 112 had benign cytopathology, and only two (1.8 %) had malignancy discovered on surgical pathology. The authors concluded that FNA cytology is an accurate method for screening nodules ≥3 cm in diameter.

In contrast, other authors found that larger nodules were more likely to yield false-negative results on FNA than were smaller ones. For example, Wharry et al. [28] found in a prospective study of 361 patients with 382 nodules greater than or equal to 4 cm by ultrasound who all underwent FNA and thyroidectomy that the false-negative rate on biopsy was 10.4 %. Whether ultrasound guidance was used for the biopsies was not indicated. There was no comparison group of smaller nodules in this study. Carillo et al. [29] studied 159 patients who had thyroidectomy for thyroid nodules. Nodules were biopsied by palpation, not with ultrasound guidance. Of those nodules, 35 were ≥4 cm in diameter. They found seven (20 %) of the 35 nodules ≥4 cm in diameter had false-negative cytology. McCoy et al. [30] studied patients who had undergone biopsy with ultrasound guidance. In their cohort there were 223 patients with nodules ≥4 cm in diameter who had a thyroidectomy. They found a 13 % false-negative rate for thyroid biopsy among the nodules measuring ≥4 cm. Meko et al. [31] studied 90 patients who underwent biopsy without ultrasound guidance. After thyroidectomy they found that larger nodules (≥3 cm) had a 17 % false-negative rate for cytopathology. More impressive was a 30 % false-negative rate for larger cystic and solid nodules. Pinchot et al. [32] studied 155 patients who underwent thyroidectomy for thyroid nodules ≥4 cm. They found 4/52 (8 %) had false-negative preoperative cytopathology.

A related question is whether larger nodules are more likely to harbor malignancy just based on their size. Some investigators found no association between nodule size and risk of malignancy [20, 21, 26, 33]. Other investigators found larger nodules were more likely to be malignant. For example, Carillo et al. [29] found that of their cohort of 61 nodules with malignant pathology, 63.9 % were ≥4 cm in diameter. Kuru et al. [22] found an incidence of thyroid cancer in nodules ≥4 cm of 24 % versus 12 % for smaller nodules. McCoy et al. [30] found thyroid cancer in 26 % of thyroid nodules measuring ≥4 cm. Finally, Wharry et al. [28] found an incidence of malignancy in thyroid nodules ≥4 cm of 22 %.

The investigators who found a higher false-negative rate for FNA in larger nodules, and those that found a higher risk of thyroid cancer in larger nodules, recommend surgery for thyroid nodules measuring 4 cm or greater. Those authors who found no relationship between size and false-negative biopsy or malignancy risk do not recommend routine surgery for all nodules greater than 4 cm. With the numbers of studies relatively equal on the two sides of this debate, it is difficult to know what to do. Methodology for most of the studies is similar, with retrospective review of patients who went to surgery after FNA cytology. Sample sizes vary from 90 to more than 600. Sample sizes did not dictate the outcome of the studies regarding whether large nodules are more likely to be malignant or more likely to have false-negative biopsy results. In one study, all patients with nodules greater than or equal to 4 cm went to surgery regardless of cytopathology results [25]. In this report, 22.5 % of patients had malignant histology, and the negative predictive value of cytology was a relatively high 96.4 %. Shin et al. [34] performed a review with statistical analysis of 15 studies including 13,180 patients. Their conclusion was that larger nodules have a higher pretest probability of malignancy and cited a reduced accuracy of biopsy in nodules measuring 3–4 cm or larger. They concluded that thyroidectomy is a reasonable approach for nodules greater than 3 cm in diameter.

In conclusion, whether larger thyroid nodules are more likely than their smaller counterparts to yield false-negative biopsy results remains controversial. The current ATA guidelines [1] concluded that based on available evidence, it is currently uncertain whether nodules ≥4 cm with benign cytology are more likely to be malignant and need to be managed differently than their smaller counterparts.

Role of Molecular Testing for Benign Thyroid Nodules

Molecular testing for indeterminate thyroid nodules has been embraced as a way to gain additional information about an indeterminate nodule thereby avoiding thyroidectomy. For indeterminate nodules this has been a way to reduce the need for what often turns out to be unnecessary surgical procedures to obtain definitive pathology. The use of molecular testing for cytologically benign nodules is less well recognized but still is possible and may be appropriate in some situations.

A retrospective study by Proietti et al. [35] studied 1347 consecutive papillary thyroid cancers at a single center where cytopathology and histology results were available. They found a false-negative rate for FNA diagnosis of 4.8 %. Those with false-negative FNA were subjected to molecular testing for BRAF mutations and RAS alterations. BRAF mutations were found in 11 % of cases, and RAS alterations were found in 29.6 % of cases. In conclusion, molecular testing would have considerably lowered the false-negative rate in this cohort. In a prospective study by Nikiforov et al. [36], 470 FNA samples were collected from 328 patients and subjected to cytopathology analysis as well as molecular analysis for mutations in BRAF, RAS, RET/PTC, and PAX8/PPARγ. Of those who had a thyroidectomy, there were 12 that tested negative for malignancy by cytopathology. Of these, one tested positive for BRAF mutation and proved to be a papillary carcinoma. Three tested positive for RAS mutations and proved to be papillary thyroid carcinoma in one case, follicular thyroid carcinoma in one case, and follicular adenoma in one case. Of those that were negative by cytopathology and molecular testing but went to surgery ($N=8$), there was one papillary thyroid cancer and one follicular thyroid cancer. Thus, molecular testing on cytologically benign nodules may provide additional information that would lead to the clinician to recommend thyroidectomy. However, even with molecular testing, some nodules will be incorrectly classified as benign. Currently, it is not standard of practice to proceed to molecular testing for nodules with cytologically benign FNAs.

In the future we may see more use of molecular testing on cytologically benign biopsy samples. For example, the cytologically benign nodule with suspicious ultrasound characteristics is appropriate for molecular testing as another means of looking for evidence of malignancy. Nodules that are benign by both cytopathology and molecular testing may not need to be followed longitudinally by ultrasound in the same way as nodules evaluated by cytopathology alone currently are. Furthermore, in the future we may see all nodules with suspicious ultrasound characteristics evaluated by both cytopathology and molecular testing as a more complete way to evaluate the risk of malignancy.

References

1. Haugen BR, et al. 2015 American Thyroid Association management guidelines for adult patients with thyroid nodules and differentiated thyroid cancer. Thyroid. 2015;26(1):1–133.
2. Brauer VFH, et al. Interobserver variation for ultrasound determination of thyroid nodule volumes. Thyroid. 2005;15(10):1169–75.
3. Durante C, et al. The natural history of benign thyroid nodules. JAMA. 2015;313(9):926–35. doi:10.1001/jama.2015.0956.
4. Papini E, et al. Long-term changes in nodular goiter: a 5-year prospective randomized trial of levothyroxine suppressive therapy for benign cold thyroid nodules. J Clin Endocrinol Metab. 1998;83(3):780–3.
5. Erdogan MF, et al. Natural course of thyroid nodules in a moderately iodine deficient area. Clin Endocrinol. 2006;65:767–71.
6. Amrikachi M, et al. Accuracy of fine-needle aspiration of thyroid a review of 6226 cases and correlation with surgical or clinical outcome. Arch Pathol Lab Med. 2001;125:484–8.
7. Gharib H. Fine-needle aspiration biopsy of thyroid nodules: advantages, limitations, and effect. Mayo Clin Proc. 1994;69:44–9.
8. Dwarakanathan AA, et al. Importance of repeat fine-needle biopsy in the management of thyroid nodules. Am J Surg. 1993;166:350–2.
9. Flanagan MB, et al. Repeat thyroid nodule fine-needle aspiration in patients with initial benign cytologic results. Am J Clin Pathol. 2006;125:698–702. doi:10.1309/4AXLDMN1JRPMTX5P.
10. Furlan JC, et al. Single versus sequential fine-needle aspiration biopsy in the management of thyroid nodular disease. Can J Surg. 2005;48(1):12–8.
11. Illouz F, et al. Usefulness of repeated fine-needle cytology in the follow-up of non-operated thyroid nodules. Eur J Endocrinol. 2007;156:303–8.
12. Nou E, et al. Determination of the optimal time interval for repeat evaluation after a benign thyroid nodule aspiration. J Clin Endocrinol Metab. 2014;99(2):510–6. doi:10.1210/jc.2013-3160.
13. Oertel YC, et al. Techniques in thyroidology value of repeated fine needle aspirations of the thyroid: an analysis of over ten thousand FNAs. Thyroid. 2007;17(11):1061–6.
14. Orlandi A, et al. Repeated fine-needle aspiration of the thyroid in benign nodular thyroid disease: Critical evaluation of long-term follow-up. Thyroid. 2005;15(3):274–8.

15. Rosário PW, Purisch S. Ultrasonographic characteristics as a criterion for repeat cytology in benign thyroid nodules. Arq Bras Endocrinol Metab. 2010;54(1):52–5.
16. Erdogan MF, et al. Value of re-aspirations in benign nodular thyroid disease. Thyroid. 1998;8(12):1087–90.
17. Alexander EK, et al. Natural history of benign solid and cystic thyroid nodules. Ann Intern Med. 2003;138:315–8.
18. Albuja-Cruz MB, et al. Reliability of fine-needle aspiration for thyroid nodules greater than or equal to 4 cm. J Surg Res. 2013;181:6–10.
19. Porterfield JR, et al. Reliability of benign fine needle aspiration cytology of large thyroid nodules. Surgery. 2008;144:963–9.
20. Bohacek L, et al. Diagnostic accuracy of surgeon-performed ultrasound-guided fine-needle aspiration of thyroid nodules. Ann Surg Oncol. 2012;19:45–51. doi:10.1245/s10434-011-1807-z.
21. Kamran SC, et al. Thyroid nodule size and prediction of cancer. J Clin Endocrinol Metab. 2013;98:564–70.
22. Kuru B, et al. The false-negative rate of fine-needle aspiration cytology for diagnosing thyroid carcinoma in thyroid nodules. Langenbecks Arch Surg. 2010;395:127–32. doi:10.1007/s00423-009-0470-3.
23. Mehanna R, et al. False negatives in thyroid cytology: impact of large nodule size and follicular variant of papillary carcinoma. Laryngoscope. 2013;123:1305–9.
24. Raj MD, et al. Diagnostic lobectomy is not routinely required to exclude malignancy in thyroid nodules greater than four centimetres. ANZ J Surg. 2012;82:73–7. doi:10.1111/j.1445-2197.2011.05667.x.
25. Rosario PW, et al. Low false-negative rate of cytology in thyroid nodules ≥ 4 cm. Arq Bras Endocrinol Metab. 2009;53(9):1143–5.
26. Shrestha M, et al. The impact of thyroid nodule size on the risk of malignancy and accuracy of fine-needle aspiration: a 10-year study from a single institution. Thyroid. 2012;22(12):1251–6. doi:10.1089/thy.2012.0265.
27. Yoon JH, et al. The diagnostic accuracy of ultrasound-guided fine-needle aspiration biopsy and the sonographic differences between benign and malignant thyroid nodules 3 cm or larger. Thyroid. 2011;21(9):993–1000. doi:10.1089/thy.2010.0458.
28. Wharry LI, et al. Thyroid Nodules (≥4 cm): can ultrasound and cytology reliably exclude cancer? World J Surg. 2014;38:614–21. doi:10.1007/s00268-013-2261-9.
29. Carrillo JF, et al. Accuracy of fine-needle aspiration biopsy of the thyroid combined with an evaluation of clinical and radiologic factors. Otolaryngol Head Neck Surg. 2000;122:917–21.
30. McCoy KL, et al. The incidence of cancer and rate of false-negative cytology in thyroid nodules greater than or equal to 4 cm in size. Surgery. 2007;142:837–44.
31. Meko JB, Norton JA. Large cystic/solid thyroid nodules: a potential false-negative fine-needle aspiration. Surgery. 1995;118:996–1004.
32. Pinchot SN, et al. Accuracy of fine-needle aspiration biopsy for predicting neoplasm or carcinoma in thyroid nodules 4 cm or larger. Arch Surg. 2009;144(7):649–55. doi:10.1001/archsurg.2009.116.
33. McHenry CR, et al. Is nodule size an independent predictor of thyroid malignancy? Surgery. 2008;144:1062–9.
34. Shin JJ, et al. Impact of thyroid nodule size on prevalence and post-test probability of malignancy: a systematic review. Laryngoscope. 2015;125:263–72.
35. Proietti A, et al. Molecular characterization of 54 cases of false negative fine needle aspiration among 1347 papillary thyroid carcinomas. Cancer (Cancer Cytopathol). 2014;122:751–9.
36. Nikiforov YE. Molecular testing for mutations in improving the fine needle aspiration diagnosis of thyroid nodules. J Clin Endocrinol Metab. 2009;94:2092–8.

Part II
Management of Nodular Hyperthyroidism

Chapter 8
The Role of Medical Management for Nodular Hyperthyroidism

Ana E. Espinosa De Ycaza and Marius N. Stan

Abbreviations

AFTN	Autonomously functioning thyroid nodule
ATDs	Antithyroid drugs
CVD	Cardiovascular disease
PEI	Percutaneous ethanol injection
PLA	Percutaneous laser ablation
RAI	Radioactive iodine
RFA	Radiofrequency ablation
TMNG	Toxic multinodular goiter

Introduction

Hyperthyroidism occurs in 1.3 % of the population [1]. The most common cause of hyperthyroidism is Graves' disease, followed by toxic multinodular goiter (TMNG) and autonomously functioning thyroid nodules (AFTN). The co-occurrence of autonomously functioning thyroid nodule(s) or TMNG with Graves' disease is termed Marine-Lenhart syndrome or nodular Graves'. It is a rare presentation of hyperthyroidism that occurs in around 1–2.7 % of Graves' disease cases [2, 3].

The standard therapy for TMNG and AFTN is either thyroid surgery or radioactive iodine (^{131}I) therapy. However, in certain circumstances, such as patients with high surgical risk or patients not interested in surgery who also have a low radioac-

A.E.E. De Ycaza, MD • M.N. Stan, MD (✉)
Endocrinology, Diabetes, Metabolism and Nutrition, Mayo Clinic,
200 First Street SW, Rochester, MN 55905, USA
e-mail: espinosadeycaza.ana@mayo.edu; stan.marius@mayo.edu

S.A. Roman et al. (eds.), *Management of Thyroid Nodules and Differentiated Thyroid Cancer*, DOI 10.1007/978-3-319-43618-0_8

tive iodine uptake, among others, alternative medical therapies can be considered. Herein we will discuss the nonsurgical management of toxic multinodular goiter, toxic thyroid nodules, and Marine-Lenhart syndrome.

Role of Radioactive Iodine (^{131}I)

Since the discovery of artificial radioactivity in 1934, there has been growing interest of the potential applications of radioactive isotopes for the diagnosis and treatment of diseases. In regard to the thyroid gland, ^{128}iodine(I) was the first isotope used to evaluate thyroid gland uptake in rabbits, but with a decay half-life of only 25 min, its use was not practical [4]. In the late 1930s, the radioactive isotopes ^{130}I, ^{126}I, and ^{131}I were used for the study of thyroid iodine uptake and metabolism using a Geiger counter. In 1941, ^{131}I was used for the first time to treat hyperthyroidism in humans. ^{131}I is now widely used for treatment of hyperthyroidism; it is a radionuclide taken up by thyroid tissue, and it has predominantly β-emissions, thus causing cell death. It has a decay half-life of about 8 days.

Efficacy

The ideal goal of therapy with radioactive iodine (RAI) is to achieve euthyroidism. However, in some cases hypothyroidism may develop after treatment with RAI. The cure rate defined as the development of hypothyroidism or euthyroidism after one dose of RAI varies among studies. It ranges between 60 and 93 % for TMNG [5–9] and between 71 and 97 % for AFTN [6, 8, 9]. Hyperthyroidism resolves at a mean time of 5.4 months [8]. RAI is also safe and efficacious in elderly individuals, with a reported cure rate of 80 % for TMNG and 86 % for AFTN at 12 months [9].

After RAI there is usually reduction in size of the goiter or of the toxic nodule. In TMNG the gland decreases in volume by 43 % at 24 months [7]. For AFTN, the nodule reduces in size by 35 % after 3 months and by 45 % at 24 months [10]. Ideally one dose of RAI should cure hyperthyroidism. However, if there is persistence of hyperthyroidism 6 months after RAI [11] or recurrence of hyperthyroidism, a second dose can be given. On occasions it can take up to 24 months for hyperthyroidism to completely resolve after RAI [9]; therefore, the use of antithyroid drugs (ATDs) can be considered with periodic monitoring of thyroid tests to evaluate for cure. In the case of severe refractory hyperthyroidism, surgery should be considered, specifically thyroid lobectomy for AFTN or near-total/total thyroidectomy for TMNG.

Treatment with RAI is also indicated for the rare patients with TMNG or AFTN that failed surgical therapy (<1 %) and are thus still hyperthyroid [12, 13].

Factors Associated with RAI Efficacy

Certain clinical and laboratory factors were thought to affect the response to RAI therapy such as size of the goiter, gender, age at diagnosis of thyrotoxicosis, TSH value, and pretreatment with antithyroid drugs. Of these factors, gender and age at time of diagnosis are not clearly associated with RAI therapy response in observational studies [5, 7]. However, larger goiters have been associated with lower cure rates [6]. Patients with low but detectable TSH values had a higher cure rate and hypothyroidism than those with undetectable TSH values before RAI [14]. The potential effect of pretreatment with antithyroid drugs and the response to RAI therapy will be discussed later.

Dose and Regimen

Even though RAI have been used for the treatment of hyperthyroidism since the 1940s [15], there is still debate on the appropriate dose or regimen used to cure hyperthyroidism while avoiding permanent hypothyroidism.

Dose and regimens used for RAI are often institution dependent, but in general, treatment with RAI can be given either as (1) a standard fixed activity or (2) as a calculated dose based on nodule size (for AFTN) or gland size (for TMNG) corrected for the RAI uptake. Fixed activities can be given as a standard fixed activity for everybody or by adapting the standard activity to the thyroid gland size. Usual fixed doses of ^{131}I range between 10 and 30 mCi. For toxic adenoma and TMNG, higher fixed doses (20–30 mCi) are associated with higher cure rates and higher rates of hypothyroidism compared to lower doses (around 10 mCi). In a study comparing 2 doses of RAI, hypothyroidism occurred in 26 % of patients who received a higher dose of RAI compared to 11 % of those who received a lower dose [16].

Calculated doses of RAI are given with the goal of controlling hyperthyroidism and minimizing hypothyroidism. The premise is that a larger nodule (for AFTN) or larger goiter (for TMNG) requires higher RAI activity, and a higher RAI uptake, which means the tissue will more avidly take iodine, will require a lower RAI activity to achieve euthyroidism. Therefore, the dose of RAI administered can be calculated as follows:

$$\text{Activity } (\mu\text{Ci or MBq}) = \frac{\text{Gland weight}(\text{g}) \times \text{desired dose per gram of thyroid tissue}}{\text{Percentage of 24} - \text{h thyroid uptake}} \times 100$$

The gland weight in grams can be estimated by palpation, by ultrasound, or by nuclear imaging; in practice the first two methods are most commonly used. The desired dose to the thyroid tissue is expressed as the activity desired per gram of tissue (μCi/g or MBq/g), and it has ranged in studies between 90 and 200 μCi/g or 3.33–7.4 MBq/g. An activity of radioiodine between 150 and

200 μCi is usually recommended [11]. Several studies have reported outcomes of RAI given as fixed doses or calculated doses in hyperthyroidism [16, 17]; however, head-to-head trials comparing both methods are scarce. A study comparing different protocols of RAI therapy in toxic adenoma found a higher cure rate in the calculated high-dose protocol compared to a calculated low-dose, fixed high-dose, or fixed low-dose protocol [18]. At the same time, the rate of hypothyroidism was higher in the calculated and fixed high-dose groups compared to the lower-dose groups. A systematic review and meta-analysis of studies comparing fixed doses or estimated doses, based on thyroid size, to calculated doses in patients with hyperthyroidism showed no significant differences in cure of hyperthyroidism between the two methods. They included in the analysis patients with Graves' disease, TMNG, and AFTN [19].

Pretreatment with Antithyroid Drugs

The antithyroid drugs (ATDs), methimazole, propylthiouracil, and carbimazole, inhibit the synthesis of new thyroid hormone from the thyroid gland, thus controlling the hyperthyroidism of TMNG, AFTN, or Graves' disease. In the case of TMNG and toxic adenoma, they are frequently used before definite therapy with RAI.

In theory, RAI therapy can exacerbate signs and symptoms of thyrotoxicosis; therefore, the use of ATDs depletes thyroid hormone stores and can potentially ameliorate or prevent exacerbation of hyperthyroidism induced by RAI therapy. The benefit of this approach has not been thoroughly investigated in RCTs, and the use of ATDs in this setting is controversial with some advocating against the use of ATDs given the lack of evidence of benefit. Still some institutions use them routinely before administration of RAI. It is thought that RAI therapy exacerbates symptoms of thyrotoxicosis through induction of radiation thyroiditis. In a study of 34 patients with hyperthyroidism (11 with TMNG, 2 with AFTN, and 21 with Graves' disease) who didn't receive ATDs, all patients with TMNG had elevations of thyroid hormones after RAI compared to only 29 % of those with Graves' disease. However, none had worsening symptoms of thyrotoxicosis [20]. Despite these findings there are reports in the literature of thyroid storm and severe hyperthyroidism after RAI [21, 22].

When considering pretreatment with ATDs, three main factors need to be addressed: (1) the severity of hyperthyroidism; (2) the patient's comorbidities such as cardiovascular disease, cardiac arrhythmias, patient's age, and overall health; and (3) the risk of decreasing the effectiveness of RAI in patients taking ATDs.

Patients with severe hyperthyroidism, elderly patients, or patients with cardiac disease are at higher risk of developing complications from exacerbation of the hyperthyroid state. Consequently these are the patients in which pretreatment with ATDs should be considered.

If ATDs are continued at the time of RAI, there is clear evidence that the cure rate in TMNG and AFTN is significantly lower compared to when no ATDs are given [23]. However, whether ATDs reduce the efficacy of ^{131}I if they are stopped a few days before therapy is controversial. A systematic review and meta-analysis of 14 randomized controlled trials of the effect of ATDs on RAI found that the adjunctive use of ATDs was associated with higher RAI failure rates compared to no ATDs [24]. However, only 5/14 studies included patients with TMNG or AFTN, and 5 of the included studies gave ATDs concomitantly with RAI.

The most common practice is to discontinue ATDs before RAI, and the time interval between discontinuation of ATD and RAI therapy varies among studies between 2 and 7 days. If carbimazole is stopped 3 days before RAI, the cure rates were similar than if no ATDs were given [25].

If ATDs are given before RAI, it is preferred to use either methimazole or carbimazole instead of propylthiouracil (PTU) given the higher risk of liver dysfunction [26] and evidence from observational studies, suggesting radioresistance of the thyroid gland with PTU [27].

ATDs can be given for several weeks until hyperthyroidism is controlled; however, TSH should not be normalized to avoid the inadvertent therapy of the normal thyroid tissue, thus increasing the long-term risk of hypothyroidism. ATDs should be discontinued 3–7 days before RAI [11] and reinitiated 7 days later if there are concerns about risks associated with transient increase in thyroid hormone values. The dose of ATDs should be gradually decreased with the goal to discontinue them 1 month after RAI.

Should rhTSH Be Used to Augment RAI Uptake and Efficacy?

Recombinant human TSH (rhTSH) is commonly used with RAI ablative therapy after thyroidectomy for thyroid cancer. In the case of TMNG, the use of rhTSH has been considered in cases of low RAI uptake to increase the uptake and potentially increase the efficacy of RAI and the thyroid absorbed dose. Observational studies [28, 29] and one RCT [30] using rhTSH before RAI have included patients with nontoxic multinodular goiter and a subset of patients with TMNG with subclinical hyperthyroidism or mild hyperthyroidism. The RAI uptake increased two- to fourfold 24 h and 72 h after rhTSH, respectively. No clinical worsening of hyperthyroidism was reported after 0.1 or 0.3 mg of rhTSH. However, thyroid hormone levels increase after rhTSH, and exacerbation of hyperthyroidism can occur [31]. Consequently, more studies evaluating the safety and efficacy of rhTSH augmented RAI in TMNG compared to RAI alone are needed before recommending its use.

Risk of Hypothyroidism

The risk of hypothyroidism persists years after treatment with ^{131}I. Rates of subclinical hypothyroidism or overt hypothyroidism as high as 72 % have been reported 8 years after RAI [32]. Higher doses of RAI are more likely to cause hypothyroidism [18, 32]. For TMNG the rate of hypothyroidism 5 years after treatment is between 7 % and 14 % for lower and higher doses of RAI, respectively [7, 33, 34]. The average rate of hypothyroidism is 2.7 %/year with 64 % of patients hypothyroid 24 years after RAI [35].

For autonomously functioning thyroid nodules, the rate of hypothyroidism is between 7 % and 55 % when lower and higher doses of RAI are given, respectively [17, 36], and the cumulative incidence of hypothyroidism is 7 % at 1 year, 28 % at 5 years, and up to 60 % at 20 years [37]. Besides the dose of RAI administered, other risk factors associated with higher rates of hypothyroidism include the presence of thyroid antibodies, a smaller or non-palpable thyroid gland, and the use of ATDs before ^{131}I [6, 34, 38].

To prevent hypothyroidism, ATDs combined with thyroid hormone were used in 149 patients, with a reported rate of overt hypothyroidism of 3.3 %, 6.8 years after RAI [39]. The idea of this approach was to first control hyperthyroidism with ATDs and then give enough thyroid hormone to suppress TSH to avoid RAI uptake by normal thyroid tissue. This approach has not been validated and is therefore not recommended. Because the risk of hypothyroidism after RAI in TMNG and AFTN is significant, thyroid function tests should be periodically monitored even after clinical and biochemical evidence of euthyroidism.

Contraindications to RAI

Absolute contraindications to RAI therapy for hyperthyroidism from TMNG or toxic adenomas are pregnancy, concomitant diagnosis of thyroid cancer (for which surgery is the most appropriate therapy), women planning pregnancy within the next few months of therapy with RAI, or people unable to comply with radiation safety procedures [11].

Risks of RAI

Cancer Risk

The Cooperative Thyrotoxicosis Therapy Follow-Up Study has followed patients treated for hyperthyroidism in 26 medical centers in the United States and England. At 6 years of follow-up, the incidence of thyroid cancer mortality and leukemia was not increased in the patients treated with ^{131}I compared to the patients treated with other modalities [40, 41]. At a mean follow-up of 21 years, there was no difference in overall cancer mortality in the ^{131}I-treated patients compared to the general population. However, there was a small but significant increase in thyroid cancer deaths (SMR 3.94. CI: 2.52–5.86) in the ^{131}I-treated patients [42]. Patients who died from thyroid cancer were more likely to have had toxic nodular goiter, suggesting that the increased risk in thyroid cancer might be related to nodular goiter itself and not to RAI.

Mortality and CVD Mortality Risk

Population-based studies have found an increased risk in CVD and all-cause mortality in patients with hyperthyroidism treated with ^{131}I when compared to mortality estimates in the general population [43, 44]. A major limitation in these studies is the inability to differentiate the contribution of the RAI treatment itself to the increased mortality which could be solely explained by hyperthyroidism.

Induction of Thyroid Autoimmunity

Appearance of Graves-like disease after RAI for TMNG or AFTN has been repeatedly reported. Its occurrence is rare between 1 and 4% [45, 46]. It usually manifests 3–6 months after RAI with elevation of thyroid hormone levels, appearance of thyrotropin receptor antibodies (TRAB), and a thyroid scan showing diffuse radioiodine uptake.

Thyroglobulin, a protein synthesized solely by follicular cells in the thyroid gland, is released to the systemic circulation after RAI. Therefore, it is thought that an increase in thyroid antigens following RAI may stimulate an immune response toward the TSH receptor.

In a study evaluating the risk to develop Graves' disease after RAI, the phenotype occurred more commonly for TMNG than for toxic adenoma with rates of 2% and 0.3%, respectively, but none of those with toxic nodular goiter that didn't receive ^{131}I developed the disease [46]. This finding suggests that RAI therapy induces the thyroid autoimmune response. If a patient with TMNG or toxic adenoma develops recurrence of hyperthyroidism months after RAI therapy, it is much more likely to be from recurrence of autonomy than Graves' disease. However, we recommend getting a thyroid ^{121}I uptake and scan, and if there is diffuse uptake throughout the gland, Graves' disease is more likely, and treatment with ATDs or retreatment with RAI should be considered.

Marine-Lenhart Syndrome

The diagnosis of this entity is usually made by the presence of hyperthyroidism, positive thyrotropin receptor antibodies, and thyroid nodules seen on ultrasound and thyroid uptake and scan. The treatment for Marine-Lenhart syndrome follows the same principles discussed. Radioactive iodine and surgery are the most commonly used therapies. The dose of RAI required for cure is usually similar to the dose required for TMNG or AFTN, which is higher than the dose required for Graves'.

Role of Antithyroid Drugs

Mechanism of Action

The thionamide compounds available in the United States are methimazole (MMI) and propylthiouracil (PTU). Carbimazole (CBZ) is another thionamide available and commonly used in some European and Asian countries. These compounds alleviate hyperthyroidism by inhibiting thyroid hormone synthesis. They inhibit the oxidation from iodide to iodine and iodine organification catalyzed by thyroperoxidase, a necessary step for the incorporation of iodine into thyroglobulin. Thionamides also inhibit coupling of iodotyrosines and alter the structure of thyroglobulin [47]. Carbimazole is metabolized to methimazole in serum. Propylthiouracil, but not methimazole or carbimazole, inhibits the conversion from T4 to T3 in extrathyroidal tissues.

Efficacy

ATDs control hyperthyroidism but don't cause remission in toxic nodular goiter. After 12 months of therapy with ATDs, 95 % of patients with TMNG have recurrence of hyperthyroidism when ATDs are discontinued [48]. If ATDs are chosen as the main treatment, lifelong therapy will be required. Accordingly, surgery, radioactive iodine, or other ablative therapies are usually preferred over ATDs in the treatment of TMNG and AFTN (see Table 8.1). A study evaluating the effects of long-term therapy with methimazole in diffuse toxic goiter compared to RAI showed that methimazole therapy for 10 years is overall safe. Euthyroidism was achieved in 93 % of patients on MMI [49]. There were more thyroid test abnormalities at follow-up in the group that received RAI. However, there was a high number loss to follow up over all.

Nevertheless, long-term therapy with ATDs can be considered in elderly individuals with cardiac disease or other significant comorbidities when the risk for radioactive iodine or surgery is high. This is of particular importance for TMNG, because other therapeutic modalities to be discussed later, such as radiofrequency or thermal ablation, are effective in toxic adenomas but less so in TMNG.

Side Effects

Allergic reactions such as pruritus, rash, urticaria, and arthralgias occur in 5 % of people taking these medications and are the most common side effects. Agranulocytosis, polyarthritis, vasculitis, and hepatitis are rare but serious side effects. Agranulocytosis, which is an idiosyncratic reaction, occurs in 0.2–0.5 % with MMI, CBZ, or PTU [50]. Polyarthritis, vasculitis, and fulminant hepatitis are more commonly reported with PTU than MMI (frequency <1 %) [50]. Fulminant hepatitis occurs in 1:10,000 adults on PTU and is more common in children [26]. Liver dysfunction can also occur with MMI and is usually a cholestatic pattern [51].

Table 8.1 Preferred treatment option for toxic multinodular goiter (TMNG) or autonomously functioning thyroid nodule (AFTN) according to specific clinical factors

	Therapy options			
Clinical factors	Surgery	Radioactive iodine (RAI)	Ablative therapies[a]	Antithyroid drugs
Contemplating pregnancy within few months	✓✓✓	–[b]	✓OK to consider for AFTN	–
Goiter with compressive symptoms	✓✓✓	✓✓	✓OK to consider for AFTN	–
Short life expectancy	–	✓	✓✓✓	✓✓✓
Multiple comorbidities	✓	✓✓✓	✓✓✓	✓
Previous neck/thyroid surgery	✓	✓✓✓	✓	✓
Severe hyperthyroidism[c]	✓✓✓	✓✓✓	–	✓

✓✓✓ most recommended therapy, ✓✓ recommended, ✓ can be considered, – not recommended

[a]Include RFA and PLA. Ablative therapies are preferred for toxic adenomas and not TMNG

[b]Pregnancy should be avoided within 6 months after RAI and until euthyroidism is achieved

[c]Pretreatment with antithyroid drugs should be strongly considered before surgery or RAI

Given the concern of significant hepatitis with PTU associated with deaths and liver transplantation, in most circumstances, MMI and CBZ are the first-line drug therapies for hyperthyroidism.

Role of Ablative Therapies

A large number of patients with nodular thyroid disease are advanced in age and have non-thyroidal comorbidities that increase the risk of a surgical intervention. It is also not uncommon for these patients to have large nodules without a very high uptake of radioactive iodine which leads to the need to use large doses of RAI (by comparison with Graves' disease patients). On this background the developments of ultrasonography over the last couple decades has allowed the creation of procedures that target the thyroid nodules percutaneously with delivery of high energy or chemical agents in the nodular tissue under direct ultrasound visualization. The main area of use for these procedures has been the benign, nontoxic thyroid nodules. However, these procedures have also been employed in patients with toxic nodules that for cultural or other nonmedical issues have refused surgery or RAI. In almost all studies, the targeted nodules have been large nodules, many with documented compressive symptoms or at risk of producing such symptoms. The ultrasound-based procedures targeting thyroid nodules are radiofrequency ablation (RFA), percutaneous laser ablation (PLA), and percutaneous ethanol injection (PEI). Table 8.1 summarizes the clinical situations where the interventions described here could be considered.

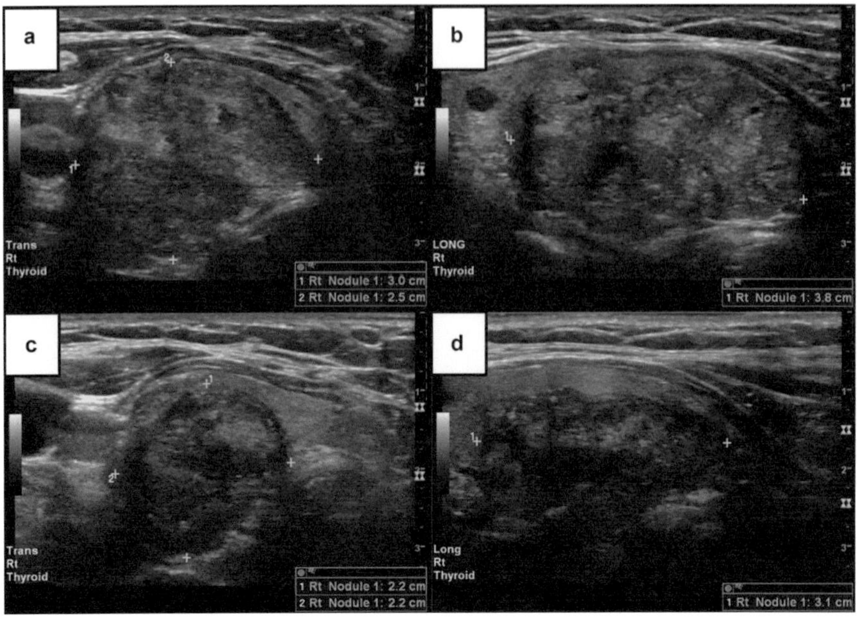

Fig. 8.1 Ultrasound images of thyroid nodule before and after radiofrequency ablation (RFA). Pre-RFA (**a**, **b**) and 3 months post-RFA (**c**, **d**) images of thyroid nodule in transverse (**a**, **c**) and longitudinal (**b**, **d**) views. Three months after RFA (**c**, **d**), the nodule volume decreased by 52 %

Radiofrequency Ablation

Radiofrequency ablation or radiofrequency thermal ablation (RFA) is the most utilized of the ablative therapies. Its use is based on the principle that ultrasound-based energy delivery into the thyroid tissue will raise the local temperature to about 101–105°C which will lead to local thrombosis followed by ischemia and fibrosis and subsequent shrinkage of the treated tissue volume (see Fig. 8.1). The needles employed are 14–18 G, some allowing further deployment of one to four expandable hooks that are then making contact with multiple portions of the targeted nodule. The procedure in all cases is performed under continuous ultrasound guidance. There are at least two techniques in practice: fixed-needle technique and "moving-shot" technique which are distinguished by the degree of manipulating the needle during the procedure. The energy delivered per nodule is a variable between reports, and it has been delivered for most patients in multiple sessions (mean is about two sessions/nodule from combining multiple studies data). The sessions were repeated based on thyroid function and/or nodule size response and performed 1–2 months apart. Local anesthesia with 2 % lidocaine has been employed for the superficial cervical tissue and the thyroid capsule. In most cases the cystic content, if present, is aspirated before the energy is delivered. No significant side effects or hospitalization was noted in these patients. A sensation of heat in the neck was reported by patients. That did not affect the course of the procedure. If pain developed the power was decreased or ablation stopped completely for few seconds. Some reports described repeat biopsies prior to procedure to ensure the benign character of the treated lesions.

The efficacy of the procedure has been tested in a number of clinical studies. One of the early series [52] reported on 94 patients that included both toxic (28 patients) and nontoxic nodules (66 patients). They have utilized the 14G needles with four expandable hooks. Thyroid function normalized in all those with subclinical hyperthyroidism and in about 50 % of patients with overt hyperthyroidism. Added benefit was the decrease in the size of thyroid nodule in 50 % of patients. The discomfort was minimal and always local and there was no need for additional therapy for this side effect. There were no hospitalizations, local infections, nerve injuries, or any injuries to the neck vital structures. The authors followed with a more rigorous assessment of RFA [53] comparing ten patients with solid toxic nodules (<30 % cystic component) that they compared with a similar group of patients followed with observation only. Nontoxic nodules were evaluated the same way. Reassuringly 40 % of patients reached euthyroidism and another 40 % experienced a reduction in the dose of methimazole needed to control their hyperthyroidism. More importantly none developed worsening of their thyroid parameters. All the treated nodules shrank and the process was already noticeable at 1 month and continued for the 12 months of observation. The average decrease in volume was 86 % over that period. A simple symptom scoring system (no symptoms = 0, severe symptoms = 6) was employed reflecting compressive symptoms and esthetic complaints, and it was very encouraging to find the score improving in treated patients (from 3.4/6 to 0.6 at 12 months), while it worsened in the control group (3.0 to 4.1 at 12 months).

While one might wonder if these results are population specific, similar data emerged at about the same time from Korea. Those researchers [54] reported initially on 9 patients with toxic nodules that were treated with RFA. They have utilized 18G electrodes without additional prongs and used local anesthesia for pain control. A mean of 2.2 sessions were performed (range 1–4). The volume reduction was a mean of 36.4 % at 1 month and 70.7 % at 6 months. TSH level normalized in five out of nine patients, improved yet still suppressed in three, and remained elevated in one patient. Encouragingly no patient reported aggravation of hyperthyroid symptoms after therapy. Symptom and cosmetic scores improved in all but one patient. No adverse effects except for local heat and neck discomfort were reported, and no procedure had to be discontinued because of such symptoms. Most recently the same group reported on a multicenter study that evaluated the outcome of RFA for autonomously functioning thyroid nodules at five Korean institutions [55]. Following 44 patients they noticed again a rapid decline in the volume of the nodule (from 46 % at 1 month to 82 % at the last follow-up, mean of 20 months). The thyroid function normalized in 36/44 patients (82 %), but 18 % of patients still had a suppressed TSH despite repeat RFA. No case of hypothyroidism developed. The score for symptoms and cosmetic appearance improved significantly, while no patient reported deterioration of local symptoms or symptoms of hyperthyroidism.

RFA was repeated if TSH did not normalize, and thus a mean of 1.8 sessions/nodule was performed (maximum up to 6). Their results are thus consistent with the other studies on RFA.

It thus appears that the thyroid function is normalized in half to three quarters of these patients. It also appears that the moving-shot technique is slightly superior regarding volume reduction to the fixed-needle technique with expandable electrodes. It is also purported to be easier to perform given the difficulty with tracking and moving 2–4 separate electrodes. Clearly both techniques require a significant amount of expertise, and all the radiologists involved in these studies were trained specifically in this procedure. This is an essential component in order to replicate these results in other practices, both regarding efficacy and minimizing the side effects. Volume reduction was significantly correlated with the vascularity of the lesion at the initial ultrasound in one report but not described on the others.

Reassuringly no adverse effects were noted except for local pain which was fairly straightforward to control. It should be noted that none of these reports list any negative impact of RFA on subsequent thyroid surgery, but it is not clear that such sequence has been followed in any of the RFA-treated patients. Another practical issue to be considered is that of cost. We are not aware of any report of cost comparisons with surgery or radioactive iodine, but based on our experience, RFA will be of significantly lower cost compared with surgery but probably more expensive than RAI in the USA. Combining the efficacy and safety data with patients' medical limitations and cultural preferences will be an ongoing process to understand the potential role for this procedure in clinical practice. As is, RFA evolves into an attractive approach for the therapy of AFTN.

Percutaneous Laser Ablation (PLA)

This procedure is very similar to the technique utilized for RFA. It has also similar side-effect profile with maybe slightly inferior efficacy. The protocol utilized in various trials has varied. The needles employed have been between 14 and 21G, and the number of fibers utilized to deliver the energy has been up to four, depending on the size and shape of the nodule. The treatments were delivered usually in 1–2 sessions spaced 1 month apart, preceded by local anesthesia with lidocaine. The total energy delivery per treatment was about 1800 J, but this also varied between reports. To prevent local pain and limit injection site edema, an injectable steroid can be used intramuscularly. Still local pain is reported but it appears to rarely require therapy, and when if it does so, it responds to NSAIDs. Occasionally repositioning of the needle away from the capsule is required in order to diminish pain. One of the early PLA series was completed in Italy [56] and treated both patients with isolated toxic nodules and patients with toxic MNG. After a median of three PLA sessions, they noted normalization of thyroid levels in all patients with toxic nodules and in 50 % of those with toxic MNG. Reassuringly there was only a mild and transient increase in T3/T4 values after the therapy session. The median decrease in nodule volume was 59 % at 1 year (range 24–72 %), and the nodules had a nonhomogeneous appearance on ultrasound. As RAI is a standard treatment modality for AFTN and toxic MNG, another Italian trial went further [57] and included 15 patients with large toxic nodules that received laser ablation followed by RAI 1 month later and compared them with RAI-alone therapy. Interestingly in 60 % of patients, TSH normalized at 1 month after PLA, and in 20 % of patients, RAI therapy was no longer employed. Nodule shrinkage was evident at 1 month post-therapy and at 2 years post-therapy reached 71 % reduction in the combination therapy compared with 47 % in the RAI-alone group.

Local compressive symptoms improved rapidly post-PLA, but at 2 years they were not different between the groups. From a nuclear medicine perspective, it is pertinent that the dose of RAI required for therapy was 21 % lower in the combination therapy group. This also led to outpatient therapy in all such patients as opposed to only 50 % of the RAI-only group (based on the RAI therapy regulations at the time in Italy). Similar data was obtained in other trials as well [58, 59], while only one early trial reported lack of significant benefit of PLA on AFTN [60].

The available data suggests that PLA is better suited for one or at most two autonomous nodules while being less effective for MNG. It is important to note the expected changes in the ultrasound appearance of nodules treated by PLA, to avoid raising unnecessary concerns. Thus, at 1 week post-procedure, ultrasound reveals a central area of cavitation (which is anechoic), surrounded by a rim of charred tissue (appearing hyperechoic on ultrasound), and at the periphery there is a hypoechoic area thought to represent coagulative necrosis [56].

PLA of TMNG has also been studied in some of the studies mentioned earlier. However, given the limited targeting of this procedure, it is to be expected that other toxic nodules can continue hypersecreting thyroid hormones and likely patients will remain hyperthyroid after one to two PLA sessions. The factors that influence the ultimate response in nodule size are not well defined, but it is presumed that the composition of the nodule (i.e., colloid vs. water content) and, like with RFA, the vascularity of the lesion are playing a significant role in the overall response [56]. Unfortunately no head-to-head trials between the RFA and PLA have been performed, and given the costs of the equipment involved and the training required to achieve sufficient expertise in each of these procedures, it is unlikely that such a trial will take place.

Alcohol Ablation

Alcohol ablation for solid nodules is to be distinguished from alcohol injection into a thyroid cyst. The ablation of solid nodules, also known as percutaneous ethanol injection (PEI), has been employed since 1990. The procedure was being done under anesthesia or sedation at some centers or without any such support at others. It employed 95 % alcohol that is injected using a 20–22G needle directly in the nodule in question. The volume injected varied with some centers using 1/3 of the volume of the nodule and other using a variable dose between 1 and 5 ml administered slowly over 2–5 min [61–63]. There are usually multiple injections that allow targeting different areas in the nodule. The side-effect profile, as reported initially, was largely represented by a burning sensation noted in ~ 30 % of sessions that was reported to last 30–60 min and radiate to the jaw or sides of the neck.

Early studies [61, 64] reported the effectiveness of PEI alone or followed by RAI as similar to RAI alone. It controlled hyperthyroidism in almost 100 % of patients but offered additionally a significant reduction in nodule size combined with the ability to use a lower dose of RAI.

These encouraging initial efficacy results were followed by slightly different reports more recently [65] in which 45 % of individuals either did not reach euthyroidism or had recurrence of it within 3 years. When the procedure was employed in TMNG, all patients had persistent hyperthyroidism.

After the procedure started to be employed by a larger number of medical centers, a number of reports started to surface that redefined the adverse event rate and profile of PEI. It thus was found that the local discomfort rate and intensity was higher than reported initially. Also it appeared that the alcohol could infiltrate the surrounding extranodular and occasionally extrathyroidal tissue [66, 67]. This pro-fibrotic effect could clearly be a complicating factor for subsequent surgery needed in case of PEI failure. Also reports of subcutaneous hematoma and temporary hoarseness surfaced [68], while a more detailed profile of the adverse effects associated with PEI was depicted by Bennedbaek and Hegedus [69] as they described additional problems that followed the procedure: transient thyrotoxicosis, permanent ipsilateral facial dysesthesia, increased tear flow, and para-nodular fibrosis impeding subsequent surgery in few patients but various degrees of pain and tenderness in majority of PEI-treated patients. A severe case of toxic laryngitis and dermatitis [70] showed the possibility for the alcohol to flow back from the nodule into the surrounding tissues with significant consequences. These reports led to a departure from the view of PEI as a routine procedure and started to limit its subsequent use. As some of these cases have occurred even with experienced operators, the use of the procedure has declined rapidly over the last few years, and it is now mainly used for sclerosing cystic thyroid lesions and for therapy of small thyroidal or lymphatic foci of papillary thyroid carcinoma [71].

Of note, all these procedures are known to distort the histology of the nodule and thus limit the usefulness of subsequent fine-needle aspiration. While toxic nodules are not usually subjected to cytological evaluation before therapy, it is possible that an FNA would be pursued at a later time, and the clinicians should be aware of the possible atypical results brought on by the procedure-induced tissue damage.

Based on the available evidence regarding ablative procedures, as a practical approach, in a select subgroup of patients, such as individuals who refuse surgery, or are at high surgical risk and have access to centers with excellent expertise in these procedures, RFA (or PLA) could be offered first, followed by RAI in patients that are persistently hyperthyroid.

References

1. Hollowell JG, Staehling NW, Flanders WD, Hannon WH, Gunter EW, Spencer CA, et al. Serum TSH, T(4), and thyroid antibodies in the United States population (1988 to 1994): National Health and Nutrition Examination Survey (NHANES III). J Clin Endocrinol Metab. 2002;87(2):489–99.

2. Charkes ND. Graves' disease with functioning nodules (Marine-Lenhart syndrome). J Nucl Med. 1972;13(12):885–92.
3. Carnell NE, Valente WA. Thyroid nodules in Graves' disease: classification, characterization, and response to treatment. Thyroid. 1998;8(8):647–52.
4. Becker DV, Sawin CT. Radioiodine and thyroid disease: the beginning. Semin Nucl Med. [Historical Article Research Support, Non-U.S. Gov't]. 1996;26(3):155–64.
5. Goncalves E, Castro JA, Gross JL. Standard dose 131I therapy for toxic multinodular goiter in an endemic goiter region. Braz J Med Biol Res. 1986;19(6):723–9.
6. Erem C, Kandemir N, Hacihasanoglu A, Ersoz HO, Ukinc K, Kocak M. Radioiodine treatment of hyperthyroidism: prognostic factors affecting outcome. Endocrine. 2004;25(1):55–60.
7. Nygaard B, Hegedus L, Ulriksen P, Nielsen KG, Hansen JM. Radioiodine therapy for multinodular toxic goiter. Arch Intern Med. [Research Support, Non-U.S. Gov't]. 1999;159(12): 1364–8.
8. Kang AS, Grant CS, Thompson GB, van Heerden JA. Current treatment of nodular goiter with hyperthyroidism (Plummer's disease): surgery versus radioiodine. Surgery. [Comparative Study]. 2002;132(6):916–23; discussion 23.
9. Erkan ME, Demirin H, Asik M, Celbek G, Yildirim M, Aydin Y, et al. Efficiency of radioactive I-131 therapy in geriatric patients with toxic nodular goiter. Aging Clin Exp Res. 2012;24(6):714–7.
10. Nygaard B, Hegedus L, Nielsen KG, Ulriksen P, Hansen JM. Long-term effect of radioactive iodine on thyroid function and size in patients with solitary autonomously functioning toxic thyroid nodules. Clin Endocrinol (Oxf). [Research Support, Non-U.S. Gov't]. 1999;50(2): 197–202.
11. Bahn RS, Burch HB, Cooper DS, Garber JR, Greenlee MC, Klein I, et al. Hyperthyroidism and other causes of thyrotoxicosis: management guidelines of the American Thyroid Association and American Association of Clinical Endocrinologists. Endocr Pract. [Practice Guideline]. 2011;17(3):456–520.
12. Erickson D, Gharib H, Li H, van Heerden JA. Treatment of patients with toxic multinodular goiter. Thyroid. [Clinical Trial Comparative Study]. 1998;8(4):277–82.
13. Vidal-Trecan GM, Stahl JE, Eckman MH. Radioiodine or surgery for toxic thyroid adenoma: dissecting an important decision. A cost-effectiveness analysis. Thyroid. 2004;14(11):933–45.
14. Pedersen-Bjergaard U, Kirkegaard C. Serum TSH and the response to radioiodine treatment of toxic multinodular goitre. Eur J Endocrinol. 1997;137(4):365–9.
15. Kaplan MM, Meier DA, Dworkin HJ. Treatment of hyperthyroidism with radioactive iodine. Endocrinol Metab Clin North Am. [Comparative Study Review]. 1998;27(1):205–23.
16. Sonmez B, Erem C, Dogan I, Ersoz HO, Sonmez M. Efficacy of low and high fixed dose radioactive iodine therapy in patients with toxic nodular goiter. Minerva Endocrinol. 2011;36(2):117–21.
17. Ross DS, Ridgway EC, Daniels GH. Successful treatment of solitary toxic thyroid nodules with relatively low-dose iodine-131, with low prevalence of hypothyroidism. Ann Intern Med. [Research Support, U.S. Gov't, P.H.S.]. 1984;101(4):488–90.
18. Zakavi SR, Mousavi Z, Davachi B. Comparison of four different protocols of I-131 therapy for treating single toxic thyroid nodule. Nucl Med Commun. [Comparative Study Controlled Clinical Trial Randomized Controlled Trial Research Support, Non-U.S. Gov't]. 2009;30(2):169–75.
19. de Rooij A, Vandenbroucke JP, Smit JW, Stokkel MP, Dekkers OM. Clinical outcomes after estimated versus calculated activity of radioiodine for the treatment of hyperthyroidism: systematic review and meta-analysis. Eur J Endocrinol. [Comparative Study Meta-Analysis Review]. 2009;161(5):771–7.
20. Koornstra JJ, Kerstens MN, Hoving J, Visscher KJ, Schade JH, Gort HB, et al. Clinical and biochemical changes following 131I therapy for hyperthyroidism in patients not pretreated with antithyroid drugs. Neth J Med. 1999;55(5):215–21.
21. Thyroid storm shortly after 131 I therapy of a toxic multinodular goiter? Am J Med. [Case Reports]. 1972;52(6):786–96.

22. McDermott MT, Kidd GS, Dodson LE, Jr., Hofeldt FD. Radioiodine-induced thyroid storm. Case report and literature review. Am J Med. [Case Reports Review]. 1983;75(2):353–9.
23. Clerc J, Izembart M, Dagousset F, Jais JP, Heshmati HM, Chevalier A, et al. Influence of dose selection on absorbed dose profiles in radioiodine treatment of diffuse toxic goiters in patients receiving or not receiving carbimazole. J Nucl Med. 1993;34(3):387–93.
24. Walter MA, Briel M, Christ-Crain M, Bonnema SJ, Connell J, Cooper DS, et al. Effects of antithyroid drugs on radioiodine treatment: systematic review and meta-analysis of randomised controlled trials. Bmj. [Meta-Analysis Research Support, Non-U.S. Gov't Technical Report]. 2007;334(7592):514.
25. Walter MA, Christ-Crain M, Schindler C, Muller-Brand J, Muller B. Outcome of radioiodine therapy without, on or 3 days off carbimazole: a prospective interventional three-group comparison. Eur J Nucl Med Mol Imaging. [Controlled Clinical Trial]. 2006;33(6):730–7.
26. Cooper DS, Rivkees SA. Putting propylthiouracil in perspective. J Clin Endocrinol Metab. [Evaluation Studies]. 2009;94(6):1881–2.
27. Imseis RE, Vanmiddlesworth L, Massie JD, Bush AJ, Vanmiddlesworth NR. Pretreatment with propylthiouracil but not methimazole reduces the therapeutic efficacy of iodine-131 in hyperthyroidism. J Clin Endocrinol Metab. 1998;83(2):685–7.
28. Duick DS, Baskin HJ. Utility of recombinant human thyrotropin for augmentation of radioiodine uptake and treatment of nontoxic and toxic multinodular goiters. Endocr Pract. 2003;9(3):204–9.
29. Duick DS, Baskin HJ. Significance of radioiodine uptake at 72 hours versus 24 hours after pretreatment with recombinant human thyrotropin for enhancement of radioiodine therapy in patients with symptomatic nontoxic or toxic multinodular goiter. Endocr Pract. [Clinical Trial Multicenter Study]. 2004;10(3):253–60.
30. Nielsen VE, Bonnema SJ, Boel-Jorgensen H, Veje A, Hegedus L. Recombinant human thyrotropin markedly changes the 131I kinetics during 131I therapy of patients with nodular goiter: an evaluation by a randomized double-blinded trial. J Clin Endocrinol Metab. [Clinical Trial Randomized Controlled Trial Research Support, Non-U.S. Gov't]. 2005;90(1):79–83.
31. Magner J. Problems associated with the use of thyrogen in patients with a thyroid gland. N Engl J Med. [Comment Letter]. 2008;359(16):1738–9; author reply 9.
32. Kahraman D, Keller C, Schneider C, Eschner W, Sudbrock F, Schmidt M, et al. Development of hypothyroidism during long-term follow-up of patients with toxic nodular goitre after radioiodine therapy. Clin Endocrinol (Oxf). [Research Support, Non-U.S. Gov't]. 2012;76(2):297–303.
33. Huysmans DA, Hermus AR, Corstens FH, Kloppenborg PW. Long-term results of two schedules of radioiodine treatment for toxic multinodular goitre. Eur J Nucl Med. 1993;20(11):1056–62.
34. Khanna CM, Magdum M, Ravishankar L, Dham DN, Chugh P. Evaluation of long-term results of two schedules of treatment for toxic multinodular goitre with radioiodine therapy (I 131). J Assoc Physicians India. [Clinical Trial Comparative Study]. 1996;44(2):102–5.
35. Holm LE, Lundell G, Israelsson A, Dahlqvist I. Incidence of hypothyroidism occurring long after iodine-131 therapy for hyperthyroidism. J Nucl Med. [Comparative Study Research Support, Non-U.S. Gov't]. 1982;23(2):103–7.
36. Tzavara I, Tzanela M, Vlassopoulou B, Kouyioumoutzakis G, Kyriazopoulou V, Alevizaki C, et al. Long term thyroid function after (131)I treatment for toxic adenoma. Hormones (Athens). 2002;1(2):99–103.
37. Ceccarelli C, Bencivelli W, Vitti P, Grasso L, Pinchera A. Outcome of radioiodine-131 therapy in hyperfunctioning thyroid nodules: a 20 years' retrospective study. Clin Endocrinol (Oxf). 2005;62(3):331–5.
38. Ahmad AM, Ahmad M, Young ET. Objective estimates of the probability of developing hypothyroidism following radioactive iodine treatment of thyrotoxicosis. Eur J Endocrinol. 2002;146(6):767–75.

39. Paghera B, Panarotto MB, Maira G, Magri GC, Bertagna F, Bosio G, et al. (1)(3)(1)I treatment of toxic nodular goiter under combined thyrostatic-thyromimetic medication is at low risk of late hypothyroidism. Q J Nucl Med Mol Imaging. 2010;54(3):341–7.
40. Dobyns BM, Sheline GE, Workman JB, Tompkins EA, McConahey WM, Becker DV. Malignant and benign neoplasms of the thyroid in patients treated for hyperthyroidism: a report of the cooperative thyrotoxicosis therapy follow-up study. J Clin Endocrinol Metab. 1974;38(6):976–98.
41. Saenger EL, Thoma GE, Tompkins EA. Incidence of leukemia following treatment of hyperthyroidism. Preliminary report of the Cooperative Thyrotoxicosis Therapy Follow-Up Study. JAMA. 1968;205(12):855–62.
42. Ron E, Doody MM, Becker DV, Brill AB, Curtis RE, Goldman MB, et al. Cancer mortality following treatment for adult hyperthyroidism. Cooperative Thyrotoxicosis Therapy Follow-up Study Group. Jama. [Research Support, Non-U.S. Gov't Research Support, U.S. Gov't, P.H.S.]. 1998;280(4):347–55.
43. Franklyn JA, Maisonneuve P, Sheppard MC, Betteridge J, Boyle P. Mortality after the treatment of hyperthyroidism with radioactive iodine. N Engl J Med. [Comparative Study Research Support, Non-U.S. Gov't]. 1998;338(11):712–8.
44. Metso S, Jaatinen P, Huhtala H, Auvinen A, Oksala H, Salmi J. Increased cardiovascular and cancer mortality after radioiodine treatment for hyperthyroidism. J Clin Endocrinol Metab. [Research Support, Non-U.S. Gov't]. 2007;92(6):2190–6.
45. Nygaard B, Faber J, Veje A, Hegedus L, Hansen JM. Transition of nodular toxic goiter to autoimmune hyperthyroidism triggered by 131I therapy. Thyroid. [Research Support, Non--U.S. Gov't]. 1999;9(5):477–81.
46. Meller J, Siefker U, Hamann A, Hufner M. Incidence of radioiodine induced Graves' disease in patients with multinodular toxic goiter. Exp Clin Endocrinol Diabetes. [Comparative Study]. 2006;114(5):235–9.
47. Werner SC, Ingbar SH, Braverman LE, Utiger RD. Werner & Ingbar's the thyroid: a fundamental and clinical text. 9th ed. Philadelphia: Lippincott Williams & Wilkins; 2005.
48. van Soestbergen MJ, van der Vijver JC, Graafland AD. Recurrence of hyperthyroidism in multinodular goiter after long-term drug therapy: a comparison with Graves' disease. J Endocrinol Invest. [Comparative Study]. 1992;15(11):797–800.
49. Azizi F, Ataie L, Hedayati M, Mehrabi Y, Sheikholeslami F. Effect of long-term continuous methimazole treatment of hyperthyroidism: comparison with radioiodine. Eur J Endocrinol. [Clinical Trial Comparative Study Randomized Controlled Trial]. 2005;152(5):695–701.
50. Watanabe N, Narimatsu H, Noh JY, Yamaguchi T, Kobayashi K, Kami M, et al. Antithyroid drug-induced hematopoietic damage: a retrospective cohort study of agranulocytosis and pancytopenia involving 50,385 patients with Graves' disease. J Clin Endocrinol Metab. [Evaluation Studies]. 2012;97(1):E49–53.
51. Arab DM, Malatjalian DA, Rittmaster RS. Severe cholestatic jaundice in uncomplicated hyperthyroidism treated with methimazole. J Clin Endocrinol Metab. [Case Reports]. 1995;80(4):1083–5.
52. Spiezia S, Garberoglio R, Milone F, Ramundo V, Caiazzo C, Assanti AP, et al. Thyroid nodules and related symptoms are stably controlled two years after radiofrequency thermal ablation. Thyroid. [Clinical Trial]. 2009;19(3):219–25.
53. Faggiano A, Ramundo V, Assanti AP, Fonderico F, Macchia PE, Misso C, et al. Thyroid nodules treated with percutaneous radiofrequency thermal ablation: a comparative study. J Clin Endocrinol Metab. [Comparative Study Controlled Clinical Trial Research Support, Non–U.S. Gov't]. 2012;97(12):4439–45.
54. Baek JH, Moon WJ, Kim YS, Lee JH, Lee D. Radiofrequency ablation for the treatment of autonomously functioning thyroid nodules. World J Surg. 2009;33(9):1971–7.
55. Sung JY, Baek JH, Jung SL, Kim JH, Kim KS, Lee D, et al. Radiofrequency ablation for autonomously functioning thyroid nodules: a multicenter study. Thyroid. [Multicenter Study]. 2015;25(1):112–7.

56. Barbaro D, Orsini P, Lapi P, Pasquini C, Tuco A, Righini A, et al. Percutaneous laser ablation in the treatment of toxic and pretoxic nodular goiter. Endocr Pract. [Clinical Trial]. 2007;13(1):30–6.
57. Chianelli M, Bizzarri G, Todino V, Misischi I, Bianchini A, Graziano F, et al. Laser ablation and 131-iodine: a 24-month pilot study of combined treatment for large toxic nodular goiter. J Clin Endocrinol Metab. [Clinical Trial]. 2014;99(7):E1283–6.
58. Dossing H, Bennedbaek FN, Bonnema SJ, Grupe P, Hegedus L. Randomized prospective study comparing a single radioiodine dose and a single laser therapy session in autonomously functioning thyroid nodules. Eur J Endocrinol. [Comparative Study Randomized Controlled Trial Research Support, Non-U.S. Gov't]. 2007;157(1):95–100.
59. Spiezia S, Vitale G, Di Somma C, Pio Assanti A, Ciccarelli A, Lombardi G, et al. Ultrasound-guided laser thermal ablation in the treatment of autonomous hyperfunctioning thyroid nodules and compressive nontoxic nodular goiter. Thyroid. 2003;13(10):941–7.
60. Pacella CM, Bizzarri G, Spiezia S, Bianchini A, Guglielmi R, Crescenzi A, et al. Thyroid tissue: US-guided percutaneous laser thermal ablation. Radiology. [Clinical Trial]. 2004;232(1):272–80.
61. Del Prete S, Russo D, Caraglia M, Giuberti G, Marra M, Vitale G, et al. Percutaneous ethanol injection of autonomous thyroid nodules with a volume larger than 40 ml: three years of follow-up. Clin Radiol. 2001;56(11):895–901.
62. Monzani F, Caraccio N, Goletti O, Lippolis PV, Casolaro A, Del Guerra P, et al. Five-year follow-up of percutaneous ethanol injection for the treatment of hyperfunctioning thyroid nodules: a study of 117 patients. Clin Endocrinol (Oxf). 1997;46(1):9–15.
63. Guglielmi R, Pacella CM, Bianchini A, Bizzarri G, Rinaldi R, Graziano FM, et al. Percutaneous ethanol injection treatment in benign thyroid lesions: role and efficacy. Thyroid. 2004;14(2):125–31.
64. Zingrillo M, Modoni S, Conte M, Frusciante V, Trischitta V. Percutaneous ethanol injection plus radioiodine versus radioiodine alone in the treatment of large toxic thyroid nodules. J Nucl Med. [Clinical Trial Comparative Study Randomized Controlled Trial]. 2003;44(2):207–10.
65. Yano Y, Sugino K, Akaishi J, Uruno T, Okuwa K, Shibuya H, et al. Treatment of autonomously functioning thyroid nodules at a single institution: radioiodine therapy, surgery, and ethanol injection therapy. Ann Nucl Med. 2011;25(10):749–54.
66. Gharib H, Papini E. Thyroid nodules: clinical importance, assessment, and treatment. Endocrinol Metab Clin North Am. [Review]. 2007;36(3):707–35, vi.
67. Hegedus L. Clinical practice. The thyroid nodule. N Engl J Med. [Review]. 200421;351(17):1764–71.
68. Brkljacic B, Sucic M, Bozikov V, Hauser M, Hebrang A. Treatment of autonomous and toxic thyroid adenomas by percutaneous ultrasound-guided ethanol injection. Acta Radiol. 2001;42(5):477–81.
69. Bennedbaek FN, Hegedus L. Percutaneous ethanol injection therapy in benign solitary solid cold thyroid nodules: a randomized trial comparing one injection with three injections. Thyroid. [Clinical Trial Comparative Study Randomized Controlled Trial Research Support, Non-U.S. Gov't]. 1999;9(3):225–33.
70. Mauz PS, Maassen MM, Braun B, Brosch S. How safe is percutaneous ethanol injection for treatment of thyroid nodule? Report of a case of severe toxic necrosis of the larynx and adjacent skin. Acta Otolaryngol. [Case Reports]. 2004;124(10):1226–30.
71. Hay ID, Lee RA, Davidge-Pitts C, Reading CC, Charboneau JW. Long-term outcome of ultrasound-guided percutaneous ethanol ablation of selected "recurrent" neck nodal metastases in 25 patients with TNM stages III or IVA papillary thyroid carcinoma previously treated by surgery and 131I therapy. Surgery. 2013;154(6):1448–54; discussion 54–5.

Chapter 9
The Role of Surgery for Nodular Hyperthyroidism

Dawn M. Elfenbein and David F. Schneider

Introduction

Patients with thyroid nodules and hyperthyroidism may present in a number of ways. Often, thyroid nodules are discovered incidentally on imaging obtained for other indications, or they are found on physical exam. If a thyroid nodule is found, even in the absence of hyperthyroid symptoms, one should always screen for abnormal thyroid function with a serum TSH level. Most patients with thyroid nodules will have normal or low thyroid function, but it is important to know if patients have hyperthyroidism in order to determine the best treatment. Alternatively, hyperthyroidism may be diagnosed first, and in the absence of a clear underlying reason for the hyperthyroidism (such as obvious Graves' disease with ophthalmopathy or positive antibodies), a search for nodules should be performed since one etiology of hyperthyroidism is a functional or "hot" nodule. Treatment of a single hyperfunctioning nodule is different than diffuse toxic nodular goiter or Graves' disease with nodules, so it is important to distinguish between these entities.

When a patient is discovered to have a thyroid nodule and hyperthyroidism, further clarification can be achieved with a nuclear medicine scan known as radionuclide scintigraphy. The scan is obtained after administering a low dose of radioactive iodine orally to a patient since the thyroid gland is unique in its ability to absorb and organify iodide. If a nodule is hyperfunctioning, it should take up more

D.M. Elfenbein, MD, MPH
Department of Surgery, University of California, Irvine, Irvine, CA, USA

D.F. Schneider, MD, MS (✉)
Section of Endocrine Surgery, Department of Surgery, University of Wisconsin, Madison, WI, USA
e-mail: schneiderd@surgery.wisc.edu

S.A. Roman et al. (eds.), *Management of Thyroid Nodules and Differentiated Thyroid Cancer*, DOI 10.1007/978-3-319-43618-0_9

iodide and appear "hot" on the image. These hot nodules are almost always benign and may be treated with either ablative doses of radioactive iodine or surgery to remove the half of the thyroid gland containing the hyperfunctioning nodule. Other ablative therapies are discussed in Chap. 9. If the surrounding thyroid is hyperfunctioning, and the nodule has lost the ability to absorb iodide, this is known as a "cold" nodule. If a cold nodule meets other criteria (such as size or concerning ultrasound features) for fine needle aspiration (FNA) biopsy, it should be performed, as cold nodules may represent malignancy. With the excellent resolution of ultrasound today, the role of diagnostic radioactive iodine imaging should be limited only to those patients who are hyperthyroid with nodules to distinguish a single functioning nodule from bilateral disease. In patients who are euthyroid or hypothyroid with nodules, there is no added value to getting this nuclear medicine study [1]. Even in hyperthyroid patients, radioactive iodine uptake scanning probably only becomes cost-effective if used selectively when the diagnosis is unclear or the results will alter management [2].

The remainder of this chapter focuses on the various treatment options, especially surgery, for a solitary hyperfunctioning nodule, toxic multinodular goiter, and nodular Graves' disease.

Nodular Graves' Disease

Robert James Graves wrote about a disease that presented with goiter, palpitations, and exophthalmos in 1835, and although Caleb Perry first published a similar constellation of symptoms 10 years prior, we now commonly refer to this autoimmune thyroid condition as Graves' disease [3]. Activating antibodies to the TSH receptor cause hyperthyroidism. Today, a diagnosis of Graves' disease is made in a patient with biochemical hyperthyroidism and at least one of the following: (1) ophthalmopathy or obvious dermopathy such as pretibial myxedema, (2) detectable serum TSH receptor antibodies (TRAb), or (3) diffuse, increased thyroid uptake on a radioiodine scan. Thyroid nodules are common, however, and 12–33 % of patients with Graves' disease may also have a nodule or nodules within their abnormally functioning thyroid gland [4, 5]. Graves' disease with nodules can be difficult to distinguish from toxic multinodular goiter in some cases, particularly if no other extra-thyroidal manifestations of Graves' are present. On a thyroid uptake scan, toxic multinodular goiter would have high uptake within nodules surrounded by thyroid parenchyma with less uptake, while Graves' disease with nodules would show increased uptake in the thyroid parenchyma outlining the circular nodules (Fig. 9.1), although in reality it is not always straightforward to interpret these uptake scans.

Three treatment options exist for Graves' disease: antithyroid medications such as methimazole or propylthiouracil, radioactive iodine (RAI) ablation, and surgical thyroidectomy. One randomized clinical trial directly compared these three treatment modalities and concluded that they are all equally effective in eventually

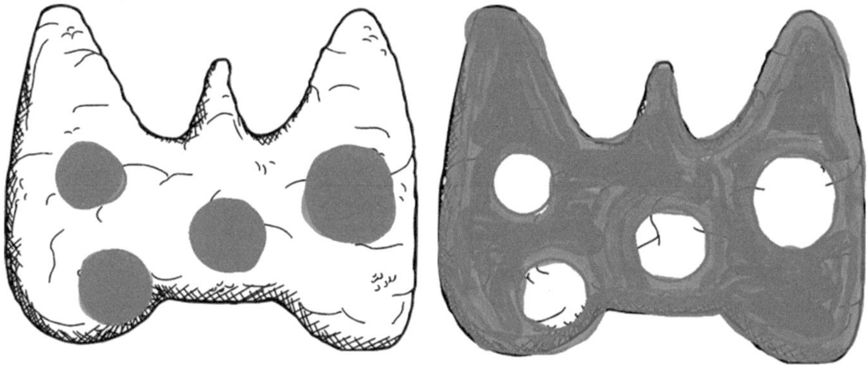

Fig. 9.1 Radioactive iodine scans. The appearance of a radioactive uptake scan for both toxic multinodular goiter (*left*) and Graves' disease (*right*) is shown, with the shaded or gray areas indicating increased uptake. In Graves' disease (*right*), the thyroid parenchyma has diffuse uptake, while the nodules have slightly less uptake

achieving a euthyroid state [6], although there are clinical situations when one treatment modality should be considered more or less strongly than the others. For example, RAI is contraindicated during pregnancy. The current published and accepted guidelines for the treatment of hyperthyroidism stress the importance of active discussion between patients and their providers before deciding on a treatment plan [7]. Those discussions should include details about the speed of recovery, risks and benefits, side effects and costs of each treatment, as well as discussions about certain clinical scenarios where one treatment is clearly favored.

Once a diagnosis of Graves' disease is established through biochemical evidence of hyperthyroidism along with clinical extra-thyroidal manifestations, positive antibodies, or diffuse, or increased thyroid uptake on a radioiodine scan, treatment should be tailored to the individual patient's clinical situation and his or her personal preferences and goals of therapy. No treatment yet exists that addresses the specific underlying autoimmune condition. Therefore, the goal of treatment for Graves' disease is to correct the end-organ thyroid dysfunction. With rare exception, at the time of diagnosis, patients should be initiated on an antithyroid medication to restore euthyroidism [7]. This is usually achieved in 6–8 weeks, during which time more information can be gathered to help the patient and provider decide on a more definitive treatment plan. Antithyroid drugs pose long-term toxicities on the bone marrow and liver. For this reason, antithyroid medications cannot serve as a lifelong solution.

If palpable nodules are present on exam of a patient with newly diagnosed Graves' disease, a formal ultrasound of the thyroid and lateral neck should be performed. Some groups advocate performing thyroid ultrasound in all patients newly diagnosed with Graves' disease, since the incidence of differentiated thyroid cancer seems to be higher than in the general population [8, 9]. Newer data suggest that only patients with palpable nodules should undergo ultrasound imaging prior to definitive treatment [10], which may be more prudent in the current era where we are starting to recognize the economic effect of overdiagnosing and treating small thyroid cancers [11]. In some surgical practices, all patients referred for thyroid surgery undergo in-office surgeon-performed neck ultrasound for surgical planning, looking at gland size and anatomic position, vascularity, or presence of extra-thyroidal abnormalities that may need to be addressed, and incidental nodules may be found at this time. Whether palpable or incidentally discovered, fine needle aspiration should be performed for nodules according to the updated guidelines for the management of thyroid nodules, particularly if it will change management. The newest guidelines recommend biopsy of high or intermediate suspicion nodules based on ultrasound characteristics if the nodule is >1 cm, but for low suspicion waiting until the nodule is >1.5 cm, and very low suspicion nodules should be >2 cm [12]. One should keep in mind that the hyperplasia associated with hyperthyroidism may increase the likelihood for cytologic interpretation as follicular neoplasm or atypia due to the increased cellularity and inflammation.

Patients with Graves' disease and nodules that are indeterminate or suspicious for thyroid cancer should be referred to an experienced thyroid surgeon for consideration of a total thyroidectomy for treatment of both conditions. Any patient with Graves' disease and a nodule that is causing compressive symptoms, even if it is biopsy proven to be benign, should also be referred for surgical treatment, as neither antithyroid medications nor RAI will be effective in treating the symptomatic nodule, and RAI may make subsequent surgery more difficult. RAI leads to a fibrotic reaction similar to scar tissue that can increase operative difficulty and complications. Several surgical series have reported an increased incidence of thyroid cancer in Graves' patients who underwent surgery, but this is most likely due to surgical series biases – more patients with suspicious nodules will be referred for surgery, so there will appear to be an increased incidence of cancer among those who have surgery. A recent series comparing cytology specimens to surgical specimens suggests that this is the case [13].

Regardless of this bias, patients with any suspicion of cancer at the time of diagnosis of nodular Graves' disease should strongly consider thyroidectomy as their definitive treatment option, and such procedure should be performed by an experienced thyroid surgeon. Although the increased vascularity and inflammation of a Graves' gland make the operation more challenging, the complication rate remains extremely low when done by high-volume centers [14].

We do not have a good estimate of the number of patients with Graves' disease and nodules who undergo RAI treatment only to have their nodule turn out to be cancer and require further treatment. One study performed over 30 years ago reported on 11 patients who had previously undergone RAI for hyperthyroidism and then subsequently presented with thyroid cancer [15]. All of these 11 patients had their cancer diagnosis made more than 1 year after RAI, but there was no way of knowing whether the cancer was present prior to or as a result of the treatment. They did not report an increased number of surgical complications when operating on these patients with previous RAI therapy, though surgeons may find operating on a previously irradiated thyroid gland to be challenging due to the increased fibrosis and scarring as mentioned earlier. In the modern era where many patients undergo thyroid ultrasound or other imaging, we may be better at selecting patients with Graves' disease and nodules who may be better suited for surgery over the other treatment options.

Historically, surgeons would perform subtotal thyroidectomy for Graves' disease, with the goal of leaving enough thyroid tissue behind to render the patient euthyroid. Such approach is associated with unacceptably high recurrence risks and potentially more dangerous repeat surgery. Surgery for Graves' disease today consists of a total thyroidectomy followed by lifelong levothyroxine administration [16, 17]. One recent meta-analysis of 3,242 patients found that subtotal thyroidectomy was associated with a tenfold higher risk of recurrence, although subtotal thyroidectomy did have lower rates of postoperative hypoparathyroidism [18]. Because Graves' disease itself plays a role in a patient's metabolism of calcium, even temporary hypoparathyroidism is not an insignificant complication, sometimes manifesting in very low calcium levels causing severe symptoms. One recent study suggests that pretreatment with calcium carbonate can decrease these symptoms in the postoperative period for patients with Graves' disease [19], and this low-cost intervention may be something that surgeons should consider adding to their regimen for preparing patients for the operating room.

The treatment for thyroid cancer is also total thyroidectomy, so any patient with suspicious nodules and Graves' disease is well suited to this treatment modality. With any suspicious nodule, a preoperative ultrasound including an examination of the lateral compartment lymph nodes should be performed [20], and this recommendation holds true for patients with Graves' disease and nodules. Any abnormal appearing lymph nodes that are amenable to FNA biopsy should be sampled prior to surgery to determine the extent of surgery. The first surgical procedure is always the best time to do a complete nodal basin dissection, and the underlying diagnosis of Graves' disease should not distract a surgeon from doing a thorough workup of coexisting nodules.

The technical aspects of thyroidectomy for Graves' disease are no different than thyroidectomy for other indications, but the vascularity and friability of the gland can make it challenging [21]. Adding large or adherent nodules to an already challenging operation can increase the complexity. It is important that a surgeon remember a few important pearls when operating on patients with Graves' disease in an attempt to reduce both surgical complications and recurrence rates. The surgeon and anesthesiologist must communicate frequently regarding the possibility and manifestations of thyroid storm (such as tachycardia or fever) and be able to appropriately manage this condition should it occur. It is best to have medications immediately available (beta-blockers – specifically esmolol due to its rapid onset and steroids) in case they are needed, but thoughtful preoperative preparation is the best way to prevent this. In any patient with hyperthyroidism or suspicious nodules, a surgeon must be vigilant about the presence of a pyramidal lobe and to entirely resect it to reduce recurrence risk. Finally, the inflammation of the gland and the possible presence of reactive lymph nodes can make parathyroids difficult to identify, and they can be densely adherent to the thyroid gland. The large surface vessels and overall vascularity of a Graves' thyroid gland may make it additionally challenging to identify and preserve the blood supply to the parathyroid glands. A close capsular dissection is important to preserve the parathyroid glands. After the thyroid gland has been removed, the surgeon should carefully examine it to be sure that no parathyroid glands were inadvertently removed with the specimen. This is a step many surgeons may forget, particularly if the dissection was difficult and lengthy, but this step may prove critical in preventing long-term hypocalcemia. If a parathyroid gland is seen on the specimen or its blood supply is compromised, then the parathyroid gland should be placed in cold saline and autotransplanted at the end of the case. One recent study found that parathyroid tissue identified by the pathologist was associated with a higher incidence of temporary and permanent hypoparathyroidism [22].

Toxic Multinodular Goiter

Nodular thyroid disease is extraordinarily common. High-resolution ultrasound can detect nodules in up to two-thirds of adults [23]. Since nodule growth and formation is a hyperplastic process, some of these nodules can develop autonomous hormone production over time. Somatic, activating mutations in the genes regulating follicular cell growth and hormone production contribute to the slow growth of the nodules over time [24, 25]. In the setting of a multinodular goiter, autonomous hormone secretion usually presents in a subclinical fashion with suppressed TSH and normal T3 and T4 levels. Although subclinical disease can progress to overt hyperthyroidism, subclinical disease can manifest the outward signs and symptoms of hyperthyroidism. Furthermore, long-term subclinical disease can impair bone and cardiovascular health [26]. The incidence of toxic nodular disease increases with age. The only other risk factor for the development of toxic multinodular goiter is iodine deficiency, an extremely rare condition in the United States.

Much of the diagnostic workup for toxic nodular goiter proceeds as it does for any form of hyperthyroidism. After establishing the biochemical diagnosis through laboratory testing, a radioactive iodine scan can distinguish the various etiologies of hyperthyroidism, especially in the presence of thyroid nodular disease. Toxic multinodular goiter displays increased or normal uptake. Unlike Graves' disease, the uptake may show focal areas of increased uptake and suppression. However, when the uptake becomes very high, it may become difficult to distinguish the images from that of Graves' disease. Nonfunctioning or "cold" nodules seen on the radioactive iodine scan should undergo the same workup as any newly discovered thyroid nodule [12]. The size of the nodule (>1 cm) and its ultrasonographic characteristics should help guide the decision for fine needle aspiration (FNA) biopsy (see Chap. 4). In the setting of multiple nodules, ultrasound features can help determine which nodules have suspicious features that warrant biopsy [27, 28]. Evaluation of nodules via FNA should occur prior to any decision on treatment with RAI or surgery as any potential thyroid cancer should not be treated with RAI.

Historically, the prevalence of cancer in toxic multinodular goiter was estimated at 3 % or less [29]. More recent series have demonstrated the cancer rate to be 10–15 % or even as high as 20 % [30, 31]. In a recent large, multi-institutional surgical study of toxic nodular goiter, the rate of cancer was 18.3 %, and significantly more cancers occurred in the toxic multinodular goiter group (21 %) compared to the toxic adenoma patients (4.5 %) [31]. The inclusion of microcarcinomas obviously drives the reported cancer rate higher. In this series, only 23 % of the cancers were greater than 1 cm in size [31]. Nonetheless, the incidence of thyroid cancers found within toxic multinodular goiters is much higher than previously reported. Surgery obviously removes any potential cancer, whereas RAI leaves the tumor in situ. The cancer risk should certainly factor into the risk-benefit discussion when considering surgery versus RAI with patients.

As with any multinodular goiter, completely ruling out cancer becomes challenging for several reasons. First, it is difficult to track nodules over time when there are multiple present in each lobe. In this setting, FNA of up to four nodules greater than 1 cm in size can help rule out cancer [32], but cytology from hyperthyroid patients must be interpreted with caution. Often, the hyperplasia from hyperfunctioning nodules and the associated inflammation can cause increased cellularity and/or atypia. Hence, an FNA of such a nodule may end up diagnosed as a follicular neoplasm or a follicular lesion of undetermined significance (FLUS), even though the nodule is just a benign, hyperplastic nodule. Limiting FNAs to "cold" nodules on uptake scans or suspicious appearing nodules by ultrasound should help reduce this type of diagnostic confusion.

Since we do not truly understand the natural history of cytologically benign nodules, a patient may choose surgery over RAI in order to avoid surveillance of the nodules and the possibility of future biopsy or surgery. The thyroid surgeon should also embrace this idea since RAI often results in a fibrotic reaction around the gland that makes surgery more risky. Finally, if the goiter extends beneath the clavicles (substernal goiter), then this portion of the gland cannot be evaluated with either ultrasound or FNA, making the exclusion of cancer impossible [33].

Another reason to pursue surgery as the definitive treatment for toxic multinodular goiter is that these glands can become quite large and cause compressive symptoms. The natural history of toxic multinodular goiter is not well defined, but many do continue to grow over time. A large thyroid can cause a variety of compressive symptoms. Patients can experience pain and pressure in the neck, either directly in the central neck or as referred pain to the ears. Dysphagia and odynophagia can occur from the thyroid pressing down on the esophagus; this is especially true for large goiters or nodularity on the left since the esophagus runs behind the thyroid in the left central neck. A large thyroid or posteriorly located nodules can also place pressure onto the recurrent laryngeal nerves, leading to voice changes. However, true vocal cord paresis should trigger concern for malignancy and encasement of the recurrent nerve. Large glands with a substernal component compress or deviate the trachea at the thoracic inlet, resulting in dyspnea. Many of these symptoms are positional, and patients will avoid lying completely flat as the thyroid will pressurize the trachea and esophagus in this position. Classically, patients describe a "choking" or "strangled" sensation when lying flat [34]. In a large series of patients with toxic multinodular goiter, all those with compressive symptoms undergoing total thyroidectomy experienced resolution of these symptoms, whereas only 46 % of those treated with radioactive iodine reported improvement in these symptoms [35].

In terms of patient satisfaction, those undergoing surgery experience equivalent levels of long-term satisfaction when compared to those treated with RAI [36], but these data exist only for patients with Graves' disease. For patients with toxic goiters, there are a few additional caveats to receiving RAI that are somewhat unique to this population. Like Graves' disease, patients with toxic multinodular goiters treated with RAI may relapse. In one series that included patients with toxic goiters, the failure rate after RAI was nearly 23 %. Higher doses of RAI reduce the chance for relapse, and ablating a larger gland will certainly require a higher RAI dose [37, 38]. This poses additional radiation exposure for the patient and their family. Much of the literature on cancer risk after RAI exists for either thyroid cancer or Graves' disease. However, if we extrapolate those data to patients with toxic multinodular goiter, then RAI likely increases the risk of developing secondary cancers in a dose-dependent fashion. For toxic multinodular goiter, there is an association between treatment with RAI and thyroid cancer, but this may reflect the nature of this disease and the thyroid nodules themselves rather than the radiation exposure [31, 39, 40].

Radiation exposure remains one of the few known risk factors for the development of thyroid cancer. While most of this literature comes from data on external beam radiation or radiation exposure from nuclear disasters, RAI by definition creates sustained radiation within the gland. Modern dosing strategies aim to destroy all thyroid tissue, and this is difficult to accomplish in a large goiter with multiple nodules. Any surviving thyroid tissue will therefore have been radiated with a theoretical risk of developing thyroid carcinoma in the future. For this reason, younger patients may prefer surgery over RAI.

As with surgery for Graves' disease, total thyroidectomy carries a low rate of complications when performed by experienced surgeons. Nonetheless, toxic multinodular goiter and Graves' disease probably represent the highest risk thyroidectomies due to the inflammation, vascularity, and, in some cases, fibrosis, associated with hyperthyroidism. The two main complications of total thyroidectomy are recurrent laryngeal nerve paresis and hypoparathyroidism. Both are classified as either temporary (<6 months postoperatively) or permanent (>6 months postoperatively).

Hence, there are several reasons patients and providers faced with a toxic multinodular goiter may opt for total thyroidectomy over RAI. Thyroidectomy addresses current and future cancer thyroid cancer risk; it can alleviate local symptoms from the size of the gland and/or nodules; and total thyroidectomy provides an immediate cure for hyperthyroidism with minimal to none chance for relapse.

Toxic Solitary Nodule

Toxic solitary nodule constitutes the least common etiology for hyperthyroidism in the United States. However, the signs and symptoms remain similar to other types of hyperthyroidism. A thyroid uptake scan can differentiate between Graves' disease, toxic multinodular goiter, and solitary toxic nodule. A toxic single adenoma will demonstrate intense uptake with suppression of the remaining thyroid tissue.

Once diagnosed, guidelines recommend either radioactive iodine or thyroid lobectomy as definitive treatment options. Surgery carries a much lower risk of persistent or recurrent hyperthyroidism in the setting of solitary toxic adenoma (<1 %). However, hyperthyroidism persists in 6–18 % of cases following radioactive iodine, and 5.5 % of cases will experience a recurrence after radioactive iodine [41, 42]. Overall, radioactive iodine has a 75 % response rate by 3 months posttreatment [42] (see Chap. 8).

Similar to Graves' disease and toxic multinodular goiter, surgery for a solitary toxic nodule provides the most expedient mechanism for definitive resolution of hyperthyroidism. After radioactive iodine, the patient must undergo surveillance with lab checks and medication adjustment as they transition from a hyperthyroid to hypothyroid state. For toxic adenomas, surgical treatment only involves removal of half the thyroid (thyroid lobectomy) containing the toxic nodule. Hyperthyroidism resolves within days of surgery. Additionally, the patient keeps functioning thyroid tissue, with a much lower chance of requiring thyroid hormone replacement. Following lobectomy for a toxic adenoma, only 2.3 % of patients required thyroid hormone replacement [43]. The incidence of hypothyroidism becomes even lower after isthmusectomy. However, performance of isthmusectomy is somewhat controversial and only appropriate for toxic nodules located in the isthmus over the trachea. This is in contrast to treatment with radioactive iodine. In one series of 684 patients with solitary toxic nodules who were treated with radioactive iodine, the incidence of hypothyroidism increased progressively over time with a 7.6, 28, 46, and 60 % incidence at 1, 5, 10, and 20 years, respectively [44].

Due to the lesser extent of surgery required to treat a solitary toxic nodule, complication rates are quite low. Because only half the thyroid is removed, hypoparathyroidism is not likely, and the risk of permanent recurrent laryngeal nerve injury is under 2 % [45, 46]. Similar to other forms of hyperthyroidism, compressive symptoms of the nodule or the need for rapid correction of hyperthyroidism also make surgery an attractive option. Radioactive iodine rarely destroys the nodule completely, and therefore the need for continued surveillance with ultrasounds and/or FNA remains [47]. Hence, surgery offers rapid, definitive correction of hyperthyroidism due to a toxic solitary nodule with a very low complication rate.

Conclusions

Thyroid nodular disease presents a unique set of challenges for the clinician when working up patients with hyperthyroidism. Since RAI will never completely eliminate a nodule, the need for surveillance always remains, even for nodules that are benign. The risk of any current or future thyroid cancer makes the use of RAI somewhat unsettling for patients and clinicians. For these reasons, surgery becomes an attractive treatment option for patients who have both nodules and hyperthyroidism. Surgery also offers the quickest and most definitive option to resolve their hyperthyroid state, with the lowest chance for relapse.

Sometimes, the decision to opt for surgery is clear, for example, the patient with a large toxic, multinodular goiter, compressive symptoms, and nodules with indeterminate cytology. In other cases, RAI may be more attractive, especially for patients with lots of comorbidities. A knowledgeable clinician can and should lead a comprehensive, tailored discussion of the risks and benefits of surgery or RAI for each patient with nodular hyperthyroidism.

References

1. Panneerselvan R, Schneider DF, Sippel RS, Chen H. Radioactive iodine scanning is not beneficial but its use persists for euthyroid patients. J Surg Res. 2013;184(1):269–73.
2. Okosieme OE, Chan D, Price SA, Lazarus JH, Premawardhana LD. The utility of radioiodine uptake and thyroid scintigraphy in the diagnosis and management of hyperthyroidism. Clin Endocrinol (Oxf). 2010;72(1):122–7.
3. Weetman AP. Grave's disease 1835–2002. Horm Res. 2003;59 Suppl 1:114–8.
4. Carnell NE, Valente WA. Thyroid nodules in Graves' disease: classification, characterization, and response to treatment. Thyroid. 1998;8(8):647–52.
5. Tam AA, Kaya C, Kilic FB, Ersoy R, Cakir B. Thyroid nodules and thyroid cancer in Graves' disease. Arq Bras Endocrinol Metabol. 2014;58(9):933–8.
6. Torring O, Tallstedt L, Wallin G, Lundell G, Ljunggren JG, Taube A, et al. Graves' hyperthyroidism: treatment with antithyroid drugs, surgery, or radioiodine--a prospective, randomized study. Thyroid Study Group. J Clin Endocrinol Metab. 1996;81(8):2986–93.
7. Bahn RS, Burch HB, Cooper DS, Garber JR, Greenlee MC, Klein I, et al. Hyperthyroidism and other causes of thyrotoxicosis: management guidelines of the American Thyroid Association and American Association of Clinical Endocrinologists. Endocr Pract. 2011;17(3):456–520.
8. Kim WB, Han SM, Kim TY, Nam-Goong IS, Gong G, Lee HK, et al. Ultrasonographic screening for detection of thyroid cancer in patients with Graves' disease. Clin Endocrinol (Oxf). 2004;60(6):719–25.
9. Lee J, Nam KH, Chung WY, Soh EY, Park CS. Clinicopathologic features and treatment outcomes in differentiated thyroid carcinoma patients with concurrent Graves' disease. J Korean Med Sci. 2008;23(5):796–801.
10. Nys P, Cordray JP, Sarafian V, Lefort-Mosse E, Merceron RE. Screening for thyroid cancer according to French recommendations with thyroid ultrasound in newly diagnosed Graves' disease without palpable nodule is not useful. Ann Endocrinol (Paris). 2015;76(1):13–8.
11. Ahn HS, Kim HJ, Welch HG. Korea's thyroid-cancer "epidemic"–screening and overdiagnosis. N Engl J Med. 2014;371(19):1765–7.

12. Cooper DS, Doherty GM, Haugen BR, Kloos RT, Lee SL, Mandel SJ, et al. Revised American Thyroid Association management guidelines for patients with thyroid nodules and differentiated thyroid cancer. Thyroid. 2009;19(11):1167–214.
13. Castagna MG, Belardini V, Memmo S, Maino F, Di Santo A, Toti P, et al. Nodules in autoimmune thyroiditis are associated with increased risk of thyroid cancer in surgical series but not in cytological series: evidence for selection bias. J Clin Endocrinol Metab. 2014;99(9):3193–8.
14. Liu J, Bargren A, Schaefer S, Chen H, Sippel RS. Total thyroidectomy: a safe and effective treatment for Graves' disease. J Surg Res. 2011;168(1):1–4.
15. Ozaki O, Ito K, Mimura T, Sugino K, Kitamura Y, Iwabuchi H, et al. Thyroid carcinoma after radioactive iodine therapy for Graves' disease. World J Surg. 1994;18(4):518–21.
16. Wilhelm SM, McHenry CR. Total thyroidectomy is superior to subtotal thyroidectomy for management of Graves' disease in the United States. World J Surg. 2010;34(6):1261–4.
17. Al-Adhami A, Snaith AC, Craig WL, Krukowski ZH. Changing trends in surgery for Graves' disease: a cohort comparison of those having surgery intended to preserve thyroid function with those having ablative surgery. J Otolaryngol. 2013;42:37.
18. Feroci F, Rettori M, Borrelli A, Coppola A, Castagnoli A, Perigli G, et al. A systematic review and meta-analysis of total thyroidectomy versus bilateral subtotal thyroidectomy for Graves' disease. Surgery. 2014;155(3):529–40.
19. Oltmann SC, Brekke AV, Schneider DF, Schaefer SC, Chen H, Sippel RS. Preventing postoperative hypocalcemia in patients with Graves disease: a prospective study. Ann Surg Oncol. 2015;22(3):952–8.
20. Elfenbein DM, Scheri R, Roman S, Sosa JA. Detection and management of cervical lymph nodes in papillary thyroid cancer. Expert Rev Endocrinol Metabol. 2013;8(4):365–78.
21. Mok VM, Oltmann SC, Chen H, Sippel RS, Schneider DF. Identifying predictors of a difficult thyroidectomy. J Surg Res. 2014;190(1):157–63.
22. Ritter K, Elfenbein D, Schneider DF, Chen H, Sippel RS. Hypoparathyroidism after total thyroidectomy: incidence and resolution. J Surg Res. 2015;197(2):348–53.
23. Tan GH, Gharib H. Thyroid incidentalomas: management approaches to nonpalpable nodules discovered incidentally on thyroid imaging. Ann Intern Med. 1997;126(3):226–31.
24. Berghout A, Wiersinga WM, Smits NJ, Touber JL. Interrelationships between age, thyroid volume, thyroid nodularity, and thyroid function in patients with sporadic nontoxic goiter. Am J Med. 1990;89(5):602–8.
25. Gozu HI, Lublinghoff J, Bircan R, Paschke R. Genetics and phenomics of inherited and sporadic non-autoimmune hyperthyroidism. Mol Cell Endocrinol. 2010;322(1–2):125–34.
26. Martin FI, Deam DR. Hyperthyroidism in elderly hospitalised patients. Clinical features and treatment outcomes. Med J Aust. 1996;164(4):200–3.
27. American Thyroid Association Guidelines Taskforce on Thyroid N, Differentiated Thyroid C, Cooper DS, Doherty GM, Haugen BR, Kloos RT, et al. Revised American Thyroid Association management guidelines for patients with thyroid nodules and differentiated thyroid cancer. Thyroid. 2009;19(11):1167–214.
28. Bahn Chair RS, Burch HB, Cooper DS, Garber JR, Greenlee MC, Klein I, et al. Hyperthyroidism and other causes of thyrotoxicosis: management guidelines of the American Thyroid Association and American Association of Clinical Endocrinologists. Thyroid. 2011;21(6):593–646.
29. Kang AS, Grant CS, Thompson GB, van Heerden JA. Current treatment of nodular goiter with hyperthyroidism (Plummer's disease): surgery versus radioiodine. Surgery. 2002;132(6):916–23; discussion 23.
30. Cerci C, Cerci SS, Eroglu E, Dede M, Kapucuoglu N, Yildiz M, et al. Thyroid cancer in toxic and non-toxic multinodular goiter. J Postgrad Med. 2007;53(3):157–60.
31. Smith JJ, Chen X, Schneider DF, Nookala R, Broome JT, Sippel RS, et al. Toxic nodular goiter and cancer: a compelling case for thyroidectomy. Ann Surg Oncol. 2013;20(4):1336–40.
32. Frates MC, Benson CB, Doubilet PM, Kunreuther E, Contreras M, Cibas ES, et al. Prevalence and distribution of carcinoma in patients with solitary and multiple thyroid nodules on sonography. J Clin Endocrinol Metab. 2006;91(9):3411–7.

33. Chen AY, Bernet VJ, Carty SE, Davies TF, Ganly I, Inabnet 3rd WB, et al. American Thyroid Association statement on optimal surgical management of goiter. Thyroid. 2014;24(2):181–9.
34. Stang MT, Armstrong MJ, Ogilvie JB, Yip L, McCoy KL, Faber CN, et al. Positional dyspnea and tracheal compression as indications for goiter resection. Arch Surg. 2012;147(7):621–6.
35. Porterfield Jr JR, Thompson GB, Farley DR, Grant CS, Richards ML. Evidence-based management of toxic multinodular goiter (Plummer's Disease). World J Surg. 2008;32(7):1278–84.
36. Abraham-Nordling M, Torring O, Hamberger B, Lundell G, Tallstedt L, Calissendorff J, et al. Graves' disease: a long-term quality-of-life follow up of patients randomized to treatment with antithyroid drugs, radioiodine, or surgery. Thyroid. 2005;15(11):1279–86.
37. Sztal-Mazer S, Nakatani VY, Bortolini LG, Boguszewski CL, Graf H, de Carvalho GA. Evidence for higher success rates and successful treatment earlier in Graves' disease with higher radioactive iodine doses. Thyroid. 2012;22(10):991–5.
38. Schneider DF, Sonderman PE, Jones MF, Ojomo KA, Chen H, Jaume JC, et al. Failure of radioactive iodine in the treatment of hyperthyroidism. Ann Surg Oncol. 2014;21(13):4174–80.
39. Ron E, Doody MM, Becker DV, Brill AB, Curtis RE, Goldman MB, et al. Cancer mortality following treatment for adult hyperthyroidism. Cooperative Thyrotoxicosis Therapy Follow-up Study Group. JAMA. 1998;280(4):347–55.
40. Metso S, Auvinen A, Huhtala H, Salmi J, Oksala H, Jaatinen P. Increased cancer incidence after radioiodine treatment for hyperthyroidism. Cancer. 2007;109(10):1972–9.
41. Vidal-Trecan GM, Stahl JE, Eckman MH. Radioiodine or surgery for toxic thyroid adenoma: dissecting an important decision. A cost-effectiveness analysis. Thyroid. 2004;14(11):933–45.
42. Nygaard B, Hegedus L, Nielsen KG, Ulriksen P, Hansen JM. Long-term effect of radioactive iodine on thyroid function and size in patients with solitary autonomously functioning toxic thyroid nodules. Clin Endocrinol (Oxf). 1999;50(2):197–202.
43. Vaiman M, Nagibin A, Hagag P, Kessler A, Gavriel H. Hypothyroidism following partial thyroidectomy. Otolaryngol Head Neck Surg. 2008;138(1):98–100.
44. Goldstein R, Hart IR. Follow-up of solitary autonomous thyroid nodules treated with 131I. N Engl J Med. 1983;309(24):1473–6.
45. Wahl RA, Rimpl I, Saalabian S, Schabram J. Differentiated operative therapy of thyroid autonomy (Plummer's disease). Exp Clin Endocrinol Diabetes. 1998;106 Suppl 4:S78–84.
46. van Soestbergen MJ, van der Vijver JC, Graafland AD. Recurrence of hyperthyroidism in multinodular goiter after long-term drug therapy: a comparison with Graves' disease. J Endocrinol Invest. 1992;15(11):797–800.
47. Bonnema SJ, Bertelsen H, Mortensen J, Andersen PB, Knudsen DU, Bastholt L, et al. The feasibility of high dose iodine 131 treatment as an alternative to surgery in patients with a very large goiter: effect on thyroid function and size and pulmonary function. J Clin Endocrinol Metab. 1999;84(10):3636–41.

Part III
The Indeterminate Thyroid Nodule

Chapter 10
Surgical Intervention for Indeterminate Thyroid Nodules

Snehal G. Patel and Linwah Yip

Introduction

Thyroid nodules are a common clinical problem particularly with the recent increased use of imaging such as computed tomography and ultrasonography. Several studies have demonstrated that thyroid nodules are found in 4–8 % of the general population with the use of palpation [1–4], in 19–67 % of patients with the use of ultrasound, and in 50 % of autopsies [5]. The clinical importance of thyroid nodules is that ~5 % are potentially malignant [6].

Initial evaluation of thyroid nodules using ultrasound-guided fine-needle aspiration (FNA) is now well established since its introduction in the 1970s. Its routine use has decreased the number of patients requiring surgery and has increased the yield of thyroid malignancy in those patients who undergo surgery [7]. FNA has proven to be a rapid, cost-effective, safe, and reliable method of investigation [8]. In 2007, the Bethesda System for Reporting Thyroid Cytopathology (BSRTC) was established to standardize the reporting of thyroid cytopathology and includes six distinct categories. The indeterminate category includes (1) atypia of undetermined significance/follicular lesion of undetermined significance (AUS/FLUS); (2) follicular neoplasm/suspicious for follicular neoplasm (FN/SFN), a category that also

S.G. Patel, MD
Department of Surgery, Division of Endocrine Surgery and Surgical Oncology, University of Pittsburgh, Pittsburgh, PA, USA

L. Yip, MD (✉)
Department of Surgery, Division of Endocrine Surgery and Surgical Oncology, University of Pittsburgh, Pittsburgh, PA, USA

University of Pittsburgh School of Medicine,
Suite 101-3471 Fifth Avenue, Pittsburgh, PA 15213, USA
e-mail: yipl@upmc.edu

S.A. Roman et al. (eds.), *Management of Thyroid Nodules and Differentiated Thyroid Cancer*, DOI 10.1007/978-3-319-43618-0_10

encompasses the diagnosis of Hürthle cell neoplasm/suspicious for Hürthle cell neoplasm; and (3) suspicious for malignancy (SUSP) [8]. The rate of malignancy within each category varies with a predicted probability of cancer of 5–15 % for AUS/FLUS, 15–30 % for FN/SFN, and 60–75 % for SUSP [9]. Because of these variable malignancy rates, the management of patients with cytologically indeterminate thyroid nodules can be problematic.

The diagnostic difficulty is due to the nonspecific follicular pattern identified by cytologic evaluation that can be found in nodules with benign hyperplastic changes, follicular adenomas, follicular thyroid carcinomas (FTC), and follicular variant of papillary carcinoma (FV-PTC) [10]. Other rare lesions, which can also present with follicular-patterned cytology, include medullary thyroid cancer, parathyroid glands, and metastatic malignancies to the thyroid. The histologic malignancies associated with preoperative indeterminate FNA biopsy results are usually conventional papillary thyroid cancer (PTC), but up to 30 % are either FV-PTC or FTC [11–13]. FTC requires capsular and/or vascular invasion which is not readily apparent on cytology analysis. FV-PTC is the second most common variant of PTC and is associated with the multifocal and heterogeneous distribution of the characteristic nuclear features seen in PTC such as elongation, enlargement, chromatin clearing, intranuclear grooves, and inclusions [14]. FV-PTC is the most frequent histology associated with false-negative cytology and intraoperative frozen section results [15, 16]. To further complicate interpretation of diagnostic testing, interobserver variability for cancer type is up to 30 % even among expert thyroid pathologists [11]. A Hürthle cell neoplasm is the oncocytic variant of follicular-patterned lesions and may correspond to the histology of Hürthle cell adenoma, Hürthle cell carcinoma, or PTC with Hürthle cell/oncocytic features which also all require histology for diagnosis [17].

Treatment Options

Management of the indeterminate nodule includes consideration of clinical, sonographic, and molecular risk factors (Table 10.1). Depending on these factors, indeterminate nodules may undergo repeat FNA or surgical excision for definitive diagnosis. Repeat biopsies are typically reserved for nodules with initial cytology classified as AUS/FLUS. An AUS/FLUS biopsy has a low risk of cancer (5–20 %), and a repeat FNA can result in a benign cytology diagnosis in up to 50 % of nodules [18–20]. For low-risk lesions without any concomitant risk factors and/or for AUS/FLUS nodules in patients who are poor surgical candidates, active surveillance can be considered. However, the majority of patients with cytologically indeterminate thyroid nodules will undergo diagnostic surgery with the primary goals of thyroidectomy being to safely establish a histological diagnosis and to limit the need for two-stage thyroidectomy.

Surgical options include diagnostic thyroid lobectomy with isthmusectomy or total thyroidectomy (Table 10.2). Nodulectomy is not indicated. Voice changes are a risk of thyroid surgery, have been reported in 30–80 % of post-thyroidectomy

Table 10.1 Risk factors associated with thyroid cancer in cytologically indeterminate nodules

Clinical	Rapid nodule growth
	Family or personal history of predisposition syndrome (e.g., *PTEN* hamartoma tumor, *APC*-associated polyposis, *RET* associated)
	Childhood exposure to ionizing radiation
	Younger (<18 years) or older (>50 years) age
	Men
	Larger nodule size
Imaging	Ultrasound features (especially taller-than-wide shape, microcalcifications, increased intranodular vascularity)
	FDG-PET avidity
Molecular	Galectin-3- or HBME-1-positive on immunocytological analysis
	TSHR mRNA detectable in peripheral blood
	Gene expression classifier or micro-RNA panel testing of biopsy is "suspicious"
	Detection of somatic mutation or rearrangement (e.g., *BRAF* V600E, *RAS*) in preoperative biopsy using conventional sequencing or next-generation sequencing

FDG-PET fluorodeoxyglucose-positron emission tomography, *RNA* ribonucleic acid, *TSHR mRNA* thyroid-stimulating hormone receptor messenger RNA

Table 10.2 Initial surgical options for indeterminate nodule

	Pros	Cons	Indication
Thyroid lobectomy	Limits risks of hypoparathyroidism and bilateral recurrent laryngeal nerve injury	Second operation for completion thyroidectomy necessary if histology indicates	Preoperative concern for low-risk thyroid cancer
	70–85 % avoid permanent hypothyroidism		Patient preference
Total thyroidectomy	Provides initial oncologic surgery in preparation for radioactive iodine ablation when indicated	Permanent hypothyroidism	Preoperative concern for high-risk thyroid cancer and need for post-op radioactive iodine ablation/ treatment
		Increased operative risks including risk of permanent hypoparathyroidism and bilateral recurrent laryngeal nerve injury	Concurrent clinical features such as contralateral dominant nodule, existing hypothyroidism, family, or personal history of predisposition syndrome
			Patient preference

patients, and are usually transient [21, 22]. There is a 1–5 % risk of recurrent laryngeal nerve palsy and 1–2 % risk of recurrent laryngeal nerve paralysis following thyroidectomy [7, 23]. Total thyroidectomy is associated with the rare (likelihood of ~1 in 1000) risk of bilateral recurrent laryngeal nerve injury necessitating tracheostomy. After total thyroidectomy, the risk of temporary hypocalcemia is 1–14 % and can be permanent in 1–6 % of patients [23]. Postoperative cervical hematoma requiring reoperation can be life-threatening and cause airway compromise but is infrequent occurring in ~1 % of post-thyroidectomy patients [24–26]. The type and incidence of risks following completion thyroidectomy are similar to that of a near-total or total thyroidectomy [27, 28]. L-Thyroxine supplementation is required in all patients following total thyroidectomy and in 15–30 % of patients following thyroid lobectomy [29, 30]. Surgeon experience influences the risks of thyroidectomy, and in population-level analysis, higher-volume surgeons have lower overall complication rates [31, 32].

The decision regarding extent of initial surgery is influenced by a number of clinical factors including preexisting thyroid dysfunction, presence of a contralateral dominant thyroid nodule, and patient preference [7]. The presurgical likelihood of malignancy is also an essential component in deciding the extent of initial surgery. Due to the decreasing use of radioactive iodine ablation, the 2015 American Thyroid Association guidelines now recommend thyroid lobectomy for thyroid cancers <1 cm without extrathyroidal extension or lymph node metastasis. Total thyroidectomy or lobectomy can be considered for thyroid cancers 1–4 cm that do not have extrathyroidal extension or lymph node metastasis, while total thyroidectomy is definitively indicated for cancer >4 cm or for cancer of any size with gross extrathyroidal extension, clinically apparent nodal, or distant metastases. Therefore, counseling patients on the appropriate extent of initial surgery requires accurate preoperative assessment of malignancy risk in addition to consideration for the likelihood that the malignancy may be associated with more aggressive biologic behavior.

After lobectomy, completion thyroidectomy is recommended for patients with histologic malignancy who would have required total thyroidectomy if the diagnosis was known preoperatively. Completion thyroidectomy and radioactive iodine ablation should be performed for malignancies with a higher risk of structural recurrence such as patients with American Joint Committee on Cancer advanced stage III/IV disease or patients with incomplete tumor resection or bulky clinical lymphadenopathy [7, 33]. Preoperative vocal fold assessment with either direct laryngoscopy or transcutaneous laryngeal ultrasound should be performed prior to any reoperative surgery [7, 34, 35].

Clinical Risk Factors

Clinical variables such as age, gender, and the presence of unique symptoms or examination findings have been examined with regard to their ability to predict malignancy. Traditionally, an elevated concern for cancer has been associated with a history of rapid nodule growth; family history of thyroid cancer or inherited predisposition syndrome such as *RET* associated, *PTEN* hamartoma tumor, or *APC*-associated polyposis syndromes; or childhood exposure to ionizing radiation. On physical exam, fixation of nodule to surrounding neck structures and palpable lymphadenopathy are also concerning features.

The ability of clinical characteristics of patients with indeterminate FN/SFN cytology to predict malignancy was examined by Baloch et al., and factors associated with malignancy included age >40 years, nodule size >3 cm, and male gender [36]. The association between gender and an increased risk of malignancy has been inconsistent, but in a meta-analysis inclusive of 19 studies with "indeterminate" nodules, men had a 1.5-fold higher risk for malignancy compared to women [37]. In the subset of nodules with Hürthle cell neoplasm cytology, men have been shown more consistently to have a higher risk of cancer [38–40]. Interestingly, in one of the larger published series of 603 follicular and Hürthle cell neoplasms from Italy, gender was not associated with cancer risk but women compared to men had a higher incidence of histologic malignancy with extrathyroidal extension [38].

The association between age and malignancy has also been variable, and increased risk has been seen with both younger and older patients [41]. In another large single institution series of 639 patients with indeterminate nodules, Banks et al. observed that age was an independent predictor of malignancy on multivariate analysis; patients' age <50 years had a 3 % increase in risk of cancer for each year younger in age, and patients' age >50 years had a 3.4 % increase in cancer risk for each year older in age [42]. An age of 50 years has also been shown to be the threshold for increased cancer risk in other studies [39, 43]. Pediatric patients (age ≤18 years) have an overall higher risk of malignancy associated with thyroid nodules (15–30 %), and the risk can be up to 50 % in nodules with indeterminate cytology [44, 45]. The 2015 American Thyroid Association guidelines for pediatric patients recommend surgery for all indeterminate FNA results in children [46].

Larger nodule size has been reported to be associated with a higher risk of malignancy especially for follicular neoplasms and Hürthle cell neoplasms [47]. In a study of 149 nodules with FN/SFN cytology, Tuttle et al. found that the risk of malignancy was ~threefold higher in nodules >4 cm as measured by palpation [48], while Baloch et al. found that ≥3 cm was associated with a twofold greater risk of malignancy in a single institution series of 184 follicular neoplasm nodules [36]. In a consecutive series of 55 patients with Hürthle cell neoplasms, malignancy increased with nodule size and older patient age [49]. Nodule size was another predictor of malignancy in Banks et al., and indeterminate nodules that were 2.5 cm had the lowest risk of cancer. A higher risk of cancer was associated with smaller indeterminate nodules (53 % increase in risk for every 1 cm decrease in size) and with larger nodules (39 % increase in risk for every 1 cm increase in size) [42]. Surgery for relief of compressive symptomatology may also be indicated for nodules >3 cm as these have been associated with globus symptoms on multivariate analysis [50].

Imaging Risk Factors

Thyroid ultrasound has been widely used for nodule risk stratification and is used to identify non-palpable nodules, define nodule features, and characterize cervical lymph nodes. In studies inclusive of all thyroid nodules, ultrasound features that increase concern for cancer includes marked hypoechogenicity, spiculated or ill-defined margin, taller-than-wide shape, and microcalcifications [51]. However, whether these features are useful in nodules with indeterminate cytology remains unclear. In a study of 180 patients who had thyroid nodules with indeterminate cytology (follicular neoplasm, Hürthle cell neoplasm, and SUSP), a taller-than-wide shape was associated with 99 % specificity and 92 % positive predictive value for malignancy. When ≥2 concerning ultrasound features were present, the risk of malignancy was >70 % [52]. Taller-than-wide shape was also shown to be associated with cancer in a series of 61 patients who all had thyroidectomy for AUS/FLUS cytology [53]. But in another study of 505 follicular and Hürthle cell neoplasms, malignancy was associated with only microcalcifications [54].

In a meta-analysis by Brito et al., nodules with indeterminate cytology were evaluated in a subset analysis; they found that suspicious features did not accurately predict malignancy with the exception of increased intranodular vascularity, which was likely due to the increased frequency of follicular neoplasms in the study population [55]. Use of color Doppler to evaluate intranodular vascularity may be helpful for evaluating follicular neoplasms as it is theorized that these contain higher cellularity and variation in echogenicity and internal vascularity compared to PTC [56] (Fig. 10.1). However, interpretation of flow on color Doppler may be associated with up to 30 % interobserver variability, limiting its utility.

Improving preoperative risk stratification has also been studied using other imaging modalities such as fluorodeoxyglucose-positron emission tomography (FDG-PET) (Fig. 10.1). In a systematic review inclusive of six articles that examined accuracy of FDG-PET to diagnose thyroid cancer, the pooled specificity and sensitivity were 95 % and 48 %, respectively [57]. Thus, an FDG-avid indeterminate nodule is not always malignant, but malignant nodules are rarely non-FDG avid. Broad applicability of FDG-PET scans is complicated by inconsistent definitions for FDG avidity, low imaging resolution for small nodules, and selection bias. Furthermore, FDG-PET scanning is costly overall, although a cost-effectiveness study using reimbursement rates from the Netherlands demonstrated that routine use of PET could reduce unnecessary surgeries and was associated with lower costs than other diagnostic adjuncts such as molecular testing [58].

Real-time elastography measures the tissue displacement when external force is applied to the thyroid nodule of interest. The imaging relies on the assumption that thyroid cancers are firmer than benign nodules, and as a result, calcifications and cystic nodules can cause diagnostic inaccuracies. Although small single institution studies have demonstrated high sensitivity (up to 96 %) and specificity (up to 95 %) in detecting cancer, high interobserver variability in addition to non-standardized

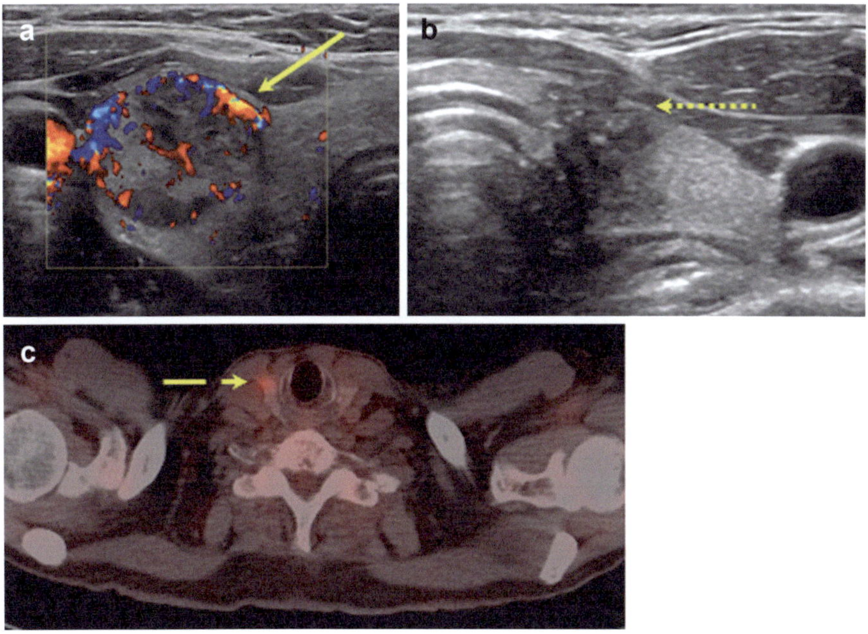

Fig. 10.1 Imaging features that increase concern for malignancy in indeterminate nodules. Ultrasound features including intranodular hypervascularity (**a**, *solid line*) and taller-than-wide shape (**b**, *dotted line*) have been associated with an increased risk of malignancy in nodules with indeterminate cytology. Avidity on fluorodeoxyglucose-positron emission tomography (FDG-PET) (**c**, *dashed line*) may also increase cancer risk, but the high cost of FDG-PET scans limits their widespread use as part of diagnostic evaluation

methodologies has limited its use. In a multi-institutional study inclusive of 498 nodules, the addition of elastography to ultrasound appeared to increase sensitivity for malignancy which could potentially better identify nodules that do not require FNA biopsy. For nodules with indeterminate cytology, elastography results appear to be poorly predictive of histology [59, 60].

Molecular Risk Factors

A number of adjunctive molecular tests have been evaluated to determine their utility in diagnosing malignancy in indeterminate nodules. Immunocytochemical analysis of markers expressed predominantly in PTC such as CK-19, galectin-3, and HBME-1 have been studied [61]. Galectin-3 staining in preoperative cytology was specifically evaluated in a multi-institutional study of 465 follicular neoplasms and accuracy was 88 % [62]. Serum markers such as thyroid-stimulating hormone receptor (TSHR) mRNA or thyroglobulin (Tg) can be measured in peripheral blood and are another area of investigation. When *TSHR* mRNA is detected in patients with follicular neoplasm nodules, accuracy for predicting malignancy was 85 %. In an algorithm that incorporated *TSHR* mRNA positivity, nodule size (<3.5 cm or ≥3.5 cm), and number of suspicious ultrasound characteristics (hypervascularity, microcalcifications, irregular shape, and indistinct margins), the diagnostic discrimination for indeterminate FNA results was increased to 91 % accuracy, 97 % sensitivity, 95 % negative predictive value, 84 % specificity, and 88 % positive predictive value. In a series of 164 indeterminate nodules, elevated preoperative basal serum Tg levels were an independent predictor of malignancy [63]. These results have not been consistent, and in another smaller study of 39 patients with follicular or Hürthle cell neoplasms, Tg levels were poorly predictive [63]. Preoperative Tg levels are difficult to interpret especially in the presence of detectable Tg antibodies and should not be routinely used to assess malignancy risk.

The Afirma diagnostic test is a gene expression classifier (GEC) that measures the expression of 167 gene transcripts. The expression pattern was selected to be predictive of benign nodules and in a prospective, multicenter trial demonstrated a relatively high sensitivity (92 %) that translated into a negative predictive value of 93 % [64]. However, in nodules with SUSP cytology, the high malignancy rate resulted in an unreliable negative predictive value of 85 %, and thus GEC was not recommended for cytologically SUSP nodules. The GEC panel has a low specificity of 52 %, and diagnostic thyroidectomy is still needed when cytology results are "suspicious" even though many such nodules will be histologically benign. In Marti et al., GEC test performance was evaluated at two separate tertiary care centers with different cancer prevalences [65]. With the goal of obtaining a calculated negative predictive value >94 % and using the sensitivity and specificity data from the Alexander et al. multi-institutional study [64], Marti et al. determined that the pre-test cancer risk of an indeterminate nodule should be 15–21 % for GEC to be clinically useful [65]. In this range, the cancer risk when GEC is "suspicious" is only 25–32 %. These findings further underscored the evolving observation that published negative and positive predictive values are not uniformly applicable across institutions or practices and vary according to cancer prevalence and risk of malignancy for each BSRTC category [66].

The second molecular testing modality frequently evaluated is the identification of somatic mutations and rearrangements. Activation of MAPK and PI3K-AKT pathways via cell-membrane receptor tyrosine kinases (RET, NTRK1) and intracellular signal transducers (BRAF, RAS) are known initiators of thyroid carcinogenesis [67, 68]. In PTC, *BRAF* V600E is the most common somatic mutation with an incidence that varies geographically in the USA from 40 to 50 % but up to 80 % of PTCs in Asia. Identification of *BRAF* V600E in indeterminate nodules can improve preoperative detection for PTC, and in a meta-analysis inclusive of 47 studies reporting use of *BRAF* V600E analysis in FNA biopsy specimens, a pooled specificity could not be calculated for the meta-analysis, but was 100 % when reported by selected studies. Pooled sensitivity in the indeterminate category inclusive of AUS/FLUS, FN/SFN, and SUSP nodules was 30 % (range 11–50 %) [69]. Therefore, *BRAF* V600E testing alone was not sufficient to reduce the need for diagnostic surgery altogether.

An alternative to single gene testing is to use a multigene panel such as the 7-gene panel inclusive of *RAS* (*H-*, *N-*, *K-RAS* codons 12, 13, and 61), *BRAF* (V600E and K601E), *RET*/*PTC*, and *PAX8*/*PPAR* rearrangements. In a validation study by Nikiforov et al., 513/1056 nodules with indeterminate cytology and histology had correlative molecular results using such panel. All *BRAF*-, *RET*/*PTC*-, and *PAX8-*/*PPARG*-positive cytology specimens were histologically thyroid cancers (specificity 100 %); however, *RAS* positivity was associated with an 85 % risk of malignancy [70]. A subsequent prospective study evaluating the clinical and real-time utility of the 7-gene panel demonstrated that the added specificity associated with using mutation testing was helpful for guiding extent of initial surgery such as total thyroidectomy for thyroid cancers that on histology were >1 cm in size. Therefore, the need for two-stage thyroidectomy was reduced in 30 % of patients [71]. However, the low sensitivity associated with the 7-gene panel resulted in a rate of malignancy associated with "negative" results that were too high to allow for surveillance only.

Newer multigene panels utilizing next-generation sequencing have incorporated additional genetic alterations that have since been identified in thyroid cancer. For example, one such panel (ThyroSeq) evaluates 14 genes, 42 gene rearrangements, and additional expression analysis of 8 genes used to assess for quantity and type of cells. Nikiforov et al. described the use of this broad panel in 143 follicular neoplasm nodules; 91 were studied retrospectively, and 52 were studied prospectively. Malignancy was diagnosed in 27 %, including 26 FV-PTC and 6 FTC. The overall sensitivity and specificity were 90 % and 92 %, respectively [72]. These performance parameters were replicated in a series of 98 AUS/FLUS nodules from the same institution [73]. Another test combines the 7-gene panel with a panel of 10 micro-RNAs (ThyGenX and ThyraMir), and in a study of 109 nodules with AUS/FLUS or FN/SFN cytology (32 % cancer prevalence), the combined panel sensitivity and specificity were 89 % and 85 %, respectively [74]. Independent validation studies for all of these newer molecular tests are still needed.

The detection of a genetic mutation or rearrangement may be helpful in predicting the presence of thyroid cancer, but the type of genetic alteration may also provide information on the thyroid cancer type and biologic behavior. The presence of *BRAF* V600E has been shown in some studies to be associated with an increased risk of PTC recurrence due to its association with lymph node metastasis and advanced stage disease [75]. However, these results have not been consistent in all studies [76, 77]. In a study inclusive of 1,510 patients who had 7-gene panel testing and treatment for thyroid cancer, *RET*/*PTC* rearrangement had the highest association with distant metastases. *RAS*-positive tumors were usually encapsulated FV-PTC, however; some aggressive tumor types were also seen with *RAS* mutations including medullary thyroid cancer and poorly differentiated/anaplastic cancers [78]. The multigene panel ThyroSeq has additional markers that may be associated with more aggressive variants of thyroid cancer including *TERT* and *p53*, and refinement of thyroid cancer phenotype may be obtained with this test although this is still being evaluated [79, 80].

The use of molecular testing for indeterminate nodules should consider the test strengths and planned clinical management. For example, the GEC can help identify nodules that may be more likely to be benign. Therefore, GEC does not provide any added utility if active surveillance is not a clinical consideration due to patient preference, associated symptoms, or presence of other concerning clinical or radiographic features. The 7-gene panel may help identify nodules with a higher risk of cancer and guide extent of thyroidectomy. Thus, such panel will not add to clinical decision-making if total thyroidectomy is already indicated due to preexisting thyroid dysfunction, contralateral dominant nodule, or patient preference. No study to date has yet determined the clinical or cost efficacy when using >1 molecular test on the same nodule.

Clinical Management Recommendations

AUS/FLUS The incidence of an AUS/FLUS diagnosis ranges from 5 to 20 %, and the risk of cancer in an AUS/FLUS nodule is 15.9 % but ranges in studies from 5 to 40 % [8]. AUS/FLUS nodules with cellular atypia compared to a predominant microfollicular pattern have been observed to have a higher risk of malignancy [81]. Because of the highly variable incidence and malignancy rates associated with this cytology category, consideration of institutional and geographical rates should be incorporated into patient management recommendations. Repeat FNA can be benign in 40–50 % of nodules and should be considered in nodules that lack concerning clinical or imaging features [18, 19]. A repeated AUS/FLUS biopsy carries a 30–50 % risk of cancer, and either thyroid lobectomy or total thyroidectomy should be considered.

Molecular testing can certainly be considered if clinically indicated, and its accuracy is dependent on the prevalence of cancer in the tested population of nodules [66]. When AUS/FLUS biopsy results are GEC benign or ThyroSeq negative, the risk of cancer has been reported to be 3–4 %. According to recent National Comprehensive Cancer Network guidelines, if the cancer risk of an indeterminate nodule can be lowered to be equivalent to that of a cytologically benign nodule, then active surveillance can be considered [82]. GEC-suspicious or gene-positive nodules should undergo either thyroid lobectomy or total thyroidectomy.

FN/SFN The incidence of an FN/SFN biopsy is 5–20 %, and nodules within the FN/SFN category were found to have a risk of cancer after removal of 20–30 % [8]. Therefore, diagnostic surgical excision has been the standard of care for the management of FN/SFN cytology nodules. Molecular testing may help assessment of malignancy risk. Although the risk varies according to cancer prevalence, when follicular neoplasms are GEC benign, the risk of cancer has been reported to be ~6 %, while ThyroSeq-negative follicular neoplasms have a 3–4 % risk of cancer. Molecular-negative follicular neoplasms can be considered for active surveillance, but long-term follow-up studies are still needed to determine natural history of these lesions. If molecular testing is positive or GEC suspicious, then either thyroid lobectomy or total thyroidectomy should be considered.

Hürthle cell neoplasms are also included in this cytology category, and specific study to evaluate if molecular testing results can be extrapolated to this subset is still needed. Brauner et al. evaluated GEC results for 43 Hürthle cell neoplasms, and 60–65 % were classified as GEC suspicious although only 14 % were histologic malignancies. Other studies have shown that Hürthle cell carcinomas have a different molecular signature compared to PTC or FTC which may impact the predictive ability of 7-gene panel or ThyroSeq in nodules with this histology.

SUSP This is the highest risk category of indeterminate cytology in the BSRTC system, with an estimated cancer risk of 60–75 % [8]. According to the American Thyroid Association guidelines, cytologically SUSP nodules should be managed with oncologic preoperative evaluation and thyroidectomy, due to the high risk of cancer [7]. GEC testing has a positive predictive value that is similar to cytology alone (76 %) and a negative predictive value of 85 % [64]. Therefore, molecular testing is unlikely to contribute to the management of this cytological diagnosis. When 7-gene panel testing is negative, a lower rate of cancer is observed (20–25 %) and lobectomy can be considered for diagnostic purposes.

Conclusion

The optimal management of the indeterminate thyroid nodule continues to evolve. Clinical and sonographic risk factors are important preoperative variables used to guide initial recommendations. Current molecular testing modalities were specifically developed to resolve the diagnostic uncertainty associated with these nodules, and initial studies of their use have been promising in improving preoperative risk stratification. Clinical presentation and patient preferences remain important considerations in decision-making.

References

1. Harach HR, Franssila KO, Wasenius VM. Occult papillary carcinoma of the thyroid. A "normal" finding in Finland. A systematic autopsy study. Cancer. 1985;56(3):531–8. Epub 1985/08/01. eng.
2. Brander A, Viikinkoski P, Nickels J, Kivisaari L. Thyroid gland: US screening in a random adult population. Radiology. 1991;181(3):683–7. Epub 1991/12/01. eng.
3. Tan GH, Gharib H. Thyroid incidentalomas: management approaches to nonpalpable nodules discovered incidentally on thyroid imaging. Ann Intern Med. 1997;126(3):226–31. Epub 1997/02/01. eng.
4. Frates MC, Benson CB, Charboneau JW, Cibas ES, Clark OH, Coleman BG, et al. Management of thyroid nodules detected at US: Society of Radiologists in Ultrasound consensus conference statement. Radiology. 2005;237(3):794–800. Epub 2005/11/24. eng.
5. Mortensen JD, Woolner LB, Bennett WA. Gross and microscopic findings in clinically normal thyroid glands. J Clin Endocrinol Metab. 1955;15(10):1270–80. Epub 1955/10/01. eng.

6. Gharib H, Papini E, Paschke R, Duick DS, Valcavi R, Hegedus L, et al. American Association of Clinical Endocrinologists, Associazione Medici Endocrinologi, and European Thyroid Association Medical guidelines for clinical practice for the diagnosis and management of thyroid nodules: executive summary of recommendations. Endocr Pract Off J Am Coll Endocrinol Am Assoc Clin Endocrinologists. 2010;16(3):468–75. Epub 2010/06/17. eng.
7. Haugen BR, Alexander EK, Bible KC, Doherty GM, Mandel SJ, Nikiforov YE, et al. 2015 American Thyroid Association Management Guidelines for adult patients with thyroid nodules and differentiated thyroid cancer: the American Thyroid Association Guidelines Task Force on thyroid nodules and differentiated thyroid cancer. Thyroid. 2016;26(1):1–133. Pubmed Central PMCID: PMC4739132, Epub 2015/10/16. eng.
8. Bongiovanni M, Spitale A, Faquin WC, Mazzucchelli L, Baloch ZW. The Bethesda system for reporting thyroid cytopathology: a meta-analysis. Acta Cytol. 2012;56(4):333–9.
9. Baloch ZW, LiVolsi VA, Asa SL, Rosai J, Merino MJ, Randolph G, et al. Diagnostic terminology and morphologic criteria for cytologic diagnosis of thyroid lesions: a synopsis of the National Cancer Institute Thyroid Fine-Needle Aspiration State of the Science Conference. Diagn Cytopathol. 2008;36(6):425–37.
10. Carling T, Udelsman R. Follicular neoplasms of the thyroid: what to recommend. Thyroid Off J Am Thyroid Assoc. 2005;15(6):583–7. Epub 2005/07/21. eng.
11. Elsheikh TM, Asa SL, Chan JK, DeLellis RA, Heffess CS, LiVolsi VA, et al. Interobserver and intraobserver variation among experts in the diagnosis of thyroid follicular lesions with borderline nuclear features of papillary carcinoma. Am J Clin Pathol. 2008;130(5):736–44.
12. Siddiqui MA, Griffith KA, Michael CW, Pu RT. Nodule heterogeneity as shown by size differences between the targeted nodule and the tumor in thyroidectomy specimen: a cause for a false-negative diagnosis of papillary thyroid carcinoma on fine-needle aspiration. Cancer. 2008;114(1):27–33.
13. Widder S, Guggisberg K, Khalil M, Pasieka JL. A pathologic re-review of follicular thyroid neoplasms: the impact of changing the threshold for the diagnosis of the follicular variant of papillary thyroid carcinoma. Surgery. 2008;144(1):80–5.
14. LiVolsi VA, Baloch ZW. Follicular neoplasms of the thyroid: view, biases, and experiences. Adv Anat Pathol. 2004;11(6):279–87.
15. Lloyd RV, Erickson LA, Casey MB, Lam KY, Lohse CM, Asa SL, et al. Observer variation in the diagnosis of follicular variant of papillary thyroid carcinoma. Am J Surg Pathol. 2004;28(10):1336–40.
16. Mehanna R, Murphy M, McCarthy J, O'Leary G, Tuthill A, Murphy MS, et al. False negatives in thyroid cytology: impact of large nodule size and follicular variant of papillary carcinoma. Laryngoscope. 2013;123(5):1305–9.
17. Kini SR, Miller JM, Hamburger JI. Cytopathology of Hurthle cell lesions of the thyroid gland by fine needle aspiration. Acta Cytol. 1981;25(6):647–52. Epub 1981/11/01. eng.
18. Chen JC, Pace SC, Chen BA, Khiyami A, McHenry CR. Yield of repeat fine-needle aspiration biopsy and rate of malignancy in patients with atypia or follicular lesion of undetermined significance: the impact of the Bethesda System for Reporting Thyroid Cytopathology. Surgery. 2012;152(6):1037–44.
19. Sullivan PS, Hirschowitz SL, Fung PC, Apple SK. The impact of atypia/follicular lesion of undetermined significance and repeat fine-needle aspiration: 5 years before and after implementation of the Bethesda System. Cancer Cytopathol. 2014;122(12):866–72.
20. Broome JT, Solorzano CC. The impact of atypia/follicular lesion of undetermined significance on the rate of malignancy in thyroid fine-needle aspiration: evaluation of the Bethesda System for Reporting Thyroid Cytopathology. Surgery. 2011;150(6):1234–41.
21. Maeda T, Saito M, Otsuki N, Morimoto K, Takahashi M, Iwaki S, et al. Voice quality after surgical treatment for thyroid cancer. Thyroid Off J Am Thyroid Assoc. 2013;23(7):847–53.
22. Stojadinovic A, Shaha AR, Orlikoff RF, Nissan A, Kornak MF, Singh B, et al. Prospective functional voice assessment in patients undergoing thyroid surgery. Ann Surg. 2002;236(6):823–32. Pubmed Central PMCID: 1422649.

23. Rosato L, Avenia N, Bernante P, De Palma M, Gulino G, Nasi PG, et al. Complications of thyroid surgery: analysis of a multicentric study on 14,934 patients operated on in Italy over 5 years. World J Surg. 2004;28(3):271–6. Epub 2004/02/13. eng.
24. Bergenfelz A, Jansson S, Kristoffersson A, Martensson H, Reihner E, Wallin G, et al. Complications to thyroid surgery: results as reported in a database from a multicenter audit comprising 3,660 patients. Langenbeck's Arch Surg/Deutsche Gesellschaft fur Chirurgie. 2008;393(5):667–73. Epub 2008/07/18. eng.
25. Burkey SH, van Heerden JA, Thompson GB, Grant CS, Schleck CD, Farley DR. Reexploration for symptomatic hematomas after cervical exploration. Surgery. 2001;130(6):914–20. Epub 2001/12/14. eng.
26. Lang BH, Yih PC, Lo CY. A review of risk factors and timing for postoperative hematoma after thyroidectomy: is outpatient thyroidectomy really safe? World J Surg. 2012;36(10):2497–502. Pubmed Central PMCID: Pmc3465547, Epub 2012/06/21. eng.
27. Untch BR, Palmer FL, Ganly I, Patel SG, Michael Tuttle R, Shah JP, et al. Oncologic outcomes after completion thyroidectomy for patients with well-differentiated thyroid carcinoma. Ann Surg Oncol. 2014;21(4):1374–8. Epub 2013/12/25. eng.
28. Pelizzo MR, Variolo M, Bernardi C, Izuzquiza M, Piotto A, Grassetto G, et al. Complications in thyroid resurgery: a single institutional experience on 233 patients from a whole series of 4,752 homogeneously treated patients. Endocrine. 2014;47(1):100–6.
29. Verloop H, Louwerens M, Schoones JW, Kievit J, Smit JW, Dekkers OM. Risk of hypothyroidism following hemithyroidectomy: systematic review and meta-analysis of prognostic studies. J Clin Endocrinol Metab. 2012;97(7):2243–55.
30. Stoll SJ, Pitt SC, Liu J, Schaefer S, Sippel RS, Chen H. Thyroid hormone replacement after thyroid lobectomy. Surgery. 2009;146(4):554–8. Pubmed Central PMCID: 2755641, discussion 8–60.
31. Sosa JA, Bowman HM, Tielsch JM, Powe NR, Gordon TA, Udelsman R. The importance of surgeon experience for clinical and economic outcomes from thyroidectomy. Ann Surg. 1998;228(3):320–30. Pubmed Central PMCID: 1191485.
32. Youngwirth LM, Adam MA, Scheri RP, Roman SA, Sosa JA. Patients treated at low-volume centers have higher rates of incomplete resection and compromised outcomes: analysis of 31,129 patients with papillary thyroid cancer. Ann Surg Oncol. 2016;23(2):403–9.
33. Carhill AA, Litofsky DR, Ross DS, Jonklaas J, Cooper DS, Brierley JD, et al. Long-term outcomes following therapy in differentiated thyroid carcinoma: NTCTCS registry analysis 1987–2012. J Clin Endocrinol Metab. 2015;100(9):3270–9.
34. Wong KP, Lang BH, Chang YK, Wong KC, Chow FC. Assessing the validity of transcutaneous laryngeal ultrasonography (TLUSG) after thyroidectomy: what factors matter? Ann Surg Oncol. 2015;22(6):1774–80.
35. Carneiro-Pla D, Solorzano CC, Wilhelm SM. Impact of vocal cord ultrasonography on endocrine surgery practices. Surgery. 2016;159(1):58–64.
36. Baloch ZW, Fleisher S, LiVolsi VA, Gupta PK. Diagnosis of "follicular neoplasm": a gray zone in thyroid fine-needle aspiration cytology. Diagn Cytopathol. 2002;26(1):41–4. Epub 2002/01/10. eng.
37. Trimboli P, Treglia G, Guidobaldi L, Saggiorato E, Nigri G, Crescenzi A, et al. Clinical characteristics as predictors of malignancy in patients with indeterminate thyroid cytology: a meta-analysis. Endocrine. 2014;46(1):52–9. Epub 2013/11/08. eng.
38. Sorrenti S, Trimboli P, Catania A, Ulisse S, De Antoni E, D'Armiento M. Comparison of malignancy rate in thyroid nodules with cytology of indeterminate follicular or indeterminate Hurthle cell neoplasm. Thyroid Off J Am Thyroid Assoc. 2009;19(4):355–60. Epub 2009/04/10. eng.
39. Giorgadze T, Rossi ED, Fadda G, Gupta PK, Livolsi VA, Baloch Z. Does the fine-needle aspiration diagnosis of "Hurthle-cell neoplasm/follicular neoplasm with oncocytic features" denote increased risk of malignancy? Diagn Cytopathol. 2004;31(5):307–12. Epub 2004/10/07. eng.

40. Chen H, Nicol TL, Zeiger MA, Dooley WC, Ladenson PW, Cooper DS, et al. Hurthle cell neoplasms of the thyroid: are there factors predictive of malignancy? Ann Surg. 1998;227(4):542–6. Pubmed Central PMCID: 1191310.
41. Nayar R, Ivanovic M. The indeterminate thyroid fine-needle aspiration: experience from an academic center using terminology similar to that proposed in the 2007 National Cancer Institute Thyroid Fine Needle Aspiration State of the Science Conference. Cancer. 2009;117(3):195–202.
42. Banks ND, Kowalski J, Tsai HL, Somervell H, Tufano R, Dackiw AP, et al. A diagnostic predictor model for indeterminate or suspicious thyroid FNA samples. Thyroid Off J Am Thyroid Assoc. 2008;18(9):933–41.
43. Sclabas GM, Staerkel GA, Shapiro SE, Fornage BD, Sherman SI, Vassillopoulou-Sellin R, et al. Fine-needle aspiration of the thyroid and correlation with histopathology in a contemporary series of 240 patients. Am J Surg. 2003;186(6):702–9; discussion 9–10. Epub 2003/12/16. eng.
44. Smith M, Pantanowitz L, Khalbuss WE, Benkovich VA, Monaco SE. Indeterminate pediatric thyroid fine needle aspirations: a study of 68 cases. Acta Cytol. 2013;57(4):341–8.
45. Norlen O, Charlton A, Sarkis LM, Henwood T, Shun A, Gill AJ, et al. Risk of malignancy for each Bethesda class in pediatric thyroid nodules. J Pediatr Surg. 2015;50(7):1147–9. Epub 2015/03/19. eng.
46. Francis GL, Waguespack SG, Bauer AJ, Angelos P, Benvenga S, Cerutti JM, et al. Management guidelines for children with thyroid nodules and differentiated thyroid cancer. Thyroid Off J Am Thyroid Assoc. 2015;25(7):716–59.
47. Kamran SC, Marqusee E, Kim MI, Frates MC, Ritner J, Peters H, et al. Thyroid nodule size and prediction of cancer. J Clin Endocrinol Metab. 2013;98(2):564–70.
48. Tuttle RM, Lemar H, Burch HB. Clinical features associated with an increased risk of thyroid malignancy in patients with follicular neoplasia by fine-needle aspiration. Thyroid Off J Am Thyroid Assoc. 1998;8(5):377–83. Epub 1998/06/12. eng.
49. Zhang YW, Greenblatt DY, Repplinger D, Bargren A, Adler JT, Sippel RS, et al. Older age and larger tumor size predict malignancy in hurthle cell neoplasms of the thyroid. Ann Surg Oncol. 2008;15(10):2842–6.
50. Nam IC, Choi H, Kim ES, Mo EY, Park YH, Sun DI. Characteristics of thyroid nodules causing globus symptoms. Eur Arch otorhinolaryngol Off J Eur Fed Otorhinolaryngol Soc (EUFOS) Affiliated Ger Soc Otorhinolaryngology – Head Neck Surg. 2015;272(5):1181–8. Epub 2015/02/01. eng.
51. Kwak JY, Jung I, Baek JH, Baek SM, Choi N, Choi YJ, et al. Image reporting and characterization system for ultrasound features of thyroid nodules: multicentric Korean retrospective study. Korean J Radiol. 2013;14(1):110–7. Pubmed Central PMCID: Pmc3542293, Epub 2013/01/17. eng.
52. Mendez W, Rodgers SE, Lew JI, Montano R, Solorzano CC. Role of surgeon-performed ultrasound in predicting malignancy in patients with indeterminate thyroid nodules. Ann Surg Oncol. 2008;15(9):2487–92.
53. Khoncarly SM, Tamarkin SW, McHenry CR. Can ultrasound be used to predict malignancy in patients with a thyroid nodule and an indeterminate fine-needle aspiration biopsy? Surgery. 2014;156(4):967–70. Epub 2014/07/31. eng.
54. Rago T, Di Coscio G, Basolo F, Scutari M, Elisei R, Berti P, et al. Combined clinical, thyroid ultrasound and cytological features help to predict thyroid malignancy in follicular and Hupsilonrthle cell thyroid lesions: results from a series of 505 consecutive patients. Clin Endocrinol (Oxf). 2007;66(1):13–20. Epub 2007/01/05. eng.
55. Brito JP, Gionfriddo MR, Al Nofal A, Boehmer KR, Leppin AL, Reading C, et al. The accuracy of thyroid nodule ultrasound to predict thyroid cancer: systematic review and meta-analysis. J Clin Endocrinol Metab. 2014;99(4):1253–63. Pubmed Central PMCID: Pmc3973781, Epub 2013/11/28. eng.
56. LiVolsi VA, Asa SL. The demise of follicular carcinoma of the thyroid gland. Thyroid Off J Am Thyroid Assoc. 1994;4(2):233–6. Epub 1994/01/01. eng.

57. Vriens D, de Wilt JH, van der Wilt GJ, Netea-Maier RT, Oyen WJ, de Geus-Oei LF. The role of [18F]-2-fluoro-2-deoxy-d-glucose-positron emission tomography in thyroid nodules with indeterminate fine-needle aspiration biopsy: systematic review and meta-analysis of the literature. Cancer. 2011;117(20):4582–94. Epub 2011/03/25. eng.
58. Vriens D, Adang EM, Netea-Maier RT, Smit JW, de Wilt JH, Oyen WJ, et al. Cost-effectiveness of FDG-PET/CT for cytologically indeterminate thyroid nodules: a decision analytic approach. J Clin Endocrinol Metab. 2014;99(9):3263–74. Epub 2014/05/31. eng.
59. Lippolis PV, Tognini S, Materazzi G, Polini A, Mancini R, Ambrosini CE, et al. Is elastography actually useful in the presurgical selection of thyroid nodules with indeterminate cytology? J Clin Endocrinol Metab. 2011;96(11):E1826–30. Epub 2011/08/26. eng.
60. Trimboli P, Treglia G, Sadeghi R, Romanelli F, Giovanella L. Reliability of real-time elastography to diagnose thyroid nodules previously read at FNAC as indeterminate: a meta-analysis. Endocrine. 2015;50(2):335–43. Epub 2014/12/24. eng.
61. de Matos LL, Del Giglio AB, Matsubayashi CO, de Lima FM, Del Giglio A, da Silva Pinhal MA. Expression of CK-19, galectin-3 and HBME-1 in the differentiation of thyroid lesions: systematic review and diagnostic meta-analysis. Diagn Pathol. 2012;7:97. Pubmed Central PMCID: 3523001.
62. Bartolazzi A, Orlandi F, Saggiorato E, Volante M, Arecco F, Rossetto R, et al. Galectin-3-expression analysis in the surgical selection of follicular thyroid nodules with indeterminate fine-needle aspiration cytology: a prospective multicentre study. Lancet Oncol. 2008;9(6):543–9.
63. Lee EK, Chung KW, Min HS, Kim TS, Kim TH, Ryu JS, et al. Preoperative serum thyroglobulin as a useful predictive marker to differentiate follicular thyroid cancer from benign nodules in indeterminate nodules. J Korean Med Sci. 2012;27(9):1014–8. Pubmed Central PMCID: Pmc3429817, Epub 2012/09/13. eng.
64. Alexander EK, Kennedy GC, Baloch ZW, Cibas ES, Chudova D, Diggans J, et al. Preoperative diagnosis of benign thyroid nodules with indeterminate cytology. N Engl J Med. 2012;367(8):705–15.
65. Marti JL, Avadhani V, Donatelli LA, Niyogi S, Wang B, Wong RJ, et al. Wide inter-institutional variation in performance of a molecular classifier for indeterminate thyroid nodules. Ann Surg Oncol. 2015;22(12):3996–4001.
66. Ferris RL, Baloch Z, Bernet V, Chen A, Fahey 3rd TJ, Ganly I, et al. American thyroid association statement on surgical application of molecular profiling for thyroid nodules: current impact on perioperative decision making. Thyroid Off J Am Thyroid Assoc. 2015;25(7):760–8. Pubmed Central PMCID: 4519104.
67. Xing M, Haugen BR, Schlumberger M. Progress in molecular-based management of differentiated thyroid cancer. Lancet. 2013;381(9871):1058–69. Pubmed Central PMCID: 3931461.
68. Nikiforov YE, Yip L, Nikiforova MN. New strategies in diagnosing cancer in thyroid nodules: impact of molecular markers. Clin Cancer Res Off J Am Assoc Cancer Res. 2013;19(9):2283–8.
69. Fnais N, Soobiah C, Al-Qahtani K, Hamid JS, Perrier L, Straus SE, et al. Diagnostic value of fine needle aspiration BRAF(V600E) mutation analysis in papillary thyroid cancer: a systematic review and meta-analysis. Hum Pathol. 2015;46(10):1443–54.
70. Nikiforov YE, Ohori NP, Hodak SP, Carty SE, LeBeau SO, Ferris RL, et al. Impact of mutational testing on the diagnosis and management of patients with cytologically indeterminate thyroid nodules: a prospective analysis of 1056 FNA samples. J Clin Endocrinol Metab. 2011;96(11):3390–7. Pubmed Central PMCID: 3205883.
71. Yip L, Wharry LI, Armstrong MJ, Silbermann A, McCoy KL, Stang MT, et al. A clinical algorithm for fine-needle aspiration molecular testing effectively guides the appropriate extent of initial thyroidectomy. Ann Surg. 2014;260(1):163–8.
72. Nikiforov YE, Carty SE, Chiosea SI, Coyne C, Duvvuri U, Ferris RL, et al. Highly accurate diagnosis of cancer in thyroid nodules with follicular neoplasm/suspicious for a follicular neoplasm cytology by ThyroSeq v2 next-generation sequencing assay. Cancer. 2014;120(23):3627–34.

73. Nikiforov YE, Carty SE, Chiosea SI, Coyne C, Duvvuri U, Ferris RL, et al. Impact of the multi-gene ThyroSeq next-generation sequencing assay on cancer diagnosis in thyroid nodules with atypia of undetermined significance/follicular lesion of undetermined significance cytology. Thyroid Off J Am Thyroid Assoc. 2015;25:1217–23.
74. Labourier E, Shifrin A, Busseniers AE, Lupo MA, Manganelli ML, Andruss B, et al. Molecular testing for miRNA, mRNA, and DNA on fine-needle aspiration improves the preoperative diagnosis of thyroid nodules with indeterminate cytology. J Clin Endocrinol Metab. 2015;100(7):2743–50. Pubmed Central PMCID: 4490308.
75. Tufano RP, Teixeira GV, Bishop J, Carson KA, Xing M. BRAF mutation in papillary thyroid cancer and its value in tailoring initial treatment: a systematic review and meta-analysis. Medicine. 2012;91(5):274–86.
76. Aragon Han P, Kim HS, Cho S, Fazeli R, Najafian A, Khawaja H, et al. Association of BRAF mutation and MicroRNA expression with central lymph node metastases in papillary thyroid cancer: a prospective study from four endocrine surgery centers. Thyroid Off J Am Thyroid Assoc. 2016;26(4):532–42.
77. Gouveia C, Can NT, Bostrom A, Grenert JP, van Zante A, Orloff LA. Lack of association of BRAF mutation with negative prognostic indicators in papillary thyroid carcinoma: the university of California, San Francisco, experience. JAMA Otolaryngol Head Neck Surg. 2013;139(11):1164–70.
78. Yip L, Nikiforova MN, Yoo JY, McCoy KL, Stang MT, Armstrong MJ, et al. Tumor genotype determines phenotype and disease-related outcomes in thyroid cancer: a study of 1510 patients. Ann Surg. 2015;262(3):519–25; discussion 24–5.
79. Melo M, da Rocha AG, Vinagre J, Batista R, Peixoto J, Tavares C, et al. TERT promoter mutations are a major indicator of poor outcome in differentiated thyroid carcinomas. J Clin Endocrinol Metab. 2014;99(5):E754–65. Pubmed Central PMCID: 4191548.
80. Nikiforova MN, Wald AI, Roy S, Durso MB, Nikiforov YE. Targeted next-generation sequencing panel (ThyroSeq) for detection of mutations in thyroid cancer. J Clin Endocrinol Metab. 2013;98(11):E1852–60. Pubmed Central PMCID: 3816258, Epub August 26, 2013.
81. Hyeon J, Ahn S, Shin JH, Oh YL. The prediction of malignant risk in the category "atypia of undetermined significance/follicular lesion of undetermined significance" of the Bethesda System for Reporting Thyroid Cytopathology using subcategorization and BRAF mutation results. Cancer Cytopathol. 2014;122(5):368–76.
82. Network NCC. Thyroid Carcinoma (Version 2.2015). Available from: http://www.nccn.org/professionals/physician_gls/pdf/thyroid.pdf.

Part IV
Papillary Thyroid Cancer

Chapter 11
Staging for Papillary Thyroid Cancer

Heather Stuart, Steven Rodgers, and Janice L. Pasieka

Staging for Papillary Thyroid Cancer

Staging systems for malignant tumors are constantly evolving and being updated based on new knowledge about each disease. The basis for developing accurate systems for staging is multifold: (1) to estimate the prognosis of patients and help develop treatment plans, (2) to standardize communication of a patient's status between health-care providers, and (3) to establish a foundation for research allowing for comparison of disease states [1]. Thyroid cancer staging has been reevaluated by many groups over time, each with the goal of identifying a model that would accurately predict disease-related mortality and recurrence risk. The large majority of models include patient age at diagnosis, tumor size, presence of metastasis, and a descriptor for tumor invasion outside the capsule (i.e., extrathyroidal extension). About half of thyroid staging systems use local lymph node status as a prognostic factor and even

H. Stuart, MD, FRCSC
Department of Surgery, Division of Surgical Oncology, University of Miami Miller School of Medicine, Miami, FL, USA

Department of Surgery, Sections of General Surgery and Surgical Oncology, University of Calgary, Cunning School of Medicine, Calgary, AB, Canada

S. Rodgers, MD, PhD, FACS
Department of Surgery, Division of Surgical Oncology, University of Miami Miller School of Medicine, Miami, FL, USA

J.L. Pasieka, MD, FRCSC, FACS (✉)
Department of Surgery, Sections of General Surgery and Surgical Oncology, University of Calgary, Cunning School of Medicine, Calgary, AB, Canada

Department of Surgery and Oncology, Faculty of Medicine, University of Calgary, Foothills Medical Centre, 1403 29th St NW, North Tower, Calgary, AB T2N 2T9, Canada
e-mail: janice.pasieka@ahs.ca

S.A. Roman et al. (eds.), *Management of Thyroid Nodules and Differentiated Thyroid Cancer*, DOI 10.1007/978-3-319-43618-0_11

fewer attempt to incorporate additional characteristics such as tumor grade and/or histological features, DNA ploidy, or completeness of surgical resection [2]. In an attempt to understand what are the most important factors in predicting thyroid cancer outcomes, the above characteristics can be globally categorized into (1) patient risk factors, (2) preoperative findings, (3) intraoperative findings, and (4) postoperative findings. The following chapter will explore some of the rationale behind the evaluation of staging systems before examining pertinent patient factors and perioperative findings that are relevant in papillary thyroid cancer (PTC) staging.

Thyroid Cancer Staging Systems

Thyroid cancer staging systems are subdivided according to their histological type. Differentiated thyroid cancers [3, 4] (papillary and follicular) were distinguished from undifferentiated thyroid cancers (medullary and anaplastic) and then further separated to have specific staging systems exclusive to papillary thyroid cancer (PTC) [5–7]. At least 17 different systems have been proposed; however, despite numerous studies to determine the most accurate system in predicting prognosis, the results are inconsistent [2]. The proportion of variance explained (PVE) is the most recognized statistical method of evaluating staging systems. PVE uses Cox proportional hazard analysis to assess how well a staging system can predict a population event. As the value approaches 100 %, the staging system is determined to be more accurate in predicting outcomes [8]. The American Joint Committee on Cancer (AJCC) TNM staging system (Table 11.2) is one of the most commonly used systems, but even this model has relatively low PVE scores (10–33 %) depending on the population it is evaluating [4, 9]. Not only are the PVE scores consistently low, but they demonstrate considerable variability when applied to comparable populations. Other well-known prognostic scoring systems for differentiated thyroid cancer (AGES [6], AMES [3], and MACIS [5]) also display low PVE scores with significant variability (23–46 %, 9–40 %, 15–48 %, respectively) [9]. It is also important to note that PVE scores are consistently low (less than 50 %) for any thyroid cancer staging system developed to date, indicating that the accuracy of predicting events, for even the best system, is limited.

The variability in PVE of a system and between systems occurs for a multitude of reasons. First, the creation of each prognostic system (with the exception of TNM) was based on a population that was reported on in the same study. This generates a bias of the system to the population it is analyzing and makes it difficult to achieve the same prognostic score when applied to a subsequent population [10]. The TNM classification has an advantage of being empirically derived; this has the potential to remove some of the bias that exists from systems created from a preexisting population. Secondly, there have been a number of models for calculating PVE proposed over time, but none have emerged as superior. The caveat to this calculation also rests on the basis that the accuracy of the prediction model increases with the risk of event occurrence in the population [8]. This makes it difficult to produce a prediction model for PTC because the indolent nature of the disease makes the overall event rate low. This factor is exacerbated for thyroid cancer over time because the increasing numbers of small tumors (<1 cm) that are discovered and treated make the proportional event rate even lower [11].

Consistently over time, the TNM staging model has emerged among the top models for predicting differentiated thyroid cancer-related death and loss of life expectancy [12]. However, when predictive models for PTC alone are evaluated, the MACIS scoring system is often the most accurate [2, 13]. The MACIS (metastases, age, completeness of resection, invasion, and size) scoring system was described at the Mayo Clinic in 1993 and uses proportions of age and tumor size in addition to resection status, presence of invasion, and/or metastases to produce a score that predicts a cause-specific survival rate (Table 11.1) [5]. While this system utilizes the completeness of resection and presence of invasion outside the thyroid capsule, it does not incorporate the presence of locally involved lymph nodes. Although regional LN metastasis have been shown in some studies to be a predictive factor for increasing the risk of local recurrence [14], they do not appear to affect long-term survival, especially in those patients that do not have local invasion or metastatic disease.

Preoperative Assessment

The initial assessment of a patient with thyroid cancer begins with a focused history for intrinsic and acquired risk factors and a physical exam, including neck ultrasound, for local, regional, and metastatic disease. Review of pathology, indicated imaging, and the possibility of genetic analysis are also parts of the preoperative assessment.

Risk Factors

The main acquired risk factor for PTC is exposure to radiation, either external or internal. External radiation exposure is typically in the form of x-rays or radiation therapy for cancer or benign disease. Internal radiation exposure in the setting of

Table 11.1 Twenty-year disease-specific survival (DSS) rates bases on MACIS (metastases, age, completeness of resection, invasion, sizes) score

MACIS score	20 year DSS (%)
<6	99
6–6.99	89
7–7.99	56
>8	24

Score = 3.1 (if aged < or = 39 years) or 0.08 × age (if aged > or = 40 years), + 0.3 × tumor size (in centimeters), +1 (if incompletely resected), +1 (if locally invasive), +3 (if distant metastases present)

radioactive particle ingestion is most commonly related to nuclear fallout (e.g., Chernobyl) or radioactive iodine treatment. The risk for developing thyroid cancer following radiation exposure is increased even with small doses, as low as 100 mGy. The relative risk of developing thyroid cancer is dose dependent initially (RR 6.8 with 2–4Gy), but then plateaus between exposures of 5–30Gy (RR14.8–15.2) and begins to decrease after 30Gy (RR 5.1–9.3) [15]. The risk is greatest in patients less than 15 years old and returns to almost baseline risk for exposures after age 20. Despite the increase in relative risk of developing thyroid cancer following radiation exposure, these cancers have similar recurrence rates following treatment (7–28 % in the short term) and similar long-term mortality (<1 % at 10 year) [16]. Therefore, a history of radiation exposure should warrant surveillance for thyroid cancer incidence but does not significantly impact prognosis or treatment [17].

The most common non-modifiable risk factors for PTC include family history, age, and sex. Familial inheritance of thyroid cancer is largely associated with medullary thyroid cancer - up to 25 % of medullary cancers are familial. However, there are some syndromes that have been linked to differentiated thyroid cancers. Familial adenomatous polyposis (FAP) is a syndrome primarily known for the development of innumerable colonic polyps that undergo malignant transformation over a short time period. Among the other extra-colonic malignancies associated with this syndrome are differentiated thyroid cancer, childhood hepatoblastoma, and medulloblastomas. These patients have a 2–12 % incidence of PTC (compared with 0.2 % in the general population), specifically a cribriform variant that is seen almost exclusively in FAP patients [18–20]. These cancers are often bilateral, occur in young female patients, and have similar prognosis to non-FAP-related PTC. Because of the increased incidence in this population and the low sensitivity of physical exam for detection, several studies suggest that screening thyroid ultrasound should be instituted in patients known to have FAP, although the age and interval to initiate this have not been determined [21, 22].

Other genetic syndromes, such as Cowden's syndrome, Carney's complex, and Werner's syndrome, have an association with thyroid cancer, but they are largely linked to follicular thyroid cancer rather than papillary. Screening for thyroid cancer is recommended for these patients, although there is no documentation of inferior outcomes based on an underlying genetic mutation [23].

Familial non-medullary thyroid cancer (FNMTC), the majority of which are PTC, account for 3.2–6.2 % of thyroid cancers and follow an autosomal dominant pattern of inheritance. The diagnosis is established in patients with non-medullary thyroid cancer, in the absence of predisposing hereditary syndromes (e.g., FAP) or environmental risk factors (e.g., radiation exposure), and two or more first-degree relatives with thyroid cancer. If three or more family members are affected, it is 94 % likely that there is a familial predisposition [24]. Thyroid tumors of affected individuals are thought to have a more aggressive biology with increased incidence of multifocality and higher risk of recurrence [25, 26]. The data to support this is mixed with other studies suggesting no difference in pathophysiology compared to nonfamilial tumors [27]. A number of genes have been linked with FNMTC, most recently a germ line mutation in the HABP2 gene. This mutation was found in all members of a kindred with FNMTC and 4.7 % of a population of patients with sporadic thyroid cancer making it a strong candidate for a susceptibility gene [28]. Currently the recommendation is to perform a total thyroidectomy with strong consideration of CLND in patients with FNMTC. Screening is generally agreed upon for family members of affected patients beginning by age 20 or 5–10 years before the age of the youngest diagnosed member [29].

Thyroid cancer staging has always uniquely included age at diagnosis as a significant prognostic indicator of survival. The large majority of staging systems include age [1, 3–7, 30] as a risk factor with studies historically showing an improved survival associated with younger age at diagnosis. This finding has extended into the AJCC/UICC TNM staging system such that patients younger than 45 years old can only be maximally staged as stage II, regardless of the presence of distant metastatic disease (Table 11.2). The exact cutoff is somewhat arbitrary, typically around age 45 years, but most systems recognize age as a prognosticator of survival. The knowledge of thyroid cancer tumor cell biology does not provide a complete understanding of the contribution of age to survival, and it does not signify that young patients cannot have poor outcomes. In fact, young patients with metastatic disease have worse outcomes than older patients with localized disease. One study demonstrated a 50 % increase in mortality in patients from age 30 to age 40 years, and this increase continued to double for each 10-year increment thereafter. This finding translated into a rise in the overall risk of mortality for patients between stage I and stage II (HR 1.38, $p=0.2$). When this is sub-stratified, the risk is ameliorated with older patients and exacerbated with younger patients (HR 11.48, $p<0.001$) [31].

Additional studies have investigated the specific age at which patients are separated into low and high risk. A recent study suggested that an age of 55 years rather than 45 years may be a more accurate predictor of disease-specific survival (DSS). For localized and metastatic disease, age was the most significant predictor of outcome, with age cutoffs of 56 and 54 years, respectively [32]. Similarly, another study investigating the effect of age and gender on DSS showed that men and women older than 55 years had similar outcomes, while women diagnosed at an age less that 55 years had improved outcomes over men [33]. Therefore, while one can be confident that age does affect survival, the relationship is complex and likely involves additional factors that have not been fully identified or quantified at this time.

Male gender has long been considered a risk factor for developing more aggressive thyroid cancer. The incidence of PTC in women is three times that of men, and men present with more advanced tumors leading to inferior outcomes [34]. However, when further evaluated, women tend to present at a younger age and with earlier-stage tumors, so when matched by stage, men have similar outcomes to women. Additionally, when survival curves for men and women are compared to the general population, the female advantage seen in thyroid cancer outcomes mimics the

Table 11.2 AJCC/UICC TNM staging system for differentiated thyroid cancer

Primary tumor (T)	
TX	Primary tumor cannot be assessed
T0	No evidence of primary tumor
T1	Tumor ≤ 2 cm in greatest dimension, limited to the thyroid
T1a	Tumor ≤ 1 cm, limited to the thyroid
T1b	Tumor > 1 cm but ≤ 2 cm, limited to the thyroid
T2	Tumor > 2 cm but ≤ 4 cm, limited to the thyroid
T3	Tumor > 4 cm in greatest dimension Limited to the thyroid or with minimal extrathyroidal extension
T4a	Moderately advanced disease Tumor of any size extending beyond thyroid capsule to invade subcutaneous soft tissue, larynx, trachea, esophagus, or RLN
T4b	Very advanced disease Tumor invades prevertebral fascia or encases carotid artery or mediastinal vessels
Regional lymph nodes (N)	
NX	Regional lymph nodes cannot be assessed
N0	No regional lymph node metastasis
N1	Regional lymph node metastasis
N1a	Metastasis to level VI (pretracheal, paratracheal, and prelaryngeal/Delphian lymph nodes)
N1b	Metastasis to unilateral, bilateral, or contralateral cervical (levels I, II, III, IV, or V) or retropharyngeal or superior mediastinal lymph nodes (level VII)

Distant metastasis (M)	
M0	No distant metastasis
M1	Distant metastasis

Anatomic stage/prognostic group			
Under 45 years old			
Stage I	Any T	Any N	M0
Stage II	Any T	Any N	M1
45 years and older			
Stage I	T1	N0	M0
Stage II	T2	N0	M0
Stage III	T3 T1 T2 T3	N0 N1a N1a N1a	M0 M0 M0 M0
Stage IVA	T4a T4a T1 T2 T3 T4a	N0 N1a N1b N1b N1b N1b	M0 M0 M0 M0 M0 M0
Stage IVB	T4b	Any N	M0
Stage IVC	Any T	Any N	M1

Adapted from Edge and American Joint Committee on Cancer [4]

survival advantage seen in the general population. When a cohort of 3572 patients was separated into those younger and older than 55 years, females younger than 55 had better DSS for PTC compared to men; however, the outcomes were similar between genders when evaluating patients older than 55 years [33]. One explanation for this is the theory of estrogen modulation of tumor biology, in which more frequent but less aggressive tumors develop during the period of estrogen exposure. Conversely, more aggressive tumors may develop in postmenopausal women [35]. There are obviously multiple factors that contribute to tumor biology and prognosis in different populations, and the excellent overall long-term survival of thyroid cancer patients makes it difficult to study treatment effects. It is currently accepted that risk factors are taken into consideration in patient management, but there are no specific guidelines for changes in treatment or surveillance.

In addition to screening for risk factors for development of PTC, patients should be asked about physical findings that would increase their risk of malignancy - rapid growth of a solitary nodule or compressive symptoms (dysphagia, dysphonia, cough/dyspnea, hoarseness). These symptoms are not diagnostic of malignancy, but their presence would increase clinical suspicion and warrant timely investigation.

Physical Examination

The physical examination for suspicious or confirmed thyroid cancer historically has relied upon manual palpation of the thyroid gland and regional lymph nodes. However, examination has expanded over time to include ultrasound of the neck (performed in clinic) and laryngoscopy. Direct examination of the thyroid should focus on the consistency of the gland, fixation to adjacent structures, and size of the nodule - nodules measuring greater than 4 cm have a 26 % chance of harboring a clinically significant thyroid cancer [36]. Fine-needle aspiration (FNA) is the recommended method of further evaluating thyroid nodules. It can be performed by palpation or under ultrasound guidance. The Bethesda system provides a framework with which to interpret FNA results, and if cytology is suspicious for or diagnostic of PTC, the patient should go on to have surgical management [37].

A thorough evaluation for enlarged cervical lymph nodes should cover levels II through VI [4]. Levels II–IV are found adjacent to and around the carotid sheath, often posterior to the sternocleidomastoid muscle, with II between the level of the base of the skull and hyoid, III being between the level of the hyoid and cricoid cartilage, and IV being between the cricoid cartilage and the clavicle. Level V consists of the transverse cervical chain and posterior triangle lymph nodes, and level VI comprises the central compartment between the carotid sheaths transversely and the hyoid and sternal notch longitudinally (Fig. 11.1). Lymphadenopathy is common in PTC - it is grossly evident in 20–50 % of cases and microscopically presents in up to 90 % [37]. Despite the necessity of the manual exam, there is a high degree of variability in exam findings even between specialists, which is improved significantly with the use of ultrasound [38].

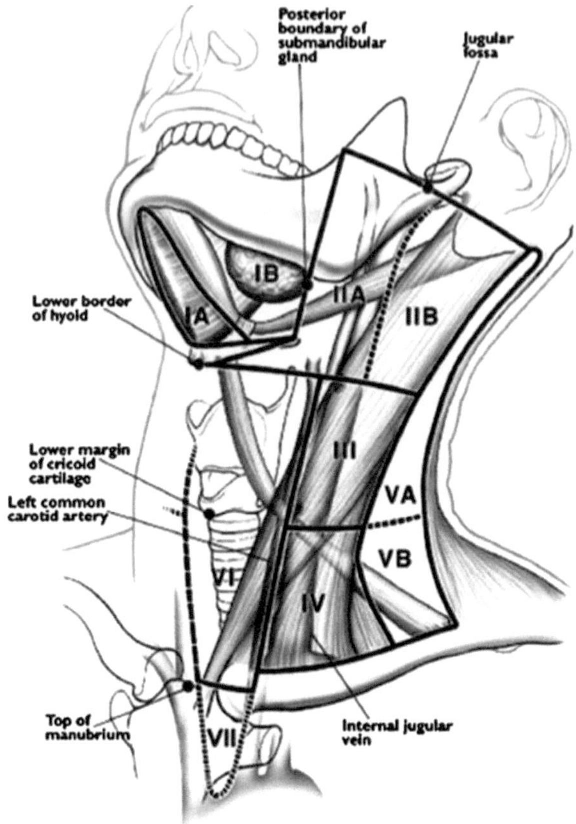

Fig. 11.1 Neck lymph node levels and compartments (With permission from Elsevier [89])

Preoperative Imaging

The use of ultrasonography significantly improved the ability of clinicians to assess for lateral and central compartment lymphadenopathy in several studies - detecting 14–20 % additional lymph nodes not detected on physical exam for patients undergoing primary surgery and 28–64 % in patients having re-operative surgery [39, 40]. The finding of non-palpable cervical chain lymph nodes on ultrasound leads to a change in the operative plan in 40 % of patients [39]. Although ultrasound cannot distinguish definitively between benign and malignant characteristics of nodules or lymph nodes, there are several findings that increase the suspicion of malignancy. Hypoechogenicity, microcalcifications, irregular margins, increased blood flow, and the absence of a halo have median sensitivities and specificities ranging from 52 to 81 % and 53 to 83 %, respectively, for malignant thyroid nodules. Sonographically, metastatic lymph nodes characteristically have a larger ratio of short to long axis (making the nodes rounder), a hyperechoic cortex, intranodal calcifications and cystic necrosis, loss of echogenic hilum, and a peripheral or diffuse vascular pattern

[41]. Suspicious lymph nodes that are identified clinically or on imaging should be biopsied with ultrasound-guided FNA and sent for cytology or thyroglobulin levels. Preoperative lymph node mapping is considered the standard of care for patients having surgery for thyroid malignancy [37].

In the past, preoperative laryngoscopy was reserved for patients presenting with complaints of voice abnormalities or clinical evidence of tumor invasion; however, several studies have shown poor correlation between patient reporting and confirmed vocal cord dysfunction [42, 43]. And while surgeon assessed voice abnormalities and a patient history of neck surgery are reasonable starting points for establishing who should have laryngoscopy, it is advocated by many that it should performed in all thyroid cancer patients preoperatively [43, 44]. Ultrasound assessment of vocal cord function may be another screening tool easily performed in the office to help select those patients for whom laryngoscopic visualization of the vocal cords is necessary [45–47].

Computed tomography (CT) and magnetic resonance imaging (MRI) are not recommended as routine modalities for preoperative imaging of the thyroid. Ultrasound is less expensive and accurate and avoids radiation exposure and is therefore generally sufficient in preoperative staging. However, there are instances when cross-sectional imaging with CT or MRI may contribute to clinical decision making, such as when there is physical evidence of invasion, incomplete evaluation of a large tumor or bulky nodes seen on ultrasound (e.g., tumor/node extension into the mediastinum), or any question about anatomic extent of disease [48]. The utilization of enhanced CT scanning preoperatively may delay the use of RAI treatment for several weeks postoperatively due to the iodine load of intravenous contrast. However, contrasted CT scans are necessary to avoid an incomplete resection; therefore, the benefit of a good preoperative imaging and planning may outweigh the mild potential delay in postoperative radioactive iodine treatment.

Positron emission tomography (PET) or PET-CT is typically reserved for evaluating patients for persistent or recurrent disease and non-RAI avid disease; its role is not established as a primary preoperative imaging modality [48]. It is most useful to assess for recurrent disease or as part of a surveillance program, and its findings have been shown to alter management in up to 30% of recurrent cases [49].

Histopathology

Preoperatively, FNA is performed to obtain a cytological diagnosis of thyroid cancer. Papillary thyroid cancer has several typical findings that are not pathognomonic but are frequently present. These include the presence of (1) papillae formed by layers of tumor cells; (2) large, overlapping, oval-shaped nuclei containing hypodense chromatin and cytoplasmic inclusion bodies (Orphan Annie eye nuclei); (3) nuclear grooves; and (4) psammoma bodies. The impact of the pathological diagnosis becomes more important when variants of PTC are identified; however, these are usually only recognized on postoperative histology. Variants associated with a poorer prognosis include tall cell, diffuse sclerosing, and insular variants. Others with a more favorable prognosis include follicular, solid, trabecular, oncocytic, microfollicular, pseudo-Warthin, and clear cell variants [50]. The incidence of the tall cell variant ranges from 1 to 19 % of PTC, and histologically this subset lives up to its name in that 30 % of cells are twice as long as they are wide. Diffuse sclerosing variant has an incidence of 2–6 %, and in addition to classic PTC features, it exhibits stromal fibrosis, lymphocytic infiltration, and squamous metaplasia. These two variants were described in a paper by Kazaure et al., which reviewed outcomes of over 43,000 cases of PTC from the SEER database. They showed increased incidence of extrathyroidal extension, multifocality, nodal and distant metastases in tall cell, and diffuse sclerosing variants when compared to classic PTC (Table 11.3). Additionally, there was a significant decrease in 5-year disease-specific survival between tall cell and classic PTC (87.5 vs. 97.4, $p<0.001$) [51]. Insular variants also

Table 11.3 Pathologic characteristics of 43,738 patients with aggressive variants and classic PTC, SEER (1988–2008)

Characteristic	DSV ($n=261$)	TCV ($n=573$)	Papillary (classic) ($n=42{,}904$)	*P*
Tumor size (cm), mean (SEM)[a]	1.7 (1.0)	2.7 (0.8)	1.8 (0.1)	<0.001
≤1.0	46.3	16.5	36.2	
1.1–2.0	27.5	28.8	31.4	
2.1–4.0	15.8	35.9	25.2	
>4.0	10.4	18.8	7.2	
Focality: multifocal	29.5	29.3	26.7	<0.001
Extrathyroidal extension	31.0	54.7	20.1	<0.001
≥1 positive lymph node[b]	72.2	66.8	56.3	<0.001
Median (IQR)	4 (1–11)	3 (1–7)	3 (1–7)	
SEER stage[c]				<0.001
Localized	48.1	28.3	58.2	
Regional	44.6	60.6	37.5	
Distant	7.3	11.1	4.3	
5-year overall survival	87.5	80.6	93.5	<0.001
5-year disease-specific survival	96.1	87.5	97.4	<0.001

With kind permission from Springer Science+Business Media: Table 11.2 [51]

Unless otherwise noted, characteristics are in percentages; percentages have been rounded and may not add up to 100

SEM standard error of mean, *IQR* interquartile range, *DSV* diffuse sclerosing variant, *TCV* tall cell variant

[a]Tumor size (*n*): data available for 88.1, 92.8, and 89.2 % of DSV, TCV, and classic PTC, respectively

[b]Analyses performed for patients who had ≥1 lymph node examined

[c]SEER stage: data missing for approximately 0.04 % DSV, 1.2 % TCV, and 2.6 % of classic PTC, respectively

have an inferior prognosis compared with classic PTC. These variants are described as existing in "nests" or insulae of tumor cells. They typically form large tumors and are prone to extrathyroidal extension (47 %), lymph node metastases (62 %), and distant metastatic disease (30 %). These patients have a decreased 5-year DSS compared with classic PTC (73 vs. 97 %, $p < 0.001$) [52].

Molecular Profiling

The preoperative assessment for papillary thyroid cancer has recently expanded from a detailed history, physical exam, and imaging to include molecular profiling. In the last two decades, many advances have been made that identify genetic mutations present in cancer with several specific mutations that are found frequently in thyroid cancer. The most frequently discussed mutation is BRAF, an isoform of the RAF (rapidly accelerated fibrosarcoma) gene. It is mutated in papillary thyroid cancer in 30–80 % of cases [53, 54]. The BRAF protein acts in the RAF/MEK/MAPK pathway and, when mutated, forms the BRAFV600E protein, which is constitutively activated. The BRAF mutation has been described in melanoma and colon cancer, but is most frequently associated with PTC. Over the last 10 years, there have been a number of studies associating BRAFV600E with invasive growth patterns, increased risk of recurrence, and higher mortality [55, 56]. However, there have also been several studies that have failed to replicate these findings and support a less aggressive tumor biology associated with mutation [57, 58]. There is also some evidence that unless there is a clinically relevant change in management based on BRAF status, the financial implications of genetic analysis might outweigh any benefit [59].

Other genes implicated in PTC that also play a role in the MAPK activation pathway are RET and RAS. The RET gene undergoes rearrangements leading to chimeric genes that are constitutively active; these are referred to as RET/PTC. Germ line mutations in RET/PTC are the cause of medullary thyroid cancer in MEN2 syndromes; however, this gene product is not expressed in normal thyroid cells, which explains why PTC is not seen in MEN2 patients. Somatic rearrangements associated with PTC are present in approximately 40 % of sporadic cases [60, 61]. RAS mutations are most commonly found in follicular adenomas, suggesting that these mutations may lead to a more benign phenotypic outcome; however, they have been described in follicular variants of papillary thyroid cancer [62].

Recently, Yip et al. reported on the correlation of clinical outcomes with specific genetic mutations in a study of 1510 patients with thyroid cancer (97 % PTC). They showed that patients with a RAS mutation had a low incidence of extrathyroidal extension (4.6 %) and lymph node metastases (LNM) (5.6 %) compared to patients with a BRAFV600E mutation that had significantly higher incidences (extrathyroidal extension 51 %, LNM 46 %). Additionally when grouped into histologically similar tumors, BRAFV600E and RET/PTC mutations were associated more often with stage III/IV disease (40 vs. 15 %, $p < 0.001$) and recurrence (10 vs. 0.7 %,

$p<0.001$) compared with tumors containing RAS or PAX8/PPARG mutations [63]. Some of the newer gene sequencing assays have been reported to have a high sensitivity (90.9 %) and specificity (92.1 %) for detecting gene mutations and classifying thyroid cancers [64]. The potential to characterize the molecular identity of tumors preoperatively may help to guide management of individuals based on tumor biology.

Intraoperative Assessment

Thyroid Gland Assessment

The main objectives intraoperatively are to perform an appropriate oncologic resection and to minimize the risk of postoperative complications. The thyroid gland and cervical lymph nodes are assessed preoperatively, but the accuracy of determining specific characteristics such as extrathyroidal extension of the primary tumor or metastatic lymph node deposits is limited (sensitivity and specificity for each was 60 and 80 % for extrathyroidal extension and 83 and 87 % for lymph node metastasis [40, 65]). Gross invasion of tumor into the strap muscles necessitate an en bloc resection of the involved muscles. Suspicion of tracheal invasion not predicted preoperatively can be difficult to confirm and may require frozen sections to establish whether resection is warranted. The reported positive and negative predictive values of frozen section evaluation of invasion were 98 % and 87 %, respectively. This works well when extrathyroidal extension is detected but runs the risk of performing an inferior resection for 13 % of patients when it is not detected [66].

The decision tree regarding surgical management of the thyroid in PTC typically leads to either a total thyroidectomy or a lobectomy. The American Thyroid Association (ATA) guidelines from 2015 recommend that for patients with tumors greater than 4 cm, gross extra thyroidal extension, or regional or distant metastases, a total thyroidectomy should be preformed. This facilitates the used of RAI postoperatively and reduces risk of recurrence in this higher risk group [37, 67, 68]. It is also generally accepted that patients with contralateral nodules, regional or distant metastases, history of radiation exposure to the head and neck, or a first-degree family member with thyroid cancer should undergo a total thyroidectomy. Age greater than 45 years is also a relative indication for total thyroidectomy [37]. Patients with low-risk tumors, between 1 and 4 cm that are intrathyroidal and clinically node negative, can be considered for either a lobectomy or a total thyroidectomy. Recent studies have demonstrated no difference in 10-year overall survival or disease-specific survival between low-risk patients having a lobectomy versus a total thyroidectomy with tumors up to 4 cm. The decision may be influenced by the requirement for postoperative RAI and/or patient preference. Thyroid lobectomy is the accepted surgical approach for tumors less than 1 cm in the absence of extrathyroidal disease [37].

Lymph Node Assessment

Central Compartment Lymph Nodes

Grossly positive central compartment lymph nodes should be removed at the time of the operation. This may also include removal of lymph nodes from level VII (mediastinal compartment), as up to 38 % are positive when the central compartment is involved [69]. The management of clinically negative lymph nodes in papillary thyroid cancer is an area of ongoing controversy. Several centers have demonstrated no clinically meaningful improvement with the addition of a prophylactic central compartment lymph node dissection (pCLND) [70, 71], whereas others have demonstrated significant impact depending on the number of lymph nodes involved [72]. The decision of whether to perform or not perform a pCLND is complicated by the high incidence of lymph node metastases in even low-risk cancers (20–90 % [39, 73]) and the uncertain impact that involved lymph nodes have on recurrence and mortality [71]. The current ATA guidelines for central compartment lymph node dissection (CLND) are based on expert consensus opinion. They recommend a bilateral CLND for patients with clinically positive central or lateral lymph nodes. The guidelines also provide a weak recommendation for prophylactic ipsilateral or bilateral CLND if the primary tumor is T3 or greater, if there are clinically positive lateral neck lymph nodes in the setting of clinically negative central neck lymph nodes. If the primary tumor is T1 or T2 and noninvasive, CLND may be avoided [37]. A number of authors have investigated the short- and long-term effects of pCLND, but no definitive evidence exists as to the benefit. In 2006, Sywak et al. reported lower thyroglobulin levels post radioactive iodine (RAI) treatment in patients that had undergone ipsilateral pCLND [74]. This is important because thyroglobulin levels are used as a marker for recurrence following surgery and ablative therapy. However, in 2010 Hughes et al. published a report saying that although prophylactic central and lateral lymph node dissections (LLND) upstaged 29 % of patients, with increased doses of RAI ablation postoperatively, thyroglobulin levels were similar at 1-year post ablation [75]. A meta-analysis published in 2010 showed no difference in local recurrence between patients having a total thyroidectomy versus a total thyroidectomy with pCLND [76]. However, a recently updated meta-analysis found a trend toward lower recurrence rates in those undergoing a pCLND with an intention to treat of 31 patients [77]. Some argue that regardless of outcome, pCLND should be used as a staging investigation; however, this needs to be balanced with the risk of complications associated with a neck dissection [68]. The advantages of pCLND would be the ability to administer RAI at a dose proportional to the number of LNM, to provide therapeutic benefit if LNM are present and to prevent further dissection in a re-operative field [78]. However, there is still a significant risk of postoperative complications, especially when performed outside of high volume centers. Transient hypocalcemia is the most commonly reported (0.6–46 %), but permanent hypocalcemia (1.8–11.8 %), temporary or permanent nerve injury (0–11.8 % and 0–5.9 %), chyle leak (<1–8.3 %), hemorrhage (0–1.8 %), and wound infection (0–1.8 %) are other possible complications [74, 75, 78–80]. Therefore, although there is no clear recurrence benefit for pCLND, it can be considered in patients with high-risk tumors as suggested by the tumor size recommendation in the ATA guidelines.

Lateral Lymph Nodes

Lateral neck lymph node dissection has a strong recommendation with moderate evidence (Table 11.4) recommendation from the ATA for biopsy-proven LNM in the lateral neck [37]. It is generally not performed in a prophylactic setting, although some groups do advocate for this on the basis of guiding RAI treatment [78]. The original radical neck dissection described by Crile in 1906 included an en bloc resection of all the lateral neck lymphatic tissue (levels I–V), as well as the internal jugular vein, the sternocleidomastoid muscle, the submandibular gland, and the spinal accessory nerve. With the recognition that radical surgery did not improve outcomes, the procedure evolved into a modified radical neck dissection that removes lymph node levels I through V, but preserves non-lymphatic structures. This was further adapted to a selective neck dissection that preserves non-lymphatic structures and selective lymph node levels depending on the site of the primary tumor and stage [81]. The approach most commonly used for PTC is a selective neck dissection that includes dissection of the lymph node levels mostly likely to harbor LNM, specifically II, III, IV, VI, and sometimes V (Fig. 11.1). Roh *et al.* reported in 2008 that for PTC with clinically positive lateral neck LNM, the distribution of positivity was 84.6 % level VI, 75.9 % level IV, 72.2 % level IIa and III, 16.7 % level IIb, 13 % level Va (inferior portion), 3.7 % level Vb, and 0 % level Va (superior portion). Eighty percent of patients had multilevel LNM and 9.6 % had lateral LNM without central LNM (skip metastases) [82]. With this understanding of nodal drainage for PTC, a lymph node dissection routinely includes levels IIa, III, IV, and Vb with levels IIb and Va selectively dissected based on the presence or close vicinity of clinically positive lymph nodes in these levels [83]. Level I is not routinely dissected for PTC. In summary, patients with PTC and clinically determined lateral LNM should undergo a selective lateral lymph node dissection of levels IIa, III, IV, and Vb with the inclusion of IIb and Va if there is increased suspicion of LNM in these regions.

Postoperative Assessment

Postoperative restaging is important because of the potential for new diagnostic information collected from the resected specimen. Tumor size, the presence of extrathyroidal extension, lymph node status, and histology all contribute not only to determining the recurrence risk but also to guide postoperative management and surveillance strategies. Recently there has been increasing evidence that the risk of

Table 11.4 Recommendations (for diagnostic intervention) based on strength of evidence

Recommendation and evidence quality	Methodologic quality of supporting evidence	Interpretation
Strong recommendation		
High-quality evidence	Evidence from one or more well-designed nonrandomized diagnostic accuracy studies (i.e., observational – cross-sectional or cohort) or systematic reviews/meta-analysis of such observations studies (with non concern about internal validity or external generalizability of the results)	Implies the test can be offered to most patients in most applicable circumstances without reservation
Moderate-quality evidence	Evidence from nonrandomized diagnostic accuracy studies (cross-sectional or cohort), with one or more possible limitations causing minor concern about internal validity or external generalizability of the results	Implies the test can be offered to most patients in most applicable circumstances without reservation
Low-quality evidence	Evidence from nonrandomized diagnostic accuracy studies with one or more important limitations causing serious concern about internal validity or external generalizability of the results	Implies the test can be offered to most patients in most applicable circumstances, but the utilization of the test may change when higher-quality evidence becomes available
Weak recommendation		
High-quality evidence	Evidence from one or more well-designed nonrandomized diagnostic accuracy studies (i.e., observational – cross-sectional or cohort) or systematic reviews/meta-analysis of such observations studies (with no concern about internal validity or external generalizability of the results)	The degree to which the diagnostic test is seriously considered may differ depending on circumstances or patients' or societal values
Moderate-quality evidence	Evidence from nonrandomized diagnostic accuracy studies (cross-sectional or cohort), with one or more possible limitations causing minor concern about internal validity or external generalizability of the results	The degree to which the diagnostic test is seriously considered may differ depending on individual patients' or societal values
Low-quality evidence	Evidence from nonrandomized diagnostic accuracy studies with one or more important limitations causing serious concern about internal validity or external generalizability of the results	Alternative options may be equally reasonable
Insufficient	Evidence may be of such poor quality, conflicting, lacking (i.e., studies not done), or not externally generalizable to the target clinical population such that the estimate of the true effect of the test is uncertain and does not permit a reasonable conclusion to be made	Insufficient evidence exists to recommend for or against routinely offering the diagnostic test

Adapted from Haugen et al. [37]

recurrence in pN1 disease varies depending on the number of positive nodes, the size of the metastatic deposit, and where extranodal extension is found [72, 84]. Since the recurrence rates for patients with less than five positive lymph nodes are significantly lower than for those with greater than five (4 vs. 19 %), the new ATA guidelines have proposed a modification in postoperative risk stratification. The recommendation includes clinical N1 disease or greater than five pathological lymph nodes (less than 3 cm) as a determinant of intermediate risk patients. This would potentially alter the use of postoperative RAI and TSH suppression targets in this population of patients [37].

The first treatment decision after surgery is whether to treat with RAI ablation. The general recommendation from the ATA is against using RAI for patients stratified as low risk and patients with unifocal or multifocal papillary microcarcinoma in the abscess of other adverse features. Radioactive iodine is weakly recommended with low level evidence for patients at intermediate risk of recurrence, specifically those with microscopic invasion, RAI-avid metastatic foci in the neck, aggressive histology, greater than five pathologically involved lymph nodes (<3 cm), and multifocal PTC with ETE and BRAFV600E mutations (Table 11.4). High-risk patients include those with macroscopic invasion, incomplete resection, distant metastatic disease, elevated serum thyroglobulin, and pathologically involved lymph nodes greater than 3 cm. This group is strongly recommended with moderate evidence to undergo postoperative RAI ablation postoperatively [37]. Therefore, thorough review of the final pathology report is warranted to restage patients postoperatively.

Following ablative therapy patients enter a surveillance program that uses imaging findings and thyroglobulin levels to routinely reassess for markers of persistent or recurrent disease. The full breadth of this topic will be reviewed in a separate chapter; however, these two modalities are used frequently in postoperative staging. The resulting information collected is used to either continue surveillance (if thyroglobulin is negligible in the setting of suppressed TSH and/or dedicated neck ultrasonography is negative) or restage the patient (if thyroglobulin is elevated and/or ultrasonography is suspicious). In the latter setting, whole body RAI scanning, CT, or PET-CT are used to determine the extent and location of disease.

Dynamic Staging

The concept of postoperative staging is a component of a more recently described concept known as dynamic staging. Most of the established staging systems attempt to predict death rather than recurrence; however, the ATA has introduced a risk of recurrence and/or persistence of disease risk stratification system [37]. The initial system that was proposed in the 2009 guidelines is still the recommended system for stratification, but a number of modifications have been proposed in the 2015 edition. The system stratifies patients into low, intermediate, and high risk of recurrence based on individual clinicopathologic features. The new modifications incorporate the extent of lymph node involvement and mutational status as additional prognostic variables, but the specific benefit of adding these has not been established. A number of studies have been able to contribute to predicting risk of recurrence based on thyroglobulin or thyroglobulin antibody levels over time and neck ultrasonography [85–87]. Tuttle et al. in 2010 described a retrospective study that reevaluated patients 2 years postoperatively, specifically looking at response to treatment. Patients were categorized following thyroidectomy and RAI as having an excellent response, acceptable response, or incomplete response based on thyroglobulin levels, neck ultrasonography, and cross-sectional or nuclear imaging. Patients that responded completely to treatment, regardless of their initial staging category, had a decreased risk of recurrence over a 7-year follow-up as compared to their original prognosis as derived from the ATA risk stratification [37]. The re-stratification was most obvious in patients originally designated intermediate risk by the ATA who went from an 18 % risk of recurrence to a 2 % risk when they exhibited an excellent response to therapy [88].

Current models for predicting recurrence provide a starting point, but fail to accommodate response to treatment as an indicator of tumor biology. Dynamic restaging for patients with PTC is becoming the standard of care and allows for more accurate risk assessment and individualization of treatment.

Conclusion

Papillary thyroid cancer is the most common histologic subtype of thyroid cancer, and its incidence is increasing. The long-term prognosis of patients diagnosed with PTC is very good; however, certain subsets of the population develop tumors with more aggressive biology. It is essential that physicians are able to accurately stage patients with this malignancy so as to guide treatment and surveillance regimens, provide patient education, and set up infrastructure for research. This chapter has outlined (1) the acquired and intrinsic risk factors from both patient history and physical exam that are gathered preoperatively, (2) the intraoperative examination techniques and options for dissection, and (3) the postoperative reevaluation necessary to stage a patient with PTC. Although none of the current staging systems definitively predicts disease course in individual patients, the AJCC/UICC TNM staging system (Table 11.2) is used most frequently and continues to be modified over time to include staging characteristics that contribute to accurate prediction models.

References

1. Sherman SI, et al. Prospective multicenter study of thyroid carcinoma treatment: initial analysis of staging and outcome. National Thyroid Cancer Treatment Cooperative Study Registry Group. Cancer. 1998;83(5):1012–21.
2. Lang BH, et al. Staging systems for papillary thyroid carcinoma: a review and comparison. Ann Surg. 2007;245(3):366–78.

3. Cady B, Rossi R. An expanded view of risk-group definition in differentiated thyroid carcinoma. Surgery. 1988;104(6):947–53.
4. Edge SB, American Joint Committee on Cancer. AJCC cancer staging manual. 7th ed. New York; London: Springer; 2010. p. xiv–648.
5. Hay ID, et al. Predicting outcome in papillary thyroid carcinoma: development of a reliable prognostic scoring system in a cohort of 1779 patients surgically treated at one institution during 1940 through 1989. Surgery. 1993;114(6):1050–7; discussion 1057–8.
6. Hay ID, et al. Ipsilateral lobectomy versus bilateral lobar resection in papillary thyroid carcinoma: a retrospective analysis of surgical outcome using a novel prognostic scoring system. Surgery. 1987;102(6):1088–95.
7. Pasieka JL, et al. Addition of nuclear DNA content to the AMES risk-group classification for papillary thyroid cancer. Surgery. 1992;112(6):1154–9; discussion 1159–60.
8. Schemper M, Henderson R. Predictive accuracy and explained variation in Cox regression. Biometrics. 2000;56(1):249–55.
9. Wong RM, Bresee C, Braunstein GD. Comparison with published systems of a new staging system for papillary and follicular thyroid carcinoma. Thyroid. 2013;23(5):566–74.
10. Hannequin P, Liehn JC, Delisle MJ. Multifactorial analysis of survival in thyroid cancer. Pitfalls of applying the results of published studies to another population. Cancer. 1986;58(8): 1749–55.
11. Vaccarella S, et al. The impact of diagnostic changes on the rise in thyroid cancer incidence: a population-based study in selected high-resource countries. Thyroid. 2015;25:1127–36.
12. Tanase K, et al. The TNM system (version 7) is the most accurate staging system for the prediction of loss of life expectancy in differentiated thyroid cancer. Clin Endocrinol (Oxf). 2016; 84:284–291.
13. Passler C, et al. Application of staging systems for differentiated thyroid carcinoma in an endemic goiter region with iodine substitution. Ann Surg. 2003;237(2):227–34.
14. Park YM, et al. Metastatic lymph node status in the central compartment of papillary thyroid carcinoma: a prognostic factor of locoregional recurrence. Head Neck. 2016;38 Suppl 1:E1172–6.
15. Ron E, et al. Thyroid cancer after exposure to external radiation: a pooled analysis of seven studies. Radiat Res. 1995;141(3):259–77.
16. Tuttle RM, Vaisman F, Tronko MD. Clinical presentation and clinical outcomes in Chernobyl-related paediatric thyroid cancers: what do we know now? What can we expect in the future? Clin Oncol (R Coll Radiol). 2011;23(4):268–75.
17. Schneider AB, Sarne DH. Long-term risks for thyroid cancer and other neoplasms after exposure to radiation. Nat Clin Pract Endocrinol Metab. 2005;1(2):82–91.
18. Cetta F, et al. Germline mutations of the APC gene in patients with familial adenomatous polyposis-associated thyroid carcinoma: results from a European cooperative study. J Clin Endocrinol Metab. 2000;85(1):286–92.
19. Herraiz M, et al. Prevalence of thyroid cancer in familial adenomatous polyposis syndrome and the role of screening ultrasound examinations. Clin Gastroenterol Hepatol. 2007;5(3):367–73.
20. Tomoda C, et al. Cribriform-morular variant of papillary thyroid carcinoma: clue to early detection of familial adenomatous polyposis-associated colon cancer. World J Surg. 2004;28(9):886–9.
21. Feng X, et al. Characteristics of benign and malignant thyroid disease in familial adenomatous polyposis patients and recommendations for disease surveillance. Thyroid. 2015;25(3):325–32.
22. Jarrar AM, et al. Screening for thyroid cancer in patients with familial adenomatous polyposis. Ann Surg. 2011;253(3):515–21.
23. Richards ML. Familial syndromes associated with thyroid cancer in the era of personalized medicine. Thyroid. 2010;20(7):707–13.
24. Mazeh H, Sippel RS. Familial nonmedullary thyroid carcinoma. Thyroid. 2013;23(9):1049–56.
25. Mazeh H, et al. In patients with thyroid cancer of follicular cell origin, a family history of nonmedullary thyroid cancer in one first-degree relative is associated with more aggressive disease. Thyroid. 2012;22(1):3–8.

26. Park YJ, et al. The long-term outcomes of the second generation of familial nonmedullary thyroid carcinoma are more aggressive than sporadic cases. Thyroid. 2012;22(4):356–62.
27. Robenshtok E, et al. Clinical characteristics and outcome of familial nonmedullary thyroid cancer: a retrospective controlled study. Thyroid. 2011;21(1):43–8.
28. Gara SK, et al. Germline HABP2 mutation causing familial nonmedullary thyroid cancer. N Engl J Med. 2015;373(5):448–55.
29. Hillenbrand A, et al. Familial nonmedullary thyroid carcinoma-clinical relevance and prognosis. A European multicenter study. ESES Vienna presentation. Langenbecks Arch Surg. 2010;395(7):851–8.
30. Shaha AR, Loree TR, Shah JP. Intermediate-risk group for differentiated carcinoma of thyroid. Surgery. 1994;116(6):1036–40; discussion 1040–1.
31. Tran Cao HS, et al. A critical analysis of the American Joint Committee on Cancer (AJCC) staging system for differentiated thyroid carcinoma in young patients on the basis of the Surveillance, Epidemiology, and End Results (SEER) registry. Surgery. 2012;152(2): 145–51.
32. Nixon IJ, et al. Defining a valid age cutoff in staging of well-differentiated thyroid cancer. Ann Surg Oncol. 2016;23:410–5.
33. Jonklaas J, et al. The impact of age and gender on papillary thyroid cancer survival. J Clin Endocrinol Metab. 2012;97(6):E878–87.
34. Society AC. Estimated new cancer cases and deaths by sex for all sites, US, 2010. 2010; Available from: http://www.cancer.org/acs/groups/content/@epidemiologysurveilance/documents/document/acspc-026210.pdf
35. Cady B, et al. Risk factor analysis in differentiated thyroid cancer. Cancer. 1979;43(3): 810–20.
36. McCoy KL, et al. The incidence of cancer and rate of false-negative cytology in thyroid nodules greater than or equal to 4 cm in size. Surgery. 2007;142(6):837–44; discussion 844.e1–3.
37. Haugen BR, et al. 2015 American Thyroid Association management guidelines for patients with thyroid nodules and differentiated thyroid cancer: American Thyroid Association Guidelines Taskforce on Thyroid Nodules and Differentiated Thyroid Cancer. Thyroid. 2016;26(1):1–133.
38. Jarlov AE, et al. Observer variation in the clinical and laboratory evaluation of patients with thyroid dysfunction and goiter. Thyroid. 1998;8(5):393–8.
39. Kouvaraki MA, et al. Role of preoperative ultrasonography in the surgical management of patients with thyroid cancer. Surgery. 2003;134(6):946–54; discussion 954–5.
40. Stulak JM, et al. VAlue of preoperative ultrasonography in the surgical management of initial and reoperative papillary thyroid cancer. Arch Surg. 2006;141(5):489–96.
41. Fish SA, Langer JE, Mandel SJ. Sonographic imaging of thyroid nodules and cervical lymph nodes. Endocrinol Metab Clin North Am. 2008;37(2):401–17, ix.
42. Lee CY, et al. Preoperative laryngoscopy in thyroid surgery: do patients' subjective voice complaints matter? Surgery. 2014;156(6):1477–82; discussion 1482–3.
43. Randolph GW, Kamani D. The importance of preoperative laryngoscopy in patients undergoing thyroidectomy: voice, vocal cord function, and the preoperative detection of invasive thyroid malignancy. Surgery. 2006;139(3):357–62.
44. Surgeons B.A.o.E.a.T. Guidelines for the surgical management of endocrine disease and training requirements for endocrine surgery. 2003; Available from: http://www.baets.org.uk/wp-content/uploads/2013/02/BAETS-Guidelines-2003.pdf.
45. Carneiro-Pla D, et al. Feasibility of surgeon-performed transcutaneous vocal cord ultrasonography in identifying vocal cord mobility: a multi-institutional experience. Surgery. 2014;156(6):1597–602; discussion 1602–4.
46. Sabaretnam M, et al. Preoperative ultrasonography assessment of vocal cord movement during thyroid and parathyroid surgery. World J Surg. 2013;37(7):1740.
47. Wong KP, et al. A prospective, assessor-blind evaluation of surgeon-performed transcutaneous laryngeal ultrasonography in vocal cord examination before and after thyroidectomy. Surgery. 2013;154(6):1158–64; discussion 1164–5.

48. Yeh MW, et al. American Thyroid Association statement on preoperative imaging for thyroid cancer surgery. Thyroid. 2015;25(1):3–14.
49. Wiebel JL, et al. Evaluating positron emission tomography use in differentiated thyroid cancer. Thyroid. 2015;25:1026–32.
50. Roman S, Sosa JA. Aggressive variants of papillary thyroid cancer. Curr Opin Oncol. 2013;25(1):33–8.
51. Kazaure HS, Roman SA, Sosa JA. Aggressive variants of papillary thyroid cancer: incidence, characteristics and predictors of survival among 43,738 patients. Ann Surg Oncol. 2012;19(6):1874–80.
52. Kazaure HS, Roman SA, Sosa JA. Insular thyroid cancer: a population-level analysis of patient characteristics and predictors of survival. Cancer. 2012;118(13):3260–7.
53. Fugazzola L, et al. Correlation between B-RAFV600E mutation and clinico–pathologic parameters in papillary thyroid carcinoma: data from a multicentric Italian study and review of the literature. Endocr Relat Cancer. 2006;13(2):455–64.
54. Xing M. BRAF mutation in thyroid cancer. Endocr Relat Cancer. 2005;12(2):245–62.
55. Kim TH, et al. The association of the BRAF(V600E) mutation with prognostic factors and poor clinical outcome in papillary thyroid cancer: a meta-analysis. Cancer. 2012;118(7):1764–73.
56. Xing M, et al. Association between BRAF V600E mutation and mortality in patients with papillary thyroid cancer. JAMA. 2013;309(14):1493–501.
57. Lim JY, et al. Clinicopathologic implications of the BRAF(V600E) mutation in papillary thyroid cancer: a subgroup analysis of 3130 cases in a single center. Thyroid. 2013;23(11):1423–30.
58. Niederer-Wust SM, et al. Impact of clinical risk scores and BRAF V600E mutation status on outcome in papillary thyroid cancer. Surgery. 2015;157(1):119–25.
59. Lee WS, et al. BRAF mutation in papillary thyroid cancer: a cost-utility analysis of preoperative testing. Surgery. 2014;156(6):1569–77; discussion 1577–8.
60. Bongarzone I, et al. RET/NTRK1 rearrangements in thyroid gland tumors of the papillary carcinoma family: correlation with clinicopathological features. Clin Cancer Res. 1998;4(1):223–8.
61. Jhiang SM, et al. Targeted expression of the ret/PTC1 oncogene induces papillary thyroid carcinomas. Endocrinology. 1996;137(1):375–8.
62. Fagin JA, Mitsiades N. Molecular pathology of thyroid cancer: diagnostic and clinical implications. Best Pract Res Clin Endocrinol Metab. 2008;22(6):955–69.
63. Yip L, et al. Tumor genotype determines phenotype and disease-related outcomes in thyroid cancer: a study of 1510 patients. Ann Surg. 2015;262(3):519–25.
64. Nikiforov YE, et al. Impact of the multi-gene ThyroSeq next-generation sequencing assay on cancer diagnosis in thyroid nodules with atypia of undetermined significance/follicular lesion of undetermined significance cytology. Thyroid. 2015;25:1217–23.
65. Kwak JY, et al. Extrathyroid extension of well-differentiated papillary thyroid microcarcinoma on US. Thyroid. 2008;18(6):609–14.
66. Park YM, et al. Intraoperative frozen section for the evaluation of extrathyroidal extension in papillary thyroid cancer. World J Surg. 2015;39(1):187–93.
67. Matsuzu K, et al. Thyroid lobectomy for papillary thyroid cancer: long-term follow-up study of 1088 cases. World J Surg. 2014;38(1):68–79.
68. Nixon IJ, et al. Thyroid lobectomy for treatment of well differentiated intrathyroidal malignancy. Surgery. 2012;151(4):571–9.
69. Wang LY, et al. Level VII is an important component of central neck dissection for papillary thyroid cancer. Ann Surg Oncol. 2013;20(7):2261–5.
70. Gyorki DE, et al. Prophylactic central neck dissection in differentiated thyroid cancer: an assessment of the evidence. Ann Surg Oncol. 2013;20(7):2285–9.
71. Schneider DF, et al. Lymph node metastases do not impact survival in follicular variant papillary thyroid cancer. Ann Surg Oncol. 2015;22(1):158–63.

72. Adam MA, et al. Presence and number of lymph node metastases are associated with compromised survival for patients younger than age 45 years with papillary thyroid cancer. J Clin Oncol. 2015;33(21):2370–5.
73. Grebe SK, Hay ID. Thyroid cancer nodal metastases: biologic significance and therapeutic considerations. Surg Oncol Clin N Am. 1996;5(1):43–63.
74. Sywak M, et al. Routine ipsilateral level VI lymphadenectomy reduces postoperative thyroglobulin levels in papillary thyroid cancer. Surgery. 2006;140(6):1000–5; discussion 1005–7.
75. Hughes DT, et al. Influence of prophylactic central lymph node dissection onpostoperative thyroglobulin levels and radioiodine treatment in papillary thyroid cancer. Surgery. 2010;148(6):1100–6; discussion 1006–7.
76. Zetoune T, et al. Prophylactic central neck dissection and local recurrence in papillary thyroid cancer: a meta-analysis. Ann Surg Oncol. 2010;17(12):3287–93.
77. Wang TS, et al. A meta-analysis of the effect of prophylactic central compartment neck dissection on locoregional recurrence rates in patients with papillary thyroid cancer. Ann Surg Oncol. 2013;20(11):3477–83.
78. Hartl DM, et al. Optimization of staging of the neck with prophylactic central and lateral neck dissection for papillary thyroid carcinoma. Ann Surg. 2012;255(4):777–83.
79. Rammal A, et al. Chyle leak: a rare complication post-hemithyroidectomy. case report and review of literature. Otolaryngol Pol. 2014;68(4):204–7.
80. Ywata de Carvalho A, Chulam TC, Kowalski LP. Long-term results of observation vs prophylactic selective level VI neck dissection for papillary thyroid carcinoma at a cancer center. JAMA Otolaryngol Head Neck Surg. 2015;141(7):599–606.
81. Myers EN, Carrau RL. Operative otolaryngology head and neck surgery. Philadelphia: Saunders/Elsevier; 2008.
82. Roh JL, Kim JM, Park CI. Lateral cervical lymph node metastases from papillary thyroid carcinoma: pattern of nodal metastases and optimal strategy for neck dissection. Ann Surg Oncol. 2008;15(4):1177–82.
83. Farrag T, et al. Is routine dissection of level II-B and V-A necessary in patients with papillary thyroid cancer undergoing lateral neck dissection for FNA-confirmed metastases in other levels. World J Surg. 2009;33(8):1680–3.
84. Randolph GW, et al. The prognostic significance of nodal metastases from papillary thyroid carcinoma can be stratified based on the size and number of metastatic lymph nodes, as well as the presence of extranodal extension. Thyroid. 2012;22(11):1144–52.
85. Castagna MG, et al. Limited value of repeat recombinant human thyrotropin (rhTSH)-stimulated thyroglobulin testing in differentiated thyroid carcinoma patients with previous negative rhTSH-stimulated thyroglobulin and undetectable basal serum thyroglobulin levels. J Clin Endocrinol Metab. 2008;93(1):76–81.
86. Kloos RT, Mazzaferri EL. A single recombinant human thyrotropin-stimulated serum thyroglobulin measurement predicts differentiated thyroid carcinoma metastases three to five years later. J Clin Endocrinol Metab. 2005;90(9):5047–57.
87. Pacini F, et al. Recombinant human thyrotropin-stimulated serum thyroglobulin combined with neck ultrasonography has the highest sensitivity in monitoring differentiated thyroid carcinoma. J Clin Endocrinol Metab. 2003;88(8):3668–73.
88. Tuttle RM, et al. Estimating risk of recurrence in differentiated thyroid cancer after total thyroidectomy and radioactive iodine remnant ablation: using response to therapy variables to modify the initial risk estimates predicted by the new American Thyroid Association staging system. Thyroid. 2010;20(12):1341–9.
89. Sakorafas GH, Sampanis D, Safioleas M. Cervical lymph node dissection in papillary thyroid cancer: current trends, persisting controversies, and unclarified uncertainties. Surg Oncol. 2010;19(2):e57–70.

Chapter 12
Importance of Surgeon Experience in the Surgical Management of Thyroid Cancer

Kathryn E. Coan and Tracy S. Wang

Introduction

Prior to the late nineteenth century, thyroidectomy was associated with an extremely high morbidity and mortality and was even banned at some institutions [1]. However, with the advent of antiseptics, improved hemostasis, and surgeon experience, thyroidectomy has transformed into a safe surgical procedure that is routinely performed worldwide. Although the mortality associated with contemporary thyroidectomy is minimal, thyroidectomy-specific complications, such as injury to the recurrent laryngeal nerve and/or hypoparathyroidism, can still lead to significant morbidity.

A direct relationship between hospital and/or surgeon volume and patient outcomes has been well documented across multiple surgical subspecialties for a variety of procedures [2–6]. While first published in cardiovascular and major oncologic procedures, such as coronary artery bypass graft surgery, abdominal aortic aneurysms, esophagectomy, and pancreatectomy, the literature now includes ample evidence for improved outcomes from thyroidectomy by high-volume surgeons for both benign and malignant disease [2–4, 7, 8].

K.E. Coan, MD
Department of Surgery, Division of Surgical Oncology, Section of Endocrine Surgery, Medical College of Wisconsin, Milwaukee, WI, USA

T.S. Wang, MD, MPH (✉)
Department of Surgery, Division of Surgical Oncology, Section of Endocrine Surgery, Medical College of Wisconsin, Milwaukee, WI, USA

Section of Endocrine Surgery, Medical College of Wisconsin, 9200 W. Wisconsin Avenue, Milwaukee, WI 53226, USA
e-mail: tswang@mcw.edu

S.A. Roman et al. (eds.), *Management of Thyroid Nodules and Differentiated Thyroid Cancer*, DOI 10.1007/978-3-319-43618-0_12

The incidence of thyroid cancer continues to increase worldwide, especially in the United States, where there was a 4.4 % increase in the diagnosis of new cases of thyroid cancer from 2007 to 2011 [9]. The American Cancer Society estimates there were over 62,000 new cases of thyroid cancer in 2015, which was the fifth most common cancer diagnosed in women [9]. As the prevalence continues to increase, the implications of improved outcomes when thyroidectomy is performed by higher-volume surgeons are significant, in decreasing morbidity and in optimizing oncologic outcomes [8–12].

Historical Perspective

Some of the most compelling evidence of the "volume-outcome" relationship can be traced to the evolution of modern-day thyroid surgery. The earliest thyroid operations were performed during the twelfth and thirteenth century using setons, hot irons, and caustic powders and were associated with significant morbidity and mortality. As a result of these crude techniques, the French Academy of Medicine enacted a total ban on thyroidectomy in 1850 [1]. In 1886, the surgeon Samuel Gross was famously quoted as saying: "Can the thyroid gland when in the state of enlargement be removed with a reasonable hope of saving the patient? Experience emphatically answers, no! … If a surgeon should be so foolhardy as to undertake it … every step he takes will be followed by a torrent of blood, and lucky will it be for him if his victim live long enough to enable him to finish his horrid butchery. … No honest and sensible surgeon would ever engage in it [1]."

It was not until the late nineteenth century when Theodor Billroth (1829–1894) and Theodor Kocher (1841–1917) demonstrated that low morbidity and mortality was possible with thyroidectomy and associated with increased surgical volume. Billroth was a distinguished surgeon of his time and, by the early 1880s, was one of the most experienced thyroid surgeons. However, in the 1860s, his first 20 thyroidectomies had a mortality of 40 %, and he abandoned thyroidectomy for a decade, until improvements in surgical instrumentation, technique, and anesthesia occurred. Subsequently, in his second series of patients in the 1880s, his mortality decreased to 8.3 %. Theodor Kocher is considered by many to be the "father of thyroid surgery." During his initial tenure at University of Bern, he excised 101 goiters with a mortality rate of 12.8 %. Following another 250 procedures, his mortality rate had declined to 2.4 %, and in 1917, a few weeks before his death, he presented his entire series of approximately 5,000 operations to the Swiss Surgical Congress with a mortality rate of approximately 0.5 % [1]. This relation of increasing surgical experience and volume and improved rates of morbidity and mortality was also seen in the United States in the experience of Charles Mayo (1865–1939), who was regarded as the most experienced thyroid surgeon of his time. His first thyroidectomy for goiter was in 1889, and for his first 16 patients, his operative mortality rate was 25 %. This decreased to 6 % after thyroidectomy in 234 patients, and he then performed 278 consecutive thyroidectomies without a single death and only one patient experienced transient tetany [1].

Complications of Thyroid Surgery

Today, mortality from thyroid surgery is uncommon. The most frequent endocrine-specific complications that contribute to patient morbidity include superior/recurrent laryngeal nerve injury, hypoparathyroidism, and postoperative neck hematoma. In general, thyroid cancer tends to affect a younger patient population with the majority of patients being diagnosed under the age of 65 [9]. These patients often do not have other comorbidities that may increase the likelihood of postoperative morbidity and mortality and, importantly, given their relatively young age and increased life expectancy of the population worldwide, recurrent laryngeal nerve injury and/or hypoparathyroidism can have significant, long-term effects on quality-of-life.

The most frequent complication associated with thyroidectomy is hypocalcemia secondary to hypoparathyroidism, which may occur from parathyroid devascularization, stunning, or incidental removal of parathyroid glands at the time of thyroidectomy. Different studies have reported a wide variation in the incidence of postoperative hypocalcemia, with transient hypoparathyroidism reported in up to 50 % of patients and permanent hypoparathyroidism reported in 0.5–2 % of patients [13–15]. The incidence of this complication has been reported to be increased in patients undergoing thyroidectomy for thyroid cancer and those undergoing reoperative cervical surgery [10, 16].

The other primary endocrine-specific complication is injury to the superior and/or recurrent laryngeal nerves. Injury to the external branch of the superior laryngeal nerve can lead to voice fatigue, lower voice range, and difficulty singing; injury to the superior laryngeal nerve may have been associated with the ending of opera singer Amelita Galli-Curci career following thyroidectomy, in 1935 [17]. Reported rates of superior laryngeal nerve injury are varied but have generally ranged from 0.9 to 3 %; these have included a wide variety of methods for detection including patient-reported symptoms, electromyography, and laryngoscopy [18].

Injury to the recurrent laryngeal nerve can be more evident and more clinically significant, particularly with bilateral recurrent laryngeal nerve injury. Unilateral injury to the recurrent laryngeal nerve may be associated with hoarseness, micro-aspiration, and cough, while bilateral injury is associated with aphonia and dyspnea and, in severe situations, may require tracheostomy [19]. The reported incidence of recurrent laryngeal nerve injury ranges from 2 to 12 % and is usually transient, although it may take up to 6–12 months to resolve; permanent injury may occur in 0.4–2 % of patients [10, 19, 20]. The incidence of recurrent laryngeal nerve injury has been reported to be higher when surgery is performed for Graves' disease, thyroid cancer, or reoperative thyroid surgery [21]. In a study of 871,644 patients that underwent thyroidectomy with routine identification of the nerve during the procedure between 1993 and 2008, the overall incidence of recurrent laryngeal nerve injury was 1 %, during the 30-day postoperative study period. In this study, the rate of injury was higher (2 %) in patients undergoing surgery for thyroid cancer, as compared to patients having surgery for benign disease (0.6 %; $p<0.001$) [10].

Hospital Volume, Surgeon Volume, and Outcomes

The inverse relationship of high hospital volume to low complication rates has been well documented [22]. In 2002, Birkmeyer et al. used the national Medicare claims database and the National Inpatient Sample (NIS) to evaluate 2.5 million procedures, including six different cardiovascular and eight major cancer operations. Overall, there was a difference in mortality of more than 12 % between very low-volume hospitals and very high-volume hospitals for both esophagectomy and pancreatectomy [3]. In a study that utilized the Surveillance, Epidemiology, and End Results (SEER) database, 5,013 patients aged 65 years or older undergoing major cancer surgery, including pancreatectomy, esophagectomy, liver resection, pneumonectomy, or pelvic exenteration, were analyzed based on hospital volume and 30-day mortality. Significant decreases in mortality rates were associated with increased hospital volume for all procedures, excluding pneumonectomy ($p<0.05$), and was most apparent for esophagectomy (17.3 % for low-volume hospitals vs. 3.4 % for high-volume hospitals). After adjusting for case mix and patient factors, low hospital volume remained strongly associated with worse mortality [2].

Studies have also shown an association between higher surgeon volume and improved patient outcomes, independent of hospital volume. In a 2003 study, Medicare claims data was used to evaluate 474,108 patients undergoing cardiovascular procedures or cancer resections. The authors found a significant inverse relationship between surgeon volume and operative mortality for all eight procedures, especially for esophagectomy and pancreatectomy. After adjustment for hospital volume, the odds ratio (OR) and 95 % confidence interval (CI) of operative death with low-volume surgeons were OR 1.8 (1.13–2.87) for esophagectomy and OR 2.31 (1.43–3.72) for pancreatectomy. For aortic valve replacement, high surgeon volume accounted entirely for improved outcomes, compared with hospital volume alone [4].

Boudourakis et al. performed a cross-sectional analysis of discharge data from the Health Care Utilization Project National Inpatient Sample (HCUP-NIS) to evaluate the utilization of high-volume surgeons for a number of procedures (colorectal procedures, esophagectomy, gastrectomy, pancreatectomy, thyroidectomy, CABG, and carotid endarterectomy) between 1999 and 2005. In this study, the thresholds for high- and low-volume surgeons were 30 and 9 procedures, respectively. There was a significant increase in the number of these procedures performed by high-volume surgeons within the 6-year time period; the most noticeable increases were seen for gastrectomy (54 %), pancreatectomy (31 %), and thyroidectomy (23 %). Overall, unadjusted mortality and length of stay were

Table 12.1 Unadjusted outcomes by surgeon volume group and year

	1999			2005		
Procedure	High	Low	*p* value[a]	High	Low	*p* value[a]
Oncology						
Colectomy						
Mortality (%)	1.3	3.5	<0.001	2.3	2.8	NS
LOS (mean days)	8.5	10.0	<0.001	8.1	9.7	<0.001
Esophagectomy						
Mortality (%)	0.0	6.8	<0.05	0.6	8.8	<0.05
LOS (mean days)	11.2	17.4	<0.001	12.5	18.5	<0.05
Gastrectomy						
Mortality (%)	4.0	6.6	NS	3.8	6.8	NS
LOS (mean days)	11.4	14.0	<0.05	13.0	14.8	<0.05
Lung lobectomy						
Mortality (%)	2.5	3.9	NS	1.4	3.3	<0.05
LOS (mean days)	7.1	9.1	<0.001	6.4	8.9	<0.001
Pancreatectomy						
Mortality (%)	2.5	10.3	<0.05	2.5	9.0	NS
LOS (mean days)	13.3	20.6	<0.001	13.6	24.1	<0.001
Thyroidectomy						
Complications (%)	2.5	7.1	<0.001	4.9	7.9	<0.001
LOS (mean days)	1.4	2.4	<0.001	1.3	2.3	<0.001
Cardiovascular						
CABG						
Mortality (%)	2.4	4.1	<0.001	2.0	2.3	NS
LOS (mean days)	8.9	9.7	<0.001	9.1	9.6	<0.001
CEA						
Mortality (%)	0.5	1.0	<0.05	0.2	0.4	NS
LOS (mean days)	2.7	4.5	<0.001	2.3	3.9	<0.001

Reprinted with permission from Ref. [5]
[a]*NS* not significant

significantly lower for high-volume surgeons (Table 12.1); following multivariate analysis, the difference in length-of-stay persisted (Table 12.2) [5]. Specifically for thyroidectomy, this study found complication rates in both 1999 and 2005 were lower for high-volume versus low-volume surgeons (2.5 % vs. 7.1 %; p <0.001) and (4.9 % vs. 7.9 %; p<0.001), respectively.

Surgical specialization also appears to be related to improved patient outcomes. A systematic review analyzed studies on hospital volume, surgeon volume, and surgeon subspecialty. This review identified 58 studies related to surgical volume and found 74 % of studies reported better outcomes with high-volume surgeons. Surgical subspecialization was specifically evaluated in 22 studies. The majority of these studies evaluated specialization in surgical oncology and vascular surgery, and two studies looked exclusively at endocrine surgery. The entire cohort included 144,421 patients. Surgical subspecialists had significantly better outcomes than general surgeons

Table 12.2 Adjusted increased length of stay for low-volume surgeons compared with high-volume surgeons, by year

	1999		2005	
Procedure	Odds ratio (CI)	*p* value[a]	Odds ratio (CI)	*p* value[a]
Oncology				
Colectomy	2.3 (1.5–3.6)	<0.001	1.0 (0.7–1.3)	NS
Gastrectomy	1.2 (0.4–4.1)	NS	1.3 (0.5–3.2)	NS
Lung lobectomy	1.2 (0.6–2.5)	NS	1.3 (0.5–3.2)	NS
Thyroidectomy	1.8 (0.9–3.6)	NS	1.4 (0.9–2.2)	NS
Cardiovascular				
CABG	1.4 (1.1–1.8)	<0.05	0.9 (0.6–1.3)	NS
CEA	1.2 (0.5–3.2)	NS	2.3 (0.6–8.1)	NS

Reprinted with permission from Ref. [5]
[a]*NS* not significant, *CI* 95 % confidence interval

performing the same procedure in 20 of 22 studies (91 %). Lower mortality rates were seen in 11 of 12 studies (92 %), and lower complications rates were observed in 14 of 17 studies (82 %). In studies that evaluated surgical subspecialization and length of stay, specialists had shorter hospital length of stay in all studies [6].

Surgeon Volume and Thyroidectomy

Sosa et al. published the earliest study addressing surgeon experience and its relationship to short-term clinical and economic outcomes specifically for thyroidectomy [8]. The authors reviewed 5,860 patients that underwent thyroidectomy for both benign and malignant disease between 1991 and 1996 in a single state. Surgeons were stratified into four groups by case volume over the 6-year period (1–9 cases, 10–29 cases, 30–100 cases, and >100 cases). Nearly two thirds of surgeons performed, on average, less than one thyroidectomy per year. The highest-volume surgeons represented less than 1 % of surgeons but performed 14 % of the cases. Thyroidectomies performed by high-volume surgeons were more complex (29 % total thyroidectomy vs. 15 % in the lowest-volume group) and the highest-volume surgeons more likely to operate on patients with thyroid cancer, compared to the lowest-volume surgeons (31 % vs. 23 %). The highest-volume surgeons also had significantly fewer complications, including both thyroidectomy-specific complications such as recurrent laryngeal nerve injury and hypoparathyroidism as well as those indirectly related to surgery such as drug reactions ($p<0.001$). Regarding length of stay, the highest-volume surgeon had the shortest length of stay 2.8 days vs. 1.7 days and 1.9 days vs. 1.4 days ($p<0.05$), before and after adjustment for differences in patient characteristics, procedure, hospital volume, and time period. When analyzed by indication for surgery, differences between surgeon volume and outcomes persisted for the 1,470 patients with thyroid cancer. The complication rate in patients with thyroid cancer was overall higher than in those with adenomas

8.1 % vs. 4.8 % ($p<0.001$). Complications occurred in 4.7 % of the patients operated on by the highest-volume surgeon versus 12.9 % in the lowest group ($p<0.001$). The length of stay was 1.4 days versus 2.1 days ($p<0.001$) (Table 12.3) [8].

A 2010 study that utilized the Maryland Health Service Cost Review Commission database evaluated trends in thyroid surgery and the relationship between surgeon volume and complications over a 19 year period (1990–2009) [7]. Over 1,000 surgeons at 51 hospitals performed a total of 21,270 thyroidectomies. Only 8 (0.8 %) of surgeons were categorized as high-volume surgeons, defined as >24 cases per year, while 888 surgeons (85.9 %) performed 3 or fewer thyroid surgery procedures per year on average. Similar to the study by Sosa et al., complications rates were significantly lower for high-volume surgeons. When surgery was performed by a high-volume surgeon, there was a lower risk of recurrent laryngeal nerve injury (OR 0.46 [0.28–0.75]; $p=0.002$) and lower risk of hypoparathyroidism (OR 0.62 [0.50–0.66]; $p<0.001$). Patients operated on by high-volume surgeons were more likely to have shorter length of stay (OR 0.44 [0.50–0.66]; $p<0.001$). Looking at trends over the time period showed that the number of thyroidectomies performed by high-volume

Table 12.3 Adjusted outcomes of surgeon volume groups by diagnosis (Reprinted with permission from Ref. [8])

Outcome, by Surgeon volume Group (case/year)	Adenoma ($n=1381$)	Diagnosis Other benign ($n=3009$)	Cancer ($n=1470$)
Complications	(%)	(%)	(%)
A (1–9 cases)	5.7NS	9.1^{a}	12.9^{c}
B (10–29 cases)	5.0 NS	6.2^{a}	8.0 NS
C (30–100 cases)	4.2 NS	6.2^{a}	9.4^{a}
D (>100 cases)	7.6 ref	6.0 ref	4.7ref
Length of stay	(Days)	(Days)	(Days)
A (1–9 cases)	1.7^{c}	2.0^{c}	2.1^{c}
B (10–29 cases)	1.6^{b}	1.8^{c}	1.8^{a}
C (30–100 cases)	1.5^{b}	1.8^{c}	1.9^{c}
D (>100 cases)	1.3 ref	1.5 ref	1.4 ref
Hospital charges	($)	($)	($)
A (1–9 cases)	3467 NS	4068 NS	4416^{c}
B (10–29 cases)	3499NS	3696 NS	4046^{c}
C (30–100 cases)	3311^{b}	3591^{b}	3978 NS
D (>100 cases)	3911 ref	4252 ref	3553 ref

Outcomes adjusted for surgeon volume and patient age, comorbidities, hospital volume, and time period

Key: *NS* not significant, *ref* reference category when dummy variables used to calculate *p* values in multivariate regression model

Ref = reference category when dummy variables used to calculate *p* values in multivariate regression model

$^{a}p<0.05$ compared to group D (ref)

$^{b}p<0.01$ compared to group D (ref)

$^{c}p<0.001$ compared to group D (ref)

surgeons increased from 15.7 % in 1990–1999 to 30.9 % in 2000–2009 (OR 3.69 [3.41–3.99]; $p<0.001$). High-volume surgeons were more likely to perform total thyroidectomy (OR 2.5 [2.29–2.73]; $p<0.001$) and neck dissections (OR 1.86 [1.52–2.27]; $p<0.001$). Interestingly, in this study cancer surgery was less likely to be performed by high-volume surgeons (OR 0.89 [0.81–0.98], $p=0.01$) [7].

Evaluating these trends on a national scale, Loya et al. used discharge data from the NIS. A total of 871,644 patients underwent thyroid surgery from 1993 to 2008; surgeons were stratified by annual case volume (<3 cases, 4–9 cases, 9–23 cases, and >23 cases). Again, a lower complication rate was seen in high-volume surgeons with respect to recurrent laryngeal nerve injury (OR 0.7 [0.53–0.95], $p=0.024$) and postoperative hypocalcemia (OR 0.7 [0.57–0.88], $p=0.002$). Compared to low-volume surgeons and after adjustment for hospital volume, high-volume surgeons were more likely to perform total thyroidectomy (OR 1.4 [1.23–1.64]; $p<0.001$) [10].

The Effect of Surgeon Volume on the Management of Patients with Thyroid Cancer

Patients diagnosed with differentiated thyroid cancer have an excellent prognosis, with only an estimated 1,950 deaths expected in 2015 [9]. As a result, focus has turned to decreasing rates of recurrent thyroid cancer after initial thyroidectomy and adjuvant treatment. In a study of over 50,000 patients using data from the National Cancer Data Base between 1985 and 1998, the overall recurrence rate was 5.7 % at 5 years and 9.4 % at 10 years [23]. The American Thyroid Association (ATA) guidelines for management of differentiated thyroid cancer (DTC) goals for initial therapy emphasize the importance of completeness of surgical resection to include all areas of tumor extension as an important determinate of outcome while stating that the extent of the surgery and surgeon experience are vital to minimize treatment-related morbidity [24].

Specific ATA treatment guidelines for DTC recommend near total or total thyroidectomy for tumors greater than 1 cm in size or in patients with other high risk features including multifocality, regional or distant metastases, history of head/neck radiation, or family history of thyroid cancer [24]. Complete resection has been shown to decrease recurrence and improve survival [23]. It also allows for adjuvant treatment with radioactive iodine ablation and improves the ability to detect recurrence with thyroglobulin levels [24]. Remnant uptake on radioactive iodine scans following thyroidectomy allows for evaluation of the quality of surgical resection [12]. Schneider et al. looked at remnant uptake on initial postoperative scan and its relation to disease recurrence and surgeon volume. High-volume surgeons were defined as performing more than 20 thyroidectomies per year. There were a total of 223 patients, of which 21 (9.4 %) developed recurrent thyroid cancer. Patients with recurrent disease had a tenfold higher remnant uptake ($p=0.001$). Remnant uptake was also significantly lower for high-volume surgeons ($p=0.001$) and rates of permanent complications remained low for this group of surgeons [12]. In a separate study, RAI remnant uptake was used to evaluate the extent of surgical resection when completion thyroidectomy after initial thyroid lobectomy, versus total thyroidectomy, was performed for cancer. This study found that remnant uptake following completion thyroidectomy was significantly higher than after total thyroidectomy (0.07 vs. 0.04 %; $p=0.04$). However, when completion thyroidectomy was performed by a high-volume surgeon, defined as greater than 20 thyroidectomies per year, there was much lower remnant uptake following completion thyroidectomy (0.06 %), as compared to low-volume surgeons (0.22 %; $p=0.04$) [25]. These data suggests that surgeon volume may influence oncologic outcomes in patients with DTC.

Reoperation may be traumatic for patients and place them at increased risk of injury to the recurrent laryngeal nerve, hypoparathyroidism, and poor cosmetic outcomes. Although some reoperations such as completion thyroidectomy for cancer following lobectomy are unavoidable, other reoperations are potentially avoidable with the use of accurate preoperative staging and adequate initial surgical resection. Mitchell et al. looked at hospital data from a single institution from 1999 to 2007 and found that cancer reoperations accounted for 134 of 189 (71 %) of reoperative thyroid cases. When stratified by a volume threshold of less than or more than 20 cases per year, low-volume centers accounted for 35 of the 43 (81 %) avoidable reoperations, such as partial thyroidectomy when total thyroidectomy was indicated, or inadequate lymph node dissection. Also noted in this study was a higher incidence of recurrent laryngeal nerve injury if the index case was performed at a low-volume center (9 %), as compared to a high-volume center (3 %; $p<0.05$) [26]. A tertiary care center evaluated 72 patients who underwent reoperation for papillary thyroid cancer between 1992 and 2003. Reoperations were performed for persistent disease (reoperation less than 6 months from initial surgery) in 17 (24 %) patients and for recurrent disease (reoperation more than 6 months after initial surgery) in 55 (76 %) patients. When reoperation was performed for persistent disease, 14 (82 %) of patients were thought by the authors to have been potentially avoidable, secondary to inadequate preoperative imaging or incomplete initial surgery. In patients with recurrent disease, 14 (25 %) reoperations may have been secondary to inadequate surgical resection at the primary surgery. This included 9 (64 %) patients who underwent only node plucking ("berry picking") at the site of recurrent disease, and 5 (36 %) patients did not undergo any form of lymph node dissection despite preoperative knowledge of lymph node metastases. Overall, reoperation in 28 of 72 (39 %) patients was deemed potentially preventable with adherence to the National Comprehensive Cancer Network (NCCN) treatment guidelines at the time of initial surgery [27].

Surgeon Experience for Pediatric Thyroid Cancer

Although rare, thyroid cancer is the most common endocrine malignancy in children [28]. Data from the Surveillance, Epidemiology, and End Results (SEER) database from 1973 to 2004 showed an annual increase of 1.1 % over the 31-year study period [29]. Pediatric patients with DTC present with more extensive disease compared to adults. At initial diagnosis, lymph node metastasis is seen in 40–80 % of children, compared to only 20–50 % of adults, and distant metastatic disease is seen in 20–30 % of children [29]. Adequate surgical resection is paramount to decreasing the risk of recurrence. In a retrospective review of 329 patients under the age of 21 diagnosed with DTC progression-free survival was directly associated with the presence of residual cervical disease following surgery ($p=0.001$) [30]. In a similar study of 235 patients diagnosed with DTC before age 18, anything less than a total thyroidectomy was associated with an increased risk of local recurrence in the thyroid bed (OR 9.5 [1.2–78.1]; $p=0.04$) [31].

Higher complication rates have also been reported in children undergoing thyroidectomy and parathyroidectomy, as compared to adults. In a study of patients age 17 years and younger utilizing the Healthcare Cost and Utilization Project Nationwide Inpatient Sample (HCUP-NIS) discharge data from 1999 to 2005, the outcomes of 1,199 operations were evaluated. Thyroidectomy was performed in 1094 (91 %) of patients, the majority 765 (70 %) for benign disease. Complications for the cohort of 1,199 children were compared with 96,002 adults who underwent the same thyroid and parathyroid procedures during the study period. Children had higher endocrine-specific complication rates than adults after thyroidectomy (9.1 % vs. 6.3 %; $p<0.01$). For both parathyroidectomy and thyroidectomy, children aged 0–6 years had higher complication. A second study evaluated a cross-sectional analysis of surgeon volume and outcomes for thyroidectomy using the HCUP-NIS data for 607 patients 17-year-old and under. Surgeons were classified as high volume (more than 30 cervical operations per year), pediatric (more than 90 % of their practice was on patients under 17 years old), and others (those who did not meet the criteria for a high-volume or pediatric surgeon). High-volume surgeons had the lowest length-of-stay (1.5 days), vs. 2.3 days for pediatric surgeons and 2.0 days for others ($p<0.05$). They also had the lowest cost ($12,474) vs. $19,594 for pediatric surgeons and $13,614 for others ($p<0.01$) [32]. For these reasons, the NCCN and ATA both recommend high-volume surgeons experienced in thyroid surgery along with collaboration of a multidisciplinary team when operating on pediatric patients [33, 34].

Conclusion

Thyroid cancer is increasing in prevalence as are the number of thyroidectomies being performed. Although many thyroidectomies are still performed by low-volume surgeons, there appears to be a trend toward referral to more experienced surgeons with high-volumes of thyroid surgery. The importance of surgeon volume to improved outcomes has been repeatedly demonstrated for thyroidectomy-specific complications, such as recurrent laryngeal nerve injury and hypoparathyroidism. It has also been shown that high-volume surgeons have improved oncologic outcomes from improved adequacy of resection to decreased need for avoidable reoperations, both in the adult and pediatric populations.

References

1. Sakorafas GH. Historical evolution of thyroid surgery: from the ancient times to the dawn of the 21st century. World J Surg. 2010;34(8):1793–804.
2. Begg CB, Cramer LD, Hoskins WJ, Brennan MF. Impact of hospital volume on operative mortality for major cancer surgery. JAMA. 1998;280(20):1747–51.
3. Birkmeyer JD, Siewers AE, Finlayson EV, Stukel TA, Lucas FL, Batista I, et al. Hospital volume and surgical mortality in the United States. N Engl J Med. 2002;346(15):1128–37.
4. Birkmeyer JD, Stukel TA, Siewers AE, Goodney PP, Wennberg DE, Lucas FL. Surgeon volume and operative mortality in the United States. N Engl J Med. 2003;349(22):2117–27.
5. Boudourakis LD, Wang TS, Roman SA, Desai R, Sosa JA. Evolution of the surgeon-volume, patient-outcome relationship. Ann Surg. 2009;250(1):159–65.
6. Chowdhury MM, Dagash H, Pierro A. A systematic review of the impact of volume of surgery and specialization on patient outcome. Br J Surg. 2007;94(2):145–61.
7. Gourin CG, Tufano RP, Forastiere AA, Koch WM, Pawlik TM, Bristow RE. Volume-based trends in thyroid surgery. Arch Otolaryngol Head Neck Surg. 2010;136(12):1191–8.
8. Sosa JA, Bowman HM, Tielsch JM, Powe NR, Gordon TA, Udelsman R. The importance of surgeon experience for clinical and economic outcomes from thyroidectomy. Ann Surg. 1998;228(3):320–30.
9. Society AC. Cancer facts & figures 2015. Atlanta: American Cancer Society; 2015. p. 2015.
10. Loyo M, Tufano RP, Gourin CG. National trends in thyroid surgery and the effect of volume on short-term outcomes. Laryngoscope. 2013;123(8):2056–63.
11. Rosato L, Avenia N, Bernante P, De Palma M, Gulino G, Nasi PG, et al. Complications of thyroid surgery: analysis of a multicentric study on 14,934 patients operated on in Italy over 5 years. World J Surg. 2004;28(3):271–6.
12. Schneider DF, Ojomo KA, Chen H, Sippel RS. Remnant uptake as a postoperative oncologic quality indicator. Thyroid. 2013;23(10):1269–76.
13. Asari R, Passler C, Kaczirek K, Scheuba C, Niederle B. Hypoparathyroidism after total thyroidectomy: a prospective study. Arch Surg. 2008;143(2):132–7; discussion 8.
14. Cayo AK, Yen TW, Misustin SM, Wall K, Wilson SD, Evans DB, et al. Predicting the need for calcium and calcitriol supplementation after total thyroidectomy: results of a prospective, randomized study. Surgery. 2012;152(6):1059–67.
15. Pattou F, Combemale F, Fabre S, Carnaille B, Decoulx M, Wemeau JL, et al. Hypocalcemia following thyroid surgery: incidence and prediction of outcome. World J Surg. 1998;22(7):718–24.
16. Lefevre JH, Tresallet C, Leenhardt L, Jublanc C, Chigot JP, Menegaux F. Reoperative surgery for thyroid disease. Langenbecks Arch Surg. 2007;392(6):685–91.
17. Marchese-Ragona R, Restivo DA, Mylonakis I, Ottaviano G, Martini A, Sataloff RT, et al. The superior laryngeal nerve injury of a famous soprano, Amelita Galli-Curci. Acta Otorhinolaryngol Ital. 2013;33(1):67–71.
18. Morton RP, Whitfield P, Al-Ali S. Anatomical and surgical considerations of the external branch of the superior laryngeal nerve: a systematic review. Clin Otolaryngol. 2006;31(5):368–74.
19. Jiang Y, Gao B, Zhang X, Zhao J, Chen J, Zhang S, et al. Prevention and treatment of recurrent laryngeal nerve injury in thyroid surgery. Int J Clin Exp Med. 2014;7(1):101–7.
20. Pisanu A, Porceddu G, Podda M, Cois A, Uccheddu A. Systematic review with meta-analysis of studies comparing intraoperative neuromonitoring of recurrent laryngeal nerves versus visualization alone during thyroidectomy. J Surg Res. 2014;188(1):152–61.
21. Chiang FY, Wang LF, Huang YF, Lee KW, Kuo WR. Recurrent laryngeal nerve palsy after thyroidectomy with routine identification of the recurrent laryngeal nerve. Surgery. 2005;137(3):342–7.
22. Luft HS, Bunker JP, Enthoven AC. Should operations be regionalized? The empirical relation between surgical volume and mortality. N Engl J Med. 1979;301(25):1364–9.

23. Bilimoria KY, Bentrem DJ, Ko CY, Stewart AK, Winchester DP, Talamonti MS, et al. Extent of surgery affects survival for papillary thyroid cancer. Ann Surg. 2007;246(3):375–81; discussion 81–4.
24. Haugen BR, Alexander EK, Bible KC, Doherty GM, Mandel SJ, Nikiforov YE, et al. 2015 American Thyroid Association Management Guidelines for adult patients with thyroid nodules and differentiated thyroid cancer: The American Thyroid Association Guidelines Task Force on thyroid nodules and differentiated thyroid cancer. Thyroid. 2016;26(1):1–133.
25. Oltmann SC, Schneider DF, Leverson G, Sivashanmugam T, Chen H, Sippel RS. Radioactive iodine remnant uptake after completion thyroidectomy: not such a complete cancer operation. Ann Surg Oncol. 2014;21(4):1379–83.
26. Mitchell J, Milas M, Barbosa G, Sutton J, Berber E, Siperstein A. Avoidable reoperations for thyroid and parathyroid surgery: effect of hospital volume. Surgery. 2008;144(6):899–906; discussion –7.
27. Kouvaraki MA, Lee JE, Shapiro SE, Sherman SI, Evans DB. Preventable reoperations for persistent and recurrent papillary thyroid carcinoma. Surgery. 2004;136(6):1183–91.
28. Dinauer CA, Breuer C, Rivkees SA. Differentiated thyroid cancer in children: diagnosis and management. Curr Opin Oncol. 2008;20(1):59–65.
29. Hogan AR, Zhuge Y, Perez EA, Koniaris LG, Lew JI, Sola JE. Pediatric thyroid carcinoma: incidence and outcomes in 1753 patients. J Surg Res. 2009;156(1):167–72.
30. Newman KD, Black T, Heller G, Azizkhan RG, Holcomb 3rd GW, Sklar C, et al. Differentiated thyroid cancer: determinants of disease progression in patients <21 years of age at diagnosis: a report from the Surgical Discipline Committee of the Children's Cancer Group. Ann Surg. 1998;227(4):533–41.
31. Handkiewicz-Junak D, Wloch J, Roskosz J, Krajewska J, Kropinska A, Pomorski L, et al. Total thyroidectomy and adjuvant radioiodine treatment independently decrease locoregional recurrence risk in childhood and adolescent differentiated thyroid cancer. J Nucl Med Off Pub Soc Nucl Med. 2007;48(6):879–88.
32. Tuggle CT, Roman SA, Wang TS, Boudourakis L, Thomas DC, Udelsman R, et al. Pediatric endocrine surgery: who is operating on our children? Surgery. 2008;144(6):869–77; discussion 77.
33. Waguespack SG, Francis G. Initial management and follow-up of differentiated thyroid cancer in children. J Natl Compr Canc Netw. 2010;8(11):1289–300.
34. Wells Jr SA, Asa SL, Dralle H, Elisei R, Evans DB, Gagel RF, et al. Revised American Thyroid Association guidelines for the management of medullary thyroid carcinoma. Thyroid. 2015;25(6):567–610.

Chapter 13
The Pediatric Thyroid Nodule and Papillary Thyroid Cancer Management

Scott A. Rivkees and Catherine A. Dinauer

Introduction

Pediatric thyroid cancer is a rare and treatable disease with an excellent prognosis [1–3]. Papillary thyroid cancer (PTC) accounts for the vast majority of cases of thyroid cancer in children and presents most commonly as thyroid nodules [2, 3]. Compared with adults, PTC presents at more advanced stages of disease in children and is associated with higher rates of recurrence, yet mortality rates are low. Fortunately, even in the presence of metastatic disease, long-term follow-up data show 30-year survival rates of 90–99 % for children with DTC [4–6]. Even with distant metastases, mortality rates are more favorable in children than adults [7], and pulmonary metastases can remain stable for extended periods [8]. The favorable prognosis reflects the fact that most young patients have well-differentiated tumor types, few have bone metastasis, and most tumors respond well to radioactive iodine (RAI) therapy. In caring for children with thyroid cancer, it is important to consider the important recently revised management guidelines of the American Thyroid Association for adults [9] and the recently published guidelines for children [2].

S.A. Rivkees, MD (✉)
Department of Pediatrics, University of Florida College of Medicine,
1600 SW Archer Road – Room R1-118, Gainesville, FL 32610-0296, USA
e-mail: srivkees@ufl.edu

C.A. Dinauer, MD
Department of Surgery, Yale University School of Medicine, New Haven, CT, USA

Department of Pediatrics, Yale University School of Medicine, New Haven, CT, USA

S.A. Roman et al. (eds.), *Management of Thyroid Nodules and Differentiated Thyroid Cancer*, DOI 10.1007/978-3-319-43618-0_13

Thyroid Cancer in Children

Data from the Surveillance, Epidemiology, and End Results (SEER) registry from 1973 to 2004 provide contemporary insights into thyroid cancer in children [1]. Thyroid cancer in the pediatric population is rare. In children less than 10 years of age, the incidence of DTC is 1 per 1,000,000 [1]. In children from 10 to 14 years of age, the incidence of DTC is 1 per 200,000 [1]. In children from 15 to 19 years, the incidence of DTC is 4.1 per 100,000 females and 0.9 per 100,000 males [1, 10]. The thyroid cancer types in children in the USA are PTC in 60 %, follicular variant of papillary in 23 %, FTC in 10 % (FTC), and medullary in 5 % (MTC) [1].

Compared with adults, children with PTC present with more extensive disease [5, 6, 11–18]. Lymph node involvement at diagnosis is seen in 40–90 % of children [5, 6, 11–19], compared with 20–50 % of adults [20]. The prevalence of distant metastases, most commonly lung, is 15–30 % in children vs. 2 % in adults [5, 6, 11–18, 21]. Multifocal disease is more common in children than adults and is seen in about 40 % of childhood PTC cases. It is believed that proliferation of individual clones, not metastases, accounts for the multifocal nature of disease [22, 23].

Risk Factors for Thyroid Cancer in Children

In most cases specific risk factors for DTC cannot be identified in children; however, risk factors are found in a subset of patients. Exposure to low level head and neck irradiation has been recognized for more than six decades as predisposing to DTC [24, 25]. Low-level radiation doses to the thyroid of less than 30 Gy (3000 cGy or Rad) increase the risk for cancer, with the risk being higher at progressively younger ages [26–28]. The latency period between the time of radiation exposure and cancer onset in children is typically 10–20 years [25, 27, 28].

One of the largest growing groups of children at risk for thyroid cancer is childhood cancer survivors who have had head and neck irradiation. Thyroid cancers are the most common second malignancy in children who have had Hodgkin's and non-Hodgkin's lymphomas [26, 29–32]. Thyroid cancer is the third most frequent malignancy in leukemia survivors [26, 29–32].

Of the children at risk for thyroid cancer, those treated for cancer before 10 years-of-age are at highest risk [30, 32]. The incidence of DTC increases linearly with radiation doses up to 30 Gy, (3,000 cGy or Rad) and declines with higher doses [26, 30–32]. Thyroid cancer in this group develops with a mean latency of 10 years, with a range of 5 to >20 years [26, 30–33].

Thyroid cancer in children can also be observed in families. Familial non-medullary differentiated thyroid cancer (FNMTC), most commonly papillary type, is diagnosed when two or more individuals in the family have DTC [34–37]. Other rare genetic syndromes are associated with an increased risk for thyroid cancer, with higher prevalence rates of both papillary and follicular thyroid cancer than is reported for the general population. Cowden syndrome is caused by mutation in the PTEN gene and is a rare autosomal dominant disorder associated with hamartomas of mucosal surfaces and both PTC and FTC [38–40]. Cowden syndrome falls under the umbrella PTEN tumor hamartoma syndromes (PTHS) which also includes Bannayan-Riley-Ruvalcaba and Proteus syndromes [41]. Gardner syndrome (familial colorectal polyposis) is an autosomal dominant condition associated with multiple polyps in the colon and other tumors including DTC [42–44]. Gardner syndrome is caused by mutation in the APC gene located in chromosome 5q21 [42, 43]. Werner syndrome, caused by a mutation in the WRN gene, a DNA helicase, is a very rare autosomal recessive disorder characterized by premature aging [40]. The syndrome is associated with DTC, melanomas, and sarcomas [40].

Nodule Evaluation

Thyroid cancer must be suspected when thyroid nodules are detected in children and adolescents. In a compilation of 16 different studies that examined the malignancy rate of thyroid nodules in children, 299 of 1134 nodules were malignant for an overall rate of 26 % [45]. When thyroid nodules are detected, serum thyrotropin (TSH), estimated free thyroxine and/or total thyroxine, and a neck ultrasound should be obtained. A calcitonin level may be measured to screen for medullary thyroid cancer, which accounts for 3–5 % of pediatric thyroid cancers [1, 46].

Ultrasound characteristics suggestive of malignancy include microcalcifications, indistinct margins, increased intranodular vascular flow, and a variable echotexture [33, 47–49]. Ultrasound can determine the intrathyroidal location of nodules, identify additional nodules, and assess if there is lateral cervical lymph node involvement [33, 47, 48]. Ultrasonographic appearance alone, though, cannot reliably distinguish between benign and malignant lesions. Thus, fine needle aspiration (FNA) is indicated for children with thyroid nodules and a normal or elevated TSH [47].

FNA is the most accurate means to evaluate if a thyroid nodule is malignant [47]. As in adults, FNA samples from pediatric thyroid nodules should be interpreted using the Bethesda System for Reporting Thyroid Cytopathology [50]. Reports of FNAs performed in children [50, 51] describe similar specificity and sensitivity as adults [52–54]. Difficulty arises when the FNA is nondiagnostic or the cytology is indeterminate (Bethesda criteria III AUS/FLUS), as malignancy can be present up to 50 % of the time with such cytological features [55]. If this occurs, the clinician may repeat the ultrasound study and FNA in 3–6 months or proceed to surgical lobectomy. Data examining the predictive value of the Bethesda system for pediatric thyroid nodules suggest that the risk of malignancy may be higher in children than adults when cytology is Bethesda criteria III or IV [2]. Thus, children may be referred for surgery (lobectomy with completion thyroidectomy if frozen section and/or surgical histology is positive for malignancy) more readily than adults.

Ultrasound-guided FNA is recommended especially in children because of the difficulty to biopsy small nodules which rarely can be palpated and to ensure an adequate sample, particularly in complex cystic lesions in which the solid component must be sampled [56]. When FNA is performed in children, because this is an uncommon procedure, special expertise outside pediatric departments may be needed [49, 57].

Surgical Options

The preoperative evaluation of pediatric patients with PTC or suspected PTC by FNA involves both a general examination to rule out comorbid conditions and a thyroid-focused evaluation [2, 47, 58, 59]. Thyroid assessment involves evaluation of the clinical and biochemical thyroid status combined with a detailed examination of the thyroid gland and cervical region. The neck exam focuses on thyroid size, nodularity, airway status, and an assessment of cervical lymph nodes. Ideally, surgical candidates should have their vocal cord function evaluated preoperatively, particularly if they have evidence of vocal cord compromise or a history of previous cervical surgery.

A neck ultrasound using a high-resolution probe (7.5 MHz or higher) should be performed to examine the contralateral thyroid lobe and the central and lateral neck compartments [60–63]. It is imperative to perform a detailed evaluation of the right and left lateral neck compartments prior to surgery and to biopsy any suspicious lymph nodes in order to determine whether unilateral or bilateral modified radical neck dissection is indicated or not. When further delineation of potential neck disease is needed, imaging using contrast-enhanced CT or MRI may be considered.

The location of lymph node compartments is important to consider in assessing the distribution of metastatic spread and operative sites. Lymph node compartments are designated I to VI [47]. The central compartment (VI) is the most common site of lymph node spread [64–66] and encompasses the region between the hyoid bone and sternum and the common carotid arteries [47].

Surgical options for PTC include total thyroidectomy near-total thyroidectomy or lobectomy [58]. A total thyroidectomy refers to a complete resection of the thyroid gland via an extracapsular dissection [67, 68]. If it is determined intraoperatively that a complete extracapsular dissection will result in irreversible damage to either the recurrent laryngeal nerve (RLN) or parathyroid glands, the capsule can be entered and a small amount of thyroid tissue can be left in situ to avoid injury to either the RLNs or parathyroid glands, a procedure referred to as a near-total thyroidectomy [67, 68]. Studies in children demonstrate increased relapse rates with lobectomy vs. total thyroidectomy [11, 69–72]. Thus, in an effort to minimize the recurrence risk, the recommended initial surgery for PTC is total thyroidectomy [2].

The extent of lymph node surgery has been the subject of attention [73, 74]. Lymph node metastasis is a pervasive component of DTC in children, as up to 90 % of children with DTC will have nodal disease. In addition, cancer recurrence most commonly occurs in lymph nodes in the laryngotracheal region [64]. Importantly, in up to 50 % of cases, PTC involvement of lymph nodes is not detectable by preoperative ultrasonography [65, 75], so intraoperative examination of the central lymph nodes by the surgeon is critical in determining the need for central compartment (VI) and ipsilateral and possibly contralateral central node (level VI) excision.

Considering data from children and adults, as such, for children with DTC, we recommend total or near-total thyroidectomy along with central compartment lymph node dissection as part of the initial operation [3]. In addition, lateral compartment dissection with en bloc lymph node removal is indicated when lymph node involvement is localized preoperatively by FNA. To minimize the risk of complications, surgery should be performed by high-volume, thyroid surgeons [2].

Thyroid Cancer Staging

There are multiple postoperative staging systems for DTC. The 2006 ATA guidelines recognize the American Joint Committee on Cancer and Union International Contre le Cancer (AJCC/UICC) classification system [47] as the system used by hospital tumor registries to describe the extent of disease and predict disease mortality [47]. Thyroid cancer patients < 45 years of age, and thus all children, are classified as stage I (any T, any N, M0) or II (any T, any N, M1) [47]. Such staging is based on mortality and does not distinguish pediatric and adult DTC that behave differently [47, 59, 76]. The 2009 ATA guidelines subsequently introduced a system which stratified patients by risk of recurrence with the intent to guide treatment recommendations and limit morbidity [2].

The newly published Pediatric ATA Thyroid Cancer guidelines propose a similar risk for recurrence stratification system for children, by considering cervical lymph node involvement and distant metastasis [2]. The ATA Pediatric Low-Risk category includes those patients with cancer confined to the thyroid and no lymph node involvement or microscopic metastases to a small number of central neck nodes. The ATA Pediatric Intermediate-Risk category encompasses patients with extensive central neck node involvement (N1a) or “minimal” lateral lymph node disease (N1b). These patients are at risk for residual or recurrent disease in the neck but considered low risk for distant spread. Patients in the ATA Pediatric High-Risk category include those with extensive lateral lymph node involvement (extensive N1b) or disease that is locally invasive (T4 tumors). These patients may have distant metastasis (most likely to the lungs) and are considered high risk for residual and recurrent thyroid cancer.

Radioactive Iodine Therapy

Radioactive iodine (RAI, ^{131}I, also referred to as radioiodine) was observed to kill thyroid tumor cells more than 60 years ago [3, 77, 78]. There are three major approaches for choosing an appropriate ^{131}I activity for DTC treatment [3]: [1]

applying activities based on the bone marrow toxicity limited approach [79, 80], [2] applying specific activities to result in tumor ablation [81], and [3] administering fixed activities [82], also referred to as empiric dosaging, that may or may not be based on a patient's weight. Although formal dosimetry is attractive, empiric dosaging is simpler and is widely used. The latter strategy, though, may result in over- or undertreatment of patients with DTC [83, 84]. Considering the risk of pulmonary fibrosis associated with high lung retention [greater than 100 mCi (3.7 GBq) at 24 h] [85], dosimetry should be considered for individuals with lung metastases and in situations of repeat treatment, especially in younger children [86, 87].

The overwhelming majority of pediatric patients will have nodal involvement [11–15, 88]. In this setting, based on studies showing the potential extent of lymph node spread [66, 89, 90], it must be assumed that there will be residual lymph tissue containing micrometastases following compartment dissection. Thus, RAI is favored in children with DTC and lymph node involvement [2].

Studies of children treated with RAI are limited to a small number of reports [16, 21, 69–72, 91–103]. These reports include those in which outcomes with and without RAI were compared in retrospective analyses [11, 69–71, 102], studies detailing outcome in patients treated in a standardized manner without comparison groups [76, 100, 104], and reviews on the subject [16, 21, 101, 103]. To date, randomized studies comparing RAI vs. no-RAI or dosage-response studies have not been performed in children.

The majority of pediatric patients with DTC present with nodal metastases, are not low risk, and should be assumed to have micrometastases. Based on the above data, we suggest that children who are intermediate or high risk [2] should be treated with RAI to ablate residual disease and reduce the risk of disease recurrence. Administered ^{131}I activities to be applied should range from 100 to 200 mCi (3.7–7.4 GBq) in physically mature children and may be corrected for body weight to 1.35–2.7 mCi/kg (50–100 MBq/kg) in younger children. Analyses show that treatment with at least 200 MBq/kg (5.4 mCi/kg), and in most patients even much higher activities, is possible without a risk of exceeding bone marrow tolerance limits [105].

Practical Issues of ^{131}I Therapy

To achieve ^{131}I uptake by remnant and residual tissue, TSH elevation is needed [106]. For patients taking levothyroxine (LT4), the medication should be discontinued 2–3 weeks before RAI in children, a process termed thyroid hormone withdrawal (THW) [106, 107]. Alternatively, patients can be treated with 0.7 ug/kg or triiodothyronine (LT3) for at least 1 month and the medication discontinued 2 weeks before treatment [106]. TSH levels greater than 30 mU/L appear to be adequate to stimulate ^{131}I uptake in thyroid remnants and functional metastatic lesions [108].

To facilitate ^{131}I uptake by remnant tissue or residual tumor, TSH elevation can be achieved with recombinant human TSH (rhTSH). Patients treated with rhTSH typically receive 0.9 mg of rhTSH on two consecutive days, and 24 or 48 h later ^{131}I is given [109]. It is important to emphasize that at present, rhTSH is not approved for children by drug regulatory agencies in the USA or Europe. Although the use of rhTSH has the potential to reduce whole-body radiation exposure associated with ^{131}I therapy, expanded use in the pediatric population should only be considered after clinical studies show comparable efficacy to THW.

A low-iodine diet should be adhered to 2 weeks before treatment with ^{131}I [106]. In the USA, iodine intake is about 160–177 ug per day [106, 110]. Following 1 week on a low-iodine diet, urinary iodine excretion can fall five–tenfold and lead to a doubling of the amount of radiation in residual tissue [106]. A low-iodine diet should be prescribed for 2 weeks prior to RAI and continued until 1 day after [106]. Several websites provide excellent details about dietary advice (http://www.thyca.org/rai.htm#diet).

Clinicians should be wary to avoid exposing the patient to iodine-containing compounds associated with clinical care. It has been recommended that the following minimal times between exposure to iodine-containing compounds and RAI treatment be observed: soaps and scrubs, 2 weeks; water-soluble intravenous contrast agents, 4 weeks; cavity-injected water-soluble contrast agents, 8 weeks; and cholecystographic agents, 12 weeks [106]. High iodine content medications, including amiodarone, should be avoided [106]. If there is a question as to whether the patient has iodine excess, iodine concentration can be measured in a spot urine sample [47, 59].

Another potential concern is retained gut ^{131}I [106]. An effective whole-body t1/2 of 22 h is observed in patients with large amounts of bowel ^{131}I as compared to 14 h when there is little activity in the gut [106]. Thus, it is important that patients have one or two bowel movements per day. Considering that thyroid hormone withdrawal is associated with constipation, laxative use may be needed [106].

Risks of RAI

The risks associated with RAI use in children and adults and relate primarily to second primary malignancies (SPM). Second primary malignancies initial studies of the SEER database of 30,000 adult US patients with DTC treated with RAI revealed no effects of ^{131}I therapy on SPM risk, but the risk of RAI exposure was only partially assessed [111]. Recent reevaluation of the SEER database, however, suggested that ^{131}I may have a small carcinogenic effect with increased rates of both hematologic and solid SPM in the irradiated cohort, but not in the nonirradiated group after a latency period of 3 years [112]. It was also recently suggested that treatment of low-risk thyroid cancer with ^{131}I is associated with an increased risk of SPMs [113].

A study by Verkooijen and co-workers revealed that the SPM risk is elevated, but similarly elevated before and after ^{131}I therapy [114]. These observations suggest a genetic predisposition for malignancies in such patients.

Rubino and colleagues evaluated SPMs in a European cohort of DTC patients [115]. 6,841 DTC patients, diagnosed from 1934 to 1995, were treated at a mean age of 44 years. 17 % were treated with external radiotherapy and 62 % received ^{131}I [115]. 576 patients were diagnosed with a SPM. Compared to the *general population*, an increased risk of SPM of 27 % was seen [115]. This risk was dosage related: a linear dose-response relationship with 1^{31}I administration was seen for all cancers combined and for leukemias. The increased risk of solid tumors and leukemia was found with ^{131}I activities > 200 mCi (7.4 GBq) and 100 mCi (3.7 GBq), respectively [115]. At lower activities, increased SPM risks were not apparent.

Very recently in a comprehensive study, Garsi and co-workers presented follow-up data of 11,007 European patients with DTC studied at an average of 14 years after treatment [116]. When individuals were older than 20 years at diagnosis, the risk of SPM was about 25 % higher than the general population; however, this risk was not related to ^{131}I therapy for most patients but rather to having DTC as the SPM risk without RAI was 25 % [116]. An RAI-related SPM risk was only seen when the cumulative dosage of ^{131}I exceeded 200 mCi (7.4 GBq) [116].

A secondary analysis of the European SPM data set was performed in a population of patients diagnosed less than 20 years of age by C. Rubino (personal communication). There was no evidence of an increased risk of SPMs following ^{131}I treatment of DTC in children. At present, we are not aware of other studies that have performed similar analyses comparing ^{131}I treated pediatric patients with a comparable population of pediatric DTC patients not treated with ^{131}I [117].

Levothyroxine Therapy

It is standard practice to treat thyroid cancer patients with levothyroxine postoperatively, as it is well recognized that TSH suppression can reduce rates of recurrence [118, 119]. The optimal degree of TSH suppression is debated in low-risk patients, as it is not clear if complete suppression of TSH secretion confers benefit [2].

In adults, the long-term impact of supraphysiologic doses of thyroid hormone on bone mineral density and cardiovascular risks is well recognized [120, 121]. In children, high levels of thyroid hormones can have effects on growth and profoundly impact on behavior and learning ability [122]. On the other hand, children generally need considerably higher doses of levothyroxine based on body weight to completely suppress TSH as compared to adults. To date, studies of effects of treatment resulting in subclinical hyperthyroidism in children treated for DTC have yet to be performed to assess impact.

In adults with low-risk disease, Biondi and colleagues recommend maintaining TSH levels in the low normal range (0.5–2.5 mU/L) [123, 124]. The ATA Pediatric Guidelines Taskforce recommends keeping TSH 0.5–1.0 mU/L in low-risk patients [2]. More aggressive suppression is recommended for intermediate- and high-risk patients (TSH 0.1–0.5 mU/L and <0.1 mU/L, respectively) [47]. One scheme, proposed by Baudin for children, is to initially suppress TSH levels to <0.1 mU/L and then allow the TSH to rise to 0.5 mU/L once the patient enters remission [125]. These recommendations seem appropriate for children when one considers that most recurrent DTC develops within 5 years after initial treatment [2, 126].

In pediatrics it is well recognized that medical compliance can be a major problem, especially for teens and young adults, including those with serious medical conditions [127–130]. Although TSH suppression is desirable, clinicians must recognize that TSH suppression may be difficult to enforce in the pediatric population.

Follow-Up

Follow-up care of the child with DTC involves the regular assessment of circulating thyroid hormone levels, ultrasonography of the neck, and measurement of Tg and, at select times, whole-body radioiodine scans. Follow-up regimens for children with DTC have been nicely proposed by Hung and Salaris [21] that are reasonable to follow with a few modifications. A very pertinent issue is the criteria used to assess if a patient is disease free. With more sensitive Tg assays, one can aim for an undetectable Tg level as indicative of a disease-free state, rather than a Tg of <2 ug/L, which had been standard practice. In general, follow-up ultrasound and TSH-suppressed Tg level assessment is recommended every 3–6 months for 2 years in low-risk patients and for at least 3 years in intermediate and high risk. Assessment of fT4 and TSH levels is indicated every 6 months and 1–2 months after dose changes [47, 131].

Thyroglobulin

Assessment of Tg levels is a mainstay of DTC follow-up [47, 59, 109]. rhTSH or THW-stimulated Tg levels had been considered the standard for assessing disease recurrence [2, 47, 59, 109]. However, with the more sensitive assays with detection limits of 0.1 ng/dl, one can assess unstimulated levels [2]. When unstimulated Tg levels are assessed, it is important to also assess TSH levels to assess if levels are indeed unstimulated. Although rhTSH has been used in children and shown to have a favorable safety profile [132], rhTSH is not FDA approved for use in children less than 16 years of age.

In adults, if the stimulated Tg is undetectable, no disease is present in most of patients [47]. If the level is 0.1–2.0 ug/L, 30 % will have residual disease and follow-up neck ultrasonography is indicated [47]. If the level is 2.0–10.0 ug/L, it is likely that residual disease is present and follow-up neck ultrasonography is indicated [47]. If the Tg is >10.0 ng/dl, follow-up neck ultrasonography and possibly CT or MRI scanning of the neck and chest is indicated. If gross cervical disease is present, reoperation is indicated [47]. If not, ^{131}I treatment with 100–150 mCi (3.7–5.5 GBq) should be considered [47].

A confounding factor in Tg measurement is the presence of TgAbs. In adults with DTC, less than 10 % of patients initially have elevated TgAb levels [133]. In pediatric cohorts, TgAbs or autoimmune thyroiditis is present in 20–80 % of individuals [5, 134, 135]. Because of this problem, the primary tool for assessing cure or recurrence may be difficult to use in the pediatric age group. However, trends in the TgAb titer can be used as a surrogate marker for disease status, although it is important to understand that the titer itself cannot be used to predict extent of disease. Although many TgAb-positive patients convert to being TgAb negative after treatment with surgery and RAI, 44 % of patients may remain TgAb positive 5 years after total thyroid ablation [133, 136].

Ultrasonography

Ultrasonography should be performed every 6 months to assess if there is residual thyroid tissue and lymph nodes [47]. As such it is important that studies not only focus on the thyroid bed, but encompass the neck in full, examining each lymph node compartment. Because children commonly have infection-related lymphadenopathy, serial studies may be needed every 3 months to assess if lymph nodes represent potential metastatic foci.

FNA of lymph nodes is indicated for persistent or enlarging lymph nodes or lymph nodes with abnormal characteristics, including loss of the fatty hilum, a round rather than oval shape, and/or calcification [47]. In addition, Tg levels should be assessed in lymph node aspirates [137, 138], as a measurable Tg in a lymph node is indicative of metastatic disease.

Diagnostic Whole-Body Scintigraphy

^{131}I diagnostic whole-body scintigraphy (dWBS) can be performed using 2–5 mCi (0.06–0.18 GBq) [139, 140]. Where in the past WBS was performed routinely, WBS is performed more selectively now, based on concern for persistent or recurrent disease using US and/or Tg results [2]. ^{131}I scanning is especially useful in the detection of lung metastases that are not apparent by chest radiographs or CT scanning [21]. In patients with TgAbs, ^{131}I scanning may be useful in identifying potential residual disease [139, 140]. The use of dWBS in patients without lymph node or distant metastases is debated. Some groups perform at least one ^{131}I dWBS and concurrent measurement of stimulated Tg levels after the last ^{131}I therapy course to ascertain complete remnant ablation and the absence of pathologic ^{131}I accumulation. Data, however, suggest that ^{131}I scanning adds only a modest amount of data to the combination of Tg assessment and ultrasonography [139, 140].

Synopsis

DTC in children is rare with an overall incidence of 1 per 100,000 individuals. DTC accounts for 95 % of cases of thyroid cancer in the pediatric population and typically presents with lymph node metastases and is associated with relatively high recurrence rates.

Ample evidence suggests that more extensive surgery is associated with lower rates of recurrence. Surgery is associated with clear and definable rates of complications that can be minimized when surgery is performed by high-volume thyroid surgeons. Evidence shows, that properly applied, RAI is associated with lower recurrence rates. Evidence also shows that DTC is associated with an increase SPM risk which reflects intrinsic factors related to having DTC itself. Evidence also suggests that relatively high doses of ^{131}I may contribute to an increased risk of SPMs. Thus, the proven benefit of ^{131}I in preventing cancer recurrence and cancer-related deaths needs to be weighed against potential long-term risks.

Based on the constellation of the above information, the following are recommended for children with DTC.

1. Total thyroidectomy and central compartment lymph node dissection are the surgical procedure of choice for DTC.
2. Surgery should be performed by high-volume thyroid surgeons.
3. RAI should be given for residual disease treatment using activities of 100–200 mCi (3.7–7.4 GBq) for adolescent patients with nodal and distant metastases or 1.5–3 mCi/kg (50–100 MBq/kg) for young children. For the treatment of distant metastases and recurrent disease, pretreatment dosimetry should be considered and activities up to 5 mCi/kg (200 MBq/kg) may be used.
4. Whereas empiric activity selection is convenient and practical, blood-dose limiting based or lesion-based dosimetry should be considered for children with metastatic disease to the lungs and other sites or for repeat dosing.
5. TSH levels should be maintained <0.1 mU/L for patients with extensive lateral nodal or distant metastatic disease until it is known that there is no evidence of active disease. For patients with intermediate risk or recurrence, TSH may be kept 0.1–0.5 mU/L. For patients with disease confined to the thyroid and minimal or no lymph node involvement, TSH may be kept 0.5–1.0 mU/L, and TSH suppression may be relaxed after several years of follow-up with no evidence of disease progression or recurrence.
6. Long-term follow-up for the child with DTC is essential, as disease can recur decades after initial diagnosis and therapy.
7. Considering the complexity of DTC management, the potential complications associated with therapy, and the intricacies of follow-up, it is important that pediatric DTC be managed by physicians with expertise in this area.
8. Expanded research in pediatric DTC treatment is indicated as disease aggressiveness, the risks of treatment, and long-term follow-up issues cannot be directly extrapolated from the care of adults.

References

1. Hogan AR, Zhuge Y, Perez EA, Koniaris LG, Lew JI, Sola JE. Pediatric thyroid carcinoma: incidence and outcomes in 1753 patients. J Surg Res. 2009;156(1):167–72.
2. Francis G, Waguespack SG, Bauer AJ, Angelos P, Benvenga S, Cerutti J, et al. Management guidelines for children with thyroid nodules and differentiated thyroid cancer the American Thyroid Association Guidelines Task Force on Pediatric Thyroid Cancer. Thyroid. 2015;25:716–59.
3. Rivkees SA, Mazzaferri EL, Verburg FA, Reiners C, Luster M, Breuer CK, et al. The treatment of differentiated thyroid cancer in children: emphasis on surgical approach and radioactive iodine therapy. Endocr Rev. 2011;32(6):798–826.
4. Powers PA, Dinauer CA, Tuttle RM, Robie DK, McClellan DR, Francis GL. Tumor size and extent of disease at diagnosis predict the response to initial therapy for papillary thyroid carcinoma in children and adolescents. J Pediatr Endocrinol Metab. 2003;16(5):693–702.
5. O'Gorman CS, Hamilton J, Rachmiel M, Gupta A, Ngan BY, Daneman D. Thyroid cancer in childhood: a retrospective review of childhood course. Thyroid. 2010;20(4):375–80.
6. Rachmiel M, Charron M, Gupta A, Hamilton J, Wherrett D, Forte V, et al. Evidence-based review of treatment and follow up of pediatric patients with differentiated thyroid carcinoma. J Pediatr Endocrinol Metab. 2006;19(12):1377–93.
7. Brink JS, van Heerden JA, McIver B, Salomao DR, Farley DR, Grant CS, et al. Papillary thyroid cancer with pulmonary metastases in children: long-term prognosis. Surgery. 2000;128(6):881–6; discussion 6–7.
8. La Quaglia MP, Black T, Holcomb 3rd GW, Sklar C, Azizkhan RG, Haase GM, et al. Differentiated thyroid cancer: clinical characteristics, treatment, and outcome in patients under 21 years of age who present with distant metastases. A report from the Surgical Discipline Committee of the Children's Cancer Group. J Pediatr Surg. 2000;35(6):955–9; discussion 60.
9. Haugen BRM, Alexander EK, Bible KC, Doherty G, Mandel SJ, Nikiforov YE, et al. 2015 American Thyroid Association management guidelines for adult patients with thyroid nodules and differentiated thyroid cancer. Thyroid. 2016;26:1–133.
10. Howlader N NA, Krapcho M, Garshell J, Neyman N, Altekruse SF, Kosary CL, Yu M, Ruhl J, Tatalovich Z, Cho H, Mariotto A, Lewis DR, Chen HS, Feuer EJ, Cronin KA (eds) SEER Cancer Statistics Review, 1975–2010. http://seer.cancer.gov/csr/1975_2010/. 2013.
11. Welch Dinauer CA, Tuttle RM, Robie DK, McClellan DR, Svec RL, Adair C, et al. Clinical features associated with metastasis and recurrence of differentiated thyroid cancer in children, adolescents and young adults. Clin Endocrinol (Oxf). 1998;49(5):619–28.
12. Reiners C, Demidchik YE. Differentiated thyroid cancer in childhood: pathology, diagnosis, therapy. Pediatr Endocrinol Rev. 2003;1 Suppl 2:230–5; discussion 5–6.
13. Chaukar DA, Rangarajan V, Nair N, Dcruz AK, Nadkarni MS, Pai PS, et al. Pediatric thyroid cancer. J Surg Oncol. 2005;92(2):130–3.
14. Okada T, Sasaki F, Takahashi H, Taguchi K, Takahashi M, Watanabe K, et al. Management of childhood and adolescent thyroid carcinoma: long-term follow-up and clinical characteristics. Eur J Pediatr Surg. 2006;16(1):8–13.
15. Thompson GB, Hay ID. Current strategies for surgical management and adjuvant treatment of childhood papillary thyroid carcinoma. World J Surg. 2004;28(12):1187–98.
16. Luster M, Lassmann M, Freudenberg LS, Reiners C. Thyroid cancer in childhood: management strategy, including dosimetry and long-term results. Hormones (Athens). 2007;6(4):269–78.
17. Dinauer C, Francis GL. Thyroid cancer in children. Endocrinol Metab Clin North Am. 2007;36(3):779–806, vii.
18. Dinauer CA, Breuer C, Rivkees SA. Differentiated thyroid cancer in children: diagnosis and management. Curr Opin Oncol. 2008;20(1):59–65.

19. Zimmerman D, Hay ID, Gough IR, Goellner JR, Ryan JJ, Grant CS, et al. Papillary thyroid carcinoma in children and adults: long-term follow-up of 1039 patients conservatively treated at one institution during three decades. Surgery. 1988;104(6):1157–66.
20. Zaydfudim V, Feurer ID, Griffin MR, Phay JE. The impact of lymph node involvement on survival in patients with papillary and follicular thyroid carcinoma. Surgery. 2008;144(6):1070–7; discussion 7–8.
21. Hung W, Sarlis NJ. Current controversies in the management of pediatric patients with well-differentiated nonmedullary thyroid cancer: a review. Thyroid. 2002;12(8):683–702.
22. Sugg SL, Ezzat S, Rosen IB, Freeman JL, Asa SL. Distinct multiple RET/PTC gene rearrangements in multifocal papillary thyroid neoplasia. J Clin Endocrinol Metab. 1998;83(11):4116–22.
23. Shattuck TM, Westra WH, Ladenson PW, Arnold A. Independent clonal origins of distinct tumor foci in multifocal papillary thyroid carcinoma. N Engl J Med. 2005;352(23):2406–12.
24. Duffy PJF. Cancer of the thyroid in children: a report of twenty-eight cases. J Clin Endocrinol Metab. 1950;10:1296–308.
25. Winship T, Rosvoll RV. A study of thyroid cancer in children. Am J Surg. 1961;102:747–52.
26. Sigurdson AJ, Ronckers CM, Mertens AC, Stovall M, Smith SA, Liu Y, et al. Primary thyroid cancer after a first tumour in childhood (the Childhood Cancer Survivor Study): a nested case–control study. Lancet. 2005;365(9476):2014–23.
27. Dolphin GW. The risk of thyroid cancers following irradiation. Health Phys. 1968;15:219–28.
28. Ron E, Lubin J, Shore RE, Mabuchi K, Modan B, Pottern LM, et al. Thyroid Cancer after exposure to external radiation: a pooled analysis of seven studies. Radiat Res. 1995;141:259–77.
29. Sankila R, Garwicz S, Olsen JH, Dollner H, Hertz H, Kreuger A, et al. Risk of subsequent malignant neoplasms among 1,641 Hodgkin's disease patients diagnosed in childhood and adolescence: a population-based cohort study in the five Nordic countries. Association of the Nordic cancer registries and the Nordic society of pediatric hematology and oncology. J Clin Oncol. 1996;14(5):1442–6.
30. Davies SM. Subsequent malignant neoplasms in survivors of childhood cancer: Childhood Cancer Survivor Study (CCSS) studies. Pediatr Blood Cancer. 2007;48(7):727–30.
31. Maule M, Scelo G, Pastore G, Brennan P, Hemminki K, Pukkala E, et al. Risk of second malignant neoplasms after childhood central nervous system malignant tumours: an international study. Eur J Cancer. 2008;44(6):830–9.
32. Tucker MA, Jones PH, Boice Jr JD, Robison LL, Stone BJ, Stovall M, et al. Therapeutic radiation at a young age is linked to secondary thyroid cancer. The late effects study group. Cancer Res. 1991;51(11):2885–8.
33. Brignardello E, Corrias A, Isolato G, Palestini N, Cordero di Montezemolo L, Fagioli F, et al. Ultrasound screening for thyroid carcinoma in childhood cancer survivors: a case series. J Clin Endocrinol Metab. 2008;93(12):4840–3.
34. Malchoff CD, Malchoff DM. Familial papillary thyroid carcinoma. Cancer Treat Res. 2004;122:381–7.
35. Ozaki O, Ito K, Kobayashi K, Suzuki A, Manabe Y, Hosoda Y. Familial occurrence of differentiated, nonmedullary thyroid carcinoma. World J Surg. 1988;12(4):565–71.
36. Korber C, Geling M, Werner E, Mortl M, Mader U, Reiners C, et al. Incidence of familial non-medullary thyroid carcinoma in the patient register of the Clinic and Polyclinic of Nuclear Medicine, University of Wurzburg. Nuklearmedizin. 2000;39(1):27–32.
37. Hillenbrand A, Varhaug JE, Brauckhoff M, Pandev R, Haufe S, Dotzenrath C, et al. Familial nonmedullary thyroid carcinoma—clinical relevance and prognosis. A European multicenter study. Langenbecks Arch Surg. 2010;395:851–8.
38. Farooq A, Walker LJ, Bowling J, Audisio RA. Cowden syndrome. Cancer Treat Rev. 2010;36:577–83.
39. Blumenthal GM, Dennis PA. PTEN hamartoma tumor syndromes. Eur J Hum Genet. 2008;16(11):1289–300.

40. Richards ML. Familial syndromes associated with thyroid cancer in the era of personalized medicine. Thyroid. 2010;20(7):707–13.
41. Hobert JA, Eng C. PTEN hamartoma tumor syndrome: an overview. Genet Med. 2009;11(10):687–94.
42. Vriens MR, Suh I, Moses W, Kebebew E. Clinical features and genetic predisposition to hereditary nonmedullary thyroid cancer. Thyroid. 2009;19(12):1343–9.
43. Half E, Bercovich D, Rozen P. Familial adenomatous polyposis. Orphanet J Rare Dis. 2009;4:22.
44. Perrier ND, van Heerden JA, Goellner JR, Williams ED, Gharib H, Marchesa P, et al. Thyroid cancer in patients with familial adenomatous polyposis. World J Surg. 1998;22(7):738–42; discussion 43.
45. Niedziela M. Pathogenesis, diagnosis and management of thyroid nodules in children. Endocr Relat Cancer. 2006;13(2):427–53.
46. Cheung K, Roman SA, Wang TS, Walker HD, Sosa JA. Calcitonin measurement in the evaluation of thyroid nodules in the United States: a cost-effectiveness and decision analysis. J Clin Endocrinol Metab. 2008;93(6):2173–80.
47. Cooper DS, Doherty GM, Haugen BR, Kloos RT, Lee SL, Mandel SJ, et al. Management guidelines for patients with thyroid nodules and differentiated thyroid cancer. Thyroid. 2006;16(2):109–42.
48. Corrias A, Einaudi S, Chiorboli E, Weber G, Crino A, Andreo M, et al. Accuracy of fine needle aspiration biopsy of thyroid nodules in detecting malignancy in childhood: comparison with conventional clinical, laboratory, and imaging approaches. J Clin Endocrinol Metab. 2001;86(10):4644–8.
49. Mussa A, De Andrea M, Motta M, Mormile A, Palestini N, Corrias A. Predictors of malignancy in children with thyroid nodules. J Pediatr. 2015;167(4):886–92 e1.
50. Cibas ES, Ali SZ. The Bethesda system for reporting thyroid cytopathology. Thyroid. 2009;19(11):1159–65.
51. Baloch ZW, LiVolsi VA, Asa SL, Rosai J, Merino MJ, Randolph G, et al. Diagnostic terminology and morphologic criteria for cytologic diagnosis of thyroid lesions: a synopsis of the National Cancer Institute thyroid fine-needle aspiration state of the science conference. Diagnostic cytopathology. 2008;36(6):425–37.
52. Moslavac S, Matesa N, Kusic Z. Thyroid fine needle aspiration cytology in children and adolescents. Coll Antropol. 2010;34(1):197–200.
53. Kapila K, Pathan SK, George SS, Haji BE, Das DK, Qadan LR. Fine needle aspiration cytology of the thyroid in children and adolescents: experience with 792 aspirates. Acta Cytol. 2010;54(4):569–74.
54. Corrias A, Mussa A, Baronio F, Arrigo T, Salerno M, Segni M, et al. Diagnostic features of thyroid nodules in pediatrics. Arch Pediatr Adolesc Med. 2010;164(8):714–9.
55. Theoharis CG, Schofield KM, Hammers L, Udelsman R, Chhieng DC. The Bethesda thyroid fine-needle aspiration classification system: year 1 at an academic institution. Thyroid. 2009;19(11):1215–23.
56. Izquierdo R, Shankar R, Kort K, Khurana K. Ultrasound-guided fine-needle aspiration in the management of thyroid nodules in children and adolescents. Thyroid. 2009;19(7):703–5.
57. Rivkees SA. Evaluating the rare and predicting the worst: lessons for thyroid nodules. J Pediatr. 2015;167(4):790–1.
58. Carty SE, Cooper DS, Doherty GM, Duh QY, Kloos RT, Mandel SJ, et al. Consensus statement on the terminology and classification of central neck dissection for thyroid cancer. Thyroid. 2009;19(11):1153–8.
59. Cooper DS, Doherty GM, Haugen BR, Kloos RT, Lee SL, Mandel SJ, et al. Revised American Thyroid Association management guidelines for patients with thyroid nodules and differentiated thyroid cancer. Thyroid. 2009;19(11):1167–214.
60. Kouvaraki MA, Shapiro SE, Fornage BD, Edeiken-Monro BS, Sherman SI, Vassilopoulou-Sellin R, et al. Role of preoperative ultrasonography in the surgical management of patients with thyroid cancer. Surgery. 2003;134(6):946–54; discussion 54–5.

61. Solorzano CC, Carneiro DM, Ramirez M, Lee TM, Irvin 3rd GL. Surgeon-performed ultrasound in the management of thyroid malignancy. Am Surg. 2004;70(7):576–80; discussion 80–2.
62. Gonzalez HE, Cruz F, O'Brien A, Goni I, Leon A, Claure R, et al. Impact of preoperative ultrasonographic staging of the neck in papillary thyroid carcinoma. Arch Otolaryngol Head Neck Surg. 2007;133(12):1258–62.
63. Stulak JM, Grant CS, Farley DR, Thompson GB, van Heerden JA, Hay ID, et al. Value of preoperative ultrasonography in the surgical management of initial and reoperative papillary thyroid cancer. Arch Surg. 2006;141(5):489–94; discussion 94–6.
64. Gimm O, Rath FW, Dralle H. Pattern of lymph node metastases in papillary thyroid carcinoma. Br J Surg. 1998;85(2):252–4.
65. Bonnet S, Hartl DM, Travagli JP. Lymph node dissection for thyroid cancer. J Visc Surg. 2010;147(3):e155–9.
66. Machens A, Hauptmann S, Dralle H. Lymph node dissection in the lateral neck for completion in central node-positive papillary thyroid cancer. Surgery. 2009;145(2):176–81.
67. Udelsman R, Lakatos E, Ladenson P. Optimal surgery for papillary thyroid carcinoma. World J Surg. 1996;20(1):88–93.
68. Udelsman R. Thyroid cancer surgery. Rev Endocr Metab Disord. 2000;1(3):155–63.
69. Demidchik YE, Demidchik EP, Reiners C, Biko J, Mine M, Saenko VA, et al. Comprehensive clinical assessment of 740 cases of surgically treated thyroid cancer in children of Belarus. Ann Surg. 2006;243(4):525–32.
70. Handkiewicz-Junak D, Wloch J, Roskosz J, Krajewska J, Kropinska A, Pomorski L, et al. Total thyroidectomy and adjuvant radioiodine treatment independently decrease locoregional recurrence risk in childhood and adolescent differentiated thyroid cancer. J Nucl Med. 2007;48(6):879–88.
71. Hay ID, Gonzalez-Losada T, Reinalda MS, Honetschlager JA, Richards ML, Thompson GB. Long-term outcome in 215 children and adolescents with papillary thyroid cancer treated during 1940 through 2008. World J Surg. 2010;34(6):1192–202.
72. Borson-Chazot F, Causeret S, Lifante JC, Augros M, Berger N, Peix JL. Predictive factors for recurrence from a series of 74 children and adolescents with differentiated thyroid cancer. World J Surg. 2004;28(11):1088–92.
73. Mazzaferri EL. A vision for the surgical management of papillary thyroid carcinoma: extensive lymph node compartmental dissections and selective use of radioiodine. J Clin Endocrinol Metab. 2009;94(4):1086–8.
74. Doherty GM. Prophylactic central lymph node dissection: continued controversy. Oncology (Williston Park). 2009;23(7):603–8.
75. Bonnet S, Hartl D, Leboulleux S, Baudin E, Lumbroso JD, Al Ghuzlan A, et al. Prophylactic lymph node dissection for papillary thyroid cancer less than 2 cm: implications for radioiodine treatment. J Clin Endocrinol Metab. 2009;94(4):1162–7.
76. Leboulleux S, Baudin E, Hartl DW, Travagli JP, Schlumberger M. Follicular-cell derived thyroid cancer in children. Eur J Cancer. 2004;40(11):1655–9.
77. Seidlin SM, Oshry E, Yalow AA. Spontaneous and experimentally induced uptake of radioactive iodine in metastases from thyroid carcinoma; a preliminary report. J Clin Endocrinol Metab. 1948;8(6):423–32.
78. Coliez R. Results of examination of 85 cases of cancer of the thyroid with radioactive iodine. J Radiol Electrol Arch Electr Medicale. 1954;32:881–95.
79. Benua RS, Cicale NR, Sonenberg M, Rawson RW. The relation of radioiodine dosimetry to results and complications in the treatment of metastatic thyroid cancer. Am J Roentgenol Radium Ther Nucl Med. 1962;87:171–82.
80. Verburg FA, Hanscheid H, Biko J, Hategan MC, Lassmann M, Kreissl MC, et al. Dosimetry-guided high-activity (131)I therapy in patients with advanced differentiated thyroid carcinoma: initial experience. Eur J Nucl Med Mol Imaging. 2010;37(5):896–903.
81. Maxon HR, Thomas SR, Hertzberg VS, Kereiakes JG, Chen IW, Sperling MI, et al. Relation between effective radiation dose and outcome of radioiodine therapy for thyroid cancer. N Engl J Med. 1983;309:937–41.

82. Beierwaltes WH. The treatment of thyroid carcinoma with radioactive iodine. Semin Nucl Med. 1978;8(1):79–94.
83. Kulkarni K, Van Nostrand D, Atkins F, Aiken M, Burman K, Wartofsky L. The relative frequency in which empiric dosages of radioiodine would potentially overtreat or undertreat patients who have metastatic well-differentiated thyroid cancer. Thyroid. 2006;16(10):1019–23.
84. Van Nostrand D, Atkins F, Moreau S, Aiken M, Kulkarni K, Wu JS, et al. Utility of the radioiodine whole-body retention at 48 hours for modifying empiric activity of 131-iodine for the treatment of metastatic well-differentiated thyroid carcinoma. Thyroid. 2009;19(10):1093–8.
85. Rall JE, Alpers JB, Lewallen CG, Sonenberg M, Berman M, Rawson RW. Radiation pneumonitis and fibrosis: a complication of radioiodine treatment of pulmonary metastases from cancer of the thyroid. J Clin Endocrinol Metab. 1957;17(11):1263–76.
86. Song H, He B, Prideaux A, Du Y, Frey E, Kasecamp W, et al. Lung dosimetry for radioiodine treatment planning in the case of diffuse lung metastases. J Nucl Med. 2006;47(12):1985–94.
87. Sgouros G, Song H, Ladenson PW, Wahl RL. Lung toxicity in radioiodine therapy of thyroid carcinoma: development of a dose-rate method and dosimetric implications of the 80-mCi rule. J Nucl Med. 2006;47(12):1977–84.
88. Scheumann GF, Gimm O, Wegener G, Hundeshagen H, Dralle H. Prognostic significance and surgical management of locoregional lymph node metastases in papillary thyroid cancer. World J Surg. 1994;18(4):559–67; discussion 67–8.
89. Dralle H, Machens A. Surgical approaches in thyroid cancer and lymph-node metastases. Best Pract Res Clin Endocrinol Metab. 2008;22(6):971–87.
90. Machens A, Hinze R, Thomusch O, Dralle H. Pattern of nodal metastasis for primary and reoperative thyroid cancer. World J Surg. 2002;26(1):22–8.
91. Samuel AM, Rajashekharrao B, Shah DH. Pulmonary metastases in children and adolescents with well-differentiated thyroid cancer. J Nucl Med. 1998;39(9):1531–6.
92. Bal CS, Kumar A, Chandra P, Dwivedi SN, Mukhopadhyaya S. Is chest x-ray or high-resolution computed tomography scan of the chest sufficient investigation to detect pulmonary metastasis in pediatric differentiated thyroid cancer? Thyroid. 2004;14(3):217–25.
93. Dottorini ME, Vignati A, Mazzucchelli L, Lomuscio G, Colombo L. Differentiated thyroid carcinoma in children and adolescents: a 37-year experience in 85 patients. J Nucl Med. 1997;38(5):669–75.
94. Giuffrida D, Scollo C, Pellegriti G, Lavenia G, Iurato MP, Pezzin V, et al. Differentiated thyroid cancer in children and adolescents. J Endocrinol Invest. 2002;25(1):18–24.
95. Chow SM, Law SC, Mendenhall WM, Au SK, Chan PT, Leung TW, et al. Papillary thyroid carcinoma: prognostic factors and the role of radioiodine and external radiotherapy. Int J Radiat Oncol Biol Phys. 2002;52(3):784–95.
96. Collini P, Mattavelli F, Spinelli C, Massimino M. Treatment of sporadic nonmedullary thyroid carcinomas in pediatric age. Expert Rev Anticancer Ther. 2007;7(1):23–30.
97. Grigsby PW, Gal-or A, Michalski JM, Doherty GM. Childhood and adolescent thyroid carcinoma. Cancer. 2002;95(4):724–9.
98. Pazaitou-Panayiotou K, Kaprara A, Boudina M, Georgiou E, Drimonitis A, Vainas I, et al. Thyroid carcinoma in children and adolescents: presentation, clinical course, and outcome of therapy in 23 children and adolescents in Northern Greece. Hormones (Athens). 2005;4(4):213–20.
99. Lazarus JH. Guidelines for the use of radioiodine in the management of hyperthyroidism: a summary. Prepared by the Radioiodine Audit Subcommittee of the Royal College of Physicians Committee on Diabetes and Endocrinology, and the Research Unit of the Royal College of Physicians. Journal of the Royal College of Physicians of London. 1995;29(6):464–9.
100. Lazar L, Lebenthal Y, Steinmetz A, Yackobovitch-Gavan M, Phillip M. Differentiated thyroid carcinoma in pediatric patients: comparison of presentation and course between pre-pubertal children and adolescents. J Pediatr. 2009;154(5):708–14.

101. Pawelczak M, David R, Franklin B, Kessler M, Lam L, Shah B. Outcomes of children and adolescents with well-differentiated thyroid carcinoma and pulmonary metastases following (1)(3)(1)I treatment: a systematic review. Thyroid. 2010;20(10):1095–101.
102. Chow SM, Law SC, Mendenhall WM, Au SK, Yau S, Mang O, et al. Differentiated thyroid carcinoma in childhood and adolescence-clinical course and role of radioiodine. Pediatr Blood Cancer. 2004;42(2):176–83.
103. Parisi MT, Mankoff D. Differentiated pediatric thyroid cancer: correlates with adult disease, controversies in treatment. Semin Nucl Med. 2007;37(5):340–56.
104. Kalemba B, Rozkosz J, Wloch J, Jarzab B. Early results of 131I therapy of differentiated thyroid carcinoma in children. Endokrynol Diabetol Chor Przemiany Materii Wieku Rozw. 1998;4(1):27–35.
105. Verburg E, Biko J, Diebl S, Demidchik Y, Drozd V, Rivkees S, et al. I-131 activities as high as safely administrable for the treatment of children and adolescents with advanced differentiated thyroid cancer. JCEM. 2011;96(8):E1268–71.
106. Maxon 3rd HR, Smith HS. Radioiodine-131 in the diagnosis and treatment of metastatic well differentiated thyroid cancer. Endocrinol Metab Clin North Am. 1990;19(3):685–718.
107. Huang SC, Wu VC, Lin SY, Sheu WH, Song YM, Lin YH, et al. Factors related to clinical hypothyroid severity in thyroid cancer patients after thyroid hormone withdrawal. Thyroid. 2009;19(1):13–20.
108. Edmonds CJ, Hayes S, Kermode JC, Thompson BD. Measurement of serum TSH and thyroid hormones in the management of treatment of thyroid carcinoma with radioiodine. Br J Radiol. 1977;50(599):799–807.
109. Pacini F, Schlumberger M, Dralle H, Elisei R, Smit JW, Wiersinga W. European consensus for the management of patients with differentiated thyroid carcinoma of the follicular epithelium. Eur J Endocrinol. 2006;154(6):787–803.
110. Caldwell KL, Jones R, Hollowell JG. Urinary iodine concentration: United States National Health and Nutrition Examination Survey 2001–2002. Thyroid. 2005;15(7):692–9.
111. Ronckers CM, McCarron P, Ron E. Thyroid cancer and multiple primary tumors in the SEER cancer registries. Int J Cancer. 2005;117(2):281–8.
112. Brown AP, Chen J, Hitchcock YJ, Szabo A, Shrieve DC, Tward JD. The risk of second primary malignancies up to three decades after the treatment of differentiated thyroid cancer. J Clin Endocrinol Metab. 2008;93(2):504–15.
113. Iyer NG, Morris LG, Tuttle RM, Shaha AR, Ganly I. Rising incidence of second cancers in patients with low-risk (T1N0) thyroid cancer who receive radioactive iodine therapy. Cancer. 2011;117:4439–46.
114. Verkooijen RB, Smit JW, Romijn JA, Stokkel MP. The incidence of second primary tumors in thyroid cancer patients is increased, but not related to treatment of thyroid cancer. Eur J Endocrinol. 2006;155(6):801–6.
115. Rubino C, de Vathaire F, Dottorini ME, Hall P, Schvartz C, Couette JE, et al. Second primary malignancies in thyroid cancer patients. Br J Cancer. 2003;89(9):1638–44.
116. Garsi JP, Rubino C, Lonn S, Schvartz C, Andruccioli M, Bardet S, et al. Impact of radioiodine treatment on the risk of second primary malignancy (SPM) following thyroid cancer: a European cohort study. 14th Annual International Thyroid Conference; Paris. 2010.
117. Zanzonico PB. Radiation dose to patients and relatives incident to 131I therapy. Thyroid. 1997;7(2):199–204.
118. Cooper DS, Specker B, Ho M, Sperling M, Ladenson PW, Ross DS, et al. Thyrotropin suppression and disease progression in patients with differentiated thyroid cancer: results from the National Thyroid Cancer Treatment Cooperative Registry. Thyroid. 1998;8(9):737–44.
119. Burmeister LA, Goumaz MO, Mariash CN, Oppenheimer JH. Levothyroxine dose requirements for thyrotropin suppression in the treatment of differentiated thyroid cancer. J Clin Endocrinol Metab. 1992;75(2):344–50.
120. Batrinos ML. The problem of exogenous subclinical hyperthyroidism. Hormones (Athens). 2006;5(2):119–25.

121. Osman F, Gammage MD, Franklyn JA. Hyperthyroidism and cardiovascular morbidity and mortality. Thyroid. 2002;12(6):483–7.
122. Rivkees SA. Pediatric Graves' disease: controversies in management. Horm Res Paediatr. 2010;74:305–11.
123. Biondi B, Cooper DS. Benefits of thyrotropin suppression versus the risks of adverse effects in differentiated thyroid cancer. Thyroid. 2010;20(2):135–46.
124. Biondi B, Filetti S, Schlumberger M. Thyroid-hormone therapy and thyroid cancer: a reassessment. Nat Clin Pract Endocrinol Metab. 2005;1(1):32–40.
125. Baudin E, Do Cao C, Cailleux AF, Leboulleux S, Travagli JP, Schlumberger M. Positive predictive value of serum thyroglobulin levels, measured during the first year of follow-up after thyroid hormone withdrawal, in thyroid cancer patients. J Clin Endocrinol Metab. 2003;88(3):1107–11.
126. Verburg FA, Stokkel MP, Duren C, Verkooijen RB, Mader U, van Isselt JW, et al. No survival difference after successful (131)I ablation between patients with initially low-risk and high-risk differentiated thyroid cancer. Eur J Nucl Med Mol Imaging. 2010;37(2):276–83.
127. Sherry NA, Levitsky LL. Management of diabetic ketoacidosis in children and adolescents. Paediatr Drugs. 2008;10(4):209–15.
128. Costello I, Wong IC, Nunn AJ. A literature review to identify interventions to improve the use of medicines in children. Child Care Health Dev. 2004;30(6):647–65.
129. Falkenstein K, Flynn L, Kirkpatrick B, Casa-Melley A, Dunn S. Non-compliance in children post-liver transplant. Who are the culprits? Pediatr Transplant. 2004;8(3):233–6.
130. Beardon PH, McGilchrist MM, McKendrick AD, McDevitt DG, MacDonald TM. Primary non-compliance with prescribed medication in primary care. BMJ. 1993;307(6908):846–8.
131. Beck-Peccoz P, Persani L, LaFranchi S. Safety of medications and hormones used in the treatment of pediatric thyroid disorders. Pediatr Endocrinol Rev. 2004;2 Suppl 1:124–33.
132. Luster M, Handkiewicz-Junak D, Grossi A, Zacharin M, Taieb D, Cruz O, et al. Recombinant thyrotropin use in children and adolescents with differentiated thyroid cancer: a multicenter retrospective study. J Clin Endocrinol Metab. 2009;94(10):3948–53.
133. Mazzaferri EL, Robbins RJ, Spencer CA, Braverman LE, Pacini F, Wartofsky L, et al. A consensus report of the role of serum thyroglobulin as a monitoring method for low-risk patients with papillary thyroid carcinoma. J Clin Endocrinol Metab. 2003;88(4):1433–41.
134. Van Savell Jr H, Hughes SM, Bower C, Parham DM. Lymphocytic infiltration in pediatric thyroid carcinomas. Pediatr Dev Pathol. 2004;7(5):487–92.
135. Somnuke PH, Pusuwan P, Likitmaskul S, Santiprabhob J, Sawathiparnich P. Treatment outcome of Graves' disease in Thai children. J Med Assoc Thai. 2007;90(9):1815–20.
136. Rubello D, Casara D, Girelli ME, Piccolo M, Busnardo B. Clinical meaning of circulating antithyroglobulin antibodies in differentiated thyroid cancer: a prospective study. J Nucl Med. 1992;33(8):1478–80.
137. Bournaud C, Charrie A, Nozieres C, Chikh K, Lapras V, Denier ML, et al. Thyroglobulin measurement in fine-needle aspirates of lymph nodes in patients with differentiated thyroid cancer: a simple definition of the threshold value, with emphasis on potential pitfalls of the method. Clin Chem Lab Med. 2010;48(8):1171–7.
138. Kim MJ, Kim EK, Kim BM, Kwak JY, Lee EJ, Park CS, et al. Thyroglobulin measurement in fine-needle aspirate washouts: the criteria for neck node dissection for patients with thyroid cancer. Clin Endocrinol (Oxf). 2009;70(1):145–51.
139. Chao M. Management of differentiated thyroid cancer with rising thyroglobulin and negative diagnostic radioiodine whole body scan. Clin Oncol (R Coll Radiol). 2010;22(6):438–47.
140. Heston TF, Wahl RL. Molecular imaging in thyroid cancer. Cancer Imaging. 2010;10(1):1–7.

Part V
Controversies in Papillary Thyroid Cancer

Chapter 14
Papillary Thyroid Microcarcinomas

Jennifer R. Cracchiolo and Ashok R. Shaha

Introduction

The incidence of thyroid carcinoma is increasing at a rapid pace. Papillary thyroid microcarcinomas (PTMCs) are central to this discussion, as they have been identified as a major contributor to the growing incidence of thyroid carcinoma. This pathologic presentation, which is defined by the World Health Organization as a papillary thyroid carcinoma <1 cm in size, represents a distinct entity with unique clinical behavior. Once referred to as "occult papillary carcinoma," these tumors are now commonly detected, owing to advances in radiographic imaging, and their clinical management is a source of significant debate. Whereas most PTMCs are indolent and follow a rather benign course, some metastasize, exhibit extracapsular spread, and harbor molecular mutations consistent with aggressive disease. In this chapter, we will look at whether this increase in the incidence of thyroid carcinoma represents an increase in detection or a true increase in disease. We will discuss the management and outcomes of PTMCs, as well as the risk factors that guide their treatment, including their molecular profiles. As technology continues to advance and find increased clinical use, PTMCs are projected to make up an even more substantial part of the thyroid surgical practice; therefore, PTMCs are a highly relevant topic in the management of differentiated thyroid cancer.

J.R. Cracchiolo, MD (✉) • A.R. Shaha, MD
Department of Surgery, Head and Neck Service, Memorial Sloan Kettering Cancer Center, 1275 York Avenue, New York, NY 10065, USA
e-mail: cracchij@mskcc.org; ShahaA@mskcc.org

S.A. Roman et al. (eds.), *Management of Thyroid Nodules and Differentiated Thyroid Cancer*, DOI 10.1007/978-3-319-43618-0_14

Increasing Incidence of PTMCs

As the incidence of papillary thyroid cancer has increased throughout the developed world [1–4], it is of significant importance to determine whether this is a real increase or whether it represents an increase in diagnostic scrutiny. Black and Welch first proposed a mechanism of overdiagnosis of cancers in 1993, which centers on increased diagnostic scrutiny leading to the detection of subclinical disease that may never result in symptoms or death [5]. They later went on to suggest two prerequisites for cancer overdiagnosis: (1) the existence of a silent disease reservoir and (2) activities leading to the detection of subclinical disease, such as screening [6]. Does the rise in papillary thyroid cancer fit with Black and Welch's mechanism of overdiagnosis? This question is more than an academic one. Examining the underlying drivers of this increase is important, as a true increase calls for efforts to address risk factors and etiology. In contrast, if diagnostic inquiry is driving this trend, then the appropriate use of screening and treatment for this disease must be discussed with the healthcare community.

PTMCs account for most of the increased incidence of thyroid carcinomas. In 1988, one-quarter of papillary thyroid cancers diagnosed were <1 cm. In 2008, this increased to almost 40 % [7]. In the last 30 years, thyroid carcinoma has doubled in incidence, with about half of these cases PTMCs [1]. During this time, death from disease has remained stable. This would suggest that these cancers do not translate into death from disease but represent a reservoir of subclinical disease, seeming to fulfill Black and Welsh's first prerequisite for overdiagnosis. Increased incidence has not been observed for other histologic types of thyroid cancer, including less common histologic categories such as follicular, medullary, and anaplastic thyroid cancer. Some researchers have questioned whether death is the correct endpoint to use in this discussion.

Are PTMCs, on the one hand, indolent enough to not result in death while, on the other, capable of being symptomatic? Autopsy studies would suggest this is not the case [8–10]. Harach et al. described occult papillary carcinoma of the thyroid as a "normal" finding among 101 systematically analyzed thyroid glands [11]. In this study, samples were sectioned into 2-–3-mm slices; 36 % of patients were found to have asymptomatic papillary thyroid cancer. They later calculated that, if thinner sections had been prepared and examined, PTMCs would have been detected in virtually all of the samples. Certainly, histologic sampling has contributed to the increased detection of thyroid carcinoma. This is particularly relevant when considering the finding of multifocal disease in total thyroidectomy specimens. Neuhold et al. reported that the detection rate of papillary thyroid cancer was determined by the accuracy of the histologic examination of postthyroidectomy specimens [12]. A discussion of the relevance of multifocal disease and PTMC will be included later in this chapter. However, collectively, this body of literature suggests that, if you look for PTMC, you will find it. This further advances the argument that the current situation is an epidemic of overdiagnosis, rather than disease.

The increased use of imaging also represents a source of incidentally found PTMCs and fulfills the second of Black and Welsh's prerequisites for overdiagnosis: activities leading to the detection of subclinical disease, such as screening. Such a phenomenon is neatly illustrated by the steep increase observed in the incidence of thyroid cancer in South Korea, where hospitals market health checkup programs that include thyroid cancer screening with ultrasonography. In this screening environment, thyroid cancer diagnoses increased 15-fold from 1993 to 2011, making thyroid cancer the most common type of cancer diagnosed in South Korea [2]. Imaging modalities other than ultrasound detect PTMCs as well. Among 101 "incidentalomas" identified by imaging in a study from Bahl et al., the modalities responsible for initial detection were CT (36 %), PET/CT (27 %), ultrasound (24 %), MRI (8 %), radiograph (3 %), octreotide scan (1 %), and echocardiogram (1 %) [13]. The high rate of detection by CT is secondary to its more common use; ultrasound, which has a higher spatial resolution, is more likely to detect a PTMC and does so in approximately half of patients who undergo it [14, 15].

After a subcentimeter nodule is found, the use of assertive biopsy can also play a role in the increased diagnosis of PTMCs. Although it is often not indicated, biopsy by fine needle aspiration (FNA) is a simple and low-risk procedure. The ease of performance, combined with the superficial location of the thyroid, lowers the threshold for performing FNA biopsy of the thyroid, despite recommendations that do not support this practice. This pattern shines even more light on the silent reservoir of PTMC, driving the number of diagnoses. The American Thyroid Association (ATA) recommends FNA evaluation only if nodules are >1 cm [16]. Specifically, nodules >1 cm with suspicious findings by sonography that carry high or intermediate risk should be biopsied by FNA. The ATA goes on to recommend that, for thyroid nodules that do not meet these criteria, diagnostic FNA is not required. Certainly, the presence of clinical features such as associated lymphadenopathy should prompt evaluation by FNA [17]. Additionally, nodules found incidentally on PET scan carry a risk of malignancy of approximately 33 % and are perhaps more aggressive; therefore, such nodules should be evaluated even if they are <1 cm [18, 19]. For nodules that do not meet the criteria for FNA, the timing of ultrasound follow-up should be based on sonographic findings. For nodules with highly suspicious findings, the ATA recommends follow-up with imaging every 6–12 months; for nodules with intermediate findings, follow-up every 12–24 months is recommended. Nodules that do not meet the criteria for FNA, are <1 cm, and have low-risk findings (including purely cystic or spongiform appearance) do not require routine sonographic follow-up [17].

Taken collectively, the literature suggests that PTMCs represent a "reservoir of subclinical cancers" [20]. Increased diagnostic scrutiny has led to the detection of many of these PTMCs, which, the evidence suggests, are unlikely to progress—and those that do are unlikely to be clinically relevant or affect the patient's survival. However, once a PTMC is found, the surgeon is faced with the question of how to manage this entity. Such considerations can be complex when the PTMC was detected incidentally. An understanding of the molecular biology of the tumor, the risk factors for aggressive disease, the available management strategies, and the outcomes of PTMC is useful in counseling these patients and will be covered in the remaining sections of this chapter.

Molecular Biology of Papillary Microcarcinoma

As discussed above, most PTMCs are indolent; however, some have a propensity for aggressive behavior and dissemination. Identifying the molecular characteristics that predict "bad actors" will help reduce overtreatment of indolent PTMCs. Nikiforov et al. detected *BRAF* V600E mutations in 77 % of aggressive PTMCs (lymph node metastasis or tumor recurrence), compared with 33 % of nonaggressive PTMCs. Although this finding was significant, the presence of a *BRAF* mutation alone is not adequate for accurate risk stratification. Of importance, in a cohort of 29 aggressive PTMCs, eight did not have *BRAF* mutations [21]. When histopathologic features—including superficial tumor location, intraglandular tumor spread/multifocality, and tumor fibrosis—were included, sensitivity improved from 77 to 96 %, and specificity increased from 68 to 80 %. Others have found *BRAF* mutations in up to 70 % of PTMCs and have shown this mutation to be associated with a high risk of local recurrence, secondary to features of extrathyroidal extension and nodal metastasis, specifically lateral cervical lymph node metastasis [22]. The high percentage of *BRAF*-positive PTMCs suggests that this mutation is an early event in thyroid carcinogenesis. Of importance, independent of the high rate of *BRAF* mutations, in general, histotypes with *BRAF* mutations have a good or even excellent prognosis, suggesting that the presence of a *BRAF* mutation alone is not an adequate basis to predict the clinical behavior of or dictate the clinical decision-making for PTMCs.

It has been reported that, for papillary thyroid carcinomas, the coexistence of *BRAF* V600E and *TERT* mutations results in a genetic background that predicts an aggressive clinical course [23]. This has not held true for PTMCs, however, as the presence of *TERT* mutations, whether alone or with *BRAF* mutations, has not been found to predict an aggressive clinical course.

At present, no one molecular aberration has been proven to be useful in directing surgical treatment to affect clinical outcomes. Next-generation sequencing panels such as ThyroseqV2 [24] may offer a more useful predictive tool to help direct management of PTMCs in the future.

Management of PTMCs

No consensus exists for the management of PTMCs, and, therefore, a wide range of management options have been described. These range from active observation without treatment [25] to thyroid lobectomy [26] to total thyroidectomy with elective neck dissection (central alone vs. lateral) plus or minus radioactive iodine treatment [27].

Surgical Management of the Primary Tumor

Total thyroidectomy is the standard treatment for papillary thyroid cancer; however, whether an operation that includes removal of less than the entire gland is acceptable for indolent PTMCs is less clear. In clinical decision-making, one must consider the risk factors associated with the small subset of aggressive PTMCs. The ATA states that lobectomy alone may be sufficient for small (<1 cm), low-risk, unifocal, intrathyroidal papillary carcinomas, in the absence of previous head and neck irradiation or radiologically or clinically involved cervical nodal metastases. This recommendation is derived from studies showing that recurrence rates do not differ between patients treated with unilateral lobectomy and those treated with total thyroidectomy [26, 28, 29]. Support for total thyroidectomy is often centered on eliminating multifocal disease. Contralateral and multifocal microscopic cancers are common in patients with papillary thyroid carcinoma. Untch et al. reported a series in which 34 % of patients were found to have contralateral cancer, with 89 % of these being micropapillary disease [30]. In this study, in which completion thyroidectomy for patients with well-differentiated thyroid carcinoma was examined, 33 % of patients who were recommended for observation instead of completion thyroidectomy had multifocal disease. This finding, taken together with the work of Nixon et al., who found that only 4 % of patients who had undergone lobectomy required completion thyroidectomy at a later time (secondary to contralateral disease becoming clinically significant), suggests that multifocal PTMC rarely becomes clinically relevant disease [29]. Others have suggested that total thyroidectomy allows for closer follow-up with thyroglobulin and radioactive iodine (RAI) scanning. There are clear benefits to retaining the contralateral lobe in low-risk patients, such as avoiding the need for lifelong hormone replacement and reducing surgical complications [29, 31].

Surgical Management of the Neck

Despite the indolent nature of most PTMCs, lymph node metastasis is found in 40–60 % of patients with PTMCs [25, 32]. This prompts a complex discussion regarding management of the neck in patients with PTMCs. Although most clinicians agree that therapeutic neck dissection is indicated for clinically positive lymph nodes, the role of prophylactic neck dissection is less clear. Significant emphasis has been placed on the central neck, in terms of proximity to the site of the primary surgery, concern for local-regional recurrence, and the suggested difficulty (with increased complications) of reoperation in the central compartment. Also, owing to the overlying thyroid gland, preoperative ultrasound carries certain limitations for the identification of positive central lymph nodes [31]. Therefore, emphasis on clinicopathologic factors that are suggestive of central neck disease may help identify patients at risk for regional metastatic disease. In a recent meta-analysis, male sex, younger age (<45 years), larger tumor size (>5 mm), multifocality, and extrathyroidal extension were independent predictors of positive central neck lymph nodes [33]. Other clinicians have also included the location of the primary tumor as a risk factor, reporting that the middle third of the gland is a risk factor for positive central neck lymph nodes [34]. A stepwise progression has been observed, with central lymph node involvement continuing to involvement of the lateral lymph nodes, with some reporting that the number of central lymph nodes involved predicts lateral lymph node involvement [35]. Skip lesions—where the central neck is negative, with the presence of lateral lymph node involvement—are rare. In the lateral neck, ipsilateral midlower sites are commonly involved, whereas posterior triangle involvement is infrequently observed [32]. Akin to the understanding that the increase in incidentally detected primary lesions is related to the increased use of diagnostic tools, a similar trend has been observed for the detection of lymph node metastasis. For approximately one-third of patients with differentiated thyroid cancer, disease was detected on ultrasound that was not apparent on physical examination [36].

Taken collectively, these studies show that nodal metastases are common in PTMCs, there are risk factors associated with nodal disease, and ultrasound commonly detects lymph node metastasis that was not detected by physical examination. However, what is less clear is whether identifying occult lymph nodes and acting on these findings alters clinical outcomes.

There is less disagreement regarding therapeutic neck dissection for clinically palpable disease, in terms of risk of regional recurrence. Nodal recurrence is more common in patients undergoing therapeutic neck dissection than in those undergoing elective neck dissection [32, 37], which supports the use of therapeutic neck dissection for local-regional control. However, whether to perform prophylactic removal of lymph nodes that appear normal by palpation and imaging studies preoperatively and intraoperatively is a matter of debate. Patients with PTMCs who undergo elective neck dissection have similar rates of regional recurrence as those who do not have any therapeutic intervention [32]. These data suggest that there is no additional benefit to elective neck dissection. Others have concluded that, in order to evaluate lymph node status and provide more accurate staging, central neck dissection should be considered, even in patients without evidence of structural disease [38, 39]. Of importance, survival benefits have not been demonstrated for patients undergoing central neck dissection [40–42]. Such discussions must also consider the risks of central neck dissection—namely, the risk of hypocalcemia and recurrent laryngeal nerve injury, which have been shown to be higher when central neck dissection is performed [41, 43].

Radioactive Iodine

The postoperative use of RAI has increased among patients with differentiated thyroid cancer [44]. Is the use of this modality justified for patients with PTMCs? First, let us consider the goals of RAI in the postoperative setting. An initial dose of RAI after surgery can be used to ablate a small amount of residual thyroid tissue (remnant ablation) after total thyroidectomy, making it easier to follow biochemical recurrence by measuring thyroglobulin levels. It may also aid in initial staging by identifying undiagnosed disease, such as disease in the lateral neck. In this setting, RAI may theoretically be considered adjuvant therapy in the setting of well-differentiated disease, eradicating residual disease after surgery, with the goal of reducing recurrence. Another use of postoperative RAI is for the treatment of known residual disease. Considering these goals in the context of PTMCs—including the excellent outcomes among patients with PTMCs, the low incidence of local and regional recurrence, and the potential of lobectomy as definitive treatment—the small minority of patients with PTMCs who may benefit from RAI can be more clearly understood.

The ATA states that RAI ablation is not recommended for patients with unifocal cancer <1 cm or multifocal cancer when all foci are <1 cm, without other high-risk features. These recommendations are derived from data from multiple studies showing no benefits of RAI in patients with tumors <1.5 cm without high-risk disease features [44, 45]. In an analysis of 900 PTMCs observed over a period of 60 years, the Mayo Clinic found no benefit of RAI for reducing rates of local or distant recurrence [28]. In this same retrospective cohort, RAI did not significantly affect rates of regional or distant recurrence among node-positive patients. Given the evidence, it is difficult to justify the use of RAI in patients with low-risk PTMCs. This perspective is supported by the ATA guidelines, as is the use of risk-benefit analysis in the consideration of RAI treatment for low-risk patients.

Active Observation

Autopsy studies have shown that many patients who die of causes other than thyroid carcinoma will have PTMCs that were never diagnosed or detected, were never symptomatic, and had no impact on the patient's quality of life. These findings prompt the question: Could these neoplasms, when detected incidentally and identified not to have high-risk features, be actively observed and acted on only when progression occurs? Yasuhiro Ito and colleagues, in Japan, have pioneered programs of active surveillance of PTMCs and have published extensively on their experience.

Their first report was in 2003. After 732 patients were diagnosed with PTMCs by means of FNA, 28 % chose active surveillance as a treatment strategy [25]. Active surveillance was offered only to patients without adverse features, including problematic tumor location, such as trachea and recurrent laryngeal nerve. Additionally, high-grade tumors and evidence of nodal disease were criteria for exclusion. In the group that underwent observation, 76 % of tumors either decreased in size or remained stable during the study period. Approximately one-third of these patients went on to be treated with surgery, owing to physician or patient preference. In addition, 11 % experienced enlargement of the primary tumor, and 6 % developed lymph nodes that were suspicious for metastasis during the period of active surveillance. In a study that sought to identify factors associated with disease progression, Ito et al. found younger age was related to various measures of progression [46]. Of importance, in this cohort, the faster progression observed in younger patients did not result in worse outcomes. In a recent update on Kuma Hospital's active surveillance program, Oda and colleagues reported on 2153 patients diagnosed with low-risk papillary thyroid cancer [47]. Of these patients, 1179 chose active surveillance, and 974 chose immediate surgery. Eight percent of patients in the active surveillance group went on to have surgery. Although the majority of these cases were owing to patient choice, 2.3 % of patients in the active surveillance group experienced an increase in primary tumor size ≥3 mm, and 0.5 % had novel lymph node development. There was no distant disease reported, and no patients died of thyroid cancer. At Memorial Sloan Kettering Cancer Center, Michael Tuttle and colleagues have been monitoring patients with PTMCs in a program of active surveillance for the last 8 years. Approximately 200 patients are under observation, with stable disease in nearly 95 %. These studies suggest that active surveillance is viable for a carefully selected group of patients with PTMCs.

When considering active surveillance as an alternative to immediate surgery, the use of a risk-stratified approach can aid patient selection [48]. In such an approach, three interrelated but distinct domains should be considered: (1) the tumor characteristics, (2) the patient characteristics, and (3) the medical team characteristics. The tumor characteristics include evaluation by ultrasound and consideration of the size and location of the primary tumor within the thyroid gland, the molecular profile of the tumor, and the status of the cervical lymph nodes. For example, a PTMC with a subcapsular location close to the recurrent laryngeal nerve would not be considered appropriate for active surveillance. Patient factors that should be considered in the risk stratification assessment include age, child-bearing potential, family history of thyroid cancer, and the willingness of the patient to undergo active surveillance and comply with follow-up. Finally, one must also consider the medical team. The availability and experience of the multidisciplinary team, the quality of neck ultrasonography, and the experience of the clinician treating thyroid cancer contribute to risk stratification. After considering these three domains, patients can be divided into categories that describe whether they are appropriate for active surveillance management: ideal candidate, appropriate candidate, and inappropriate candidate. Table 14.1, adopted from Brito, Ito, Miyauchi, and Tuttle, summarizes a risk stratification approach for decision-making in the treatment of patients with PTMCs.

The ATA guidelines now state that, although surgery is generally recommended for biopsy-proven thyroid cancer, an active surveillance management approach can be considered as an alternative to immediate surgery [16]. Whether this protocol can be implemented and be successful in other settings is currently under investigation.

Table 14.1 Risk-stratified approach to active surveillance in papillary thyroid microcarcinomas

Candidates for observation	Tumor characteristics	Patient characteristics	Medical team characteristics
Ideal	Solitary nodule, well-defined border, surrounded by thyroid normal thyroid tissue, stable on ultrasound, no ETE= Extrathyroidal extension, no evidence of metastatic disease	> 60 years old, select observation with understanding future surgical intervention possible, compliant with follow-up, support system, nonsurgical candidate secondary to comorbidities	Experienced multidisciplinary team, experienced ultrasonographer, prospective data collection, system in place to assure appropriate follow-up
Appropriate	Multifocal, subcapsular position away from RLN, features associated with difficult follow-up (thyroiditis, multiple thyroid nodules), PET-avid disease	Middle age, strong family history of thyroid cancer, child-bearing potential	Experienced thyroid surgeon or endocrinologist, neck ultrasonography available
Inappropriate	Aggressive histology, located subcapsular adjacent to RLN, ETE=extrathyroid extension, invasion into adjacent structures, metastatic disease	<18 years old, not likely to be compliant with follow-up, unwilling to select observation strategy	Limited experience with thyroid cancer management, neck ultrasonography not available

Adapted from Brito et al. [48]

Summary

PTMC is on the rise. The evidence suggests that this increase in incidence is associated with an increase in diagnostic scrutiny. Therefore, we need to examine how we manage this disease, which in most cases is indolent. Molecular markers will likely, one day, aid in the decision-making of which neoplasms need to be aggressively treated and which may be actively observed. At present, it is safe and effective to manage PTMCs conservatively, with active surveillance only, for appropriate patients, following the use of a risk-stratified, evidence-based approach. With the increased use of diagnostic modalities in the primary care setting, an in-depth understanding of the natural history of PTMC is important in the management of this now common—however, rarely deadly—clinical entity.

Disclosures The authors have no conflicts of interest or financial disclosures.

References

1. Davies L, Welch HG. Increasing incidence of thyroid cancer in the United States, 1973–2002. JAMA. 2006;295(18):2164–7.
2. Ahn HS, Kim HJ, Welch HG. Korea's thyroid-cancer "epidemic"--screening and overdiagnosis. N Engl J Med. 2014;371(19):1765–7.
3. Colonna M, et al. A time trend analysis of papillary and follicular cancers as a function of tumour size: a study of data from six cancer registries in France (1983–2000). Eur J Cancer. 2007;43(5):891–900.
4. Rego-Iraeta A, et al. Time trends for thyroid cancer in northwestern Spain: true rise in the incidence of micro and larger forms of papillary thyroid carcinoma. Thyroid. 2009;19(4):333–40.
5. Black WC, Welch HG. Advances in diagnostic imaging and overestimations of disease prevalence and the benefits of therapy. N Engl J Med. 1993;328(17):1237–43.
6. Welch HG, Black WC. Overdiagnosis in cancer. J Natl Cancer Inst. 2010;102(9):605–13.
7. Davies L, Welch HG. Current thyroid cancer trends in the United States. JAMA Otolaryngol Head Neck Surg. 2014;140(4):317–22.
8. Vanderlaan WP. The occurrence of carcinoma of the thyroid gland in autopsy material. N Engl J Med. 1947;237(7):221.
9. Bondeson L, Ljungberg O. Occult thyroid carcinoma at autopsy in Malmo. Swed Cancer. 1981;47(2):319–23.
10. Sobrinho-Simoes MA, Sambade MC, Goncalves V. Latent thyroid carcinoma at autopsy: a study from Oporto. Port Cancer. 1979;43(5):1702–6.
11. Harach HR, Franssila KO, Wasenius VM. Occult papillary carcinoma of the thyroid. A "normal" finding in Finland. A systematic autopsy study. Cancer. 1985;56(3):531–8.
12. Neuhold N, et al. Incidental papillary microcarcinoma of the thyroid--further evidence of a very low malignant potential: a retrospective clinicopathological study with up to 30 years of follow-up. Ann Surg Oncol. 2011;18(12):3430–6.
13. Bahl M, et al. Trends in incidentally identified thyroid cancers over a decade: a retrospective analysis of 2,090 surgical patients. World J Surg. 2014;38(6):1312–7.
14. Ezzat S, et al. Thyroid incidentalomas. Prevalence by palpation and ultrasonography. Arch Intern Med. 1994;154(16):1838–40.
15. Desser TS, Kamaya A. Ultrasound of thyroid nodules. Neuroimaging Clin N Am. 2008;18(3):463–78, vii.
16. Haugen BR, et al. 2015 American Thyroid Association management guidelines for adult patients with thyroid nodules and differentiated thyroid cancer: the American Thyroid Association Guidelines Task Force on thyroid nodules and differentiated thyroid cancer. Thyroid. 2016;26(1):1–133.
17. American Thyroid Association Guidelines Taskforce on Thyroid, N., et al., Revised american thyroid association management guidelines for patients with thyroid nodules and differentiated thyroid cancer. Thyroid. 2009;19(11): p. 1167–214.
18. Are C, et al. FDG-PET detected thyroid incidentalomas: need for further investigation? Ann Surg Oncol. 2007;14(1):239–47.
19. Katz SC, Shaha A. PET-associated incidental neoplasms of the thyroid. J Am Coll Surg. 2008;207(2):259–64.
20. Hoang JK, Nguyen XV, Davies L. Overdiagnosis of thyroid cancer: answers to five key questions. Acad Radiol. 2015;22(8):1024–9.
21. Niemeier LA, et al. A combined molecular-pathologic score improves risk stratification of thyroid papillary microcarcinoma. Cancer. 2012;118(8):2069–77.
22. Virk RK, et al. BRAFV600E mutation in papillary thyroid microcarcinoma: a genotype-phenotype correlation. Mod Pathol. 2013;26(1):62–70.
23. Xing M, et al. BRAF V600E and TERT promoter mutations cooperatively identify the most aggressive papillary thyroid cancer with highest recurrence. J Clin Oncol. 2014;32(25):2718–26.

24. Nikiforov YE, et al. Highly accurate diagnosis of cancer in thyroid nodules with follicular neoplasm/suspicious for a follicular neoplasm cytology by ThyroSeq v2 next-generation sequencing assay. Cancer. 2014;120(23):3627–34.
25. Ito Y, et al. An observation trial without surgical treatment in patients with papillary microcarcinoma of the thyroid. Thyroid. 2003;13(4):381–7.
26. Lee J, et al. Long-term outcomes of total thyroidectomy versus thyroid lobectomy for papillary thyroid microcarcinoma: comparative analysis after propensity score matching. Thyroid. 2013;23(11):1408–15.
27. Kucuk NO, et al. Treatment for microcarcinoma of the thyroid--clinical experience. Clin Nucl Med. 2007;32(4):279–81.
28. Hay ID, et al. Papillary thyroid microcarcinoma: a study of 900 cases observed in a 60-year period. Surgery. 2008;144(6):980–7; discussion 987–8.
29. Nixon IJ, et al. Thyroid lobectomy for treatment of well differentiated intrathyroid malignancy. Surgery. 2012;151(4):571–9.
30. Untch BR, et al. Oncologic outcomes after completion thyroidectomy for patients with well-differentiated thyroid carcinoma. Ann Surg Oncol. 2014;21(4):1374–8.
31. Leboulleux S, et al. Ultrasound criteria of malignancy for cervical lymph nodes in patients followed up for differentiated thyroid cancer. J Clin Endocrinol Metab. 2007;92(9):3590–4.
32. Wada N, et al. Lymph node metastasis from 259 papillary thyroid microcarcinomas: frequency, pattern of occurrence and recurrence, and optimal strategy for neck dissection. Ann Surg. 2003;237(3):399–407.
33. Qu N, et al. Risk factors for central compartment lymph node metastasis in papillary thyroid microcarcinoma: a meta-analysis. World J Surg. 2015;39(10):2459–70.
34. Xiang D, et al. Papillary thyroid microcarcinomas located at the middle part of the middle third of the thyroid gland correlates with the presence of neck metastasis. Surgery. 2015;157(3): 526–33.
35. Zeng RC, et al. Number of central lymph node metastasis for predicting lateral lymph node metastasis in papillary thyroid microcarcinoma. Head Neck. 2014;36(1):101–6.
36. Kouvaraki MA, et al. Role of preoperative ultrasonography in the surgical management of patients with thyroid cancer. Surgery. 2003;134(6):946–54; discussion 954–5.
37. Hughes CJ, et al. Impact of lymph node metastasis in differentiated carcinoma of the thyroid: a matched-pair analysis. Head Neck. 1996;18(2):127–32.
38. Lee SH, et al. Predictive factors for central compartment lymph node metastasis in thyroid papillary microcarcinoma. Laryngoscope. 2008;118(4):659–62.
39. Caliskan M, et al. Role of prophylactic ipsilateral central compartment lymph node dissection in papillary thyroid microcarcinoma. Endocr J. 2012;59(4):305–11.
40. Ito Y, et al. Clinical significance of metastasis to the central compartment from papillary microcarcinoma of the thyroid. World J Surg. 2006;30(1):91–9.
41. Roh JL, Park JY, Park CI. Total thyroidectomy plus neck dissection in differentiated papillary thyroid carcinoma patients: pattern of nodal metastasis, morbidity, recurrence, and postoperative levels of serum parathyroid hormone. Ann Surg. 2007;245(4):604–10.
42. Bardet S, et al. Macroscopic lymph-node involvement and neck dissection predict lymph-node recurrence in papillary thyroid carcinoma. Eur J Endocrinol. 2008;158(4):551–60.
43. Cavicchi O, et al. Transient hypoparathyroidism following thyroidectomy: a prospective study and multivariate analysis of 604 consecutive patients. Otolaryngol Head Neck Surg. 2007;137(4):654–8.
44. Hay ID, et al. Papillary thyroid carcinoma managed at the Mayo Clinic during six decades (1940–1999): temporal trends in initial therapy and long-term outcome in 2444 consecutively treated patients. World J Surg. 2002;26(8):879–85.
45. Mazzaferri EL. Thyroid remnant 131I ablation for papillary and follicular thyroid carcinoma. Thyroid. 1997;7(2):265–71.
46. Ito Y, et al. Patient age is significantly related to the progression of papillary microcarcinoma of the thyroid under observation. Thyroid. 2014;24(1):27–34.

47. Oda H, et al. Incidences of unfavorable events in the management of low-risk papillary microcarcinoma of the thyroid by active surveillance versus immediate surgery. Thyroid. 2016;26(1):150–5.
48. Brito JP, et al. A clinical framework to facilitate risk stratification when considering an active surveillance alternative to immediate biopsy and surgery in papillary microcarcinoma. Thyroid. 2016;26(1):144–9.

Chapter 15
Surgical Management of Low-Risk Papillary Thyroid Cancer

Jonathan Mark and David L. Steward

Introduction

The correct approach to surgical management of low-risk papillary thyroid carcinoma (low-risk PTC) is controversial. Investigation into the prevalence of thyroid nodules suggests a rate of 2–6 % with palpation, 19–35 % with ultrasound, and 8–65 % in autopsy data [1]. Increasing utilization and sensitivity of imaging modalities have lead to an increased number of incidental thyroid nodules being identified and a subset cytologically diagnosed as papillary thyroid carcinoma. From the surveillance epidemiology and end results program of the national cancer institute (SEER) database review, the rates for new thyroid cancer cases have been rising on average 5 % each year over the last 10 years, but death rates have not changed significantly over 2002–2012 [2]. Considering the survival and incidence data, perhaps it is possible to reduce the amount of thyroid surgery being performed on indolent disease. The specific decision point regarding the surgical approach to low-risk PTC can be distilled down to a choice between thyroid lobectomy (TL) and total thyroidectomy (TT).

For the purpose of discussion in this chapter, low-risk PTC is defined in Table 15.1 where the 2015 ATA risk stratification system is described. Papillary thyroid microcarcinoma is addressed in Chap. 14. Preoperative identification of low-risk PTC includes patients with tumors <4 cm without extrathyroidal extension (cT1 or cT2) and without clinical evidence of lymph node metastasis (cN0). In order for low-risk patients to be good candidates for TL, they must have unilateral disease. Patients that elect for TL for clinically unilateral, low-risk papillary thyroid carcinoma should be counseled and consented preoperatively for possible TT in the event that

J. Mark, MD • D.L. Steward, MD
Department of Otolaryngology, University of Cincinnati Medical Center,
Cincinnati 45267-0528, OH, USA
e-mail: stewardd@ucmail.uc.edu

S.A. Roman et al. (eds.), *Management of Thyroid Nodules and Differentiated Thyroid Cancer*, DOI 10.1007/978-3-319-43618-0_15

Table 15.1 ATA 2015 risk stratification system. The appropriateness of treating low-risk PTC with TL is largely dependent on using proper risk stratification to select the appropriate patients, where the risk of recurrence is a continuum that has been stratified into a three-tiered categorical staging system

ATA low-risk papillary thyroid cancer (with all of the following):
No local or distant metastases
All macroscopic tumor has been resected
No tumor invasion of locoregional tissues or structures
The tumor does not have aggressive histology (e.g., tall cell, hobnail variant, columnar cell carcinoma)
If 131 I is given, there are no RAI-avid metastatic foci outside the thyroid bed on the first posttreatment whole-body RAI scan
No vascular invasion
Clinical N0 or ≤5 pathologic N1 micrometastases (<0.2 cm in largest dimension)
Intrathyroidal, encapsulated follicular variant of papillary thyroid cancer
Intrathyroidal, well-differentiated follicular thyroid cancer with capsular invasion and no or minimal (<4 foci) vascular invasion
Intrathyroidal, papillary microcarcinoma, unifocal or multifocal, including BRAFV600E mutated (if known)
ATA intermediate risk
Microscopic invasion of tumor into the perithyroidal soft tissues
RAI-avid metastatic foci in the neck on the first posttreatment whole-body RAI scan
Aggressive histology (e.g., tall cell, hobnail variant, columnar cell carcinoma)
Papillary thyroid cancer with vascular invasion
Clinical N1 or>5 pathologic N1 with all involved lymph nodes<3 cm in largest dimension
Multifocal papillary microcarcinoma with ETE and BRAFV600E mutated (if known)
ATA high risk
Macroscopic invasion of tumor into the perithyroidal soft tissues (gross ETE)
Incomplete tumor resection
Distant metastases
Postoperative serum thyroglobulin suggestive of distant metastases
Pathologic N1 with any metastatic lymph node ‡ 3 cm in largest dimension
Follicular thyroid cancer with extensive vascular invasion (>4 foci of vascular invasion)

gross extrathyroidal extension and gross nodal metastasis are identified intraoperatively. Further, they must understand the possibility of needing a completion thyroidectomy in the event of pathologic evidence of higher-risk tumor or subsequent development of recurrence in the contralateral lobe or lymph nodes.

Following TL, completion thyroidectomy is not necessary for low-risk unilateral papillary thyroidectomy. Post TL, low-risk PTC meets all of the following criteria: no local or distant metastases, all macroscopic tumor has been resected, no tumor invasion of locoregional tissues or structures, the tumor does not have aggressive histology (e.g., tall cell, insular, columnar cell carcinoma), no lympho-vascular invasion, and clinical and pathologic N0 or ≤5 pathologic N1a micrometastases (<0.2 cm in largest dimension).

The primary arguments for TL include reduced perioperative morbidity and no difference in local recurrence or overall survival and less dependence upon thyroid hormone replacement. The primary arguments against TL include more dependence upon ultrasound surveillance, inability to use radioactive iodine (RAI), and potential need for completion thyroidectomy. The arguments for TT include no need for completion thyroidectomy, ease of surveillance with thyroglobulin (Tg), ability to administer RAI if needed, and treating any potential contralateral disease. The arguments against TT include increased perioperative morbidity (both recurrent nerves and all parathyroid glands at risk) and dependence upon thyroid hormone replacement.

Perioperative Morbidity

In recent studies, operative outcomes have been reported to be related to surgeon volume. Sosa et al. found that higher surgeon volume was associated with favorable patient outcomes, especially with regard to recurrent laryngeal nerve injury and wound complications [3]. This was clearly delineated for patients undergoing TT for thyroid cancer. In Sosa et al.'s cross-sectional analysis, all patients who underwent thyroidectomy in Maryland between 1991 and 1996 in a statewide hospital discharge database were included. Surgeons were stratified by thyroidectomy case volume per year, 1–9, 10–29, 30–99, and 100 or greater. High-volume surgeons performed the most total thyroidectomies of all the groups and were more likely to operate on patients with cancer. High-volume surgeons had significantly better outcomes than low-volume surgeons; they still had higher overall postoperative complication rates when performing TT compared to TL [3].

In a cross-sectional study of the Nationwide Inpatient Sample (the largest all-payer inpatient care database publicly available in the United States), 2003–2009, all adult patients who underwent TT and TL for benign or malignant conditions were included, and their surgeon volume was analyzed. Surgeon volume was categorized as low if they performed fewer than ten thyroid resections per year or high if performing >99 thyroid operations per year. 62,722 procedures were reviewed; most cases were TT (57.9 %) performed for benign disease. Undergoing TT had an increased risk of complications up to 20.4 % compared to TL, with a rate of 10.8 % ($p<0.0001$). High-volume surgeons performed only 5.0 % of the surgeries overall, but 62.6 % of their procedures were TT. High-volume thyroid surgeons had a complication rate of 7.6 % following TL, and low-volume surgeons had a complication rate of 11.8 %. Regarding TT, high-volume surgeons had a complication rate of 14.5 %, and low-volume surgeons had a complication rate of 24.1 %. This was a significant finding (odds ratio 1.53, 95 % confidence interval 1.12, 2.11, $p=0.0083$) that low-volume surgeons were more likely to have a complication after TT. Surgeons should counsel patients and should carefully consider the relative benefits and risks of TT vs. TL, even when high-volume surgeons perform surgery [4].

The surgical risks of TL followed by completion thyroidectomy are similar to those of a near-total or TT. Erdem et al. examined the outcomes of patients with differentiated thyroid carcinoma over a period of 8 years where 141 patients underwent completion thyroidectomy and 92 patients had primary surgery. The rate of permanent recurrent laryngeal nerve palsy and permanent hypoparathyroidism was similar between groups. They were 3.5 and 4.2 % in the completion thyroidectomy group, and 3.3 and 4.3 % in the primary TT group [5].

Surveillance: RAI Versus Long-Term Follow-Up with Ultrasound

Many centers are moving toward a more selective use of RAI coupled with a greater reliance on neck US and serial serum thyroglobulin (Tg) measurements for detection of recurrent disease. TT is necessary if the overall strategy is to include RAI therapy postoperatively, as would be the case for a known higher-risk tumor. However, more selective application of RAI and increased utilization of neck US have the potential to supplant the need for TT in low- and intermediate-risk patients that would have been performed in the past solely to facilitate RAI remnant ablation and follow-up. In addition, diagnostic whole-body RAI scanning is being used less and less, with a greater reliance on neck ultrasonography.

In a retrospective review by Vaisman et al. of 289 patients with mostly PTC >1 cm, patients were selected for either TL or TT without RAI remnant ablation and followed for recurrent or persistent structural disease with ultrasound. Changes in serum Tg were not helpful in identifying the presence of persistent/recurrent structural disease. Patients in this study with an identified recurrence were asymptomatic. The structural disease was identified on surveillance ultrasound, confirmed with biopsy, and did not have a corresponding increase in Tg [6]. In low-risk PTC treated surgically without RAI, ultrasound is the preferred modality for surveillance over Tg. Sonographic surveillance of the contralateral lobe is relatively straightforward; however sonographic surveillance of cervical nodes is more nuanced, and a lack of expertise in sonographic surveillance may limit utility of TL in some areas.

Overall Survival Differences Between TL and TT with Focused Selection Criteria

Applying selection factors to identify low-risk disease has demonstrated that in such patients the long-term outcomes are similar when treated with TL or TT. In the study by Bilimoria et al., data on extrathyroidal extension, completeness of resection, and other factors known to impact survival and recurrence were not available. It is unclear how often TL was done based on proper selection of low-risk PTC and how often TL was done in high-risk patients. Reasons for TL in a high-risk patient may include significant comorbid conditions, inability to obtain a complete resection, or concern over the status of the contralateral recurrent laryngeal nerve. In a study by Haigh, 7 % of TL patients had associated extrathyroidal extension, and 8 % had high-risk features as determined by the age, metastases, extent, and size (AMES) classification system. Further, 5 % of tumors were >5 cm and 1 % had distant metastasis [7]. In the TL patients analyzed by Mendelsohn, external beam radiation therapy was performed in 1–2 % [14]. In the published series by Haigh, Bilimoria, and Kiernan, 12–20 % of patients undergoing TL receive radioactive iodine therapy [7, 8, 9]. Thus, it is always difficult to generalize results from published series to individual patients. At the very least, patients interested in undergoing a less aggressive surgical approach such as TL must understand the potential need for intraoperative conversion to TT or completion thyroidectomy due to discovery of more advanced disease and potential need for radioiodine therapy.

New evidence shows that with proper patient selection, TL may be sufficient treatment in low-risk PTC patients. Adam et al. performed an updated analysis of 61,775 patients in the National Cancer Database who underwent thyroid surgery between 1998 and 2006. They demonstrated that the overall survival advantage seen for patients with 1–4 cm PTC who underwent TT in the Bilimoria study disappeared when further adjustment was made for additional variables related to complexity and severity of illness. Patient comorbidities, tumor multifocality, extrathyroidal extension, nodal disease, distant metastases, and completeness of resection were taken into account. Similarly, no overall survival advantage was seen when the group was subdivided into patients with 1–2 cm and 2–4 cm PTC [10].

Matsuzu et al. reviewed 1,088 papillary thyroid cancer patients who underwent TL in Japan between 1986 and 1995. Tumors ranged in size up to 10 cm and more than 85 % were >1 cm in diameter. None received postoperative RAI. A unique operative approach was applied where TL was performed. Patients with multiple ipsilateral tumors were treated by TL. TT was performed in patients with a tumor that involved both lobes or for bilateral disease. Patients with distant metastasis underwent TT. Interestingly, in cases where preoperative diagnosis of PTC had been made, routine dissection of the lymph nodes in the central compartment and the lateral compartment (level II–V) was performed regardless of whether there was any evidence of lymph node metastasis. For suspected papillary cancer not definitively confirmed preoperatively by cytology, only the central compartment was dissected. Lymph node dissection was not performed in patients with a preoperative diagnosis of benign disease. Central neck dissection alone was performed in 5.5, and 82.5 % underwent central and lateral neck dissection. Pathologic lymph node metastasis was found in 86 % of patients. They found the remnant thyroid recurrence-free survival rate to be 93.5 %, the regional lymph node recurrence-free survival rate was 90.6 %, and the distant recurrence-free survival rate was 93.6 %, 25 years after surgery. The cause-specific survival rate at 10 years was 99.4 %, and at 25 years it was 95.2 %. Age, sex, primary tumor size, extrathyroidal invasion, and clinical lymph node metastasis at the time of the initial surgery were not significantly associated with remnant thyroid recurrence-free survival. The recurrence rate in the remnant thyroid gland at 25 years was 6.5 %. The impact of the extent of neck dissection was not clarified perhaps due to the selection bias determined by their surgical strategy [11].

There are several studies published prior to the 2015 ATA guidelines that aimed to define a low-risk group of thyroid cancer patients for analysis of outcomes in TT versus TL. The conclusions of these papers are useful in establishing current low-risk criteria but intrinsically must be interpreted with scrutiny due to their incorporation of what may now be considered intermediate- or high-risk features.

Mendelsohn analyzed 22,724 patients that underwent papillary thyroid cancer surgery in the SEER database from 1988 to 2001. After controlling for tumor size, no survival difference was seen between TT and TL over a mean follow-up of 9.1 years. Overall 10-year survival for TL was 89.4 and 90.8 % for TT. Disease-specific survival was 98.4 % for TL and 97.5 % for TT. Some patients were noted to have undergone TL for tumors greater than 4 cm. Of the 2428 patients with tumors >4 cm, 534 had TL. In a subgroup analysis for tumors 1 cm or larger, no significant difference was found between the TL and TT groups. Additionally in this study, TL was performed in some high-risk patients. 1.6 % received external beam irradiation, 16 % had extrathryoidal extension, 9 % were greater than 4 cm, and 20 % received RAI ablation [12].

Haigh et al. analyzed the SEER database from 1988 to 1995 and classified patients with papillary thyroid cancer into low and high-risk groups by using the age, metastases, extent, and size (AMES) risk classification. The low-risk group included all younger patients (women <= 50 and men <= 40) with intrathyroidal cancers and all older patients with intrathyroidal cancers <5 cm without distant metastasis. The low-risk patients, 10-year survival after TT was 89 %, compared with 91 % after partial thyroidectomy. Older age, male sex, larger tumor, lymph node metastases, and lack of radioactive iodine were associated with higher mortality. In the high-risk patients, 10-year survival after TT was 72 %, compared with 78 % after partial thyroidectomy. They concluded that the survival of patients with PTC was not significantly influenced by the extent of thyroidectomy and was similar in both the low and high-risk prognostic groups [7].

A study by Nixon et al. from Memorial Sloan Kettering Cancer Center reviewed 889 patients with pT1 and pT2 well differentiated, intrathyroidal cancers treated surgically between 1986 and 2005. TT was performed in 528 (59 %) and TL in 361 (41 %) patients. The 10-year overall survival rate was 92 %, the disease-specific survival rate was 99 %, and the recurrence-free survival rate was 98 %. In their analysis there was no significant difference in OS by extent of surgical resection, but age over 45 years and male gender portended worse overall survival. Comparison of the TL group and the TT group showed no difference in local or regional recurrence. This cohort consisted of 90 % papillary histopathology, 6 % follicular, and 4 % Hurthle Cell. Tall cell variant of papillary was included despite it being known to have a poorer outcome. In this review, the development of malignancy in the residual thyroid lobe was considered a contralateral recurrence rather than local recurrence. Twenty-one of the 382 patients treated with initial TL had immediate completion thyroidectomy and 14 patients (4 %) required a completion thyroidectomy at a later date but only 9 patients actually (2.7 %) developed a malignancy in the contralateral lobe. If they had instead, counted the development of malignancy in the residual lobe as a local recurrence, it would give a local recurrence rate of only 2 %. The authors concluded that patients with pT1 and pT2 N0 WDTC can be safely managed by TL alone [13]. Again, while this study does include some non-low-risk patients, the results offer some insight into the current acceptance of offering TL as a definitive surgical option in selected patients.

Local Recurrence

It would seem that the multifocal nature of PTC would lead to an increase in recurrence in the contralateral lobe in cases treated with TL. This was the case in reviews performed by Grant, Hay, and Mazzaferri [14, 15, 16]. By applying selection criteria and targeting low-risk patients, rates of less than 1–4 % local recurrence and completion thyroidectomy rates of less than 10 % can be achieved following TL.

In a retrospective review by Vaisman et al. of 289 patients with mostly PTC greater than 1 cm, patients were selected for either TL or TT without RAI remnant ablation and followed for recurrent or persistent structural disease. After a 5-year median follow-up, structural disease recurrence was detected in 2.3 % (5/217) of patients treated with TT without RAI remnant ablation, and in 4.2 % (3/72) of patients treated with TL. Size of the primary tumor, the presence of cervical lymph node metastases and ATA risk category were all statistically significant predictors of recurrence [6]. As discussed above in the overall survival section, the few recurrences that develop during long-term follow-up are readily detected and treated with no impact on survival [6, 11, 13]. Further, evaluation of the risk difference and number need to treat would suggest that approximately 25 patients would have to undergo TT and subsequent increased risk to prevent one contralateral recurrence which could be salvaged with a later completion thyroidectomy.

Molecular Markers in FLUS and Follicular Neoplasm

Some clinicians use commercial molecular studies with cytological analysis to assist in determining if a patient should be observed, or undergo surgical management via unilateral thyroidectomy, or TT. A test with a rule out bias may be helpful in obviating a surgical biopsy. If the molecular marker risk stratifies the patient to an ATA low-risk category, unilateral thyroidectomy is an appropriate surgical option. If TL is considered adequate therapy for a low-risk PTC, then it may no longer be needed to assist in deciding between unilateral and TT. This would shift the utility of the test to be most helpful in determining between observation and unilateral thyroidectomy.

Patient Preference

Evidence-based medicine serves a guide assisting patients in medical decision making with their physician. Local medical resources and individual patient concerns allow for exceptions to general guidelines as delineated.

Financial Cost

Leiker et al. performed a cost analysis of TL and intraoperative frozen section compared to TT in patients with cytology suspicious for PTC. The outcome was determined by the incremental cost-utility ratio defined as US$/quality-adjusted life-year. They concluded that initial TT was more cost-effective for patients largely because of the need for completion thyroidectomy after a "benign" frozen diagnosis. They did, however, note that TL is preferred when complications reach unacceptable levels [17]. Alternatively, with new guidelines advocating for forgoing completion in cases of low-risk PTC, TL may be more cost-effective. It has been shown that patients undergoing TT were twice as likely to stay overnight compared with those undergoing TL. When stratified by the extent of thyroidectomy, the cost of same-day surgery has been shown to be consistently lower than that for overnight observation [18]. The cost of surveillance is another area that must be considered. Ultrasound surveillance may be necessary in the case of TT and TL, but the cost may be higher with TT as some of those patients may require stimulated Tg and RAI scans if treated with RAI.

Elective ipsilateral central node dissection Central neck dissection is discussed extensively in Chap. 16 but deserves mention here. In the event of intraoperative recognition of gross nodal metastasis (cN1a), therapeutic central node dissection should be performed to eradicate all clinically detectable disease with likely conversion to TT [19]. In the absence of clinically detectable nodal disease (cN0), the benefit of elective ipsilateral central node dissection is uncertain but may be worth considering for accurate pathologic nodal staging if pN1a disease would result in a decision to perform total or completion thyroidectomy to facilitate radioiodine therapy postoperatively.

Conclusion

Unilateral thyroidectomy should play an increasing role in the surgical management of low-risk unilateral papillary thyroid carcinoma. Unilateral TL offers reduced perioperative morbidity and does not compromise local recurrence rates in properly selected patients (cT1-2N0M0). There is no statistically significant difference in overall survival between unilateral TL and TT. Patients must be counseled about the potential need for conversion to TT or subsequent completion thyroidectomy depending upon the outcome. The role for elective ipsilateral central node dissection for accurate pathologic staging is uncertain, but intraoperative inspection for extrathyroidal extension and/or gross nodal metastasis is important. Post TL, there is an increased dependence upon ultrasound surveillance as thyroglobulin is insensitive and nonspecific in the presence of a contralateral thyroid lobe.

Works Cited

1. Adam MA, Pura J, Gu L, et al. Extent of surgery for papillary thyroid cancer is not associated with survival: an analysis of 61,775 patients. Ann Surg. 2014;260:601–5; discussion 605–7.
2. Bilimoria KY, Bentrem DJ, Ko CY, et al. Extent of surgery affects survival for papillary thyroid cancer. Ann Surg. 2007;246:375–81; discussion 381–4.
3. Dean DS, Gharib H. Epidemiology of thyroid nodules. Best Pract Res Clin Endocrinol Metab. 2008;22:901–11.
4. Erdem E, Gulcelik MA, Kuru B, Alagol H. Comparison of completion thyroidectomy and primary surgery for differentiated thyroid carcinoma. Eur J Surg Oncol. 2003;29:747–9.
5. Grant CS, Hay ID, Gough IR, Bergstralh EJ, Goellner JR, McConahey WM. Local recurrence in papillary thyroid carcinoma: is extent of surgical resection important? Surgery. 1988;104:954–62.
6. Haigh PI, Urbach DR, Rotstein LE. Extent of thyroidectomy is not a major determinant of survival in low- or high-risk papillary thyroid cancer. Ann Surg Oncol. 2005;12:81–9.
7. Hauch A, Al-Qurayshi Z, Randolph G, Kandil E. Total thyroidectomy is associated with increased risk of complications for low- and high-volume surgeons. Ann Surg Oncol. 2014;21:3844–52.
8. Haugen BR, Alexander EK, Bible KC, et al. 2015 American Thyroid Association Management guidelines for adult patients with thyroid nodules and differentiated thyroid cancer: the American Thyroid Association guidelines task force on thyroid nodules and differentiated thyroid cancer. Thyroid. 2016;26(1):1–133.
9. Hay ID, Grant CS, Bergstralh EJ, Thompson GB, van Heerden JA, Goellner JR. Unilateral total lobectomy: is it sufficient surgical treatment for patients with AMES low-risk papillary thyroid carcinoma? Surgery. 1998;124:958–64; discussion 964–6.
10. Leiker AJ, Yen TW, Cheung K, Evans DB, Wang TS. Cost analysis of thyroid lobectomy and intraoperative frozen section versus total thyroidectomy in patients with a cytologic diagnosis of "suspicious for papillary thyroid cancer". Surgery. 2013;154:1307–13; discussion 1313–4.
11. Marino M, Spencer H, Hohmann S, Bodenner D, Stack Jr BC. Costs of outpatient thyroid surgery from the University HealthSystem Consortium (UHC) database. Otolaryngol Head Neck Surg. 2014;150(5):762–9. doi:10.1177/0194599814521583. Epub 2014 Feb 4.
12. Matsuzu K, Sugino K, Masudo K, et al. Thyroid lobectomy for papillary thyroid cancer: long-term follow-up study of 1,088 cases. World J Surg. 2014;38:68–79.
13. Mazzaferri EL, Kloos RT. Clinical review 128: current approaches to primary therapy for papillary and follicular thyroid cancer. J Clin Endocrinol Metab. 2001;86:1447–63.
14. Mendelsohn AH, Elashoff DA, Abemayor E, St John MA. Surgery for papillary thyroid carcinoma: is lobectomy enough? Arch Otolaryngol Head Neck Surg. 2010;136:1055–61.
15. Nixon IJ, Ganly I, Patel SG, et al. Thyroid lobectomy for treatment of well differentiated intrathyroid malignancy. Surgery. 2012;151:571–9.
16. Sosa JA, Bowman HM, Tielsch JM, Powe NR, Gordon TA, Udelsman R. The importance of surgeon experience for clinical and economic outcomes from thyroidectomy. Ann Surg. 1998;228:320–30.

17. Vaisman F, Shaha A, Fish S, Michael Tuttle R. Initial therapy with either thyroid lobectomy or total thyroidectomy without radioactive iodine remnant ablation is associated with very low rates of structural disease recurrence in properly selected patients with differentiated thyroid cancer. Clin Endocrinol (Oxf). 2011;75:112–9.
18. Howlader N, Noone AM, Krapcho M, Garshell J, Miller D, Altekruse SF, Kosary CL, Yu M, Ruhl J, Tatalovich Z, Mariotto A, Lewis DR, Chen HS, Feuer EJ, Cronin KA, editors. SEER Cancer Statistics Review, 1975–2012, National Cancer Institute. Bethesda, MD. http://seer.cancer.gov/csr/1975_2012/, based on November 2014 SEER data submission, posted to the SEER web site, April 2015.
19. Kiernan CM, Parikh AA, Parks LL, etal. Use of Radioiodine after Thyroid Lobectomy in patients with differentiates Thyroid Cancer. Does it change outcome? J Am Coll Surg. 04/2015;220(4).

Chapter 16
Management of Central Compartment Lymph Nodes in Patients with Papillary Thyroid Carcinoma

Joy C. Chen and Christopher R. McHenry

Introduction

This chapter will review the management of lymph node metastases in the central compartment of the neck and their impact on disease recurrence and survival in patients with papillary thyroid cancer (PTC). The anatomic boundaries of a central compartment neck dissection (CCND) and the controversy over whether or not a prophylactic central compartment neck dissection (pCCND) is necessary in patients with PTC and clinically node-negative disease have previously been presented [1]. One of the major trends that is evolving is a more limited use of postoperative radioiodine (RAI). An assessment of the efficacy, risks, and benefits of postoperative RAI is presented, and the results seem to favor foregoing RAI administration in patients with low-risk PTC. This provides further support for treatment of clinically node-negative PTC with thyroidectomy alone rather than thyroidectomy and pCCND.

J.C. Chen, MD, MS
Department of Surgery, Stanford University Medical Center,
300 Pasteur Drive, H3591, Stanford, CA 94305, USA

C.R. McHenry, MD (✉)
Case Western Reserve University School of Medicine, Department of Surgery, MetroHealth Medical Center, 2500 Metrohealth Drive, Cleveland, OH 44109, USA
e-mail: cmchenry@metrohealth.org

S.A. Roman et al. (eds.), *Management of Thyroid Nodules and Differentiated Thyroid Cancer*, DOI 10.1007/978-3-319-43618-0_16

Central Compartment Neck Dissection

The anatomic boundaries of a CCND include the right and left common carotid arteries from the hyoid bone superiorly to the innominate artery inferiorly as defined by the American Thyroid Association (ATA) Surgery Working Group [2] (Fig. 16.1). A CCND consists of removal of the prelaryngeal, pretracheal, and paratracheal lymph nodes (level VI) and the lymph nodes along the innominate artery (level VII). The inferior border of dissection has not been uniformly defined in the literature, with variable use of the sternal notch, the innominate artery, and the innominate vein. It has been recommended that level VII nodes routinely be removed along with level VI nodes in order to achieve a better oncologic outcome, and it has been shown that this can be performed with no increase in morbidity [3]. This is best accomplished by performing routine transcervical thymectomy and skeletonizing the innominate artery.

A therapeutic CCND is defined as a CCND performed in a patient with macroscopic or clinical lymph node metastases. Macroscopic lymph node metastases in patients with PTC are associated with higher recurrence rates [4]. In a large population-based, case–control study, Lundgren and colleagues demonstrated an increased mortality rate in patients 45 years and older with regional lymph node metastases [5]. There is evidence that for patients with macroscopic nodal disease, lymphadenectomy reduces recurrence and mortality [4, 6, 7]. As a result, there is general agreement that patients with clinically involved lymph nodes in the central

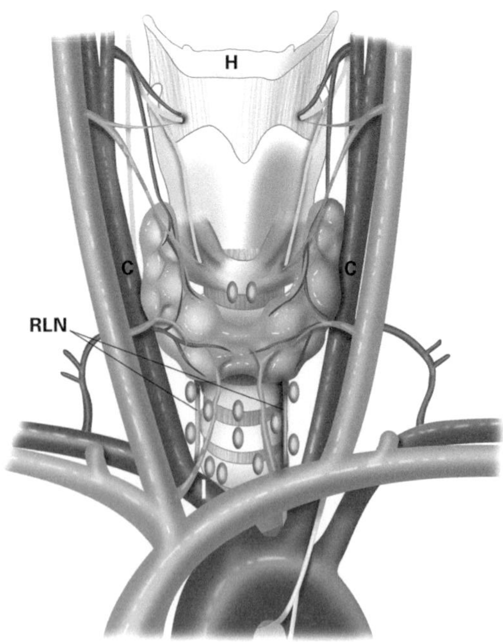

Fig. 16.1 Anatomic landmarks for performing a central compartment neck dissection. The lymph nodes removed include the prelaryngeal (superior to the isthmus of the thyroid gland), pretracheal (inferior to the isthmus and anterior to the trachea), paratracheal (along the recurrent laryngeal nerves), and the lymph nodes along the innominate artery. *H* hyoid bone, I innominate (brachiocephalic) artery, *C* carotid artery, *RLN* recurrent laryngeal nerve

compartment of the neck should be managed with a CCND preferably at the time of thyroidectomy.

Prophylactic CCND (pCCND) is a compartment-oriented lymph node dissection performed in a patient with thyroid cancer who has no evidence of lymph node metastases on preoperative clinical examination, imaging studies, or intraoperative assessment. The rationale that has been proposed for performing a pCCND is to: (1) reduce recurrence in the central compartment of the neck and to help avoid the need for reoperation in the central compartment of the neck and its associated potential for increased morbidity, (2) lower postoperative serum thyroglobulin (Tg) levels, and (3) improve selection of patients for postoperative radioiodine therapy and optimization of doses of iodine-131. The rationale against performing a pCCND is that there is no proven oncologic benefit and the associated morbidity is higher than a total thyroidectomy alone.

Some experts preferentially recommend an ipsilateral pCCND in patients with clinically node-negative disease [8]. An ipsilateral pCCND consists of removal of the pretracheal, the prelaryngeal, and the paratracheal lymph nodes from the side of the cancer. The contralateral paratracheal lymph nodes are not removed. The rationale for an ipsilateral CCND is to remove the lymph nodes in the central compartment of the neck that are most likely to be involved with cancer and, at the same time, reduce the potential for recurrent laryngeal nerve injury and hypoparathyroidism.

Preoperative Sonographic Staging of the Central and Lateral Neck

Macroscopic lymph node metastases are metastases detected on physical examination, intraoperative exploration, or ultrasound exam. Macroscopic lymph node metastases occur in approximately 35 % of patients with PTC [9–12]. In contrast, microscopic lymph node metastases refer to metastases that are undetectable on physical examination, imaging studies, or intraoperative assessment. Thirty-eight to 80 % of patients with PTC have occult microscopic lymph node metastases [13, 14]. The mean size of metastatic lymph nodes removed during a pCCND has been reported as 0.35 cm [15, 16].

An ultrasound examination of the central and lateral compartments of the neck is obtained prior to performing a thyroidectomy for PTC as recommended by the ATA [17]. Up to 40 % of macroscopic lymph node metastases in patients with PTC will be missed by physical examination [18, 19], making ultrasonography an important part of the management of patients with PTC. Stulak and colleagues evaluated the use of ultrasound in patients with PTC and identified nonpalpable, macroscopic lymph node metastases in 14 % of patients [20].

Microscopic and macroscopic lymph node metastases have different implications for recurrence and mortality. Microscopic metastases do not affect patient survival and are associated with much lower rates of recurrence compared to macroscopic metastases. Macroscopic lymph node metastases are associated with higher recurrence rates [5] as well as higher disease-specific mortality in patients 45 years or older [5, 21, 22].

Sonographic features of abnormal lymph nodes include diameter greater than 1 cm, loss of normal fatty hilum, irregular rounded contour with long-axis to short-axis ratio of less than 1.5, heterogeneous echogenicity, microcalcifications, hypervascularity, and cystic change [23–25]. The sensitivity of ultrasonography is better for detecting metastatic lymph nodes in the lateral neck compared to the central compartment of the neck (82–94 % vs. 30–60 %, respectively) [26–29]. With respect to the TNM staging system, preoperative sonographic staging of PTC offers an overall accuracy of 71.3 % for N staging [26].

Ultrasound can also be used to guide fine needle aspiration biopsy of suspicious cervical lymph nodes. Cytology specimens can be analyzed for the presence of malignant cells. In cases of inconclusive cytology, thyroglobulin can be measured in the aspirate to reliably identify metastatic lymph nodes in the preoperative setting [30].

Indications for CCND: Recommendations and Controversies

Therapeutic CCND is indicated for patients with biopsy-proven macroscopic lymph node metastases in the central compartment of the neck identified on physical examination, imaging studies, or intraoperative assessment. Compartment-oriented lymphadenectomy in patients with macroscopic disease minimizes the risk of recurrence and mortality [6]. All major endocrine societies recommend a therapeutic CCND for patients with clinically node-positive PTC, whereas recommendations differ for pCCND [2, 17, 19, 31–34].

Prophylactic CCND is an operation that was historically reserved for treatment of patients with sporadic and hereditary medullary thyroid carcinoma. The recommendation for pCCND for patients with PTC was introduced in 2006 with the publication of the ATA management guidelines for patients with thyroid nodules and differentiated thyroid cancer, which recommended that CCND be considered for all patients with PTC [17]. Prior to 2006, pCCND was not a consideration in the treatment of patients with PTC. This recommendation was said to be based on fair evidence that pCCND may improve health outcomes, and thus the strength of the recommendation was given a B rating. At the same time that the ATA guidelines were published, a consensus statement by the European Thyroid Association (ETA) for the management of patients with differentiated thyroid cancer was published stating that "there is no evidence that pCCND improves recurrence or mortality rates for PTC, but it does allow an accurate staging of the disease that may guide subsequent treatment and follow-up" [35]. Hence, this became an extremely controversial issue.

Modifications appeared in the revised ATA guidelines published in 2009 [33]. The new proposed recommendation was that "pCCND (ipsilateral or bilateral) may be performed in patients with PTC with clinically uninvolved central neck lymph nodes, especially for advanced primary tumors (T3 or T4)." This new recommendation was formulated based on expert opinion alone, so the strength of the recommendation was lowered to C. The most recent ATA management guidelines published in 2015 state that for clinically node-negative disease, total thyroidectomy without pCCND is strongly recommended, based on moderate-quality evidence, while pCCND is a weak recommendation based on low-quality evidence [19]. It is apparent that, since 2006, we have come full circle in terms of the recommendation for pCCND in patients with clinically node-negative PTC.

Serum Thyroglobulin

Serum thyroglobulin (Tg) monitoring is recommended after thyroidectomy for thyroid cancer to help detect recurrence. It is unclear whether total thyroidectomy with pCCND will result in lower serum Tg levels compared to total thyroidectomy alone. Reduced serum Tg levels have been reported in patients who undergo pCCND [8]. However, it is unknown whether this was the result of a CCND or a more complete thyroidectomy. Other studies report no difference in serum Tg levels between patients who undergo total thyroidectomy with pCCND and total thyroidectomy alone [36, 37]. Furthermore, normalization of serum Tg is less important than the change in Tg over time for detection of recurrent disease.

Locoregional Recurrence

The reported rates of recurrence in the central compartment of the neck after surgical therapy are variable. Macroscopic lymph node metastases in patients with PTC are associated with a much higher recurrence rate than patients with microscopic lymph node metastases [4]. Recurrence rates in patients with macroscopic lymph node metastases have been reported to vary between 10 and 42 % [38–42]. Wada and colleagues described a higher risk of nodal recurrence in patients with palpable abnormal cervical lymph nodes compared to patients with undetectable lymph node metastases who underwent pCCND (17 % vs. 0.43 %) [40]. This finding of a higher nodal recurrence rate associated with clinically N1 disease has been corroborated by other studies [38, 39], with higher recurrence seen in both young and old patients [41].

In patients with clinically node-negative disease, recurrence in the central compartment of the neck occurs in 2–3 % of patients regardless of whether or not a pCCND is performed, with a range of 0–12 % following total thyroidectomy alone, compared to 0–11 % in patients undergoing total thyroidectomy with pCCND (Table 16.1) [8, 37, 39, 42–55]. There is no significant difference in the rate of recurrence in the central compartment of the neck between patients who underwent

Table 16.1 Central compartment recurrence of PTC following total thyroidectomy alone versus total thyroidectomy with pCCND

	Recurrence after thyroidectomy alone	Recurrence after thyroidectomy + pCCND	Mean* follow-up
Barcynzski et al. [43]	7.8 % (22/282)	0.6 % (2/358)	10 years
Bardet et al. [42]	5.6 % (22/391)	11.1 % (4/36)	69 months*
Besic et al. [44]	0 % (0/83)	0 % (0/6)	56 months
Costa et al. [45]	3.4 % (4/118)	3.2 % (4/126)	47 vs. 64 months
Gemsenjager et al. [39]	2.3 % (2/88)	5.6 % (4/71)	8.1 years
Hartl et al. [46]	12 % (11/91)	3 % (2/155)	6.3 years
Hughes et al. [37]	3.1 % (2/65)	2.6 % (2/78)	27.5 vs. 19.1 months
Lang et al. [47]	0 % (0/103)	0 % (0/82)	39.1 vs. 31.1 months
Lee et al. [48]	3.9 % (4/104)	3.3 % (5/153)	49 vs. 55 months
Moo et al. [49]	5.6 % (2/36)	2.2 % (1/45)	3.1 years
Moreno et al. [50]	2.3 % (3/133)	1.7 % (2/119)	71.5 months[a]
Roh et al. [51]	0 % (0/49)	0 % (0/148)	36 months
Roh et al. [52]	4.1 % (3/73)	2.5 % (1/40)	52 months
Sywak et al. [8]	1.8 % (7/391)	0 % (0/56)	70 vs. 24.5 months
Sadowski et al. [53]	1.4 % (4/281)	0 % (0/180)	38.8 months
Ywata de Carvalho et al. [54]	1.5 % (7/478)	3.9 % (4/102)	69.7 months
Zhang et al. [55]	8.3 % (9/108)	2.2 % (3/134)	66 vs. 61 months

Except median where denoted by (*)

total thyroidectomy with pCCND and patients who underwent total thyroidectomy alone. A large meta-analysis of patients with PTC reported a recurrence rate of 1.9 % in the group who underwent thyroidectomy with pCCND versus 1.7 % in the group who underwent thyroidectomy alone [56]. Two additional large meta-analyses substantiated this finding that there is no difference in locoregional recurrence with total thyroidectomy with or without pCCND [13, 14]. Based on current information available in the literature, CCND is indicated for macroscopic lymph node metastases. In contrast, the available evidence suggests that occult microscopic metastatic disease in the lymph nodes of the central compartment of the neck rarely becomes clinically apparent and is therefore of little clinical significance.

Survival

In a large, population-based, case–control study, Lundgren and colleagues demonstrated an increased mortality rate in patients 45 years of age and older with regional lymph node metastases [5]. There is evidence that for patients with macroscopic nodal disease, lymphadenectomy reduces recurrence and mortality [4, 6, 7]. As a result, there is general agreement that patients with clinically involved lymph nodes in the central compartment of the neck should be managed with a CCND.

In the past, a single Swedish study has been referenced to support the notion that pCCND may improve survival [57]. This was a retrospective study of 195 patients with PTC, 175 of whom underwent total or near-total thyroidectomy with pretracheal and paratracheal lymph node microdissection [6]. Outcomes were compared to two prior Scandinavian studies [58, 59]. The authors reported a disease-specific mortality of 1.6 %, compared to 8.4 % in a study from Norway and 11 % from a study from Finland.

There are two major limitations in the Swedish study [57]. First, it included all patients who underwent CCND, and the breakdown of therapeutic CCND versus pCCND was not specified. Second, the comparisons of mortality were problematic. In the Norwegian study, 12 of 15 patients who died from PTC only had a palliative operation because of the initial extent of disease [58]. If these 12 patients were excluded, the disease-specific mortality was 1.9 %, similar to the 1.6 % disease-specific mortality reported by Tisell and colleagues, who excluded patients who presented with distant metastases [6]. The study in Finland occurred during an earlier period (1956–1979) than the studies from Norway (1971–1989) and Sweden (1970–1989), and data regarding extent of thyroidectomy, lymph node dissection, and radioactive iodine therapy were either incomplete or not provided [59].

Radioactive Iodine Use

Retrospective studies have suggested that accurate staging of PTC using pCCND may be used to help determine the need for RAI therapy and the doses of iodine-131 to be used [37, 46]. Hughes and colleagues compared patients with clinically node-negative PTC who underwent total thyroidectomy alone versus total thyroidectomy with pCCND. Sixty-two percent of patients who underwent pCCND had lymph node metastases in the central compartment of the neck [37]. The median dose of iodine-131 given was significantly higher (150 mCi) in the group that underwent total thyroidectomy with pCCND than in the group that underwent total thyroidectomy alone (30 mCi). However, even with pCCND and higher doses of iodine-131, there were no differences in locoregional recurrence or Tg levels 1 year after treatment. Additional studies have corroborated findings that higher doses of iodine-131 are administered after pCCND. Hartl and colleagues reported that higher doses of iodine-131 were administered to patients who underwent total thyroidectomy with pCCND and level III and IV lateral neck dissection (100 mCi) versus those who underwent total thyroidectomy alone (30 mCi) [46]. In a retrospective study, Bonnet and colleagues found that lymph node staging, resulting from pCCND and ipsilateral lateral neck dissection in patients with clinically node-negative PTC, altered the decision to use iodine-131 ablation in 21.7 % of patients [60]. One might conclude from these studies that pCCND is valuable for determining doses of iodine-131. An alternative conclusion is that pCCND leads to administration of higher doses of iodine-131 with no apparent clinical benefit.

Recently, Viola and colleagues completed a prospective, randomized controlled study to investigate the role of pCCND for patients with clinically node-negative PTC [61]. Patients were randomized to treatment with total thyroidectomy alone or total thyroidectomy and CCND. The primary endpoints of the study were to evaluate the successful ablation rate and persistent and recurrent disease after 5 years of follow-up. The secondary endpoints were to evaluate the rate of surgical complications in the two groups and the effect of pCCND in the staging of the disease. After 5 years of follow-up, patients with clinically node-negative PTC randomized to treatment with total thyroidectomy alone had received a greater number of treatments with iodine-131 and had a lower rate of permanent hypoparathyroidism and no difference in outcome compared to patients randomized to total thyroidectomy and pCCND. Almost 50 % of patients had microscopic lymph node metastases. The authors concluded that the identification of micrometastases in lymph nodes from the central compartment of the neck does not improve cancer-related outcomes but that it reduces the necessity for repeated iodine-131 treatments.

The efficacy of 131-I ablation for treatment of microscopic lymph node metastases, however, remains unclear. Sawka and colleagues found no significant benefit of iodine-131 ablation in reducing recurrence or mortality in patients with lymph node micrometastases [62]. The usefulness of iodine-131 ablation is suboptimal partly because up to 30 % of PTCs do not concentrate iodine-131 [63].

Lamartina and colleagues, in a recent systematic review of the literature, examined the evidence for postoperative RAI in staging, follow-up, and recurrence for ATA low- and intermediate-risk class patients with differentiated thyroid cancer and made some important conclusions [64]. First, it is well established that RAI remnant ablation is not of value in patients with low-risk thyroid cancer since no benefit in reducing recurrence has been demonstrated. Also, ultrasound in combination with serum Tg monitoring is equivalent and probably superior to iodine-131 whole-body scanning in identifying residual disease.

Hypothetically, pCCND may be of value for selection of patients with microscopic lymph node metastases for postoperative RAI treatment. Patients with metastases in the lymph nodes of the central compartment of the neck are classified as intermediate risk for recurrence [65]. There are studies that have shown some benefit of postoperative RAI for patients with intermediate-risk PTC in reducing recurrence, but the majority of studies show no benefit. What is clear is that the recurrence rate is low, whether or not RAI is administered. It is also important to consider the potential adverse effects of RAI, which include xerophthalmia, chronic or recurrent conjunctivitis, xerostomia secondary to acute and chronic sialoadenitis, transient loss of taste and smell, nausea and vomiting, epistaxis, bone marrow suppression, transient ovarian or testicular failure, and secondary malignancies. In patients with intermediate-risk PTC – particularly those whose cancers have been upstaged due to the presence of microscopic nodal metastasis – the low recurrence rate following thyroidectomy with or without pCCND in combination with the questionable value of RAI in reducing recurrence, the higher morbidity associated with CCND, and the potential adverse consequences of RAI favor total thyroidectomy alone without pCCND.

Complications of CCND

A significantly higher incidence of transient hypocalcemia has been reported following total thyroidectomy with pCCND compared to total thyroidectomy alone [13, 14, 56]. Most studies report a higher incidence of recurrent laryngeal nerve injury and permanent hypoparathyroidism with thyroidectomy and pCCND compared to thyroidectomy alone; however, the differences have not been statistically significant. Table 16.2 shows reported rates of complications after CCND [37, 39, 48, 52, 54, 55, 61, 66, 67].

Giordano and colleagues retrospectively studied patients with clinically node-negative PTC and found a higher rate of permanent recurrent laryngeal nerve injury in patients who underwent bilateral CCND with total thyroidectomy compared to those who underwent total thyroidectomy alone, but this difference was not statistically significant [68]. They reported a higher rate of permanent hypoparathyroidism in patients who underwent total thyroidectomy and bilateral CCND (16 %) compared to those who underwent total thyroidectomy alone (6 %). Multiple other smaller series document a higher incidence of recurrent laryngeal nerve injury and permanent hypoparathyroidism with thyroidectomy and CCND compared to thyroidectomy alone [37, 39, 52, 54, 55, 61, 67]. However, the majority of these studies have been underpowered to establish significance.

A Korean group recently performed a prospective study on patients with clinically node-negative PTC. They found that patients randomized to undergo total

Table 16.2 Morbidity of central compartment neck dissection

	Recurrent laryngeal nerve paralysis		Permanent hypoparathyroidism	
	Total thyroidectomy alone	Total thyroidectomy + CCND	Total thyroidectomy alone	Total thyroidectomy + CCND
Gemsenjager et al. [39]	0 % (0/71)	5.6 % (4/88)	0 % (0/71)	1.4 % (1/88)
Hughes et al. [37]	3.1 % (2/65)	0 % (0/78)	0 % (0/65)	2.6 % (2/78)
Lee et al. [48]	1.9 % (2/104)	3.3 % (5/153)	1.9 % (2/104)	3.3 % (5/153)
Pereira et al. [66]	–	0 % (0/43)	–	4.6 % (2/43)
Roh et al. [52]	0 % (0/73)	4.9 % (4/82)	2.7 % (2/73)	3.6 % (3/82)
Rosenbaum and McHenry [67]	1.1 % (1/88)	0 % (0/22)	0 % (0/88)	4.5 % (1/22)
Viola et al. [61]	8.0 % (7/98)	4.3 % (4/98)	8.0 % (7/98)	19.4 % (18/98)
Ywata de Carvalho et al. [54]	6.1 % (29/478)	11.8 % (12/102)	2.3 % (11/478)	11.8 % (12/102)
Zhang et al. [55]	0.9 % (1/108)	1.5 % (2/134)	0 % (0/108)	1.5 % (2/134)

thyroidectomy with pCCND developed a significantly higher rate of transient hypocalcemia compared to patients who underwent total thyroidectomy alone, with no difference in recurrence rate (3.3 % vs. 3.9 %) [48]. The rates of permanent vocal cord paralysis, permanent hypoparathyroidism, bleeding, and seroma were higher in the pCCND group, although these differences were not statistically significant.

It is important to note that most studies that have examined the morbidity from pCCND are from high-volume centers or high-volume surgeons. However, in practice, the majority of thyroid surgery for PTC is performed by surgeons who are not fellowship trained and do not have a high-volume endocrine surgery practice [69, 70]. Therefore, the actual complication rate is likely to be higher than what is reported in the literature.

Reoperation in the Central Neck

Recurrent PTC has been increasingly detected as a result of serum Tg monitoring postoperatively. Surgical excision is recommended for macroscopic recurrent disease [19, 33]. The most common indication for reoperation in the central compartment of the neck after total thyroidectomy for PTC is residual metastatic disease. Disease relapse most commonly occurs in cervical lymph nodes and less commonly in the soft tissue in the operative field [71]. One study found that up to 20 % of reoperations might have been prevented with improved surgical technique or preoperative sonographic localization of disease, although 20 % of reoperations were for relapses that were attributed to the biologic aggressiveness of the disease [72]. There is concern for an increased risk of recurrent laryngeal injury and hypoparathyroidism with reoperation in the central compartment of the neck. However, specialized endocrine units such as the University of Sydney and the University of California, San Francisco, have reported that secondary central neck dissection can be performed in patients for metastatic disease after initial thyroidectomy with no additional morbidity [73, 74].

Conclusions

Patients with clinically involved lymph nodes in the central compartment of the neck should be managed with a CCND with the expectation for reduced recurrence rates and improved survival. For patients with clinically node-negative disease, the low recurrence rate in the central compartment of the neck combined with the potential for increased morbidity with CCND outweighs the potential benefits of routine pCCND. Whether or not pCCND has any value in determining the need for adjuvant radioiodine therapy has yet to be definitively established. Patients with recurrence in the central compartment of the neck are best managed by specialists in endocrine surgery.

References

1. McHenry CR, Stulberg JJ. Prophylactic central compartment neck dissection for papillary thyroid cancer. Surg Clin North Am. 2014;94(3):529–40.
2. Carty SE, Cooper DS, Doherty GM, et al. Consensus statement on the terminology and classification of central neck dissection for thyroid cancer. Thyroid. 2009;19(11):1153–8.
3. Wang LY, Versnick MA, Gill AJ, Lee JC, Sidhu SB, Sywak MS, Delbridge LW. Level VII is an important component of central neck dissection for papillary thyroid cancer. Ann Surg Oncol. 2013;20(7):2261–5.
4. Scheumann GF, Gimm O, Wegener G, Hundeshagen H, Dralle H. Prognostic significance and surgical management of locoregional lymph node metastases in papillary thyroid cancer. World J Surg. 1994;18:559–67.
5. Lundgren CI, Hall P, Dickman PW, Zedenius J. Clinically significant prognostic factors for differentiated thyroid carcinoma: a population-based, nested case-controlled study. Cancer. 2006;106:524–31.
6. Tisell LE, Nilsson B, Mölne J, et al. Improved survival of patients with papillary thyroid cancer after surgical microdissection. World J Surg. 1996;20(7):854–9.
7. White ML, Gauger PG, Doherty GM. Central neck dissection in differentiated thyroid cancer. World J Surg. 2007;31:895–904.
8. Sywak M, Cornford L, Roach P, et al. Routine ipsilateral level VI lymphadenectomy reduces postoperative thyroglobulin levels in papillary thyroid cancer. Surgery. 2006;140(6):1000–5; discussion 1005–7.
9. Schlumberger M. Papillary and follicular thyroid carcinoma. N Engl J Med. 1998;338:297–306.
10. Noguchi S, Murakami N. The value of lymph-node dissection in patients with differentiated thyroid cancer. Surg Clin North Am. 1987;67:251–61.
11. Cranshaw IM, Carnaille B. Micrometastases in thyroid cancer. An important finding? Surg Oncol. 2008;17(3):253–8.
12. Randolph GW, Duh QY, Heller KS, et al. The prognostic significance of nodal metastases from papillary thyroid carcinoma can be stratified based on the size and number of metastatic lymph nodes, as well as the presence of extranodal extension. Thyroid. 2012;22(11):1144–52.
13. Shan CX, Zhang W, Jiang DZ, et al. Routine central neck dissection in differentiated thyroid carcinoma: a systematic review and meta-analysis. Laryngoscope. 2012;122(4):797–804.
14. Wang TS, Cheung K, Farrokhyar F, et al. A meta-analysis of the effect of prophylactic central compartment neck dissection on locoregional recurrence rates in patients with papillary thyroid cancer. Ann Surg Oncol. 2013;20(11):3477–83.
15. So YK, Son YI, Hong SD, et al. Subclinical lymph node metastasis in papillary thyroid microcarcinoma: a study of 551 resections. Surgery. 2010;148(3):526–31.
16. Roh JL, Kim JM, Park CI. Central cervical nodal metastasis from papillary thyroid microcarcinoma: pattern and factors predictive of nodal metastasis. Ann Surg Oncol. 2008;15(9):2482–6.
17. Cooper DS, Doherty GM, Haugen BR, et al. Management guidelines for patients with thyroid nodules and differentiated thyroid cancer. Thyroid. 2006;16(2):109–42.
18. Kouvaraki MA, Shapiro SE, Fornage BD, Edeiken-Monro BS, Sherman SI, Vassilopoulou-Sellin R, Lee JE, Evans DB. Role of preoperative ultrasonography in the surgical management of patients with thyroid cancer. Surgery. 2003;134(6):946–54; discussion 954–5.
19. Haugen BR, Alexander EK, Bible KC, Doherty G, Mandel SJ, Nikiforov YE, Pacini F, Randolph G, Sawka A, Schlumberger M, Schuff KG, Sherman SI, Sosa JA, Steward D, Tuttle RM, Wartofsky L. 2015 American Thyroid Association Management Guidelines for adult patients with thyroid nodules and differentiated thyroid cancer. Thyroid. 2016;26:1–133 [Epub ahead of print].
20. Stulak JM, Grant CS, Farley DR, et al. Value of preoperative ultrasonography in the surgical management of initial and reoperative papillary thyroid cancer. Arch Surg. 2006;141:489–94; discussion 494–6.

21. Sugitani I, Fujimoto Y, Yamada K, Yamamoto N. Prospective outcomes of selective lymph node dissection for papillary thyroid carcinoma based on preoperative ultrasonography. World J Surg. 2008;32(11):2494–502.
22. Podnos YD, Smith D, Wagman LD, Ellenhorn JD. The implication of lymph node metastasis on survival in patients with well-differentiated thyroid cancer. Am Surg. 2005;71:731–4.
23. Lew JI, Solorzano CC. Use of ultrasound in the management of thyroid cancer. Oncologist. 2010;15(3):253–8.
24. Rosario PW, de Faria S, Bicalho L, et al. Ultrasonographic differentiation between metastatic and benign lymph nodes in patients with papillary thyroid carcinoma. J Ultrasound Med. 2005;24:1385–9.
25. Kuna SK, Bracic I, Tesic V, Kuna K, Herceg GH, Dodig D. Ultrasonographic differentiation of benign from malignant neck lymphadenopathy in thyroid cancer. J Ultrasound Med. 2006;25:1531–7; quiz 1538–40.
26. Park JS, Son KR, Na DG, Kim E, Kim S. Performance of preoperative sonographic staging of papillary thyroid carcinoma based on the sixth edition of the AJCC/UICC TNM classification system. AJR Am J Roentgenol. 2009;192(1):66–72.
27. Hwang HS, Orloff LA. Efficacy of preoperative neck ultrasound in the detection of cervical lymph node metastasis from thyroid cancer. Laryngoscope. 2011;121(3):487–91.
28. Morita S, Mizoguchi K, Suzuki M, et al. The accuracy of (18)[F]-fluoro-2-deoxy- D-glucose-positron emission tomography/computed tomography, ultrasonography, and enhanced computed tomography alone in the preoperative diagnosis of cervical lymph node metastasis in patients with papillary thyroid carcinoma. World J Surg. 2010;34(11):2564–9.
29. Choi JS, Kim J, Kwak JY, et al. Preoperative staging of papillary thyroid carcinoma: comparison of ultrasound imaging and CT. AJR Am J Roentgenol. 2009;193(3):871–8.
30. Cunha N, Rodrigues F, Curado F, Ilhéu O, Cruz C, Naidenov P, Rascão MJ, Ganho J, Gomes I, Pereira H, Real O, Figueiredo P, Campos B, Valido F. Thyroglobulin detection in fine-needle aspirates of cervical lymph nodes: a technique for the diagnosis of metastatic differentiated thyroid cancer. Eur J Endocrinol. 2007;157(1):101–7.
31. Robbins KT, Shaha AR, Medina JE, et al. Consensus statement on the classification and terminology of neck dissection. Arch Otolaryngol Head Neck Surg. 2008;134(5):536–8.
32. National Comprehensive Cancer Network. Thyroid carcinoma. 2012. Available at: http://www.nccn.org/professionals/physician_gls/. Accessed 8 July 8 2015.
33. Cooper DS, Doherty GM, Haugen BR, et al. Revised American Thyroid Association management guidelines for patients with thyroid nodules and differentiated thyroid cancer. Thyroid. 2009;19(11):1167–214.
34. Perros P, editor. British Thyroid Association, Royal College of Physicians. Guidelines for the management of thyroid cancer. In: Report of the Thyroid Cancer Guidelines Update Group. 2nd ed. London: Royal College of Physicians; 2007.
35. Pacini F, Schlumberger M, Dralle H, Elisei R, Smit JW, Wiersinga W. European consensus for the management of patients with differentiated thyroid carcinoma of the follicular epithelium. Eur J Endocrinol. 2006;154(6):787–803.
36. Yoo D, Ajmal S, Gowda S, et al. Level VI lymph node dissection does not decrease radioiodine uptake in patients undergoing radioiodine ablation for differentiated thyroid cancer. World J Surg. 2012;36(6):1255–61.
37. Hughes DT, White ML, Miller BS, Gauger PG, Burney RE, Doherty GM. Influence of prophylactic central lymph node dissection on postoperative thyroglobulin levels and radioiodine treatment in papillary thyroid cancer. Surgery. 2010;148:1100–6.
38. Ito Y, Tomoda C, Uruno T, Takamura Y, Miya A, Kobayashi K, Matsuzuka F, Kuma K, Miyauchi A. Preoperative ultrasonographic examination for lymph node metastasis: usefulness when designing lymph node dissection for papillary microcarcinoma of the thyroid. World J Surg. 2004;28:498–501.
39. Gemsenjager E, Perren A, Seifert B, et al. Lymph node surgery in papillary thyroid carcinoma. J Am Coll Surg. 2003;197(2):182–90.

40. Wada N, Duh QY, Sugino K, Iwasaki H, Kameyama K, Mimura T, Ito K, Takami H, Takanashi Y. Lymph node metastasis from 259 papillary thyroid microcarcinomas: frequency, pattern of occurrence and recurrence, and optimal strategy for neck dissection. Ann Surg. 2003;237:399–407.
41. Wada N, Masudo K, Nakayama H, Suganuma N, Matsuzu K, Hirakawa S, Rino Y, Masuda M, Imada T. Clinical outcomes in older or younger patients with papillary thyroid carcinoma: impact of lymphadenopathy and patient age. Eur J Surg Oncol. 2008;34:202–7.
42. Bardet S, Malville E, Rame JP, Babin E, Samama G, De Raucourt D, Michels JJ, Reznik Y, Henry-Amar M. Macroscopic lymph-node involvement and neck dissection predict lymph-node recurrence in papillary thyroid carcinoma. Eur J Endocrinol. 2008;158:551–60.
43. Barczyński M, Konturek A, Stopa M, Nowak W. Prophylactic central neck dissection for papillary thyroid cancer. Br J Surg. 2013;100(3):410–8.
44. Besic N, Zgajnar J, Hocevar M, Petric R. Extent of thyroidectomy and lymphadenectomy in 254 patients with papillary thyroid microcarcinoma: a single-institution experience. Ann Surg Oncol. 2009;16(4):920–8.
45. Costa S, Giugliano G, Santoro L, et al. Role of prophylactic central neck dissection in cN0 papillary thyroid cancer Il ruolo dello svuotamento profilattico del compartimento centrale del collo. Acta Otorhinolaryngol Ital. 2009;29:61–9.
46. Hartl DM, Mamelle E, Borget I, Leboulleux S, Mirghani H, Schlumberger M. Influence of prophylactic neck dissection on rate of retreatment for papillary thyroid carcinoma. World J Surg. 2013;37(8):1951–8.
47. Lang BH, Yih PC, Shek TW, et al. Factors affecting the adequacy of lymph node yield in prophylactic unilateral central neck dissection for papillary thyroid carcinoma. J Surg Oncol. 2012;106(8):966–71.
48. Lee DY, Oh KH, Cho JG, Kwon SY, Woo JS, Baek SK, Jung KY. The benefits and risks of prophylactic central neck dissection for papillary thyroid carcinoma: Prospective Cohort Study. Int J Endocrinol. 2015;2015:571480.
49. Moo TA, McGill J, Allendorf J, et al. Impact of prophylactic central neck lymph node dissection on early recurrence in papillary thyroid carcinoma. World J Surg. 2010;34(6):1187–91.
50. Moreno MA, Edeiken-Monroe BS, Siegel ER, et al. In papillary thyroid cancer, preoperative central neck ultrasound detects only macroscopic surgical disease, but negative findings predict excellent long-term regional control and survival. Thyroid. 2012;22(4):347–55.
51. Roh JL, Park JY, Park CI. Prevention of postoperative hypocalcemia with routine oral calcium and vitamin D supplements in patients with differentiated papillary thyroid carcinoma undergoing total thyroidectomy plus central neck dissection. Cancer. 2009;115(2):251–8.
52. Roh JL, Park JY, Park CI. Total thyroidectomy plus neck dissection in differentiated papillary thyroid carcinoma patients: pattern of nodal metastasis, morbidity, recurrence, and postoperative levels of serum parathyroid hormone. Ann Surg. 2007;245(4):604–10.
53. Sadowski BM, Snyder SK, Lairmore TC. Routine bilateral central lymph node clearance for papillary thyroid cancer. Surgery. 2009;146(4):696–703; discussion 703–5.
54. Ywata de Carvalho A, Chulam TC, Kowalski LP. Long-term results of observation vs prophylactic selective level VI neck dissection for papillary thyroid carcinoma at a cancer center. JAMA Otolaryngol Head Neck Surg. 2015;141(7):599–606.
55. Zhang L, Liu Z, Liu Y, Gao W, Zheng C. The clinical prognosis of patients with cN0 papillary thyroid microcarcinoma by central neck dissection. World J Surg Oncol. 2015;13:138.
56. Zetoune T, Keutgen X, Buitrago D, et al. Prophylactic central neck dissection and local recurrence in papillary thyroid cancer: a meta-analysis. Ann Surg Oncol. 2010;17(12):3287–93.
57. Mazzaferri EL, Robbins RJ, Spencer CA, et al. A consensus report of the role of serum thyroglobulin as a monitoring method for low-risk patients with papillary thyroid carcinoma. J Clin Endocrinol Metab. 2003;88(4):1433–41. Review.
58. Salvesen H, Njølstad PR, Akslen LA, Albrektsen G, Søreide O, Varhaug JE. Papillary thyroid carcinoma: a multivariate analysis of prognostic factors including an evaluation of the p-TNM staging system. Eur J Surg. 1992;158(11–12):583–9.

59. Kukkonen ST, Haapiainen RK, Franssila KO, Sivula AH. Papillary thyroid carcinoma: the new, age-related TNM classification system in a retrospective analysis of 199 patients. World J Surg. 1990;14(6):837–41; discussion 841–2.
60. Bonnet S, Hartl D, Leboulleux S, et al. Prophylactic lymph node dissection for papillary thyroid cancer less than 2 cm: implications for radioiodine treatment. J Clin Endocrinol Metab. 2009;94(4):1162–7.
61. Viola D, Materazzi G, Valerio L, et al. Prophylactic central compartment lymph node dissection in papillary thyroid carcinoma: clinical implications derived from the first prospective randomized controlled single institution study. J Clin Endocrinol Metab. 2015;100(4):1316–24.
62. Sawka AM, Rilkoff H, Tsang RW, et al. The rationale of patients with early-stage papillary thyroid cancer for accepting or rejecting radioactive iodine remnant ablation. Thyroid. 2013;23(2):246–7.
63. Durante C, Haddy N, Baudin E, et al. Long-term outcome of 444 patients with distant metastases from papillary and follicular thyroid carcinoma: benefits and limits of radioiodine therapy. J Clin Endocrinol Metab. 2006;91(8):2892–9.
64. Lamartina L, Durante C, Filetti S, Cooper DS. Low-risk differentiated thyroid cancer and radioiodine remnant ablation: a systematic review of the literature. J Clin Endocrinol Metab. 2015;100(5):1748–61.
65. Tuttle RM, Tala H, Shah J, et al. Estimating risk of recurrence in differentiated thyroid cancer after total thyroidectomy and radioactive iodine remnant ablation: using response to therapy variables to modify the initial risk estimates predicted by the new American Thyroid Association staging system. Thyroid. 2010;20(12):1341–9.
66. Pereira JA, Jimeno J, Miquel J, Iglesias M, Munné A, Sancho JJ, Sitges-Serra A. Nodal yield, morbidity, and recurrence after central neck dissection for papillary thyroid carcinoma. Surgery. 2005;138(6):1095–100; discussion 1100–1.
67. Rosenbaum MA, McHenry CR. Central neck dissection for papillary thyroid cancer. Arch Otolaryngol Head Neck Surg. 2009;135(11):1092–7.
68. Giordano D, Valcavi R, Thompson GB, et al. Complications of central neck dissection in patients with papillary thyroid carcinoma: results of a study on 1087 patients and review of the literature. Thyroid. 2012;22(9):911–7.
69. Stavrakis AI, Ituarte PH, Ko CY, et al. Surgeon volume as a predictor of outcomes in inpatient and outpatient endocrine surgery. Surgery. 2007;142(6):887–99; discussion: 887–99.
70. Saunders BD, Wainess RM, Dimick JB, et al. Who performs endocrine operations in the United States? Surgery. 2003;134(6):924–31.
71. Wang T, Dubner S, Sznyter L, et al. Incidence of metastatic well-differentiated thyroid cancer in cervical lymph nodes. Arch Otolaryngol Head Neck Surg. 2004;130:110–3.
72. Onkendi EO, McKenzie TJ, Richards ML, Farley DR, Thompson GB, Kasperbauer JL, Hay ID, Grant CS. Reoperative experience with papillary thyroid cancer. World J Surg. 2014;38(3):645–52.
73. Alvarado R, Sywak MS, Delbridge L, Sidhu SB. Central lymph node dissection as a secondary procedure for papillary thyroid cancer: is there added morbidity? Surgery. 2009;145:514–8.
74. Shen WT, Ogawa L, Ruan D, Suh I, Kebebew E, Duh QY, Clark OH. Central neck lymph node dissection for papillary thyroid cancer: comparison of complication and recurrence rates in 295 initial dissections and reoperations. Arch Surg. 2010;145(3):272–5.

Chapter 17
The Management of the Persistent and Recurrent Cervical Lymph Node Metastases

J.D. Pasternak and W.T. Shen

Introduction

Although the incidence of well-differentiated thyroid cancer (WDTC) has been increasing in the past decade, the mortality of this disease remains extremely low [1]. While it is rare for patients to die of this disease, there is a substantial risk that after initial treatment, thyroid cancer will persist or recur. For the purposes of this chapter, we will term disease found after initial treatment as recurrent although due to the indolent nature of WDTC, differentiating the entities of persistence and recurrence may be difficult. To further complicate this idea, in patients with thyroid cancer and no clinical or radiographic evidence of metastatic spread, Wada showed that most will have at least micrometastatic deposits in the regional lymph nodes [2]. Fortunately, large American datasets have shown that the overall clinical recurrence rate of WDTC ranges from 2 to 6 % in low-risk thyroid cancer [3, 4] to about 20–40 % in high-risk cancer, independent of the high micrometastatic risk (nearly 90 % present at diagnosis) [1, 5, 6]. Since about 85 % of these cancers are papillary thyroid cancer, which preferentially spreads to cervical lymph nodes, most recurrent disease is found in the neck. As mentioned, while many patients with WDTC do not die from their disease, they often undergo multiple investigations for detection of recurrence, and, if found, sometimes many interventions to control disease spread. For the purposes of this chapter, we will focus on how thyroidologists might manage a patient after initial treatment of WDTC including surveillance and treatment interventions once recurrent disease is detected.

J.D. Pasternak
Division of General Surgery, University Health Network, Toronto, Canada

W.T. Shen (✉)
Department of Surgery, Mt Zion Hospital, University of California – San Francisco, 1600 Divisadero Street, 3rd Floor Hellman Building, San Francisco, CA, USA, 94115
e-mail: wen.shen2@ucsf.edu

S.A. Roman et al. (eds.), *Management of Thyroid Nodules and Differentiated Thyroid Cancer*, DOI 10.1007/978-3-319-43618-0_17

Detecting Recurrent Disease

The American Thyroid Association initially published a framework for predicting risk of recurrence in patients with the 2009 guideline risk stratification. Those at low risk have as little as 9 % recurrence compared to 69 % in high-risk patients [7–10]. Because of this, those more likely to develop disease should be screened more frequently. Some groups have published on the best time interval for surveillance, including factoring cost-effectiveness. Wu et al. showed that for low-risk patients, after 5 years without disease, 3-year surveillance intervals could be recommended, although this would not be sufficient for higher-risk patients [11].

With the recent recommendations from the ATA [12], treatment of low-risk thyroid cancer with less than total thyroidectomy is becoming more common. While outcomes may be similar, the follow-up of patients with WDTC will substantially change. Widespread use of total thyroidectomy and radioactive iodine therapy had allowed thyroid clinicians to use serum thyroglobulin (Tg) monitoring and ultrasonography of a cleared central neck as mainstay of surveillance. As more patients will be treated with thyroid lobectomy only, clinicians will modify their thresholds. The new ATA guidelines provide good recommendations for follow-up of these patients and comments on the decreased use of RAI, a recent visible trend in North America [12].

When to Intervene

Approximately 20 % of patients will have elevated Tg levels up to 1 year after total thyroidectomy for thyroid cancer, but only one-third will have structural disease. The rest will remain free of disease and often have a decreasing Tg over time [13, 14]. Even without RAI ablation post-surgery, Durante et al. showed that Tg levels will still fall within 5–7 years after thyroidectomy. Among tools to detect recurrent disease, ultrasound remains the best method for surveillance of thyroid cancer in the neck [15]. When recurrent disease in the neck is detected, it is important for the clinician to determine if further investigation or treatment is warranted. As will be discussed, some lesions may not be treated or even sampled for diagnosis. Increased risks of reoperation in a scarred field must be balanced with the goal to locally control metastatic thyroid cancer. To this end, there have been multiple studies which recommend surgical intervention as the treatment of choice for those lesions in the central neck (Level VI) which are ≥8 mm in size and in the lateral neck (II–V) ≥10 mm in size. Even with these general size suggestions, there are many variables that the clinician will take into account. Some variables include RLN function, intact parathyroid glands, comorbidities of the patient, and bulky or distant metastatic deposits. If surgical excision is planned, however, fine-needle aspiration (FNA) biopsy of suspicious lesions is recommended when possible. In the following section, we will discuss the surgical treatment of recurrent WDTC in the neck.

Where to Intervene

Reoperative Neck Dissection

Preoperative imaging is most important when planning for reoperation for recurrent WDTC. Most surgeons use ultrasonography with lymph node mapping to ensure all areas of the neck are examined for recurrence before intervention. As mentioned in the most recent ATA guidelines, cross-sectional imaging is also useful in the preoperative evaluation of these patients. Many centers use computed tomography (CT) scan either alone or in addition to ultrasound. CT provides a cross-sectional image of the neck and surrounding structures including the trachea and clavicles, provides insight on variant anatomy, and often characterizes the upper mediastinum (Level VII). Recent studies show CT scan may be helpful as an adjunct to ultrasound for preoperative planning in recurrent thyroid cancer specifically in better localizing disease [16, 17]. Once surgery is planned, the discussion of risks associated with reoperation should be extensively addressed with the patient, and preoperative assessment of vocal function should be performed [12].

Technique

The patient is positioned on the OR table after endotracheal intubation with the neck extended and the arms tucked. In these reoperative procedures, the authors recommend using a nerve monitoring system as the anatomy is often distorted from previous dissection in the area. Once the patient is positioned, the use of surgeon-performed ultrasound is extremely helpful to appreciate disease location in real time. As previously described by Harari et al., we suggest injecting 1 cc/cm^3 of 1:5 diluted methylene blue under ultrasound guidance into the lymph nodes of concern to ensure their incorporation into the surgical specimen. If there are numerous lymph nodes, injecting into the most cephalad and caudad lymph node targets helps guide the surgeon in the excision of diseased nodes in an often densely scarred neck [18]. As described in this chapter and mentioned in the ATA guidelines in the management of WDTC, it is recommended to pursue a lymphadenectomy by level of the neck and avoid "berry picking." Using blue dye injection intraoperatively may allow the surgeon to ensure entire levels of the neck containing disease are excised (Fig. 17.1).

Central Neck

As the region of the neck encasing the thyroid gland, the central neck (Level VI) is the most common location for persistent or recurrent WDTC. Of the 20 % of patients who are found to have recurrences in their lifetime, most of them are within this anatomical region. Defined as the area bounded by the carotid sheaths laterally, the hyoid bone superiorly, and the sternal notch or brachiocephalic vessels inferiorly, in addition to the thyroid gland, it holds the recurrent laryngeal nerves, parathyroid

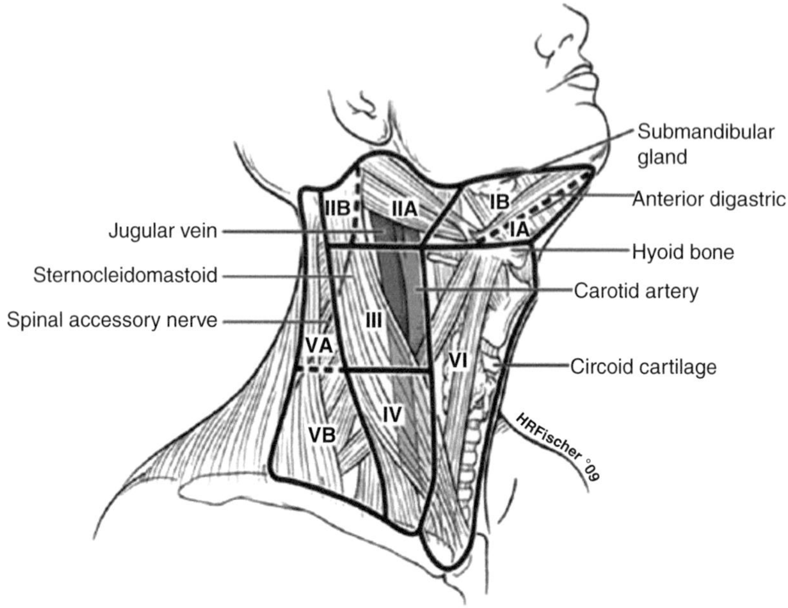

Fig. 17.1 Neck lymph nodes levels and compartments

glands, and lymph node basins. The central neck lymph nodes include prelaryngeal (Delphian), pretracheal, and paratracheal basins, in which the latter extends to the carotid sheath laterally. Recurrent thyroid cancer is most commonly found here; reoperation, while safe when performed by high-volume surgeons, carries risks of injury of the regional structures. Reoperative central neck dissection has been shown to have rates of recurrent laryngeal nerve injury from 0 % permanent risk [19–25] to 21 % transiently [20]. Postoperative hypocalcemia has been reported with a large range of 0–24 % [20–26]. Table 17.1 outlines a literature review of complications from reoperative neck dissection.

Due to the risks which are higher than first-time operations, the extent of reoperation should be dictated by disease burden. While lymph node dissection should encompass levels of the neck, specific levels and laterality should be dictated by specific recurrence patterns. If disease is limited to one side of the neck, a unilateral dissection would be recommended instead of bilateral [12]. If, however, disease is found throughout the central compartment, a bilateral procedure would be indicated, taking into consideration the recurrent laryngeal nerve and parathyroid glands which are closely related to the nodal basins.

Reoperative Lateral Neck Dissection

As mentioned, reoperative lateral neck dissection for WDTC should be performed by the neck level containing recurrent disease rather than "berry picking" single diseased lymph nodes. The most important, however, to an effective and safe

Table 17.1 Complications after reoperative central compartment (Level VI) lymph node dissection (all retrospective reviews)

		Recurrent laryngeal nerve palsy		Hypocalcemia	
Author/year	Patients (*N*)	Transient (%)	Permanent (%)	Transient (%)	Permanent (%)
Farrag et al. [20]	33 patients	21	0	6	0
Clayman et al. [19]	63 patients	2	0	19	18[a]
Alvarado et al. [23]	193 patients	3	0.6	11	2
Shen et al. [26]	106 patients	4.7	1.9	23.6	0.9
Tufano et al. [24]	120 patients		14.2[a]	10	2.5
Shah et al. [22]	82 patients	2	2	20	7
Lang et al. [25]	50 patients	6	1	14	0
Onkendi et al. [21]	410 patients		2[b], 0.5[c]		3

Reference [19–26]
[a]Permanent + persistent
[b]Recurrent laryngeal nerve resected due to tumor burden
[c]Unintentional injury

dissection is the experience and judgment of the surgeon, weighing risks and benefits of the extent of surgery. Similar to the central neck, reoperation in the lateral neck carries higher operative risks than first-time surgery. Structures in the lateral neck of concern in reoperations include the carotid sheath containing the vagus nerve proximal to the recurrent laryngeal nerve, spinal accessory nerve, and other neurovascular structures surrounding the disease. Overall, compartmental neck dissection decreases structural disease burden in 80 % of patients, including lowering Tg up to 90 % of the time even though Tg levels often do not fall to negligible levels [27, 28].

Nonsurgical Therapies for Recurrent WDTC

Aside from formal surgical neck dissection, there has been an increased experience of clinicians treating recurrent WDTC with alternative local therapies. Two main modalities which have been described with good results are ethanol and radiofrequency ablation (RFA). Recent large series have been published showing treatment with ethanol and RFA can be safe and effective in recurrent WDTC. The largest study from Norway described the treatment of 109 lymph nodes with ethanol showing sustained ablation of recurrent disease in 84 % of cases at 38 months of follow-up [29]. Although many in this study needed to be retreated with ethanol, it was done as an outpatient without general anesthetic, and they described no significant adverse effects. Studies using RFA have also showed good results, with some studies showing up to 60 % disappearance of treated lymph nodes. A complication seen specifically in RFA however is heat damage to skin [30]. Some results have been promising although long-term studies are needed to evaluate the clinical effectiveness and impact on survival of these ablative therapies.

Distant Recurrence

Due to the favorable prognosis of WDTC, distant metastatic spread is rare, especially for lower-risk thyroid cancer. Unfortunately, it is sometimes difficult to predict distant metastasis, and ultimately it is up to the clinician to decide when investigation is warranted [31]. Cross-sectional imaging is most helpful in determining metastasis, specifically contrast-enhanced CT scan. As the lungs are the most common site of distant metastasis, CT scan of the neck and chest is helpful for quantifying disease burden in these patients. FDG-PET has been used also to help quantify distant disease. Recent publications suggest that those thyroid cancers which do not take up radioactive iodine due to dedifferentiation may be best seen by this method [32, 33]. Patients with distant metastasis may still have good long-term survival, depending on the differentiation of the thyroid cancer. Referral to a multidisciplinary team consisting of surgeons, endocrinologists, radiation oncologists, medical oncologists, nuclear medicine, and radiologists will facilitate optimal outcomes [34].

Conclusion

Fortunately, WDTC has a very favorable prognosis; however, patients may have recurrent disease. Most commonly, recurrence occurs in the neck and is best treated by surgical excision with low morbidity. While there are new treatment options described in the local treatment of thyroid cancer, larger longer-term studies are needed to correlate these treatments with survival. Patients with high-risk cancer or clinical symptoms of widespread disease should be worked up with cross-sectional imaging to rule out distant spread and treated accordingly. Overall, the best care for patients with recurrent thyroid cancer occurs when a multidisciplinary team is involved in a patient-centered treatment plan.

References

1. Ahn HS, Kim HJ, Welch HG. Korea's thyroid-cancer "epidemic"–screening and overdiagnosis. N Engl J Med. 2014;371(19):1765–7.
2. Wada N, Duh QY, Sugino K, Iwasaki H, Kameyama K, Mimura T, Ito K, Takami H, Takanashi Y. Lymph node metastasis from 259 papillary thyroid microcarcinomas: frequency, pattern of occurrence and recurrence, and optimal strategy for neck dissection. Ann Surg. 2003;237(3):399–407.
3. Mazzaferri EL. Management of low-risk differentiated thyroid cancer. Endocr Pract. 2007;13:498–512.
4. Hay ID. Management of patients with low-risk papillary thyroid carcinoma. Endocr Pract. 2007;13:521–33.
5. Qubain SW, Nakano S, Baba M, Takao S, Aikou T. Distribution of lymph node micrometastasis in pN0 well-differentiated thyroid carcinoma. Surgery. 2002;131:249–56.

6. Arturi F, Russo D, Giuffrida D, Ippolito A, Perrotti N, Vigneri R, Filetti S. Early diagnosis by genetic analysis of differentiated thyroid cancer metastases in small lymph nodes. J Clin Endocrinol Metab. 1997;82:1638–41.
7. Tuttle RM, Tala H, Shah J, Leboeuf R, Ghossein R, Gonen M, Brokhin M, Omry G, Fagin JA, Shaha A. Estimating risk of recurrence in differentiated thyroid cancer after total thyroidectomy and radioactive iodine remnant ablation: using response to therapy variables to modify the initial risk estimates predicted by the new American Thyroid Association staging system. Thyroid. 2010;20:1341–9.
8. Vaisman F, Momesso D, Bulzico DA, Pessoa CH, Dias F, Corbo R, Vaisman M, Tuttle RM. Spontaneous remission in thyroid cancer patients after biochemical incomplete response to initial therapy. Clin Endocrinol (Oxf). 2012;77:132–8.
9. Castagna MG, Maino F, Cipri C, Belardini V, Theodoropoulou A, Cevenini G, Pacini F. Delayed risk stratification, to include the response to initial treatment (surgery and radioiodine ablation), has better outcome predictivity in differentiated thyroid cancer patients. Eur J Endocrinol. 2011;165:441–6.
10. Pitoia F, Bueno F, Urciuoli C, Abelleira E, Cross G, Tuttle RM. Outcomes of patients with differentiated thyroid cancer risk-stratified according to the American thyroid association and Latin American thyroid society risk of recurrence classification systems. Thyroid. 2013;23:1401–7.
11. Wu JX, Beni CE, Zanocco KA, Sturgeon C, Yeh MW. Cost-effectiveness of long-term every three-year versus annual postoperative surveillance for low-risk papillary thyroid cancer. Thyroid. 2015;25(7):797–803.
12. Haugen BR, Alexander EK, Bible KC, Doherty G, Mandel SJ, Nikiforov YE, Pacini F, Randolph G, Sawka A, Schlumberger M, Schuff KG, Sherman SI, Sosa JA, Steward D, Tuttle RM, Wartofsky L. 2015 American Thyroid Association Management guidelines for adult patients with thyroid nodules and differentiated thyroid cancer. Thyroid. 2015; 26(1):1–133.
13. Baudin E, Do CC, Cailleux AF, Leboulleux S, Travagli JP, Schlumberger M. Positive predictive value of serum thyroglobulin levels, measured during the first year of follow-up after thyroid hormone withdrawal, in thyroid cancer patients. J Clin Endocrinol Metab. 2003;88:1107–11.
14. Padovani RP, Robenshtok E, Brokhin M, Tuttle RM. Even without additional therapy, serum thyroglobulin concentrations often decline for years after total thyroidectomy and radioactive remnant ablation in patients with differentiated thyroid cancer. Thyroid. 2012;22:778–83.
15. Torlontano M, Crocetti U, Augello G, D'Aloiso L, Bonfitto N, Varraso A, Dicembrino F, Modoni S, Frusciante V, Di Giorgio A, Bruno R, Filetti S, Trischitta V. Comparative evaluation of recombinant human thyrotropin-stimulated thyroglobulin levels, 131I whole-body scintigraphy, and neck ultrasonography in the follow-up of patients with papillary thyroid microcarcinoma who have not undergone radioiodine therapy. J Clin Endocrinol Metab. 2006; 91(1):60–3.
16. Kim E, Park JS, Son KR, Kim JH, Jeon SJ, Na DG. Preoperative diagnosis of cervical metastatic lymph nodes in papillary thyroid carcinoma: comparison of ultrasound, computed tomography, and combined ultrasound with computed tomography. Thyroid. 2008;18:411–8.
17. Lesnik D, Cunnane ME, Zurakowski D, Acar GO, Ecevit C, Mace A, Kamani D, Randolph GW. Papillary thyroid carcinoma nodal surgery directed by a preoperative radiographic map utilizing CT scan and ultrasound in all primary and reoperative patients. Head Neck. 2014;36(2):191–202.
18. Harari A, Sippel RS, Goldstein R, Aziz S, Shen W, Gosnell J, Duh QY, Clark OH. Successful localization of recurrent thyroid cancer in reoperative neck surgery using ultrasound-guided methylene blue dye injection. J Am Coll Surg. 2012;215(4):555–61.
19. Clayman GL, Shellenberger TD, Ginsberg LE, et al. Approach and safety of comprehensive central compartment dissection in patients with recurrent papillary thyroid carcinoma. Head Neck. 2009;31:1152–63.
20. Farrag TY, Agrawal N, Sheth S, et al. Algorithm for safe and effective reoperative thyroid bed surgery for recurrent/persistent papillary thyroid carcinoma. Head Neck. 2007;29:1069–74.

21. Onkendi EO, McKenzie TJ, Richards ML, Farley DR, Thompson GB, Kasperbauer JL, Hay ID, Grant CS. Reoperative experience with papillary thyroid cancer. World J Surg. 2014;38(3):645–52. doi:10.1007/s00268-013-2379-9.
22. Shah MD, Harris LD, Nassif RG, et al. Efficacy and safety of central compartment neck dissection for recurrent thyroid carcinoma. Arch Otolaryngol Head Neck Surg. 2012;138:33–7.
23. Alvarado R, Sywak MS, Delbridge L, et al. Central lymph node dissection as a secondary procedure for papillary thyroid cancer: is there added morbidity? Surgery. 2009;145:514–8.
24. Tufano RP, Bishop J, Wu G. Reoperative central compartment dissection for patients with recurrent/persistent papillary thyroid cancer: efficacy, safety, and the association of the BRAF mutation. Laryngoscope. 2012;122:1634–40.
25. Lang BH, Lee GC, Ng CP, et al. Evaluating the morbidity and efficacy of reoperative surgery in the central compartment for persistent/recurrent papillary thyroid carcinoma. World J Surg. 2013;37:2853–9.
26. Shen WT, Ogawa L, Ruan D, et al. Central neck lymph node dissection for papillary thyroid cancer: comparison of complication and recurrence rates in 295 initial dissections and reoperations. Arch Surg. 2010;145:272–5.
27. Urken ML, Milas M, Randolph GW, Tufano R, Bergman D, Bernet V, Brett EM, Brierley JD, Cobin R, Doherty G, Klopper J, Lee S, Machac J, Mechanick JI, Orloff LA, Ross D, Smallridge RC, Terris DJ, Clain JB, Tuttle M. A review of the management of recurrent and persistent metastatic lymph nodes in well differentiated thyroid cancer: a multifactorial decision making guide created for the Thyroid Cancer Care Collaborative. Head Neck. 2015;37:605–14.
28. Steward DL. Update in utility of secondary node dissection for papillary thyroid cancer. J Clin Endocrinol Metab. 2012;97:3393–8.
29. Heilo A, Sigstad E, Fagerlid KH, Haskjold OI, Groholt KK, Berner A, Bjoro T, Jorgensen LH. Efficacy of ultrasound-guided percutaneous ethanol injection treatment in patients with a limited number of metastatic cervical lymph nodes from papillary thyroid carcinoma. J Clin Endocrinol Metab. 2011;96:2750–5.
30. Baek JH, Kim YS, Sung JY, Choi H, Lee JH. Locoregional control of metastatic well-differentiated thyroid cancer by ultrasound-guided radiofrequency ablation. AJR Am J Roentgenol. 2011;197:W331–6.
31. Hay ID, Hutchinson ME, Gonzalez-Losada T, McIver B, Reinalda ME, Grant CS, Thompson GB, Sebo TJ, Goellner JR. Papillary thyroid microcarcinoma: a study of 900 cases observed in a 60-year period. Surgery. 2008;144:980–7.
32. Palmedo H, Bucerius J, Joe A, et al. Integrated PET/CT in differentiated thyroid cancer: diagnostic accuracy and impact on patient management. J Nucl Med. 2006;47:616–24.
33. Schreinemakers JM, Vriens MR, Munoz-Perez N, et al. Fluorodeoxyglucose-positron emission tomography scan-positive recurrent papillary thyroid cancer and the prognosis and implications for surgical management. World J Surg Oncol. 2012;10:192.
34. Rosenthal MS, Angelos P, Cooper DS, Fassler C, Finder SG, Hays MT, Tendler B, Braunstein GD. Clinical and professional ethics guidelines for the practice of thyroidology. Thyroid. 2013;23:1203–10.

Chapter 18
Thyroid Nodular Disease and Thyroid Cancer During Pregnancy

Trevor E. Angell and Erik K. Alexander

Thyroid nodules are common, though the prevalence is markedly influenced by age and sex. Most analyses of patients presenting for initial nodule evaluation confirm a female to male predominance greater than 4:1 [1]. While the formation of new and multiple thyroid nodules is influenced by advancing age, the burden of disease on young women remains substantial. The principle purpose for thyroid nodule evaluation is to identify thyroid cancer and, more specifically, to guide treatment for those patients in whom thyroid cancer may pose a future risk to good health. Pregnancy itself has a profound influence on thyroid physiology [2], and thus the impact of gestation upon nodule formation, malignant transformation, and cancer behavior must be considered. Clinically, the risks and potential contraindications associated with any intervention performed on pregnant women also must be taken into account. This chapter will focus upon thyroid nodular disease and thyroid cancer in women planning pregnancy or those currently pregnant. Thyroid nodular disease will first be discussed, focusing upon the prevalence, clinical evaluation, and treatment specific to the pregnant patient. Thereafter, discussion will focus on thyroid cancer care.

Thyroid nodules are estimated to occur in 20–50 % of the adult population [3], and new and multiple nodules are more frequent with advancing age [4]. Iodine deficiency can increase the prevalence of thyroid nodules in a population, though iodine supplementation strategies have improved in the United States and worldwide over the last half century. Given the slow growth rate of thyroid nodules [5], most newly detected nodules during pregnancy can be assumed to have been present before conception. Though both benign and malignant thyroid nodules grow with

T.E. Angell, MD • E.K. Alexander, MD (✉)
The Thyroid Section, Department of Medicine, Brigham & Women's Hospital and Harvard Medical School, 75 Francis Street, Building PBB-B4, Room 415, Boston, MA 02115, USA
e-mail: ekalexander@partners.org

S.A. Roman et al. (eds.), *Management of Thyroid Nodules and Differentiated Thyroid Cancer*, DOI 10.1007/978-3-319-43618-0_18

time, growth is most often slow, occurring over years. An exception to this can be the rapid expansion of a cystic nodule when internal hemorrhage has occurred. Demographically, it is important to note that the average age of pregnancy in the United States has been increasing over the last four decades, with the fastest growing demographic being women seeking pregnancy after the age of 30 years [6]. This, combined with the age-associated increase in nodularity, suggests the frequency of this illness among pregnant women will increase in the future.

Physiologically, pregnancy may modestly impact thyroid nodule formation and growth, albeit to a clinically insignificant degree. Kung and colleagues studied 221 newly pregnant patients, performing serial ultrasound examination throughout gestation. The proportion of patients with thyroid nodules increased by nearly 10 % from the first to the third trimester [7]. However, newly detected thyroid nodules were very small, most measuring less than 5 mm in diameter. Similar case-control analyses demonstrate an increased prevalence of nodularity among women previously pregnant in comparison to nulliparous controls [8]. It should be emphasized again that the clinical impact of such nodule formation is minimal and that these findings should not prompt routine monitoring of patients with nonmalignant nodules during gestation.

Evaluation of the Thyroid Nodule During Pregnancy

The evaluation of a thyroid nodule in a pregnant patient is similar to that of a non-pregnant patient, with select exceptions [9]. A thorough medical history should be performed and should seek to identify rare, high-risk findings such as persistent hoarseness of voice, neck pain, or new neck lymphadenopathy. Patients should be queried about exposure to ionizing radiation as a child, or the presence of thyroid cancer in the family, as both can increase the probability that a thyroid nodule may prove cancerous. The physical examination should illustrate the size, location, and characteristics of a thyroid nodule. Attention should be given to firm (or "rock-hard") nodules, fixation to surrounding structures, new choking or aspiration when swallowing, or the presence of new, persistent lymphadenopathy. Following clinical risk assessment, pregnant women with suspected thyroid nodules should undergo ultrasound examination. As ultrasound does not transmit ionizing radiation, this test is safe during pregnancy and without contraindication. The ultrasound evaluation should include sonographic risk assessment of any nodules identified, such as cystic content, echogenic pattern, microcalcifications, and irregular margins, as these findings help assess risk of malignancy [10]. Measurement of serum thyrotropin (TSH) should also be obtained. Thereafter, patients with non-suppressed TSH values should be considered for ultrasound-guided fine needle aspiration (UG-FNA) of clinically relevant nodules. The decision to aspirate should be guided by clinical guidelines [9] and informed by the published literature. In general, solid nodules with abnormal sonographic findings should be aspirated when larger than 1 cm, while nodules with low or very low risk findings should be aspirated when larger than 1.5–2.0 cm, respectively. Purely cystic nodules should not be aspirated, as they are benign. UG-FNA is a safe procedure during pregnancy and is usually performed with subcutaneous lidocaine. Side effects of UG-FNA, beyond mild bruising, are very rare, while the information gained from cytologic analysis significantly improves thyroid cancer risk assessment.

There are no high-quality data suggesting that the cytologic analyses of thyroid nodule aspirations are affected by pregnancy. As most nodules have been present before (yet detected during) pregnancy, the distribution of FNA cytology results should mimic those seen in a young, nonpregnant population [11]. Approximately 70 % of thyroid nodules will be cytologically benign, while 5–10 % will be cytologically malignant, and ~5 % will be nondiagnostic. However, ~15–20 % of nodule aspirates are classified as cytologically indeterminate. Such aspirates demonstrate abnormal features concerning for malignancy, but are not sufficient to be called cytologically malignant. These nodules should be classified per the Bethesda system [12] and reported as atypia of undetermined significance (AUS), follicular neoplasm (FN), or suspicious for papillary carcinoma (SUSP). Such nodules prove malignant in 20–70 % of cases following histopathologic analysis.

The management of thyroid nodules detected during pregnancy should be guided by the sonographic and cytologic findings. In general, most cases of thyroid cancer detected during pregnancy behave in an indolent fashion [8, 13]. Therefore, a conservative approach to cytologically indeterminate or malignant nodules is often considered. Moosa and colleagues studied 589 patients with newly diagnosed thyroid cancer, performing a case-control study comparing 61 patients diagnosed during pregnancy with 528 patients diagnosed while not pregnant [14]. The time to treatment was delayed by 15 months in pregnant patients. Despite this delay in treatment, no attributable harm was demonstrated. Some studies have reported contradictory findings, though they remain difficult to interpret. Messuti and colleagues noted a high rate of persistent or recurrent disease when thyroid cancer was diagnosed during or shortly following pregnancy [15]. However, serum thyroglobulin levels were commonly >10 ng/ml at the time of I131 ablation, raising questions regarding the extent of initial resection and whether this might influence the finding of a biochemically incomplete response. Similar questions apply to a study by Vannucchi [16]. Given the possibility that such findings could be attributable to incomplete initial treatment, these findings should not refute previous, larger analyses demonstrating general safety. However, further research into this area remains important. It should separately be noted that thyroid surgery during pregnancy imparts an increased operative and hospital risk in comparison to nonpregnant patients. Kuy et al. investigated 31,356 women undergoing thyroid or parathyroid surgery between the years of 1999 and 2004 [17]. In women pregnant at time of surgery, operative complications (23.9 % vs 10.4 %), length of stay (2 days vs. 1 day), and total cost ($6873 vs. $5963) were all increased in comparison to nonpregnant controls.

Management of the Indeterminate Thyroid Nodule During Pregnancy

Thyroid nodules with indeterminate cytology are not definitely benign nor cancerous and remain a diagnostic dilemma. Recent data suggests that Bethesda classification can provide prognostic information well beyond simply implying the percentage risk of malignancy. Liu and colleagues studied nearly 1000 consecutive malignancies, retrospectively comparing preoperative cytology classification to final malignant histopathology [18]. Lower risk indeterminate categories such as atypia of undetermined significance (AUS) or suspicious for malignancy (SUSP) signal a likelihood of identifying lower risk variants of papillary thyroid carcinoma, as well as a reduced risk of metastatic disease or recurrence. This is in contrast to cytology classified as malignant, where the risk of tall-cell variant of PTC or distant metastatic spread is more likely. Together these data provide support for a more cautious and conservative approach to pregnant women with indeterminate thyroid nodule cytology. Furthermore, many such lesions prove benign following surgical removal. However, even if malignant, nodules with AUS cytology are much more likely to represent low-risk thyroid carcinoma. The potential harm attributable to delayed treatment until after delivery for low-risk, well-differentiated malignancy in a pregnant patient is generally minimal, while the risk of operative complications during pregnancy is increased.

In nonpregnant women, molecular diagnostic testing of cytologically indeterminate thyroid nodules has proven useful toward improvement preoperative cancer risk assessment [19, 20]. However, such tests are not recommended for use in pregnant women at this time, given the paucity of data currently available and the potential for misleading results. Most notable, the available RNA-based gene expression test (i.e., Afirma GEC) measures the expression of >160 genes. While some of the gene expression is directly related to the local tumor environment, it is also possible that other gene expressions may be influenced by hormonal changes of pregnancy. Thus, Afirma GEC test performance should be viewed as uncertain in the unique scenario of pregnancy and generally avoided. A separate molecular test is a panel of single gene (DNA) mutations. This test is made clinically available through many commercial vendors (e.g., miRInform Thyroid, Thyroseq). Mutations in oncogenes such as BRAF, RAS, and others, as well as fusion products of RET:PTC and PPAX8:PPARγ, have been investigated for their ability to predict benign or malignant disease in nonpregnant patients [21]. While such somatic mutations are less likely to be influenced by pregnancy, there have been no investigations of these DNA-based tests in pregnant women.

In practice, BRAF V600E mutations have proven to be the most predictive of malignancy in nonpregnant cohorts. Thus, one could hypothetically rationalize testing for the presence of this mutation in scenarios where the presence of the BRAF V600E mutation would impact the extent of the surgery performed. Caution should be raised however, with regard to the interpretation of other gene mutations, most notably that of the RAS oncogenes (i.e., KRAS, NRAS, and HRAS). While somatic RAS mutations increase the risk that affected nodules are malignant, recent data demonstrate that RAS mutations frequently occur in benign thyroid nodules. In a small study, Medici and colleagues showed that many RAS-positive yet cytologically benign nodules do not behave as cancerous during close sonographic follow-up over many years [22]. Furthermore, repeat FNA cytology confirms no evidence of tissue transformation from benign to malignant disease. Therefore, at a minimum, these data suggest that a finding of a new genetic mutation in a thyroid nodule should not universally imply that such a nodule is malignant. In summary, due to the paucity of available investigative data as well as the concerns regarding accuracy, the use of molecular testing in pregnant women with indeterminate FNA cytology cannot be recommended at this time.

Cancer of the Thyroid and Pregnancy

For most patients with papillary thyroid carcinoma discovered by cytology in early pregnancy, the cancer should be initially assessed and regularly monitored sonographically [9]. If sonographic evidence of substantial growth, tracheal or vessel invasion, or lymph node involvement are detected, surgery should be considered. If elected, surgery should generally occur before 24–26 weeks of gestation to minimize the risk of miscarriage. However, for most patients with low-risk, contained, well-differentiated disease that does not appear to be progressing, surgery can be safely deferred until after delivery. Data confirm that papillary thyroid carcinoma discovered during pregnancy appears to behave no differently than disease detected in nonpregnant women [13, 23]. Patients in whom well-differentiated thyroid cancer is detected in the second half of pregnancy should similarly consider delaying surgery until after delivery for identical reasons. Separate data demonstrate that delays of up to 1 year appear to show no adverse impact upon recurrence and survival rates [13]. An exception to these recommendations is the rare findings of a more aggressive thyroid malignancy, such as medullary, poorly differentiated, or anaplastic thyroid carcinoma. In such circumstances, more aggressive therapy is often warranted during pregnancy, and care must be individualized. If a low-risk cancerous nodule is being followed with a nonoperative approach during pregnancy, serum TSH levels should be targeted <2 mU/L [24]. If TSH concentrations are elevated beyond this target, initiation of levothyroxine is generally recommended, often at a starting dose of 50–75mcg daily. Repeat testing of serum TSH should be performed in 4 weeks. The rationale for these recommendations is twofold. First, TSH is a stimulating factor for thyroid tissue growth, including thyroid nodules and thyroid cancer, and lowering serum TSH therefore reduces the stimulus for cancer growth. Separately, data demonstrate the importance of maintaining normal maternal thyroid function during pregnancy as it relates to fetal and pregnancy harm [25], with TSH values ideally targeted below 2.5–3.0 mIU/L.

For many nonpregnant patients with well-differentiated thyroid carcinoma, adjunctive radioactive iodine (^{131}I) is administered following surgical resection [9]. Importantly, such radiopharmaceuticals are contraindicated during gestation and should not be administered, as radiation can directly impart teratogenic risk to the developing fetus. Furthermore, late in pregnancy the fetus has a functional thyroid gland, and maternally administered ^{131}I readily crosses the placenta where it may ablate the fetal thyroid tissue. Patients who have recently undergone surgery for well-differentiated thyroid cancer and are newly pregnant should be followed conservatively with regular monitoring and TSH suppressive therapy. If radioactive iodine therapy is indicated, this should be delayed until the postpartum period, ideally following cessation of lactation.

In monitoring the status of thyroid carcinoma in a pregnant woman, maternal serum thyroglobulin is usually the most sensitive marker for detecting recurrent or residual disease. In patients who have not undergone I131 ablation, a maternal serum concentration generally <2 IU/L supports the conclusion of no active disease. In contrast, thyroglobulin concentrations >2 IU/L, or concentrations which are rising over time, often signal concern for thyroid cancer recurrence [26]. In such cases, a thorough physical examination should be performed in conjunction with a neck ultrasound, which may identify an anatomic source. Approximately 20 % of patients are found to harbor interfering antibodies to thyroglobulin [27]. Such antibodies are not pathogenic, but most often interfere with the analytic assay for thyroglobulin making measurement unreliable. In nearly all laboratories, initial screening for thyroglobulin antibodies occurs whenever serum thyroglobulin testing is requested. If interfering antibodies are detected, serum thyroglobulin itself may not be assessed, avoiding the risk of a false-negative reading.

Changes in Thyroid Hormone During Pregnancy

It is also important that healthcare providers understand the changes in thyroid hormone physiology during pregnancy, especially when surgical resection is considered. Importantly, thyroid hormone production increases by an average of 40 % during gestation [28]. This increase often occurs seamlessly, as both maternal TSH and pregnancy-specific human chorionic gonadotropin (hCG) stimulate increased thyroxine production. In patients with impaired thyroid function (requiring levothyroxine therapy), or in whom the thyroid gland has been removed surgically, this stimulated increase in thyroxine production cannot occur endogenously, and the increasing demand of thyroxine during gestation will induce maternal and fetal hypothyroidism unless increasing doses of levothyroxine are administered and frequently monitored to ensure an appropriate serum TSH concentration. The pattern of increasing demand during gestation has been carefully studied and begins very early in gestation [28]. Demand thereafter increases linearly through approximately 16–20 weeks of gestation, where the maximal requirement is often identified. From midgestation to delivery, the increased requirement for thyroxine plateaus, but is sustained. Upon delivery, thyroxine requirements return to pregestational levels.

In the clinic, it is therefore important that all pregnant women with thyroid nodules have serum thyroid function assessed [25]. Similarly, all patients should have their medications reviewed to identify use of levothyroxine. If thyroid dysfunction is identified, or if thyroid removal is impending, levothyroxine should be given with the goal of maintaining normal thyroid function. If dysfunction is identified or surgery planned in the first half of pregnancy, maternal serum TSH should be assessed every 3–4 weeks thereafter until 20 weeks gestation. The dose of levothyroxine should be adjusted at each assessment with the goal of maintaining a serum TSH concentration <2.5 mIU/L. For euthyroid patients undergoing thyroidectomy during pregnancy, levothyroxine should be administered postoperatively at the full estimated replacement dose, typically following a weight-based estimation that is approximately 1.7 mcg of levothyroxine per kilogram of body weight. Once initiated, repeat serum TSH concentrations should be assessed in 2–3 weeks and adjusted regularly as stated previously.

In conclusion, the identification of clinically relevant thyroid nodules occurs frequently during pregnancy. Most nodules are asymptomatic and simply detected during a time of increased medical care. Initial evaluation of clinically relevant thyroid nodules identified during pregnancy should not differ from that recommended in a nonpregnant individual, excepting the use of diagnostic molecular tests and the administration of radiopharmaceuticals, such as ^{131}I. Ultrasound and UG-FNA can be safely performed during pregnancy and provide important information regarding overall cancer risk assessment. In contrast, the approach to thyroid surgery during pregnancy is more conservative. Most thyroid nodules with malignant or indeterminate cytology detected during pregnancy will not grow or pose substantial risk to the patient or fetus during a 6–12 month delay in treatment. In contrast, thyroid surgery in a pregnant woman entails increased risks. Therefore, the decision to pursue thyroidectomy must be individualized, weighing the risks and benefits of any intervention against those of conservative monitoring. In rare circumstances, high-risk scenarios necessitate thyroidectomy during pregnancy. When required, thyroid surgery is generally recommended before 24–26 weeks of pregnancy and should be performed by thyroid surgeons with a high degree of experience. Thyroid hormone concentrations should be assessed preoperatively and monitored closely postoperatively, acknowledging the increasing demand for thyroxine that occurs throughout gestation itself. Maternal serum TSH concentrations should be regularly assessed during the first half of pregnancy, with levothyroxine doses adjusted upward to maintain a TSH concentration less than 2.5 mIU/L. In conclusion, through a balanced and informed approach to the clinical care of this unique population, outcomes can be optimized for both the pregnant mother and the developing fetus.

Disclosures Dr. Angell receives research support through a grant provided to the Brigham and Women's Hospital by Veracyte, Inc. Dr. Alexander has served as a consultant to Asuragen, Inc., and Veracyte, Inc.

References

1. Frates MC, Benson CB, Doubilet PM, Kunreuther E, Contreras M, Cibas ES, Orcutt J, Moore FD, Larsen PR, Marqusee E, Alexander EK. Prevalence and distribution of carcinoma in patients with solitary and multiple thyroid nodules on sonography. J Clin Endocrinol Metab. 2006;91(9):3411–7.
2. Burrow GN, Fisher DA, Larsen PR. Maternal and fetal thyroid function. N Engl J Med. 1994;331(16):1072–8.
3. Guth S, Theune U, Aberle J, Galach A, Bamberger CM. Very high prevalence of thyroid nodules detected by high frequency (13 MHz) ultrasound examination. Eur J Clin Invest. 2009;39:699–706.
4. Kwong N, Medici M, Angell TE, Liu X, Marqusee E, Cibas ES, Krane JF, Barletta JA, Kim MI, Reed Larsen P, Alexander EK. The influence of patient age on thyroid nodule formation, multinodularity, and thyroid cancer risk. J Clin Endocrinol Metab. 2015;100:4434–40.
5. Durante C, Costante G, Lucisano G, Bruno R, Meringolo F, Paciaroni A, Puxeddu E, Torlontano M, Tumino S, Attard M, Lamartina L, Nicolucci A, Filetti S. The natural history of benign thyroid nodules. JAMA. 2015;313(9):926–35.
6. Martin JA, Hamilton BE, Osterman MJK, Curtin SC, Mathews TJ. National vital statistics report. Vol 64(1). January 15, 2015. Accessed online at: http://www.cdc.gov/nchs/data/nvsr/nvsr64/nvsr64_01.pdf.
7. Kung AW, Chau MT, Lao TT, Tam SC, Low LC. The effect of pregnancy on thyroid nodule formation. J Clin Endocrinol Metab. 2002;87(3):1010–4.
8. Karger S, Schötz S, Stumvoll M, Berger F, Führer D. Impact of pregnancy on prevalence of goitre and nodular thyroid disease in women living in a region of borderline sufficient iodine supply. Horm Metab Res. 2010;42(2):137–42.
9. Haugen BR, Alexander EK, Bible KC, Doherty G, Mandel SJ, Nikiforov YE, Pacini F, Randolph G, Sawka A, Schlumberger M, Schuff KG, Sherman SI, Sosa JA, Steward D, Tuttle RM, Wartofsky L. 2016 American Thyroid Association Management Guidelines for adult patients with thyroid nodules and differentiated thyroid cancer. Thyroid. 2016;1:1–133. [Epub ahead of print].
10. Moon HJ, Sung JM, Kim EK, Yoon JH, Youk JH, Kwak JY. Diagnostic performance of gray-scale US and elastography in solid thyroid nodules. Radiology. 2012;262:1002–13.
11. Yassa L, Cibas ES, Benson CB, Frates MC, Doubilet PM, Gawande AA, Moore FD, Kim BW, Nose V, Marqusee E, Larsen PR, Alexander EK. Long-term assessment of a multidisciplinary approach to thyroid nodule diagnostic evaluation. Cancer Cytopathology. 2007;111(6):508–16.
12. Crippa S, Mazzucchelli L, Cibas ES, Ali SZ. The Bethesda System for reporting thyroid fine-needle aspiration specimens. Am J Clin Pathol. 2010;134:343–4.
13. Rosen IB, Korman M, Walfish PG. Thyroid nodular disease in pregnancy: current diagnosis and management. Clin Obstet Gynecol. 1997;40:81–9.
14. Moosa M, Mazzaferri EL. Outcome of differentiated thyroid cancer diagnosed in pregnant women. J Clin Endocrinol Metab. 1997;82:2862–6.
15. Messuti I, Corvisieri S, Bardesono F, Rapa I, Giorcelli J, Pellerito R, Volante M, Orlandi F. Impact of pregnancy on prognosis of differentiated thyroid cancer: clinical and molecular features. Eur J Endocrinol. 2014;170:659–66.
16. Vannucchi G, Perrino M, Rossi S, Colombo C, Vicentini L, Dazzi D, Beck-Peccoz P, Fugazzola L. Clinical and molecular features of differentiated thyroid cancer diagnosed during pregnancy. Eur J Endocrinol. 2010;162:145–51.
17. Kuy S, Roman SA, Desai R, Sosa JA. Outcomes following thyroid and parathyroid surgery in pregnant women. Arch Surg. 2009;144(5):399–406.
18. Liu X, Medici M, Kwong N, Angell TE, Marqusee E, Kim MI, Larsen PR, Cho NL, Nehs MA, Ruan DT, Gawande A, Moore Jr F, Barletta J, Krane JF, Cibas ES, Yang T, Alexander EK. Bethesda categorization of thyroid nodule cytology and prediction of thyroid cancer type and prognosis. Thyroid. 2016;26(2):256–61.

19. Beaudenon-Huibregtse S, Alexander EK, Guttler RB, Hershman JM, Babu V, Blevins TC, Moore P, Andruss B, Labourier E. Centralized molecular testing for oncogenic gene mutations complements the local cytopathologic diagnosis of thyroid nodules. Thyroid. 2014;10:1479–87.
20. Alexander EK, Kennedy GC, Baloch ZW, Cibas ES, Chudova D, Diggans J, Friedman L, Kloos RT, LiVolsi VA, Mandel SJ, Raab SS, Rosai J, Steward DL, Walsh PS, Wilde JI, Zeiger MA, Lanman RB, Haugen BR. Preoperative diagnosis of benign thyroid nodules with indeterminate cytology. N Engl J Med. 2012;367:705–15.
21. Nikiforov YE, Ohori NP, Hodak SP, Carty SE, LeBeau SO, Ferris RL, Yip L, Seethala RR, Tublin ME, Stang MT, Coyne C, Johnson JT, Stewart AF, Nikiforova MN. Impact of mutational testing on the diagnosis and management of patients with cytologically indeterminate thyroid nodules: a prospective analysis of 1056 FNA samples. J Clin Endocrinol Metab. 2011;96(11):3390–7.
22. Medici M, Kwong N, Angell TE, Marqusee E, Kim MK, Frates MC, Benson CB, Cibas ES, Barletta JA, Krane JF, Ruan DT, Cho NL, Gawande AA, Moore Jr FD, Alexander EK. The variable phenotype and low-risk nature of RAS-positive thyroid nodules. BMC Med. 2015;13:184–9.
23. Herzon FS, Morris DM, Segal MN, Rauch G, Parnell T. Coexistent thyroid cancer and pregnancy. Arch Otolaryngol Head Neck Surg. 1994;120:1191–3.
24. McLeod DS, Watters KF, Carpenter AD, Ladenson PW, Cooper DS, Ding EL. Thyrotropin and thyroid cancer diagnosis: a systematic review and dose-response meta-analysis. J Clin Endocrinol Metab. 2012;97:2682–92.
25. Stagnaro-Green A, Abalovich M, Alexander EK, Azizi F, Mestman J, Negro R, Nixon A, Pearce EN, Soldin OP, Sullivan S, Wiersinga W. Guidelines of the American Thyroid Association for the diagnosis and management of thyroid disease during pregnancy and postpartum. Thyroid. 2011;21:1081–125.
26. Webb RC, Howard RS, Stojadinovic A, Gaitonde DY, Wallace MK, Ahmed J, Burch HB. The utility of serum thyroglobulin measurement at the time of remnant ablation for predicting disease-free status in patients with differentiated thyroid cancer: a meta-analysis involving 3947 patients. J Clin Endocrinol Metab. 2012;97:2754–63.
27. Latrofa F, Ricci D, Montanelli L, Rocchi R, Piaggi P, Sisti E, Grasso L, Basolo F, Ugolini C, Pinchera A, Vitti P. Lymphocytic thyroiditis on histology correlates with serum thyroglobulin autoantibodies in patients with papillary thyroid carcinoma: impact on detection of serum thyroglobulin. J Clin Endocrinol Metab. 2012;97:2380–7.
28. Alexander EK, Marqusee E, Lawrence J, Jarolim P, Fischer GA, Larsen PR. Timing and magnitude of increases in levothyroxine requirements during pregnancy in women with hypothyroidism. N Eng J Med. 2004;351(3):25–33.

Chapter 19
The Perioperative Management of the Voice and Serum Calcium Levels

David T. Hughes and Paul G. Gauger

There are nearly 100,000 thyroid surgeries each year in the United States. Thyroid surgery performed by experienced surgeons is associated with low complication rates and relatively short recovery period. The most common complications related to thyroidectomy include postoperative bleeding, surgical site infection, hypoparathyroidism, and injury to the recurrent laryngeal nerve and/or external branch of the superior laryngeal nerve. Published rates of complications with thyroid surgery range from <1 to 5 % in most series of high-volume surgical centers. Complications with lasting effects on patient quality of life include nerve injury resulting in voice dysfunction and hypoparathyroidism leading to hypocalcemic symptoms. This chapter discusses the perioperative management of the voice and serum calcium levels after thyroidectomy.

D.T. Hughes, MD (✉)
Division of Endocrine Surgery, Department of Surgery, University of Michigan, Ann Arbor, MI, USA

University of Michigan Hospitals and Health Centers, 2920 Taubman Center, SPC 5331, 1500 East Medical Center Drive, Ann Arbor, MI 48109-5331, USA
e-mail: davhughe@umich.edu

P.G. Gauger, MD
Division of Endocrine Surgery, Department of Surgery, University of Michigan, Ann Arbor, MI, USA

S.A. Roman et al. (eds.), *Management of Thyroid Nodules and Differentiated Thyroid Cancer*, DOI 10.1007/978-3-319-43618-0_19

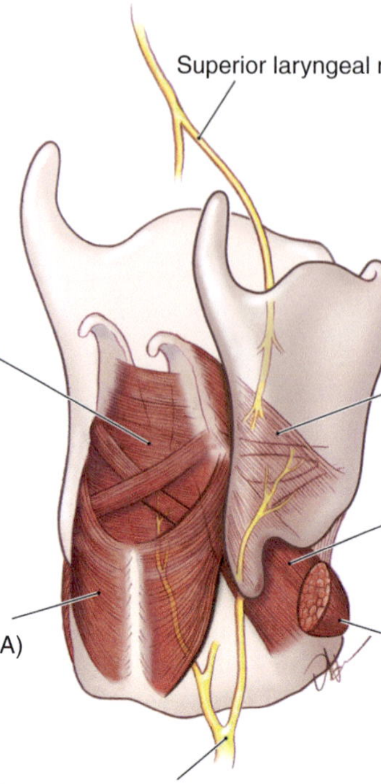

Fig. 19.1 Anatomy of the larynx (Permission granted from *Operative techniques in Laryngology* by Clark A. Rosen and C. Blake Simpson. Published by Springer. See enclosed permission)

Perioperative Management of the Voice in Thyroidectomy

Anatomy

The human voice is produced by movement of exhaled air across the membranous portion of vocal cords leading to wave-generating oscillations which produce sound. The membranous or true vocal folds adduct and abduct to differing degrees and with differing tension to produce various frequencies and intonations of sound. The medial and lateral movement of the vocal folds is produced by the intrinsic laryngeal muscles which are innervated by the recurrent laryngeal nerve (RLN) and the superior laryngeal nerve. The adductor muscles of the vocal folds include the thyroarytenoid, the lateral cricoarytenoid, and the interarytenoid muscles, while the posterior cricoarytenoid muscle provides abduction, all of which are innervated by the RLN through different neurons (Fig. 19.1 – Laryngeal anatomy). The oblique arytenoid muscles act to close the laryngeal inlet during swallowing and also innervated by the RLN, thus explaining association of aspiration with RLN injury. The cricothyroid muscle produces variations in pitch by changing the tension of the true vocal fold and is innervated by the external branch of the superior laryngeal nerve (EBSLN).

Knowledge of the anatomy of the RLN and EBSLN is of upmost importance to avoid injury during thyroid surgery. The vagus nerve exits the cranial cavity via the jugular foramen along with the glossopharyngeal and hypoglossal nerves. It descends in the carotid sheath just deep to and between the internal jugular vein and carotid artery. The right RLN branches from the vagus in the upper mediastinum and recurs around the right subclavian artery before traveling cranially in the tracheoesophageal groove toward its laryngeal insertion. The left RLN branches from the left vagus at the level of the aortic arch and recurs around the ligamentum arteriosum and travels cranially in the tracheoesophageal groove to insert into the larynx (Fig. 19.2 – Anatomy of recurrent laryngeal and superior laryngeal nerves). The cervical portion of the right RLN tends to have a slightly more oblique course from the mediastinum toward the laryngeal insertion point compared to the left RLN which travels more directly in the tracheoesophageal groove posterior to the left thyroid lobe. The RLN inserts into the larynx by passing under the inferior constrictor of the pharynx to innervate the intrinsic laryngeal muscles.

A non-recurrent RLN is an embryological anomaly present in approximately 0.5 % right RLNs and 0.04 % left RLNs. A non-recurrent right RLN is associated with the arteria lusoria vascular abnormality whereby the innominate artery is absent and the right common carotid and right subclavian arteries originate directly from the aortic arch. In this anomaly the right subclavian artery is the most distal branch of the aortic arch and travels in a retroesophageal course. This may be associated with dysphagia due to compression of the posterior esophagus (dysphagia lusoria). A left non-recurrent RLN is a rarer anomaly and is associated with a right-sided aortic arch as seen in situs inversus with displacement of the ligamentum arteriosum to the right side.

Identification of the RLN during thyroidectomy should be considered a necessity in order to prevent injury. The typical diameter of the RLN ranges from 1 to 3 mm. Identification of the RLN inferior to the lower pole of the thyroid gland allows for visualization as dissection progresses from the lower pole toward the tubercle of Zuckerkandl and the ligament of Berry. Large thyroid goiters or those with retrosternal extension can make identification of the RLN difficult, and identification of the nerve from a cranial to caudal direction after ligating the superior pole vessels can be useful. The association of the RLN to the inferior thyroid artery can vary significantly and care should be taken during ligation of the inferior thyroid artery and its braches near the ligament of Berry (Fig. 19.3). The tubercle of Zuckerkandl is a posterior extension of thyroid tissue near the ligament of Berry which often has close association with the RLN, and in cases of enlargement or nodules, the nerve can often course anterior to the tubercle and is prone to injury. The RLN frequently will bifurcate near its insertion point into the larynx into posterior and anterior branches which typically have a sensory and motor function, respectively [1]. Both of these branches need to be fastidiously followed and preserved.

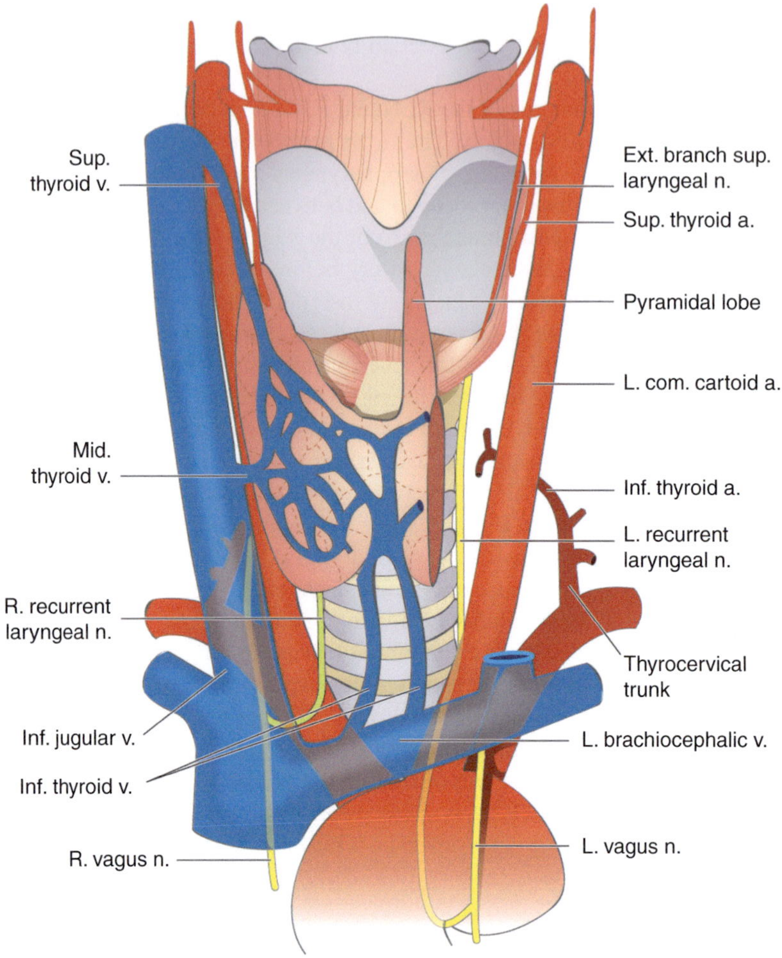

Fig. 19.2 Anatomy of recurrent laryngeal and superior laryngeal nerves (Permission granted from *Color atlas of thyroid surgery* by Yeo-kyu Youn, Kyu Eun Lee and June Young Choi. Published by Springer. See enclosed permission)

Intraoperative Considerations

Operations commonly associated with a risk of RLN injury include thyroidectomy, parathyroidectomy, anterior approach cervical spine procedures, cervical esophageal surgery, and upper mediastinal surgery. Most series of thyroidectomy in high-volume centers report an injury rate ranging from 1 to 5 %; however, RLN injury may be unrecognized in patients with minimal voice changes following surgery, and therefore actual injury rates are likely higher due to under reporting. This is one argument for routine perioperative laryngoscopy.

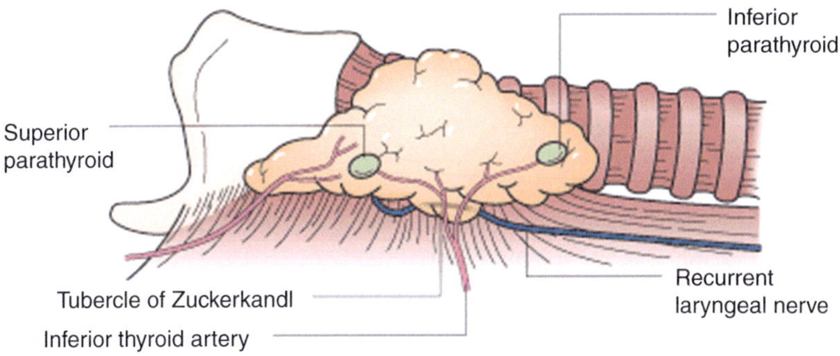

Fig. 19.3 Recurrent laryngeal nerve anatomic association with ligament of Berry (Permission granted from *Greenfield's surgery: scientific principles and practice 5th ed.* See enclosed permission)

Neuropraxia or stretch injuries to the RLN typically occur during dissection in the area of the tubercle of Zuckerkandl and the ligament of Berry near the insertion of the RLN into the larynx. Traction of the RLN due to medial and anterior retraction of the thyroid can occur due to the close association of the inferior thyroid artery and its distal branches to the RLN near the ligament of Berry. Should a neuropraxia occur and an anatomically intact RLN in confirmed, neural function typically will return in a matter of weeks to months after surgery. Intraoperative nerve monitoring can allow for recognition of such an injury manifesting as a loss of RLN function with nerve stimulation proximal to the site of injury whereas without nerve monitoring observation of an anatomically intact nerve would erroneously presume normal nerve function. The decision to proceed with contralateral thyroidectomy in the setting of a neuropraxia injury should be carefully considered, and in some cases a staged procedure which would allow the RLN function to recover can prevent bilateral nerve injury. Continuous vagal nerve stimulation may be useful in detecting real-time impending neuropraxia which is evident as decreasing nerve waveform amplitude and latency and loss of nerve signal [2]. Gentle dissection of the RLN, constant attention to tissue or iatrogenic tension on the nerve, avoidance of cautery or energy devices in close proximity of the nerve, and avoidance of constricting ligatures will avoid traumatic injury in most cases.

Transection of the RLN during thyroidectomy can occur unintentionally or intentionally in the setting of invasive thyroid cancer. Recognized unintentional transection of the RLN without loss of nerve length should be addressed intraoperatively with an attempt at neural repair. Neural repair is performed by adequate mobilization of the distal and proximal segments of the RLN with reanastomosis and epineural repair in an attempt to preserve neural tone. Canine models of recurrent laryngeal transection and reanastamosis report restoration of laryngeal adduction function in around 50 % [3]. A long segment transection which would not allow for direct neural anastomosis has been treated with anastomosis of the distal RLN to the ipsilateral ansa cervicalis nerve with some success [4, 5]. A *preoperative* paralyzed vocal cord associated with malignant infiltration should be sacrificed at the time of surgery in an attempt to achieve an oncologic complete resection since postoperative recovery of function would not be expected. However, in the setting of a normally functioning RLN preoperatively with the discovery of tumor involvement from differentiated thyroid cancer at the time of thyroidectomy, attempts should be made to anatomically preserve the nerve with resection of all gross disease. A grossly negative margin with persistent microscopic disease can often be adequately treated with postoperative therapy with radioiodine, TSH suppression and in some cases external beam radiation therapy. Magnification for sharp neurolysis and separation from the tumor can be very helpful in this situation.

Intraoperative Nerve Monitoring

Intraoperative neural monitoring of the RLN and EBSLN during thyroidectomy can be implemented with severally commercially available nerve monitoring systems. Nerve monitoring involves measurement of vocal cord movement or laryngeal muscle action potentials with either electrodes on the external surface of the endotracheal tube or with needle electrodes implanted intraoperatively into the cricothyroid muscle. Nerve stimulation of the RLN with 0.3–3 mA stimulation current will produce adduction of the true vocal cord and an evoked potential measured by the electrodes. Stimulation of the EBSLN will produce a muscular twitch of the cricothyroid muscle and can variably produce an evoked potential measured by endotracheal tube electrodes. Nerve monitoring can aid in identification of the RLN and EBSLN during thyroidectomy; however, it cannot replace surgical skill and knowledge of normal anatomy and anatomic variants which is required to consistently identify the nerves and preserve vocal cord function. Neuropraxia and subsequent loss of function of the RLN in the setting of an anatomically intact nerve can be accurately determined with intraoperative nerve monitoring. Intraoperative stimulation of the RLN that produces an evoked potential above 200 μV correlates with normal postoperative vocal cord function in nearly 100 % of patients (true negative), while loss of signal intraoperative can be related either to nerve dysfunction to technical failures of the monitoring system commonly due to malposition of the endotracheal monitoring tube, and therefore loss of intraoperative signal correlates with vocal fold paresis in about 72 % of patients [6]. Knowledge of a neuropraxic injury provided by nerve monitoring (after troubleshooting the system of confirm true loss of signal) can be important in intraoperative decision making as to whether to proceed with contralateral thyroidectomy and risk bilateral nerve dysfunction or completing the hemithyroidectomy with plans for completion thyroidectomy after nerve function has recovered [7]. The suspected pathology (i.e., benign vs. malignant) is important in this decision making.

Multiple studies and meta-analyses have shown no difference in nerve injury rates with intraoperative neural monitoring; however, it may improve recognition of nerve injury with subsequent change in intraoperative management and decision making as discussed previously [8–12]. Most advocates also suggest the technology that allows the operation to move forward more confidently and expeditiously as well as being a valuable teaching aid. The use of nerve monitoring can be especially helpful in reoperative thyroid procedures given the increased risk of nerve injury and the altered anatomic planes present in reoperative cases.

Diagnosis of Nerve Dysfunction

Unilateral RLN dysfunction generally presents as hoarseness (dysphonia) with a weak and "breathy" voice. This is often accompanied with patient complaints of running out of air during speech due to lack of complete adduction of the vocal folds during phonation. The cough has a "bovine" quality without a sharp percussive initiation since the vocal cords cannot tightly approximate. Aspiration most commonly with drinking of liquids is also common especially in the acute phase of unilateral vocal cord dysfunction or in older patients. The contralateral vocal cord compensation in its degree of adduction can often result in a nearly normal voice despite unilateral RLN palsy, and therefore the reliance of symptoms and subjective voice quality alone can often be inaccurate in elucidating nerve function. Other etiologies of dysphonia with normal nerve function including viral illnesses, reflux pharyngitis, laryngeal polyps or cancer, and voice overuse should be considered in cases of confirmed of normal vocal fold movement on laryngoscopy.

There are three primary modalities for visual inspection of the vocal cords: direct laryngoscopy, indirect mirror laryngoscopy, and flexible laryngoscopy. Direct laryngoscopy typically requires general anesthesia but can be combined with rigid scopes for interventional purposes to treat cord pathology. Indirect mirror laryngoscopy can visualize the larynx in about 50 % of patients using a dental mirror, flashlight, and anterior retraction of the tongue. Flexible laryngoscopy, either with or without video, provides consistent and complete visualization of the vocal cords without need for sedation, but with the added cost of equipment. Flexible nasolaryngoscopy is easily taught and can be accomplished in the office setting with nasal application of aerosolized topical anesthetic often combined with oxymetazoline or phenylephrine for their vasoconstrictive properties.

The typical findings on laryngoscopy in unilateral RLN paralysis include a true vocal fold in the paramedian position with anterior displacement of the arytenoid cartilage and lack of movement with vocalization (Fig. 19.4 – Flexible laryngoscopy). EBSLN dysfunction results in some bowing of the involved true vocal fold with loss of tension and is somewhat more difficult to elucidate. Bilateral RLN paralysis will result in medialization of both the right and the left true vocal folds with a narrow orifice between the immobile cords, leading to stridor and airway compromise in some patients.

Stroboscopy (phonoscopy) is a visualization of the vocal cords during vibration and may increase the diagnostic sensitivity of laryngoscopy especially in the evaluation of EBSLN injury. During stroboscopy light flashes just below or above the frequency at which the object is vibrating, therefore making the object appear at a standstill or as if it is vibrating in slow motion. High-speed digital recordings have

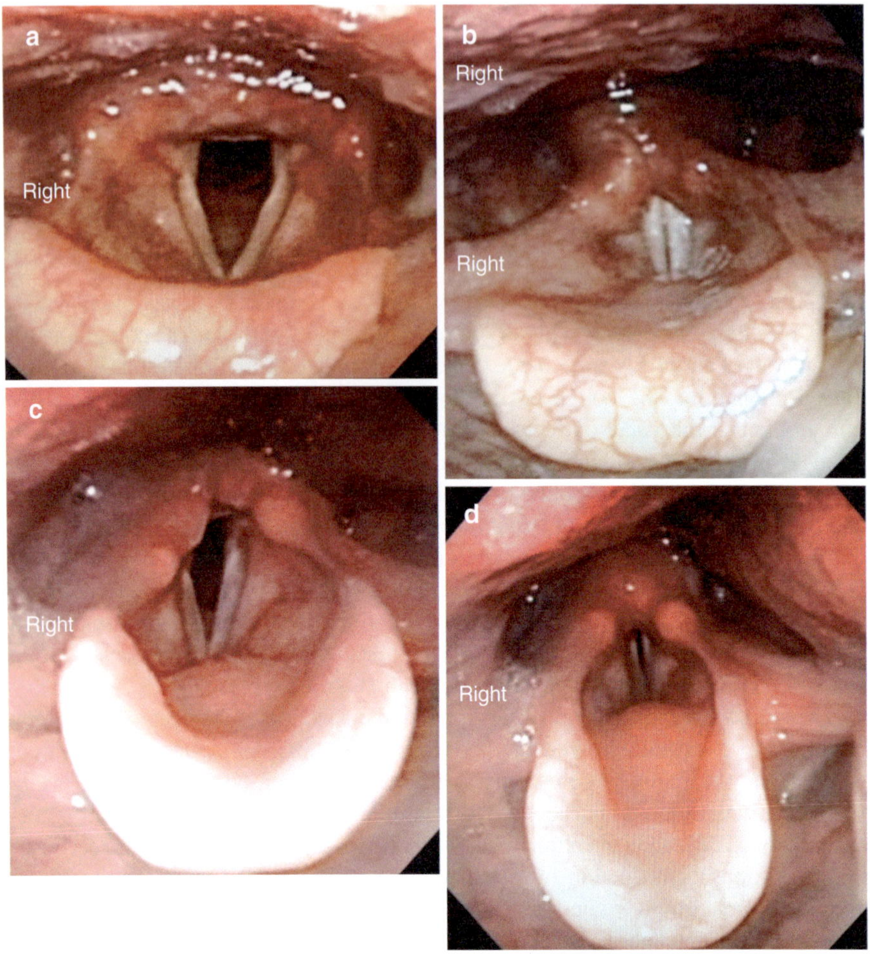

Fig. 19.4 Flexible laryngoscopy demonstrating normal vocal cord positioning (**a**, **b**) and paralyzed right vocal cord (**c**, **d**) with quite respiration (**a**, **c**) and phonation (**b**, **d**). Note the paramedian position of the paralyzed right vocal cord, the anterior positioned arytenoid, the shortened vocal cord, and the glottic gap with right recurrent laryngeal nerve paralysis. (**a**). Normal with respiration. (**b**) Normal with phonation. (**c**) Right RLN paralysis with respiration. (**d**) Right RLN paralysis with phonation

increased the capability of stroboscopy to allow for diagnostic analysis. In cases of EBSLN injury, the affected true vocal cord appears flaccid, bowed, and shortened compared to the functional contralateral cord.

Transcutaneous laryngeal ultrasound has recently been described as an additional modality useful in assessing vocal cord function. Using a linear ultrasound probe similar to that used for thyroid ultrasound, but at lower frequency (8–10 mHz) and increased gain settings, the true and false vocal cords can be visualized in static and active motion with ultrasound (Fig. 19.5 – Transcutaneous laryngeal ultrasound). Visualization of the TVC's is necessary to judge vocal fold movement appropriately. The sensitivity of ultrasound is notably lower than laryngoscopy and is unlikely to replace laryngoscopy; however, ultrasound may be a useful, non-invasive method of screening for RLN function in the perioperative period for thyroidectomy patients [13, 14].

Preoperative confirmation of vocal cord function can be applied on a routine or on a case-by-case basis. Patients with evident preoperative voice dysfunction, a risk of invasive thyroid malignancy or a past history of neck surgery, where the RLN was at risk for injury are situations where preoperative vocal cord assessment can be especially useful. Generally, patient reported voice complaints have a poor predictive value for nerve dysfunction, whereas experienced surgeons documenting voice abnormalities may be more specific as a screening method for selecting patients for laryngoscopic examination [15].

Treatment of Vocal Cord Dysfunction

Treatment modalities for vocal cord dysfunction related to RLN or EBSLN injury include voice therapy and operative treatments. Voice therapy is typically provided by speech language pathologists and includes interventions that help with pitch alteration, increasing breath support and loudness, and techniques finding the correct head and neck position for optimal voice production such as turning head to one side or manipulating the thyroid cartilage. Voice therapy can be especially useful in the immediate postoperative period in cases of neuropraxia and allow time for spontaneous recovery of the injured nerve. In patients who have not achieved acceptable voice quality with speech therapy and have persistent vocal cord paralysis after an appropriate period of time to allow for recovery of neuropraxia (typically 6 months), an operative approach can be considered. Swallowing therapy may also be necessary if the tendency for aspiration is apparent.

Operative treatment options for vocal cord paralysis include injection laryngoplasty and laryngeal framework surgery. The primary goal of these treatments is to correct the phonatory gap between the paramedian paralyzed vocal cord and the contralateral functioning vocal cord. Medialization of the paralyzed cord to a near median position can improve the phonatory gap and help produce more normal voice and can improve aspiration due to laryngeal incompetence. Thyroplasty (injection laryngoplasty) is an injection of material laterally into the vocal fold which acts to displace the cord medially thus improving the glottic gap during phonation (Fig. 19.6). Injection materials can be temporary (hyaluronic acid, acellular human cadaveric dermis, gelfoam, and collagen) or permanent (calcium hydroxyapatite, fat, Teflon). Injection laryngoplasty can often be accomplished with local anesthesia and a flexible laryngoscope in a clinical office setting. Medialization thyroplasty (laryngeal framework surgery) involves operative placement of a Silastic or Gore-tex implant lateral to the vocal fold via a window cut in

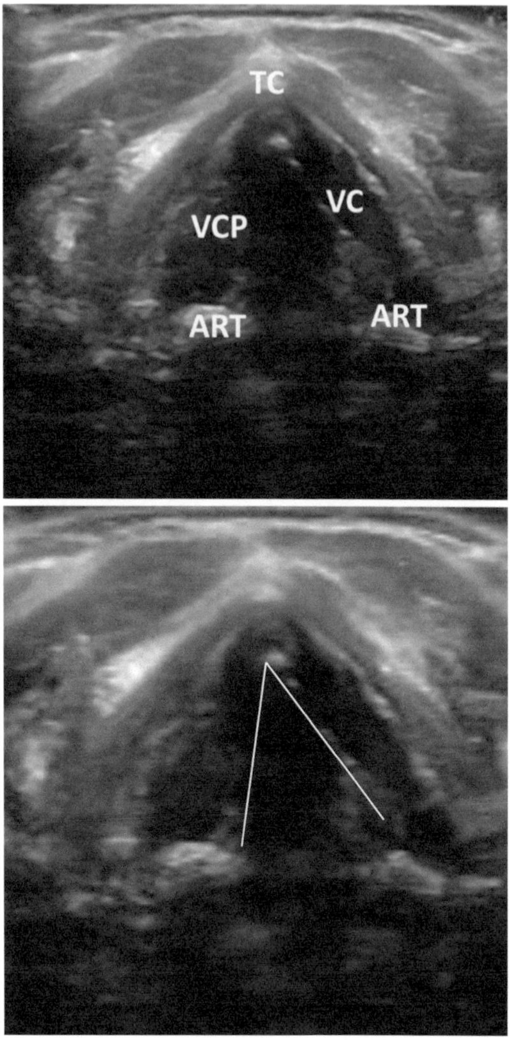

Fig. 19.5 Transcutaneous laryngeal ultrasound. Right vocal cord paralysis during respiration with paramedian location of the right true vocal fold. *TC* thyroid cartilage, *VC* vocal cord, *ART* arytenoid, *VCP* vocal cord paresis (Permission granted from Carneiro-Pla et al. [14]. See enclosed permission from Elsevier)

the thyroid cartilage (Fig. 19.7). This acts to displace the paralyzed vocal fold medially, ensuring adequate glottic closure. Some will add medialization and anterior rotation of the ipsilateral arytenoid to address the vocal cord gap at the posterior aspect of the vocal cords. Thyroplasty procedures result in a vocal cord in the medial position with improved vocal cord length which then generates a more normal voice. Thyroplasty should not be considered until surgical treatment of the thyroid pathology is complete (i.e., not before completion thyroidectomy if that is necessary).

In cases of bilateral vocal cord paralysis, the primary problem to address is the small airway opening between the bilateral paramedian paralyzed vocal cords. Tracheostomy should be considered the standard of care, especially in the early postoperative period,

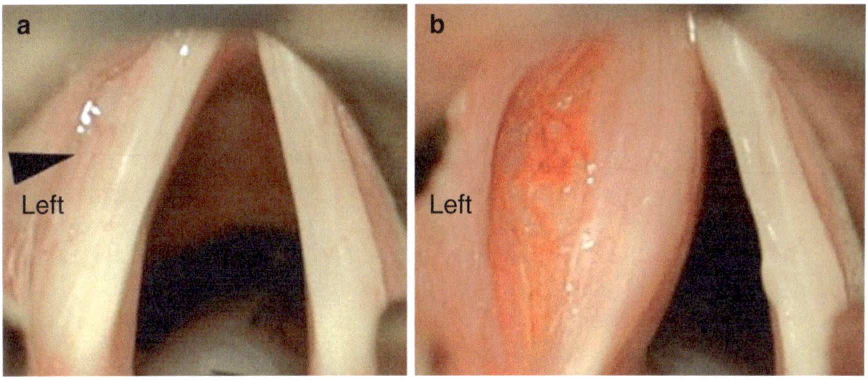

Fig. 19.6 Injection thyroplasty (**a**) *Arrowhead* indicates paralyzed left vocal cord with bowed appearance. (**b**). After injection thyroplasty the paralyzed cord has a more medial location to allow for improved glottic closure with phonation

Fig. 19.7 Type 1 thyroplasty – A right-sided thyroplasty implant with medialization of the right vocal fold

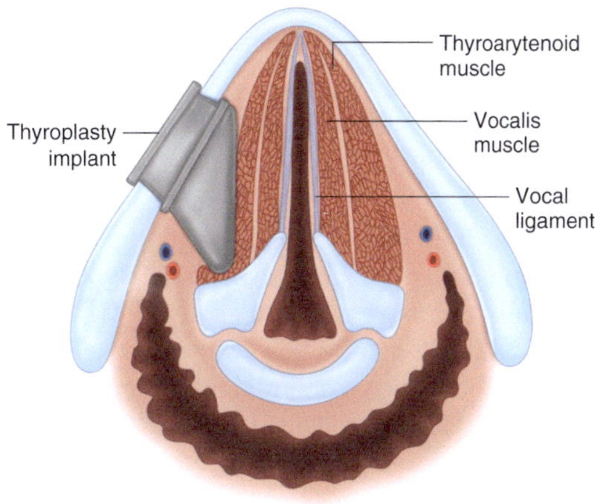

as many nerve injuries which are neuropraxic in nature will recover over time, and patients will recover normal cord function and eventually be able to be decannulated. For patients with persistent bilateral vocal cord paralysis with persistent stridor, operative intervention directed at the airway obstruction should be considered. Cordotomy involves incising the paralyzed vocal cord with a transverse, curvilinear incision resulting in traction away from the arytenoid process resulting in enlargement of the airway through tissue retraction. Cordotomy should aim to provide both respiratory and phonatory function with a goal of tracheostomy tube decannulation with some level of preserved phonatory function. Cordotomy can be used in the acute nerve injury setting as no significant vocal cord tissue is removed.

Thyroidectomy in experienced hands is a safe procedure with low rates of RLN or EBSLN injuries; however, when injuries do occur, optimal treatment requires a multidisciplinary approach for improved outcomes.

Calcium Management After Thyroid Surgery

Postoperative hypoparathyroidism occurs transiently in 10–40 % of patients after bilateral thyroid surgery and, however, is permanent in only around 1–3 % [16]. The true incidence of hypoparathyroidism following thyroid surgery is difficult to clearly define, and the definition of hypoparathyroidism varies in the literature: the presence of hypocalcemic symptoms, biochemical evidence of hypoparathyroidism (low calcium with/without low parathyroid hormone [PTH]), and need for calcium and/or vitamin D supplementation. Recommendations for increased calcium intake for osteoporosis prevention also complicate this definition. Preservation of viable parathyroid tissue during total thyroidectomy or completion thyroidectomy after prior hemithyroidectomy can prevent postoperative hypoparathyroidism. Inadvertent damage to the blood supply to parathyroids causing ischemia or inadvertent removal of parathyroids can lead to low levels of parathyroid hormone (PTH) postoperatively and subsequent lead to hypocalcemic symptoms. The incidence of hypoparathyroidism is influenced by patient factors, disease states, and surgical technique.

Hypocalcemia and Associated Abnormalities

Hypocalcemia is biochemically defined as a serum or ionized calcium level below the lower limit of the normal range (typically <8.5 mg/dL for serum calcium and <1.1 mmol/L for ionized calcium). Hypocalcemia after bilateral thyroidectomy generally occurs when postoperative PTH levels fall into the low or below normal range of 12–65 pg/mL; however, hypocalcemia often presents in a delayed fashion 12–72 h following parathyroid insult during surgery. The very short half-life of PTH (3–5 min) allows for detection of low PTH levels immediately following surgery which has led some groups to routinely check PTH levels in the immediate postoperative period in order to determine risk of hypocalcemia and therefore modify postoperative calcium and vitamin D supplementation, as discussed in detail later [17, 18]. Serum calcium levels are influenced by protein binding and therefore corrected calcium levels can be significantly higher in cases of hypoalbuminemia (Corrected calcium = [0.8 × (normal albumin-patient's albumin {g/dL})] + serum calcium level (mg/dL)). Ionized calcium is not protein bound and therefore is unaffected by serum protein levels.

Symptoms of hypocalcemia typically occur with serum and ionized calcium levels below the normal range; however, individual patients may have varying degrees of symptoms or even lack of symptoms across the range of calcium levels. Symptoms of hypocalcemia generally begin with neuromuscular irritability causing numbness and tingling (paresthesias) of the perioral area and the hands and, occasionally, feet. Neuropsychiatric symptoms often include fatigue, hyperirritability, anxiety, and depression and are often difficult to define in the acute postoperative setting. In severe cases of hypocalcemia (typically serum calcium <7.0 mg/dL or ionized calcium <0.8 mmol/L), carpopedal spasms, muscle tetany, laryngospasm, and focal or generalized seizures can occur. Cardiac dysrhythmias such as torsades de pointes can result from QT interval prolongation. Two traditional provocative tests for hypocalcemia include Chvostek's sign, contraction of the facial muscles by tapping on the facial nerve anterior to the ear, and Trousseau's sign, carpopedal spasms induced by ischemia from inflation of a blood pressure cuff on the upper arm. Most mild symptoms of hypocalcemia can be managed with oral regimens of calcium either with or without additional vitamin D supplementation, though most available supplements have both. Progressive symptoms from paresthesias to tetany which do not respond to oral calcium and vitamin D supplementation require hospitalization for parenteral calcium administration often in a semi-emergent manner.

Hypocalcemia due to hypoparathyroidism results in associated electrolyte abnormalities including hyperphosphatemia and in some cases hypomagnesemia. Hyperphosphatemia will generally resolve with correction of calcium levels in patients with intact renal function. Hypomagnesemia can cause refractory hypocalcemia due to induction of PTH resistance and should be treated with magnesium replacement along with calcium supplementation. Magnesium replacement acts to rapidly correct both hypocalcemia and can lead to an increase in PTH suggesting that magnesium may affect the release of PTH. Treatment of hypomagnesemia is often a key factor in improving severe postoperative hypocalcemia.

Preoperative Considerations

Patient factors including Graves' disease, Hashimoto's thyroiditis, history of gastric bypass surgery, childhood age, pregnancy, lactation, and remedial surgery are associated with an increased risk of postoperative hypoparathyroidism [19]. If these risk factors are multiple, they can be additive. The hyperthyroidism associated with Graves' disease can increase bone turnover which then can result in hungry bone syndrome similar to that seen after parathyroidectomy for secondary hyperparathyroidism. Hashimoto's thyroiditis is often associated with reactive central neck lymphadenopathy which can make identification and preservation of parathyroid tissue more difficult during surgery thereby increasing the risk of postoperative hypoparathyroidism. Addition of central neck dissection also may increase the risk of hypoparathyroidism due to increased manipulation and in some cases reimplantation of the inferior parathyroid glands required after lymphadenectomy [20]. Childhood age, pregnancy, and lactation may increase calcium turnover and calcium demand leading to increased rates of hypocalcemia following thyroidectomy. Reoperative central neck surgery for recurrent thyroid goiter or for recurrent thyroid cancer can make identification of parathyroid tissue difficult while prior surgery may have injured the parathyroids.

There is conflicting data about the influence of preoperative vitamin D deficiency on postoperative hypoparathyroidism. While some retrospective single-center studies have shown no increased rates of post-thyroidectomy hypocalcemia [21, 22], other studies have demonstrated significantly higher rates of hypocalcemia when preoperative serum 25-hydroxyvitamin D levels were deficient (<25 nmol/L) [23–25]. Replacement therapy for recognized vitamin D deficiency prior to thyroidectomy seems reasonable given its low risk to possible benefit profile. Cholecalciferol (D3) seems to be slightly more effective than ergocalciferol (D2) in increasing serum 25-hydroxyvitamin D levels [26]. Vitamin D deficiency can be corrected with 8–12 week cholecalciferol regimens of 1000–2000 IU/day for 25-hydroxyvitamin D levels of 12–30 or 30,000–50,000 IU/week for levels <12, but treatment should not necessarily delay surgery.

Intraoperative Considerations

Identification of parathyroid glands and their vascular supply during thyroidectomy is important to the preservation of postoperative parathyroid function. The superior parathyroid glands are derived from the fourth branchial pouches and during normal fetal development descend posterior to the upper thyroid pole before coming to rest just above the inferior thyroidal artery, posterior, and lateral to the RLN. The inferior parathyroid glands derive from the third branchial pouches and descend to a final destination near the lower pole of the thyroid gland in close association with the thyrothymic tract and can sometimes descend into the superior mediastinum. The symmetry of superior parathyroid gland location is approximately 80 % while the inferior parathyroid glands share a common contralateral location in about 70 % of cases. Both the superior and inferior parathyroid glands typically derive their vascular supply from branches of the inferior thyroid artery and care should be taken to avoid proximal ligation of the artery during thyroidectomy so as to prevent parathyroid ischemia. Superior parathyroid glands may have some contribution of blood flow from the superior thyroid artery distribution as well. Capsular dissection during thyroidectomy can help avoid injury to the parathyroids and in some cases will act to preserve small pedicle blood vessels that course along the thyroid capsule. Ectopic parathyroid glands are typically not encountered during routine thyroidectomy except in the case of intrathyroidal parathyroid glands which are often identified by the pathologist during specimen exam.

Autotransplantation of devascularized or inadvertently removed parathyroid glands during thyroidectomy is a well-described technique which is intended to preserve parathyroid function. While the overall rates of viability of reimplanted parathyroid tissue are poorly understood, reimplanted tissue can regain the ability to produce PTH when adequately revascularized. Parathyroid glands that appear pale or dark after thyroidectomy may be ischemic and should be examined closely for an intact vascular pedicle and if not intact these parathyroid glands should be reimplanted. If the gland is swollen and dark, this may be from venous congestion which can improve once the capsule is sharply incised. The techniques for implantation vary. One technique involves mincing the parathyroid into <1 mm-sized pieces and then implanting these into a well-vascularized muscle belly such as the sternocleidomastoid, strap, pectoralis, or brachioradialis. Another technique involves morcellation of the parathyroid tissue in saline solution followed by injection of the suspension into well-vascularized muscle belly. Morphologically normal parathyroid glands can be reimplanted into any easily accessible, well-vascularized muscle, typically through the thyroidectomy incision, whereby adenomatous or hyperplastic parathyroid glands should be reimplanted into more easily accessible muscles, such as the brachioradialis or pectoralis muscle in case of a need for reresection at a later date. Higher rates of *temporary* hypoparathyroidism may occur when increasing numbers of parathyroid glands are reimplanted in a single patient; however, the benefit of reimplantation may be to decrease risk of *permanent* hypoparathyroidism, and therefore there seems to be a long-term benefit despite a short-term increased incidence of hypocalcemia [27]. Patients requiring more than two autotransplanted parathyroid glands may be considered for higher doses of calcium and/or vitamin D supplementation after surgery due to this increased risk of transient hypocalcemia. There are no good data about how frequently autotransplanted parathyroid glands are functionally viable; therefore, every attempt should be made to preserve viable parathyroid tissue in situ during thyroidectomy.

Postoperative Considerations

Monitoring for hypocalcemia following thyroidectomy takes on various forms from simple symptom recognition, to defined treatment algorithms of calcium and vitamin D supplementation based on postoperative calcium and PTH levels. Generally the nadir of calcium levels following bilateral thyroidectomy occurs 12–36 h following surgery which means many patients have onset of symptoms after being discharged from the hospital. Management of temporary hypoparathyroidism with calcium and vitamin D supplementation includes two broad categories: universal supplementation and defined supplementation based on calcium and/or PTH levels. The general goal of supplementation is to avoid symptoms during the period of transient parathyroid function which typically occurs during the first few weeks after thyroidectomy. Because most hypocalcemic symptoms can be adequately addressed with enough calcium and vitamin D intake the overall goal of supplementation is to maintain eucalcemia while avoiding hypocalcemia and hypercalcemia.

Calcium and Vitamin D Supplementation

The prophylaxis and treatment for postoperative hypocalcemia due to hypoparathyroidism center on adequate calcium administration, enteral absorption, and mobilization of bone calcium. Options for calcium supplementation include various forms of calcium with or without vitamin D. The side effects of higher doses of calcium supplementation can include constipation, abdominal bloating, nausea, and in some cases hypercalcemia due to over-supplementation causing symptoms of excessive thirst and urination, muscle pain, arrhythmias, and fatigue. Thyroid hormone absorption can be hindered when taken with calcium, and therefore thyroid hormone should be taken separately from calcium on an empty stomach. Calcium supplements often report the amount of total calcium and elemental calcium which varies based on the preparation. Elemental calcium is the calcium available for absorption, and in the case of calcium carbonate, 40 % is elemental calcium; therefore, 600 mg of calcium carbonate provides 240 mg of elemental calcium; calcium citrate is 20 % elemental calcium and 600 mg will provide 120 mg of elemental calcium. Calcium and vitamin D supplementation comes in a variety of regimens:

Calcium carbonate (os-Cal, Tums): It contains 40 % elemental calcium, is readily available over the counter in many forms, and is the least expensive. Calcium carbonate may be more constipating than other forms of calcium. Is better absorbed with food and in cases of lower gastric acid may be poorly absorbed. Dosing ranges from 100 to 3000 mg daily.

Calcium citrate (Citracal): It contains 20 % elemental calcium, is readily available over the counter in many forms, and is generally slightly more expensive than calcium carbonate. Calcium citrate is equally well absorbed with or without food and may be better absorbed in those with low gastric acidity, such as those taking proton-pump inhibitors or postgastric bypass patients. Dosing ranges from 1000 to 3000 mg daily.

Calcium gluconate (intravenous): In cases of hypocalcemia not responsive to oral supplementation, parenteral infusion of calcium gluconate rapidly corrects hypocalcemia and alleviates its associated symptoms. Calcium chloride is not recommended as an infusion through peripheral lines given the risk of tissue necrosis with infiltrated IV's. Calcium gluconate contains 9 % elemental calcium and dosing ranges from 1 to 2 g generally administered in 50 mL of 5 % dextrose solution infused over 20 min. Calcium gluconate continuous infusions can be used in conjunction with oral regimens and be titrated based on serum calcium levels until adequate amounts of calcium can be taken orally.

Vitamin D3 (cholecalciferol): Vitamin D3 supplementation can be used to improve absorption of calcium either as an additive to calcium or as cholecalciferol alone. Patients with vitamin D deficiency should be treated with adequate amounts of vitamin D3 (generally 1000–2000 IU/day or 50,000 IU/week for 8–12 weeks) either prior to thyroidectomy or postoperatively. Dosing ranges from 200 to 400 IU per dose when combined with calcium supplementation to 1000–200,000 IU when used as cholecalciferol alone. Ergocalciferol (vitamin D2) is available in similar dosing ranges; however, some studies have demonstrated inferiority of this preparation in maintaining serum 25-hydroxyvitamin D levels compared to cholecalciferol [26, 28].

Calcitriol (1,25-dihyroxycholecalciferol): Calcitriol is the hormonally active metabolite of vitamin D and acts to increase the uptake of calcium from the gut, increase the renal tubular reabsorption of calcium, and possibly increase the release of calcium from the bones through osteoclas t activation. Significant hypercalcemia can occur when combining higher doses of calcium with calcitriol in the setting of transient postoperative hypoparathyroidism. However, because of calcitriol's relatively short half-life of 5–8 h, its effects can be reversed in a few days after discontinuation. Calcitriol's effect on serum calcium can be delayed after first administration up to 72 h and in some cases a loading dose of 1–2 μg are employed. Dosing ranges from 0.25 to 2 μg daily in single or divided doses. Calcitriol is available in oral or intravenous forms.

Routine Calcium and Vitamin D Supplementation

Administration of calcium with or without vitamin D3 or calcitriol on a routine basis for all patients following bilateral thyroidectomy aims to avoid hypocalcemia and its associated symptoms during the period of transient hypoparathyroidism. As the initial ischemic insult to the parathyroid glands resolves, typically over the first few weeks, the supplementation regimen is weaned. Advantages to routine supplementation include that is generally cost-effective, it avoids symptoms in most patients and is easy to use without a need for PTH determination in the early postoperative period. The disadvantages include a relatively low risk of hypercalcemia seen with use of calcium and higher doses of calcitriol and the side effects of calcium doses including most commonly the gastrointestinal complaints of constipation and nausea. Arguments that permissive hypocalcemia during the period of transient hypoparathyroidism will stimulate parathyroid tissue recovery are speculative, and there are no data to support this; therefore there appears to be no risk of routine supplementation on parathyroid recovery.

Hypocalcemia Treatment Algorithms

As an alternative to routine supplementation following bilateral thyroidectomy, several groups have proposed algorithms based on postoperative calcium and PTH levels in the immediate postoperative period to guide appropriate supplementation. In general these studies have demonstrated that PTH levels in the immediately post-thyroidectomy period less than 10–15 pg/mL are predictive of hypocalcemia and thus indicate a need for supplementation [17, 18, 29, 30] (Fig. 19.8). The advantages of these algorithms are a more specific application of supplementation to only those patients at risk for hypocalcemia as well as an ability to titrate the dose of calcium and calcitriol to avoid hypocalcemic symptoms in those with the lowest PTH levels and therefore the highest risk of developing hypocalcemia.

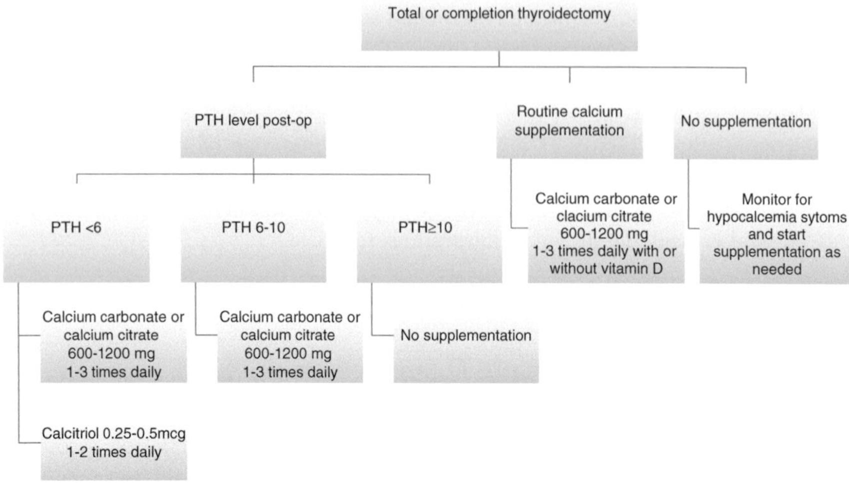

Fig. 19.8 Algorythim for post-operative calcium management after thyroidectomy

Management of Permanent Hypoparathyroidism

The definition of permanent hypoparathyroidism is the continued requirement of calcium supplementation to maintain serum calcium levels in the setting of low parathyroid hormone levels more than 6–12 months following thyroid surgery. Rates of permanent hypoparathyroidism remain low at around 1–3 % of patients after bilateral thyroidectomy even with the relatively high frequency of temporary hypoparathyroidism of 20–40 % [16]. This suggests that despite the frequent transient dysfunction of parathyroids following surgery, parathyroid functionality is rather resilient in the face of surgical trauma. The goal of treatment for permanent hypoparathyroidism is to prevent symptoms of hypocalcemia while avoiding the complications of over-supplementation including hypercalcemic symptoms, nephrolithiasis related to hypercalciuria, and heterotopic tissue calcification. The goal serum calcium levels should range in the low normal to slightly below normal range, typically 8–8.5 mg/dL. Some have suggested a goal 24-h urine calcium excretion <7.5 mmol/day and a calcium-phosphorus product <55 mg^2/dL^2 [31]. Avoidance of hypocalcemia symptoms requires calcium supplementation in the form of calcium carbonate or calcium citrate in doses to administer 1000–2000 mg of elemental calcium daily in addition to that taken in through the diet. Calcitriol 0.25–2 μg daily or in twice daily divided doses allows for a decrease in the amount of elemental calcium required to maintain adequate serum calcium levels and is required in most patients with permanent hypoparathyroidism. Hydrochlorothiazide 12.5–50 mg daily can be used to control hypercalciuria by enhancing renal tubular calcium reabsorption and is also effective at reducing daily elemental calcium requirements. In cases of hyperphosphatemia not well controlled with adequate calcium supplementation and correction of hypocalcemia, intestinal phosphate binders may prove useful.

Injectable recombinant PTH 1–84 may be useful in patients who cannot maintain stable calcium and urinary calcium levels with standard therapy with calcium, calcitriol, and hydrochlorothiazide. Recombinant PTH is given once daily as subcutaneous injection with close monitoring and adjustment of oral calcium, and vitamin D dosing is effective in reducing oral supplementation requirements, decreasing urinary calcium and serum phosphate levels, and may improve bone metabolism [32]. Recombinant PTH 1–84 (Natpara®) is currently only recommended for those patients not well controlled on calcium and vitamin D supplementation alone with dosing recommendation of 25–100 μg injection daily with close monitoring of calcium levels after starting the drug.

Patients managed for long-term hypoparathyroidism should be followed closely as acute events such as gastroenteritis, altered volume status, and pregnancy can disrupt calcium levels despite a stable regimen. Associated abnormalities including nephrolithiasis, tissue or organ calcification, and defects in bone metabolism should be considered during follow-up.

Complications with thyroidectomy are infrequent and center on the effects of injury to the recurrent laryngeal nerve and the parathyroid glands. Transient complications related to neuropraxia or temporary hypoparathyroidism effect around 5 % and 30 % of patients, respectively, while lasting effects occur in only around 2 % of patients. Avoidance of voice and parathyroid dysfunction with thyroidectomy is significantly influenced by surgeon expertise, patient factors, and thyroid disease states.

References

1. Kandil E, Abdelghani S, Friedlander P, Alrasheedi S, Tufano RP, Bellows CF, Slakey D. Motor and sensory branching of the recurrent laryngeal nerve in thyroid surgery. Surgery. 2011;150:1222–7.
2. Phelan E, Schneider R, Lorenz K, Dralle H, Kamani D, Potenza A, Sritharan N, Shin J, Randolph G. Continuous vagal IONM prevents recurrent laryngeal nerve paralysis by revealing initial EMG changes of impending neuropraxic injury: a prospective, multicenter study. Laryngoscope. 2014;124:1498–505.
3. Paniello RC, Rich JT, Debnath NL. Laryngeal adductor function in experimental models of recurrent laryngeal nerve injury. Laryngoscope. 2015;125:E67–72.
4. Li M, Chen S, Wang W, Chen D, Zhu M, Liu F, Zhang C, Li Y, Zheng H. Effect of duration of denervation on outcomes of ansa-recurrent laryngeal nerve reinnervation. Laryngoscope. 2014;124:1900–5.
5. Wang W, Chen D, Chen S, Li D, Li M, Xia S, Zheng H. Laryngeal reinnervation using ansa cervicalis for thyroid surgery-related unilateral vocal fold paralysis: a long-term outcome analysis of 237 cases. PLoS One. 2011;6:e19128.
6. Genther DJ, Kandil EH, Noureldine SI, Tufano RP. Correlation of final evoked potential amplitudes on intraoperative electromyography of the recurrent laryngeal nerve with immediate post-operative focal fold function after thyroid and parathyroid surgery. JAMA Otolaryngol Head Neck Surg. 2014;140:124–8.
7. Fontenot TE, Randolph GW, Setton TE, Alsaleh N, Kandil E. Does intraoperative nerve monitoring reliably aid in staging of total thyroidectomies? Laryngoscope. 2015;125(9):2232–5.

8. Higgins TS, Gupta R, Ketcham AS, Sataloff RT, Wadsworth JT, Sinacori JT. Recurrent laryngeal nerve monitoring versus identification alone on post-thyroidectomy true vocal fold palsy: a meta-analysis. Laryngoscope. 2011;121:1009–17.
9. Pisanu A, Porceddu G, Podda M, Cois A, Uccheddu A. System review with meta-analysis of studies comparing intraoperative neuromonitoring of recurrent laryngeal nerves versus visualization alone during thyroidectomy. J Surg Res. 2014;188:152–61.
10. Sari S, Erbil Y, Sumer A, Agcaoglu O, Bayraktar A, Issever H, Ozarmagan S. Evaluation of recurrent laryngeal nerve monitoring in thyroid surgery. Int J Surg. 2010;8:474–8.
11. Barczynski M, Konturek A, Cichon S. Randomized clinical trial of visualization versus neuromonitoring of recurrent laryngeal nerves during thyroidectomy. Br J Surg. 2009;96:240–6.
12. Dionigi G, Boni L, Rovera F, Bacuzzi A, Dionigi R. Neuromonitoring and video-assisted thyroidectomy: a prospective randomized case–control evaluation. Surg Endosc. 2009;23:996–1003.
13. Wong KP, Lang BH, Ng SH, Cheung CY, Chan CT, Lo CY. A prospective, assessor-blind evaluation of surgeon-performed transcutaneous laryngeal ultrasonography in vocal cord examination before and after thyroidectomy. Surgery. 2013;154:1158–64.
14. Carneiro-Pla D, Miller BS, Wilhelm SM, Milas M, Gauger PG, Cohen MS, Hughes DT, Solorzano CC. Feasibility of surgeon-performed transcutaneous vocal cord ultrasonography in identifying vocal cord mobility: a multi-institutional experience. Surgery. 2014;156:1597–602.
15. Lee CY, Long KL, Eldridge RJ, Davenport DL, Sloan DA. Preoperative laryngoscopy in thyroid surgery: do patients' subjective voice complaints matter? Surgery. 2014;156:1477–82.
16. Reeve T, Thompson NW. Complications of thyroid surgery: how to avoid them, how to manage them, and their possible effect on the whole patient. World J Surg. 2000;24:971–5.
17. Selberherr A, Scheuba C, Riss P, Niederle B. Postoperative hypoparathyroidism after thyroidectomy: efficient and cost-effective diagnosis and treatment. Surgery. 2015;157:349–53.
18. Cayo AK, Yen TW, Misustin SM, Wall K, Wilson SD, Evans DB, Wang TS. Predicting the need for calcium and calcitriol supplementation after total thyroidectomy: results of a prospective, randomized study. Surgery. 2012;152:1059–67.
19. Mckenzie TJ, Chen Y, Hodin RA, et al. Recalcitrant hypocalcemia after thyroidectomy in patients with previous Roux-en-Y gastric bypass. Surgery. 2013;154:1300–6; discussion 1306.
20. Hughes DT, White ML, Miller BS, Gauger PG, Burney RE, Doherty GM. Influence of prophylactic central lymph node dissection on postoperative thyroglobulin levels and radioiodine treatment in papillary thyroid cancer. Surgery. 2010;148:1100–6; discussion 1006–7.
21. Nhan C, Dolev Y, Mijovic T, Rivera JA, Kallai-Sanfacon MA, Mlynarek AM, Payne RJ. Vitamin D deficiency and the risk of hypocalcemia following total thyroidectomy. J Otolaryngol Head Neck Surg. 2012;41:401–6.
22. Lang BH, Wong KP, Cheung CY, Fong YK, Chan DK, Hung GK. Does preoperative 25-hyroxyvitamin D status significantly affect the calcium kinetics after total thyroidectomy? World J Surg. 2013;37:1592–8.
23. Al-Khatib T, Alhubaiti AM, Althubaiti A, Mosli HH, Alwasiah RO, Badawood LM. Severe vitamin D deficiency: a significant predictor of early hypocalcemia after total thyroidectomy. Otolaryngol Head Neck Surg. 2015;152:424–31.
24. Erbil Y, Bozbora A, Ozbey N, Issever H, Aral F, Ozarmagan S, Tezelman S. Predictive value of age and serum parathromone and vitamin d3 levels for postoperative hypocalcemia after total thyroidectomy for nontoxic multinodular goiter. Arch Surg. 2007;142:1182–7.
25. Kirkby-Bott J, Markogiannakis H, Slandarajah A, Cowan M, Fleming B, Palazzo F. Preoperative vitamin D deficiency predicts post-operative hypocalcemia after total thyroidectomy. World J Surg. 2011;35:324–30.
26. Binkley N, Gemar D, Engelke J, Gangnon R, Ramamurthy R, Krueger D, Drezner MK. Evaluation of ergocalciferol or cholecalciferol dosing, 1,600 IU daily or 50,000 IU monthy in older adults. J Clin Endocrinol Metab. 2011;96:981–8.

27. Palazzo FF, Sywak MS, Sidhu SB, Barraclough BH, Delbridge LW. Parathyroid auto transplantation during total thyroidectomy – does the number of glands transplanted affect outcome? World J Surg. 2005;29:629–31.
28. Armas LA, Hollis BW, Heaney RP. Vitamin D2 is much less effective than vitamin D3 in humans. J Clin Endocrinol Metab. 2004;89:5387–91.
29. Carr A, Yen T, Fareau G, Cayo A, Misustin S, Evans D, Wang T. A single parathyroid hormone level obtained 4 hours after total thyroidectomy predicts the need for postoperative calcium supplementation. J Am Chem Soc. 2014;219:757–64.
30. Wiseman JE, Mossanen M, Ituarte PH, Bath JM, Yeh MW. An algorithm informed by the parathyroid hormone level reduces hypocalcemic complications of thyroidectomy. World J Surg. 2010;34:532–7.
31. Bilezikian JP, Khan A, Potts Jr JT, et al. Hypoparathyroidism in the adult: epidemiology, diagnosis, pathophysiology, target-organ involvement, treatment, and challenges for future research. J Bone Miner Res. 2011;26:2317–37.
32. Mannstadt M, Clarke BL, Vokes T, Brandi ML, Ranganath L, Fraser WE, Lakatos P, Bajnok L, Carceau R, Mosekilde L, Lagast H, Choback D, Bilezikian JP. Efficacy and safety of recombinant human parathyroid hormone (1–84) in hypoparathyroidism (REPLACE): a double-blind, placebo-controlled, randomized, phase 3 study. Lancet Diabetes Endocrinol. 2013;1:275–83.

Part VI
Post-thyroidectomy Radioiodine Therapy, Hormonal Therapy and Surveillance

Chapter 20
Initial Radioiodine Ablation

Rebecca L. Weiss and Angela M. Leung

Introduction

Iodine was first discovered in the early nineteenth century by the French scientists, Bernard Courtois and Joseph-Louis Gay-Lussac [1]. Subsequent work by many others during the nineteenth century demonstrated the relationship between iodine nutrition and the formation of goiter. In 1896, Bauman et al. showed that iodine is concentrated in the thyroid [2]. Although external radiation has historically been used to treat a variety of metastatic tumors, it was not until the 1940s when physicians began to use ^{131}I (radioactive iodine [RAI]) to treat thyroid cancers. Frantz et al. first reported a case of a woman with metastatic thyroid cancer treated with radiation therapy (initially external beam radiation, then later RAI) in 1944 [3]. Using a Geiger counter, the physicians were able to identify that the radiation concentrated in the thyroid bed and one of her many bony metastases. An autopsy of the patient found that high uptake of RAI was seen in the well-differentiated thyroid carcinoma (WDTC) tissues in the thyroid and in the metastases, but not in the poorly differentiated carcinoma metastatic tissues [3].

There has been a steady increase in the use of RAI over the past several decades. In the United States, RAI use in all tumor sizes has increased from 40.5 % in 1990 to 65 % in 2008 [4]. In low-risk patients, the use of RAI has increased from 3.3 % in 1973 to 38.1 % in 2006 [5, 6]. According to the US Surveillance, Epidemiology, and End Results (SEER) cancer registry, in young patients (less than 25 years of age) who received a total thyroidectomy for thyroid cancer, RAI ablation use increased from 4 % in 1973 to 62 % in 2008 [7]. In contrast, the SEER database reports that only 20 % of elderly patients received adjuvant RAI treatment between 1988 and 2007 [8].

R.L. Weiss, MD • A.M. Leung, MD, MSc (✉)
Division of Endocrinology (111D), VA Greater Los Angeles Healthcare System, UCLA David Geffen School of Medicine, 11301 Wilshire Blvd, Los Angeles, CA 90073, USA
e-mail: rweiss@mednet.ucla.edu; AMLeung@mednet.ucla.edu

S.A. Roman et al. (eds.), *Management of Thyroid Nodules and Differentiated Thyroid Cancer*, DOI 10.1007/978-3-319-43618-0_20

Sodium-Iodide Symporter (NIS)

Carrasco and colleagues identified the sodium/iodide symporter (NIS) gene in 1996 [9]. Its protein, hNIS, is a transmembrane protein with 13 transmembrane domains composed of 643 amino acids [10]. The action of NIS allows for the concentration of iodide from the bloodstream into thyroid follicles and is an important step in thyroid hormone synthesis. NIS expression is variable among thyroid cancers; some research suggests decreased expression of the transporter in papillary and follicular cancer, whereas other studies reported increased expression in papillary cancer [11]. When iodide uptake in thyroid cancers is decreased, this results in a nonfunctioning or "cold nodule" on radiolabeled imaging [11]. However, thyroid-stimulating hormone (TSH) stimulation assists in inducing NIS expression in the thyroid [11, 12], thereby increasing iodide or RAI uptake. RAI is given orally, absorbed in the stomach and small intestine, and is effectively taken up by the thyroid gland by NIS, similar to the stable element [13].

Goals of Radioactive Iodine Therapy in Thyroid Cancer

RAI is used in several ways in the management of thyroid cancer. Following initial thyroidectomy, RAI can be used to eliminate normal thyroid tissue (thyroid remnant ablation) and effectively eradicate detectable serum thyroglobulin levels, thereby improving its specificity as a tumor marker [4]. Ablating the thyroid remnant also increases the sensitivity of ^{131}I scans to detect disease recurrence [14]. Normal thyroid tissue is more iodine avid than cancerous thyroid tissue [15–17]; thus by ablating normal thyroid tissue, RAI can be taken up by tumor. RAI is also used as adjuvant therapy of micrometastatic disease to decrease the risk of tumor recurrence. Finally, in some cases, RAI is also used to treat persistent metastatic disease.

Well-Differentiated Thyroid Cancer Risk Stratification

The American Thyroid Association (ATA) recommends postoperative staging in patients with WDTC to assess the risk of mortality and to guide treatment decisions, including the use of remnant ablation and radioiodine treatment of metastatic thyroid cancer [18, 19]. This staging includes both the TNM staging, as proposed by the American Joint Cancer Committee (AJCC) [20], the MACIS system from the Mayo Clinic [21] as well as recommendations proposed by the ATA to improve prognostication. These systems are used in conjunction with one another to determine the potential benefit of RAI only in patients following a total or completion thyroidectomy [19].

Beginning in 2009, ATA guidelines also divided WDTC into three risk categories based on risk of recurrence: low, intermediate, and high [18]. The risk of recurrence is considered low if the following are met: complete resection of the macroscopic tumor, lack of invasion into locoregional tissues, absence of aggressive histology, lack of vascular invasion, and lack of ^{131}I uptake outside the thyroid bed on the post-RAI ablation whole body scan. Based on the 2015 ATA guidelines, the tumor is considered to be low risk if there are only small volume lymph node metastases (≤5 micrometastases that measure <0.2 cm) [19]. The 2015 ATA guidelines also include intrathyroidal encapsulated follicular variant of papillary thyroid cancer, follicular cancer with capsular or minor vascular invasion, and intrathyroidal papillary microcarcinomas in the low-risk category [19]. Intermediate-risk factors include the microscopic invasion of soft tissue structures, ^{131}I uptake outside of the tumor bed on the post-RAI ablation whole body scan, vascular invasion, and aggressive histology. Aggressive histologies include Hurthle cell, tall cell, columnar cell, and insular [18, 22]. The 2015 ATA guidelines modified the intermediate-risk category to also include tumors with cervical lymph node metastases (clinical N1 or >5 pathologic lymph nodes measuring less than 3 cm in largest dimension), intrathyroidal papillary thyroid cancer measuring 1–4 cm with known BRAF mutation, as well as multifocal papillary microcarcinomas with extrathyroidal extension with BRAF mutation [19]. Finally, tumors are considered at high risk of recurrence if there are known distant metastases, there is macrovascular invasion into adjacent soft tissue structures, or if there is gross residual disease after tumor resection or postoperative serum Tg is suggestive of distant metastases [18]. The 2015 guidelines also expanded the high-risk category to include patients with large volume lymph nodes measuring ≥3 cm in largest dimension and follicular thyroid carcinoma with more than four foci of vascular invasion or extracapsular vascular invasion [19].

In addition to the above classifications regarding patients' risk, the 2015 ATA guidelines also note that a specific patient's risk will change over time based on the clinical course of the patient's disease and his/her response to therapy. Tuttle et al. and Vaisman et al. both proposed a "response to therapy" risk stratification system, but neither have been validated with additional studies [19, 22, 23]. Based on the data in these studies, the ATA has proposed classifying patients' based on their response to treatment in the following manner:

- Excellent response: no biochemical, clinical, or structural evidence of disease
- Biochemical incomplete response: no localizable disease, but there is biochemical evidence of disease such as an abnormal Tg or rising anti-Tg antibody level despite no localizable disease
- Structural incomplete response: persistent or new locoregional or distant metastases
- Indeterminate response: nonspecific biochemical or structural findings which cannot be classified as either benign or malignant [19]

Patient Selection for Radioactive Iodine Treatment

The ATA currently recommends use of RAI ablation in all patients with high-risk features [19]. The ATA also recommends RAI ablation for all patients with tumor size >4 cm and in patients with tumors of intermediate size (1–4 cm) with intermediate-risk features (i.e., more aggressive histology, positive lymph nodes) [19]. If a patient has a thyroid lobectomy, the ATA does not recommend use of RAI [19].

Data supporting RAI treatment of patients with intermediate- and low-risk tumors are less clear. The ATA currently recommends against routine use of RAI for patients with multifocal papillary microcarcinoma or other low-risk DTC but states that RAI may be considered in patients with intermediate-risk disease [19]. The National Thyroid Cancer Treatment Cooperative Study Group examined 4,941 thyroid cancer patients with a median follow-up of 6 years to assess the benefit of RAI in decreasing cancer recurrence [24]. In their study, they found that only patients with AJCC stage III thyroid cancer had a statistically significant benefit for RAI. However, others purport that patients with ATA low-risk disease may also benefit from RAI use, since many of the studies from which the guidelines are drawn from only follow patients for a median of 6 years from initial therapy, and recurrence can occur much later [25].

This is in contrast to several studies, which suggest that treatment with RAI in low-risk WDTC represents overtreatment, as these patients have the same risk of recurrence regardless of RAI use [4, 26]. In a recent review, Lamartina et al. reported the lack of benefit of RAI ablation among low-risk WDTC patients [4]. This review further delineated low-risk patients into micro- and macrocarcinomas. Only one study was found examining microcarcinomas retrospectively, but there was no clinical benefit to using RAI. With regard to low-risk macrocarcinomas, there was a similar result found in a series of low-risk WDTC patients followed for 10 years [4]. Similarly, another retrospective study showed that there was no statistically significant difference between patients with low-risk DTC treated with surgery alone or surgery with RAI ablation after 10 years of follow-up [26].

A more recent retrospective study examined the benefit of RAI in more than 21,000 patients with papillary thyroid cancer associated with intermediate-risk cancers [27]. Intermediate risk in this study was defined as tumors >4 cm with no lymph node metastases or tumors <4 cm who had a lymph node metastases. Notably, the study excluded patients with aggressive histology tumors, such as Hurthle cell carcinomas or tall cell variants, which are considered to be intermediate-risk factors according to ATA guidelines. The study found that in these intermediate-risk papillary thyroid cancer patients, there was a 29 % relative risk reduction in tumor recurrence following RAI use. In a subgroup analysis, this benefit improved to a 36 % reduction in risk among patients who were <45 years old. This is notable since the ATA currently recommends RAI for patients <45 years only in select cases [19]. Thus, this study suggests that RAI may be beneficial for younger patients as well [27].

Thyroid Stimulation Prior to RAI Ablation

In order for RAI to work appropriately, thyroid-stimulating hormone (TSH) should be stimulated to optimize uptake of iodine in thyroid tissue. Although there have not been any randomized controlled studies to assess the optimal level of TSH stimulation for adequate RAI ablation, there have been several non-controlled studies which suggest that TSH should be elevated to >30 mIU/L to adequately prepare the thyroid for radioactive iodine [28, 29]. Of note, there is a paucity of trials assessing whether lower levels of TSH stimulation would result in adequate radioactive iodine uptake and/or ablation, but many articles and texts cite that the optimal level of TSH stimulation is between 25 and 30 mIU/L [18, 30–33].

There are two methods to stimulate TSH prior to RAI treatment: withdrawal of thyroid hormone or the use of recombinant human thyrotropin (rhTSH). If the withdrawal method is used, patients are either withdrawn from levothyroxine (LT4) 4–6 weeks or from triiodothyronine (T3) 2 weeks prior to therapy. If rhTSH is to be utilized, the patient is kept euthyroid (i.e., withdrawal from thyroid hormone is not necessary) until the administration of rhTSH intramuscular injection as two doses: the first dose is given 2 days prior to ablation, and the second dose is given on the day prior to ablation. In both methods, patients are instructed to follow a low-iodine diet prior to ablation, and it is most important that they adhere to this diet. Uptake of radioactive iodine is inverse to the serum concentration of stable iodine. Therefore, when the serum concentration of iodine is high, the uptake of radioactive iodine will be reduced. Following the Chernobyl nuclear reactor explosion in 1986, high doses of stable iodide were distributed to some area residents to block the thyroid from radioactive iodine exposure [13]. Thus, patients are instructed to adhere to a low-iodine diet for 2–3 weeks prior to the RAI treatment. However, more recent studies suggest that 1 week of a low-iodine diet may be sufficient [34].

Successful ablation rates can be achieved with either the thyroid hormone withdrawal (THW) or rhTSH stimulation methods. There are several prospective randomized trials examining the difference between these two options for stimulating TSH (Table 20.1). The two largest of these trials showed ablation rates ranging from 86 to 92 % with either method [35, 36]. Mallick et al. followed 421 patients in the United Kingdom treated with either THW or rhTSH administration followed by either low- or high-dose ^{131}I. Patients were then followed with both a posttreatment scan and serum thyroglobulin (Tg) measurements at 6–9 months. There were similar ablation rates achieved (defined as a negative uptake scan after ablation and stimulated serum Tg < 0.2 ng/mL) in both the rhTSH group (87.1 %) and the withdrawal method group (86.7 %) [36]. Similarly, a multicenter trial done in France by Schlumberger et al. prospectively followed 684 patients treated with either rhTSH or THW [35]. Ablation was considered successful with a negative thyroid bed ultrasound and a stimulated Tg of <0.1 ng/mL or a negative ^{131}I whole body scan [35]. Similar ablation rates were achieved in both the THW group (92.9 %) and rhTSH group (91.7 %) [35]. Neither of these studies addressed long-term outcomes with rhTSH, including the rates of disease recurrence. However, a more recent study

Table 20.1 Comparison of ablation rates using recombinant human thyrotropin (rhTSH) vs. thyroid hormone withdrawal (THW) for treatment of WDTC

Study	Year	Total subjects (*n*)	rhTSH (*n*)	THW (*n*)	Definition of successful ablation	Length of follow-up	Successful ablation from rhTSH (*n*)	Successful ablation from THW (*n*)	*p*
Lee et al. [73]	2010	291	69	222	Negative WBS, negative neck US and Tg < 1.0 ng/ml	12 months	63 (91.3 %)	203 (91.4 %)	0.2061
Mallick et al. [36]	2012	421	210	211	Negative WBS and TG <2.0 ng/ml	6–9 months	183 (87.1 %)	183 (86.7 %)	0.26
Molinaro et al. [37]	2013	120	70	50	Negative neck US, stimulated Tg < 1.0 ng/mL, and negative Tg-Ab	10 years	47 (67.1 %)	37 (74 %)	0.53
Pacini et al. [37, 74]	2005	63	32	28	Negative WBS (no uptake)	8 months	24 (75 %)	24 (85.7 %)	0.300
Schlumberger et al. [35]	2012	684	348	336	Negative neck US and Tg < 1.0 ng/mL	6–10 months	319 (91.7 %)	312 (92.9 %)	Not stated

published in 2013 followed patients for 10 years after ablation who were stimulated with either rhTSH or THW and showed no significant difference in recurrence rates between the two methods [37].

The benefits of using rhTSH include improved quality of life due to less frequent symptoms of hypothyroidism, including fatigue, lacrimation, constipation, weight gain, and cold intolerance. However, within 3 months after ablation, patients treated with either THW or rhTSH have a similar quality of life [38]. Other studies have shown that patients may be able to receive less overall radiation with rhTSH use, as the renal clearance of $^{131-}$I is faster in patients treated with rhTSH use compared with THW [29, 39]. Additionally, some suggest that using the THW method exposes the patient to prolonged duration of TSH elevation, which may promote tumor growth [31, 40]. Furthermore, even after weeks of withdrawal from LT4, adequate elevation of TSH may not be achieved due to endogenous production of thyroxine from the thyroid remnant or residual disease [41].

The limitations of rhTSH include its cost and availability, as many centers may not have access to it. In the past, some insurance companies also would not reimburse for rhTSH, but it is now easier to have rhTSH pre-authorized for patients. Side effects of rhTSH include mild headaches and nausea [31]. However, as with the withdrawal method, rhTSH can stimulate tumor growth, which may result in compression of adjacent structures, respiratory compromise, or neurologic dysfunction [41]. Furthermore, in patients with high-risk DTC or with extensive lymph node involvement, rhTSH is currently not routinely recommended for most patients due to insufficient studies measuring the risks of morbidity and mortality associated with rhTSH in this cohort of patients [19].

Pre-RAI Treatment Nuclear Imaging

Historically, a whole body ^{131}I or ^{123}I scan prior to radioiodine ablation has been used to calculate the amount of residual thyroid tissue present following thyroidectomy, detect functional metastatic disease, evaluate if treatment with ^{131}I is warranted, or assess if a two-step ablation is required [42, 43]. The ATA also recommends performing pretreatment ^{131}I scans in those patients for whom the extent of thyroid remnant cannot be ascertained from the surgical operative report or neck ultrasound, or in whom the scan would potentially change management [18]. However, some practitioners have shifted away from the use of pretreatment scans because it is thought that there may be potential "stunning" of thyroid tissue with pretreatment iodine [43]. Studies suggest that stunning occurs due to downregulating transcription of NIS on thyroid cells [44]. Additionally, some studies suggest that although stunning may not be apparent in the posttreatment scan, patients who have had a pretreatment scan have decreased successful ablation rates [45]. Others have discontinued their use of pretreatment scans using the rationale that the posttreatment scan is more sensitive to detect distant metastatic disease.

However, some retrospective studies suggest that the utility of pre-ablation scans is still clinically relevant, as it may alter management. For example, if a pretreatment scan shows lymph node involvement with focal uptake, a higher RAI dose may be considered. One retrospective trial reported that the management in more than 50 % of patients (total $n = 355$) was altered based on pretreatment ^{131}I scanning results, including 18 % with either local or distant metastatic disease, 6 % with no focal uptake, and 14 % with lymph node metastases [42]. Another study retrospectively examined patients who received pretreatment ^{123}I scans. Of 122 patients, the pretreatment scan altered management in 25 %. The pretreatment scan was able to determine if a large remnant remained and was better able to differentiate between remnant tissue and lymph node disease as well as identify iodine-avid foci away from the midline (i.e., metastatic disease) [43].

Radioactive Iodine Dosing

As with other cancers, it is important to use the lowest effective dose of radiation to ablate the thyroid remnant in order to reduce the risk of secondary cancers. In patients with high-risk features, such as vascular invasion or known metastatic disease, it is generally accepted to use a higher dose of ^{131}I as a form of adjuvant therapy. In intermediate-risk cancers, there has been shown to be up to a 29 % reduction of recurrence with use of RAI [27]. The ATA currently recommends using a lower dose of 30 mCi for low-risk or intermediate-risk disease with low-risk features [19]. However, the dose of ^{131}I used to treat intermediate papillary thyroid cancer is controversial. A retrospective study in Korea treating intermediate-risk patients with tumors <2 cm with microscopic extrathyroidal extension with either low- or high-dose RAI ablation found similar rates of successful ablation; there was no difference in recurrence rates between the two groups at follow-up intervals of up to 5 years [46]. However, another large retrospective trial of 1298 WDTC patients showed that patients older than 45 years of age had increased mortality with lower doses than with higher doses of RAI [4, 47].

Additional trials similarly show mixed results regarding whether there is a benefit to higher doses of RAI (Table 20.2). Fallahi and colleagues reported better ablation success rates with higher doses of RAI [48]. This study also noted that patients who received a low dose of RAI often required a second ablation dose, which ultimately resulted in higher cumulative dose of RAI. However, Maenpaa et al. reported similar ablation success rates in patients treated with 30 mCi or 100 mCi and no difference in recurrence rates when these patients were followed for a median of 51 months [49]. As mentioned previously, recent large studies in the United Kingdom and France showed that ablation rates were similar with 30 mCi or 100 mCi of ^{131}I [35, 36]. Similarly, there was no difference shown between low- or high-dose regimens of RAI in several other studies [46, 50, 51].

In patients with high-risk papillary thyroid cancer, such as those with distant metastatic disease or macrovascular invasion, higher doses of RAI are generally

Table 20.2 Comparison of ablation rates from high-dose RAI (≥50 mci) vs. low-dose RAI (<50 mci) for treatment of WDTC

Study	Year	Total subjects (*n*)	Number receiving high-dose RAI ≥ 50 mCi (*n*)	Number receiving low-dose RAI < 50 mCi (*n*)	Definition of successful ablation	Length of follow-up	Successful ablation from high-dose RAI (*n*)	Successful ablation from low-dose RAI (*n*)	*p*
Caglar et al. [50]	2012	108	55	53	Negative neck ultrasound, negative WBS, serum Tg < 0.2 ng/ml	6–12 months	35 (64 %)	32 (60 %)	Not significant
Fallahi et al. [48]	2012	341	170	171	Negative WBS and serum Tg < 2.0 ng/ml and anti-Tg < 100 IU/ml	12 months	117 (68.8 %)	71 (41.5 %)	Not stated
Han et al. [46]	2014	176	80	96	Negative stimulated Tg, neg Tg Ab, and absent remnant thyroid on US	12 months to 7 years (retrospectively)	72 (90 %)	93 (97 %)	0.75
Maenpaa et al. [49]	2008	151	77	81	Negative WBS and Serum Tg < 1 ng/mL	4–8 months	43 (56 %)	42 (52 %)	0.61
Mallick et al. [36]	2012	421	207	214	Negative WBS and Tg < 2.0 ng/ml	6–9 months	184 (88.9 %)	182 (85 %)	0.24

(continued)

Table 20.2 (continued)

Study	Year	Total subjects (*n*)	Number receiving high-dose RAI ≥ 50 mCi (*n*)	Number receiving low-dose RAI < 50 mCi (*n*)	Definition of successful ablation	Length of follow-up	Successful ablation from high-dose RAI (*n*)	Successful ablation from low-dose RAI (*n*)	*p*
Pilli et al. [51]	2007	72	36	36	Negative WBS and serum Tg < 1 ng/ml	6–8 months	29 (80.6 %)	31 (86.1 %)	Not stated
Schlumberger et al. [35]	2012	684	337	347	Negative neck US and Tf < 1.0 ng/ml	6–10 months	307 (91.1 %)	331 (93.5 %)	Not stated

used [52, 53]. However, the optimal dose for these patients is still unknown. Some studies have showed no significant benefit of a higher dose, as well as increased morbidity related to RAI use [54]. There are retrospective studies that do suggest that even in patients with high-risk disease, such as a tumor >4 cm in size or lymph node metastases, may do just as well with a low dose (e.g., 30 mCi) of RAI [55].

Posttreatment Follow-Up

About 1 week after radioactive iodine is given, the patient should undergo a posttreatment uptake whole body scan (WBS). This scan informs the practitioner of focal iodine uptake by the thyroid remnant and any residual tumor, as well as discloses the location of iodine-avid metastatic disease [17, 56]. If there is no uptake in the thyroid bed, this suggests that the tumor is not iodine avid and other treatments should be pursued.

Subsequent to the initial ablation, patients should be followed for the measurement of serial serum Tg concentrations and Tg antibodies titers and neck ultrasonography. Neck ultrasonography with a concurrent stimulated Tg and Tg antibody is recommended 6–12 months after ablation to determine ablation success [19]. If ablation is successful, the stimulated thyroglobulin level should be less than 1 ng/mL, and the serum thyroglobulin antibody should be negative [19, 35, 37]. Some practitioners will also obtain a WBS 6–12 months after ablation to determine if ablation is successful. In this case, ablation is deemed successful if there is less than 0.1 % uptake on the posttreatment WBS with a concurrent stimulated (either with THW or rhTSH) serum Tg level less than 1–2 ng/mL [35, 36, 50].

What Patients Should Expect After Receiving RAI

Although therapy with RAI is well tolerated by most patients, there are certain aspects of therapy that should be discussed with patients prior to treatment. Patients should be informed that the radioactivity is excreted in their bodily fluids and should therefore drink sufficient fluid after receiving a dose of radioactive iodine. Additionally, patients must also be counseled regarding the recommended physical proximity to loved ones in the immediate posttreatment phase. Patients with young children or close relationships with pregnant women should be advised to refrain from interacting with their loved ones for the immediate few days and even weeks [57]. Because this may not be feasible for patients in certain instances, many centers hospitalize patients for radioactive iodine therapy. These patients are monitored in the hospital; once radioactivity has decreased to a level that is deemed safe, patients are discharged [57, 58].

Table 20.3 Potential risks of RAI

Short-term risks	Long-term risks
Nausea	Chronic sialadenitis
Vomiting	Xerostomia
Transient sialadenitis	Secondary malignancies: Leukemia Breast cancer Testicular cancer Salivary duct cancer
Change in taste/smell	Infertility
Headache	Delayed childbearing
Bone marrow suppression	
Transient ovarian failure	
Transient testicular failure	
Epistaxis	

Complications of Treatment with RAI

Treatment with ^{131}I is generally well tolerated by most patients. However, as with all medical therapies, there are side effects and complications with ^{131}I, including salivary gland dysfunction, infertility, and possibly secondary malignancy (Table 20.3) [7, 59, 60]. Immediately following ^{131}I administration, patients may experience salivary gland dysfunction, which may occur in up to 30% of patients [61]. Iodine is concentrated in salivary glands at 7–700 times the concentration in serum, thus increasing the risks of salivary gland dysfunction following RAI [61, 62]. Salivary gland dysfunction can be temporized with the use of sour candies to stimulate the salivary glands. Patients can also report dysgeusia, nausea and vomiting, nasal irritation, or stomatitis. Cytopenias have also been reported and usually present as a subclinical lowering of leukocytes and/or platelets [25, 61]. These effects typically wear off as the kidneys excrete ^{131}I and are self-limited.

However, there are potential chronic side effects, including chronic sialadenitis, xerostomia, nasolacrimal duct dysfunction, prolonged bone marrow suppression, and earlier menopause [61, 63–65]. There have also been reports of delayed childbearing and infertility [60, 64, 66, 67]. RAI treatment for thyroid cancer has been associated with increased risk for other primary malignancies, including leukemias, renal cell carcinoma, salivary cancers, and breast cancer [7, 64, 68, 69]. In younger patients (those aged less than 25 years old at time of treatment), RAI has been associated with a 1.42 relative risk of malignancy, with the most commonly reported malignancies being renal cell carcinoma, salivary cancer, and leukemia [7]. In a recent meta-analysis of US and European studies, Sawka et al. reported a 1.19 relative risk of developing a second primary malignancy after RAI among adults using a minimum latency of 2–3 years after the thyroid cancer diagnosis [69].

RAI has also been reported to be associated with an increased risk of breast cancer when it has been used to treat hyperthyroidism [70]. However, more recent studies show that RAI for treatment of either hyperthyroidism or thyroid carcinoma was found to have no association with breast cancer development [71]. A recently published retrospective cohort analysis of more than 6,000 women in Korea found no association between patients treated for thyroid cancer with RAI and risk of subsequent breast carcinoma [72]. This held true for women who were followed for more than 10 years after their diagnosis, women who were treated with high doses of RAI, and women who very young at diagnosis of thyroid cancer (<30 years old).

Conclusion

Radioactive iodine is used for several purposes in the treatment of WDTC, including remnant ablation and treatment of metastatic disease. Although it has been a mainstay of therapy for patients with WDTC, some studies examining the use of RAI ablation to treat low-risk patients reveal no benefit. Additionally, there is continued controversy when using RAI to treat patients with intermediate-risk disease. Studies with long-term follow-up are needed to assess for recurrence in this population and to further determine the short- and long-term risks of RAI therapy.

References

1. Kaiho T. Iodine chemistry and applications. Hoboken: Wiley; 2015. p. xiv–636.
2. Portulano C, Paroder-Belenitsky M, Carrasco N. The Na+/I- symporter (NIS): mechanism and medical impact. Endocr Rev. 2014;35(1):106–49.
3. Frantz VK, Ball RP, Keston AS, Palmer WW. Thyroid carcinoma with metastases: studied with radioactive iodine. Ann Surg. 1944;119(5):668–89.
4. Lamartina L, Durante C, Filetti S, Cooper DS. Low-risk differentiated thyroid cancer and radioiodine remnant ablation: a systematic review of the literature. J Clin Endocrinol Metab. 2015;100(5):1748–61.
5. Sacks W, Wong RM, Bresee C, Braunstein GD. Use of evidence-based guidelines reduces radioactive iodine treatment in patients with low-risk differentiated thyroid cancer. Thyroid. 2015;25(4):377–85.
6. Iyer NG, Morris LG, Tuttle RM, Shaha AR, Ganly I. Rising incidence of second cancers in patients with low-risk (T1N0) thyroid cancer who receive radioactive iodine therapy. Cancer. 2011;117(19):4439–46.
7. Marti JL, Jain KS, Morris LG. Increased risk of second primary malignancy in pediatric and young adult patients treated with radioactive iodine for differentiated thyroid cancer. Thyroid. 2015;25(6):681–7.
8. Marvin K, Parham K. Differentiated thyroid cancer in people aged 85 and older. J Am Geriatr Soc. 2015;63(5):932–7.
9. Dai G, Levy O, Carrasco N. Cloning and characterization of the thyroid iodide transporter. Nature. 1996;379(6564):458–60.
10. Chung JK, Youn HW, Kang JH, Lee HY, Kang KW. Sodium iodide symporter and the radioiodine treatment of thyroid carcinoma. Nucl Med Mol Imaging. 2010;44(1):4–14.
11. Kogai T, Taki K, Brent GA. Enhancement of sodium/iodide symporter expression in thyroid and breast cancer. Endocr Relat Cancer. 2006;13(3):797–826.

12. Kogai T, Endo T, Saito T, Miyazaki A, Kawaguchi A, Onaya T. Regulation by thyroid-stimulating hormone of sodium/iodide symporter gene expression and protein levels in FRTL-5 cells. Endocrinology. 1997;138(6):2227–32.
13. Brent GA, Koenig RJ. Chapter 39. Thyroid and anti-thyroid drugs. In: Brunton LL, et al., editors. Goodman & Gilman's the pharmacological basis of therapeutics. 12th ed. New York: McGraw-Hill; 2011. p. Web.
14. Eustatia-Rutten CF, Smit JW, Romijn JA, van der Kleij-Corssmit EP, Pereira AM, Stokkel MP, et al. Diagnostic value of serum thyroglobulin measurements in the follow-up of differentiated thyroid carcinoma, a structured meta-analysis. Clin Endocrinol (Oxf). 2004;61(1):61–74.
15. Smanik PA, Ryu KY, Theil KS, Mazzaferri EL, Jhiang SM. Expression, exon-intron organization, and chromosome mapping of the human sodium iodide symporter. Endocrinology. 1997;138(8):3555–8.
16. Kollecker I, von Wasielewski R, Langner C, Müller JA, Spitzweg C, Kreipe H, et al. Subcellular distribution of the sodium iodide symporter in benign and malignant thyroid tissues. Thyroid. 2012;22(5):529–35.
17. Vaisman F, Carvalho DP, Vaisman M. A new appraisal of iodine refractory thyroid cancer. Endocr Relat Cancer. 2015;22(6):R301–10.
18. Cooper DS, Doherty GM, Haugen BR, Hauger BR, Kloos RT, Lee SL, et al. Revised American Thyroid Association management guidelines for patients with thyroid nodules and differentiated thyroid cancer. Thyroid. 2009;19(11):1167–214.
19. Haugen BR, Alexander EK, Bible KC, Doherty G, Mandel SJ, Nikiforov YE, et al. 2015 American Thyroid Association Management Guidelines for adult patients with thyroid nodules and differentiated thyroid cancer. Thyroid. 2016 Jan;26(1):1–133.
20. Tran Cao HS, Johnston LE, Chang DC, Bouvet M. A critical analysis of the American Joint Committee on Cancer (AJCC) staging system for differentiated thyroid carcinoma in young patients on the basis of the Surveillance, Epidemiology, and End Results (SEER) registry. Surgery. 2012;152(2):145–51.
21. Hay ID, Bergstralh EJ, Goellner JR, Ebersold JR, Grant CS. Predicting outcome in papillary thyroid carcinoma: development of a reliable prognostic scoring system in a cohort of 1779 patients surgically treated at one institution during 1940 through 1989. Surgery. 1993;114(6):1050–7; discussion 7–8.
22. Tuttle RM, Tala H, Shah J, Leboeuf R, Ghossein R, Gonen M, et al. Estimating risk of recurrence in differentiated thyroid cancer after total thyroidectomy and radioactive iodine remnant ablation: using response to therapy variables to modify the initial risk estimates predicted by the new American Thyroid Association staging system. Thyroid. 2010;20(12):1341–9.
23. Vaisman F, Shaha A, Fish S, Michael Tuttle R. Initial therapy with either thyroid lobectomy or total thyroidectomy without radioactive iodine remnant ablation is associated with very low rates of structural disease recurrence in properly selected patients with differentiated thyroid cancer. Clin Endocrinol (Oxf). 2011;75(1):112–9.
24. Carhill AA, Litofsky DR, Ross DS, Jonklaas J, Cooper DS, Brierley JD, et al. Long-term outcomes following therapy in differentiated thyroid carcinoma: NTCTCS registry analysis 1987-2012. J Clin Endocrinol Metab. 2015;100(9):3270–9; JC20151346.
25. Ain KB. Radioiodine-remnant ablation in low-risk differentiated thyroid cancer: pros. Endocrine. 2015;50(1):61–6.
26. Bal C, Ballal S, Soundararajan R, Chopra S, Garg A. Radioiodine remnant ablation in low-risk differentiated thyroid cancer patients who had R0 dissection is an over treatment. Cancer Med. 2015;4(7):1031–8.
27. Ruel E, Thomas S, Dinan M, Perkins JM, Roman SA, Sosa JA. Adjuvant radioactive iodine therapy is associated with improved survival for patients with intermediate-risk papillary thyroid cancer. J Clin Endocrinol Metab. 2015;100(4):1529–36.
28. Edmonds CJ, Hayes S, Kermode JC, Thompson BD. Measurement of serum TSH and thyroid hormones in the management of treatment of thyroid carcinoma with radioiodine. Br J Radiol. 1977;50(599):799–807.

29. Carvalho MR, Ferreira TC, Leite V. Evaluation of whole-body retention of iodine-131 ((131) I) after postoperative remnant ablation for differentiated thyroid carcinoma - thyroxine withdrawal versus rhTSH administration: a retrospective comparison. Oncol Lett. 2012;3(3):617–20.
30. Mazzaferri EL, Kloos RT. Using recombinant human TSH in the management of well-differentiated thyroid cancer: current strategies and future directions. Thyroid. 2000;10(9):767–78.
31. Mazzaferri EL, Massoll N. Management of papillary and follicular (differentiated) thyroid cancer: new paradigms using recombinant human thyrotropin. Endocr Relat Cancer. 2002;9(4):227–47.
32. Kronenberg H, Williams RH. Williams textbook of endocrinology. 11th ed. Philadelphia: Saunders/Elsevier; 2008. p. xix–1911.
33. Hugo J, Robenshtok E, Grewal R, Larson S, Tuttle RM. Recombinant human thyroid stimulating hormone-assisted radioactive iodine remnant ablation in thyroid cancer patients at intermediate to high risk of recurrence. Thyroid. 2012;22(10):1007–15.
34. Lee M, Lee YK, Jeon TJ, Chang HS, Kim BW, Lee YS, et al. Low iodine diet for one week is sufficient for adequate preparation of high dose radioactive iodine ablation therapy of differentiated thyroid cancer patients in iodine-rich areas. Thyroid. 2014;24(8):1289–96.
35. Schlumberger M, Catargi B, Borget I, Deandreis D, Zerdoud S, Bridji B, et al. Strategies of radioiodine ablation in patients with low-risk thyroid cancer. N Engl J Med. 2012;366(18):1663–73.
36. Mallick U, Harmer C, Yap B, Wadsley J, Clarke S, Moss L, et al. Ablation with low-dose radioiodine and thyrotropin alfa in thyroid cancer. N Engl J Med. 2012;366(18):1674–85.
37. Molinaro E, Giani C, Agate L, Biagini A, Pieruzzi L, Bianchi F, et al. Patients with differentiated thyroid cancer who underwent radioiodine thyroid remnant ablation with low-activity ^{131}I after either recombinant human TSH or thyroid hormone therapy withdrawal showed the same outcome after a 10-year follow-up. J Clin Endocrinol Metab. 2013;98(7):2693–700.
38. Tu J, Wang S, Huo Z, Lin Y, Li X, Wang S. Recombinant human thyrotropin-aided versus thyroid hormone withdrawal-aided radioiodine treatment for differentiated thyroid cancer after total thyroidectomy: a meta-analysis. Radiother Oncol. 2014;110(1):25–30.
39. Ravichandran R, Al Saadi A, Al Balushi N. Radioactive body burden measurements in (131) iodine therapy for differentiated thyroid cancer: effect of recombinant thyroid stimulating hormone in whole body (131)iodine clearance. World J Nucl Med. 2014;13(1):56–61.
40. Maini CL, Sciuto R, Tofani A, Rosito I, Franciotti G, Pisano L. Thyroid-stimulating hormone (TSH) suppression in differentiated thyroid carcinoma: combined treatment with triiodothyronine and thyroxine. Eur J Cancer. 1994;30A(14):2184–5.
41. Luster M, Lippi F, Jarzab B, Perros P, Lassmann M, Reiners C, et al. rhTSH-aided radioiodine ablation and treatment of differentiated thyroid carcinoma: a comprehensive review. Endocr Relat Cancer. 2005;12(1):49–64.
42. Van Nostrand D, Aiken M, Atkins F, Moreau S, Garcia C, Acio E, et al. The utility of radioiodine scans prior to iodine 131 ablation in patients with well-differentiated thyroid cancer. Thyroid. 2009;19(8):849–55.
43. Chen MK, Yasrebi M, Samii J, Staib LH, Doddamane I, Cheng DW. The utility of I-123 pretherapy scan in I-131 radioiodine therapy for thyroid cancer. Thyroid. 2012;22(3):304–9.
44. Nordén MM, Larsson F, Tedelind S, Carlsson T, Lundh C, Forssell-Aronsson E, et al. Down-regulation of the sodium/iodide symporter explains 131I-induced thyroid stunning. Cancer Res. 2007;67(15):7512–7.
45. Chalstrey LJ, Benjamin B. High incidence of breast cancer in thyroid cancer patients. Br J Cancer. 1966;20(4):670–5.
46. Han JM, Kim WG, Kim TY, Jeon MJ, Ryu JS, Song DE, et al. Effects of low-dose and high-dose postoperative radioiodine therapy on the clinical outcome in patients with small differentiated thyroid cancer having microscopic extrathyroidal extension. Thyroid. 2014;24(5):820–5.

47. Verburg FA, Mader U, Reiners C, Hanscheid H. Long-term survival in differentiated thyroid cancer is worse after low-activity initial post-surgical 131I therapy in both high- and low-risk patients. J Clin Endocrinol Metab. 2014;99(12):4487–96.
48. Fallahi B, Beiki D, Takavar A, Fard-Esfahani A, Gilani KA, Saghari M, et al. Low versus high radioiodine dose in postoperative ablation of residual thyroid tissue in patients with differentiated thyroid carcinoma: a large randomized clinical trial. Nucl Med Commun. 2012;33(3):275–82.
49. Mäenpää HO, Heikkonen J, Vaalavirta L, Tenhunen M, Joensuu H. Low vs. high radioiodine activity to ablate the thyroid after thyroidectomy for cancer: a randomized study. PLoS One. 2008;3(4):e1885.
50. Caglar M, Bozkurt FM, Akca CK, Vargol SE, Bayraktar M, Ugur O, et al. Comparison of 800 and 3700 MBq iodine-131 for the postoperative ablation of thyroid remnant in patients with low-risk differentiated thyroid cancer. Nucl Med Commun. 2012;33(3):268–74.
51. Pilli T, Brianzoni E, Capoccetti F, Castagna MG, Fattori S, Poggiu A, et al. A comparison of 1850 (50 mCi) and 3700 MBq (100 mCi) 131-iodine administered doses for recombinant thyrotropin-stimulated postoperative thyroid remnant ablation in differentiated thyroid cancer. J Clin Endocrinol Metab. 2007;92(9):3542–6.
52. Menzel C, Grunwald F, Schomburg A, Palmedo H, Bender H, Spath G, et al. "High-dose" radioiodine therapy in advanced differentiated thyroid carcinoma. J Nucl Med. 1996;37(9):1496–503.
53. Gao YC, Lu HK. Outcome after high-dose radioiodine therapy for advanced differentiated thyroid carcinoma in childhood. Endocr Res. 2009;34(4):121–9.
54. Haq MS, McCready RV, Harmer CL. Treatment of advanced differentiated thyroid carcinoma with high activity radioiodine therapy. Nucl Med Commun. 2004;25(8):799–805.
55. Rosário PW, Calsolari MR. Thyroid ablation with 1.1 GBq (30 mCi) iodine-131 in patients with papillary thyroid carcinoma at intermediate risk for recurrence. Thyroid. 2014;24(5):826–31.
56. Sherman SI, Tielens ET, Sostre S, Wharam MD, Ladenson PW. Clinical utility of posttreatment radioiodine scans in the management of patients with thyroid carcinoma. J Clin Endocrinol Metab. 1994;78(3):629–34.
57. Rémy H, Coulot J, Borget I, Ricard M, Guilabert N, Lavielle F, et al. Thyroid cancer patients treated with 131I: radiation dose to relatives after discharge from the hospital. Thyroid. 2012;22(1):59–63.
58. Pacilio M, Bianciardi L, Panichelli V, Argirò G, Cipriani C. Management of 131I therapy for thyroid cancer: cumulative dose from in-patients, discharge planning and personnel requirements. Nucl Med Commun. 2005;26(7):623–31.
59. Ko KY, Kao CH, Lin CL, Huang WS, Yen RF. (131)I treatment for thyroid cancer and the risk of developing salivary and lacrimal gland dysfunction and a second primary malignancy: a nationwide population-based cohort study. Eur J Nucl Med Mol Imaging. 2015;42(8):1172–8.
60. Hyer S, Vini L, O'Connell M, Pratt B, Harmer C. Testicular dose and fertility in men following I(131) therapy for thyroid cancer. Clin Endocrinol (Oxf). 2002;56(6):755–8.
61. Klein Hesselink EN, Links TP. Radioiodine treatment and thyroid hormone suppression therapy for differentiated thyroid carcinoma: adverse effects support the trend toward less aggressive treatment for low-risk patients. Eur Thyroid J. 2015;4(2):82–92.
62. Spitzweg C, Joba W, Schriever K, Goellner JR, Morris JC, Heufelder AE. Analysis of human sodium iodide symporter immunoreactivity in human exocrine glands. J Clin Endocrinol Metab. 1999;84(11):4178–84.
63. Jonklaas J. Nasal symptoms after radioiodine therapy: a rarely described side effect with similar frequency to lacrimal dysfunction. Thyroid. 2014;24(12):1806–14.
64. Edmonds CJ, Smith T. The long-term hazards of the treatment of thyroid cancer with radioiodine. Br J Radiol. 1986;59(697):45–51.

65. Alexander C, Bader JB, Schaefer A, Finke C, Kirsch CM. Intermediate and long-term side effects of high-dose radioiodine therapy for thyroid carcinoma. J Nucl Med. 1998;39(9):1551–4.
66. Mazzaferri EL. Gonadal damage from 131I therapy for thyroid cancer. Clin Endocrinol (Oxf). 2002;57(3):313–4.
67. Wu JX, Young S, Ro K, Li N, Leung AM, Chiu HK, et al. Reproductive outcomes and nononcologic complications after radioactive iodine ablation for well-differentiated thyroid cancer. Thyroid. 2015;25(1):133–8.
68. Adjadj E, Rubino C, Shamsaldim A, Le MG, Schlumberger M, de Vathaire F. The risk of multiple primary breast and thyroid carcinomas. Cancer. 2003;98(6):1309–17.
69. Sawka AM, Thabane L, Parlea L, Ibrahim-Zada I, Tsang RW, Brierley JD, et al. Second primary malignancy risk after radioactive iodine treatment for thyroid cancer: a systematic review and meta-analysis. Thyroid. 2009;19(5):451–7.
70. Metso S, Auvinen A, Huhtala H, Salmi J, Oksala H, Jaatinen P. Increased cancer incidence after radioiodine treatment for hyperthyroidism. Cancer. 2007;109(10):1972–9.
71. Verkooijen RB, Smit JW, Romijn JA, Stokkel MP. The incidence of second primary tumors in thyroid cancer patients is increased, but not related to treatment of thyroid cancer. Eur J Endocrinol. 2006;155(6):801–6.
72. Ahn HY, Min HS, Yeo Y, Ma SH, Hwang Y, An JH, et al. Radioactive iodine therapy did not significantly increase the incidence and recurrence of subsequent breast cancer. J Clin Endocrinol Metab. 2015;100(9):3486–93; JC20142896.
73. Lee J, Yun MJ, Nam KH, Chung WY, Soh EY, Park CS. Quality of life and effectiveness comparisons of thyroxine withdrawal, triiodothyronine withdrawal, and recombinant thyroid-stimulating hormone administration for low-dose radioiodine remnant ablation of differentiated thyroid carcinoma. Thyroid. 2010;20(2):173–9.
74. Pacini F, Ladenson PW, Schlumberger M, Driedger A, Luster M, Kloos RT, et al. Radioiodine ablation of thyroid remnants after preparation with recombinant human thyrotropin in differentiated thyroid carcinoma: results of an international, randomized, controlled study. J Clin Endocrinol Metab. 2006;91(3):926–32.

Chapter 21
Treatment of Recurrent/Metastatic Thyroid Cancer with Radioactive Iodine

Naykky Singh Ospina and M. Regina Castro

Introduction

The incidence of thyroid cancer in the United States has increased significantly during the last three decades, with an estimated incidence of 14 cases per 100,000 individuals, with similar trends noted worldwide [1, 2]. A significant proportion of the newly diagnosed cases represent micropapillary thyroid cancer and affect mostly women; during this time, the mortality rates for thyroid cancer have remained low and unchanged [1, 2].

The cornerstone of treatment of patients with differentiated thyroid cancer (DTC) is surgical intervention [3, 4]. Radioactive iodine (RAI) can be used for diagnostic purposes, as well as a treatment agent for ablation or adjuvant therapy. The use of RAI for the treatment and diagnosis of thyroid disease is based on the ability of the thyroid gland to concentrate iodine from the circulation into thyroid follicular cells through the action of the sodium iodine symporter, therefore providing substrate for thyroid hormone synthesis [5]. Treatment with RAI can be considered for thyroid

N. Singh Ospina, MD
Division of Endocrinology, Diabetes, Metabolism, and Nutrition and Department of Internal Medicine, Mayo Clinic, 200 First Street SW, Rochester, MN 55905, USA

Knowledge and Evaluation Research Unit, Division of Endocrinology, Mayo Clinic, Rochester, MN, USA

M.R. Castro, MD (✉)
Division of Endocrinology, Diabetes, Metabolism, and Nutrition and Department of Internal Medicine, Mayo Clinic, 200 First Street SW, Rochester, MN 55905, USA
e-mail: castro.regina@mayo.edu

S.A. Roman et al. (eds.), *Management of Thyroid Nodules and Differentiated Thyroid Cancer*, DOI 10.1007/978-3-319-43618-0_21

remnant ablation, treatment of locoregional residual or recurrent disease not amenable to surgery, and treatment of distant metastatic disease [3, 4]. As expected, with the increased incidence of thyroid cancer, the use of RAI has risen between 1990 and 2008, with 56 % of the patients with well-differentiated thyroid cancer (DTC) receiving treatment with RAI; hospital volume, in addition to clinical characteristics (including tumor size), seemed to be determinants of the use of RAI [6].

The objective of this chapter is to discuss the appropriate use of RAI in patients with recurrent/residual or metastatic thyroid cancer, how to identify such patients, and how to prepare them for successful RAI therapy and to summarize the possible complications of this treatment.

Diagnosis of Recurrent or Persistent Thyroid Cancer

Although most patients with DTC will have excellent long-term prognosis in terms of survival, approximately 5–35 % will experience locoregional recurrences [4, 7, 8]. Patients with large tumors, multifocal disease, extrathyroidal extension, or cervical nodal involvement at the time of initial surgery have increased risk of recurrence, and the majority of these recurrences (up to 70 %) will occur in the neck [4, 7–10]. In the remainder of the cases, recurrences will involve the lungs or bones [8]. Therefore, long-term surveillance of these patients is indicated to identify and treat such patients in a timely manner [4, 7].

Value of Serum Thyroglobulin in the Long-Term Surveillance of Thyroid Cancer

Thyroglobulin (Tg) is a glycoprotein normally produced by thyroid follicular cells that serves as substrate for the synthesis of thyroid hormones [11, 12]. Following successful thyroidectomy, Tg levels decrease, and in patients who have undergone successful RAI remnant ablation, Tg levels often become undetectable [4, 7, 13]. In such patients, surveillance is carried out by measurement of serum Tg levels (used as a tumor marker in patients with DTC due to its tissue-specific origin) to detect biochemical recurrence [11]. This marker can help identify patients at risk of recurrence, as there is an association between the serum Tg levels and disease progression [14, 15]. Measurement of serum Tg levels coupled with neck ultrasound has become the cornerstone of surveillance strategies [4, 7, 16]. Clinical judgment in the interpretation of Tg levels is required, given that values can be misleading in cases where Tg antibodies are present or in cases of recurrence with less differentiated tumors [4, 7, 11, 17]. Other imaging modalities to identify structural disease (iodine whole-body scan [14], CT scan, and fluorodeoxyglucose/positron emission tomography [14, 16]) are often used along with Tg to further guide treatment [4, 7]. There is still debate regarding the need for stimulated Tg measurements, as compared to the currently available highly sensitive assays [11]. A study that evaluated 122 patients with low risk of recurrence found no significant differences in the positive predictive value between the combination of thyroid ultrasound and non-stimulated Tg or stimulated Tg measurement for the detection of recurrence [18]. Similar findings were found by Persoon et al. who studied 118 patients free of recurrence with both stimulated and non-stimulated Tg and found only a nonsignificant (0.8 %) increase in the detection of recurrence in the group with stimulated Tg measurement [19]. Current management guidelines recommend the use of serum Tg measurement during the follow-up of most patients and reserved the use of Tg after TSH stimulation as a consideration in patients with indeterminate or incomplete response (biochemical or structural) after additional therapies have been performed (or as decline in Tg is noted) to assess the response to therapy [4]. As a result, the combination of Tg measurement and neck ultrasound is a noninvasive approach that allows the identification of the majority of cases of recurrence, without the need to perform iodine WBS in all patients [4]. Several studies have found that in patients with DTC who have undergone thyroidectomy and RAI ablation and who were deemed at moderate or high risk of recurrence, an iodine WBS did not provide any valuable additional information, when Tg and neck ultrasound were both negative [20, 21].

Imaging Modalities Helpful in the Follow-Up of Patients with DTC

Ultrasound of the neck should be the initial imaging modality in patients with suspected tumor recurrence (e.g., elevated Tg levels). Ultrasound is the most sensitive method to evaluate the most common sites of recurrence, the thyroid bed and cervical lymph nodes [22]. Studies have shown that in patients with an overall low risk for recurrence, a combination of low serum Tg levels and normal thyroid US has a high negative predictive value for recurrence [23]. On the other hand, when serum Tg levels are increased, further imaging studies are needed to determine the site and extent of recurrence and the presence of RAI-avid areas that could be amenable to treatment [23]. In such patients, imaging modalities such as CT scan of the chest, looking for lung metastases, or an iodine WBS should be performed, and if negative, a FDG/PET scan should follow [22]. Chest CT scan can detect pulmonary metastases in 80–90 % of the cases, being able to detect lesions between 3 and 6 mm [24, 25].

Iodine WBS is able to detect iodine-avid lesions (e.g., not useful in non-differentiated thyroid cancer) both in the thyroid bed and in metastatic locations. See Figure 21.1 (skeletal lesions) and Fig. 21.2 (lung lesions) [16]. The sensitivity and specificity of the iodine WBS are affected by the degree of residual thyroid tissue, the iodine avidity of the tumor, the dose of iodine given, and the overall burden of disease [16].

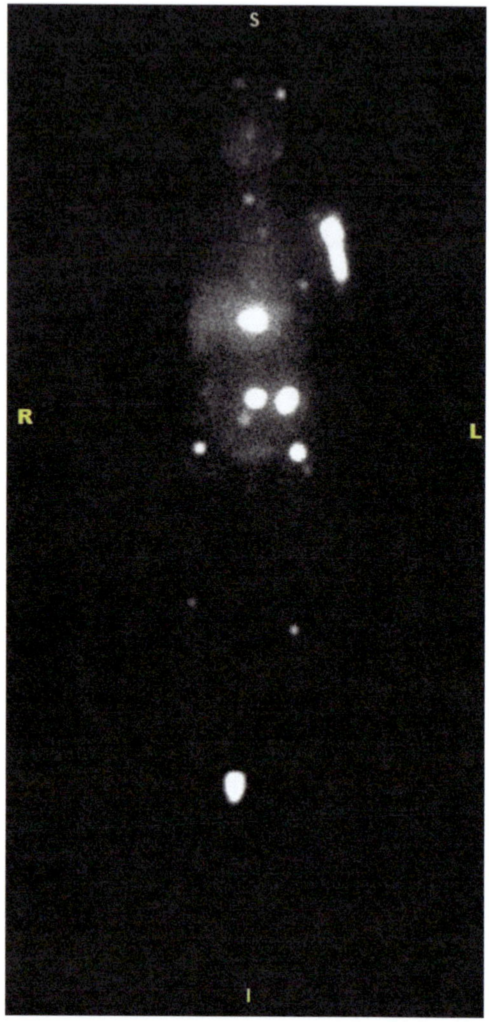

Fig. 21.1 Whole-body Iodine scan (I-123) showing extensive radioiodine uptake in the left proximal humerus. Additional metastatic foci are present in the right iliac crest, proximal left femur, the right 5th and 9th ribs, and other multiple skeletal regions

FDG/PET is usually performed in the setting of elevated Tg with a negative WBS [4, 26]. This imaging modality can offer additional information in about 10 % of these patients [26]. A review of the performance of FDG/PET for the diagnosis of recurrent/metastatic thyroid cancer showed variable sensitivity (45–100 %) but good specificity (90–100 %). Variables that can explain these wide ranges include tumor burden, previous imaging studies before the FDG/PET, and location of metastatic disease [27]. The rate of cases in which the results of FDG/PET changes clinical management is also quite variable with values between 9 and 54 %. The exact advantage of FGD/PET when compared to other diagnostic modalities and the most cost-effective diagnostic algorithm for recurrent or metastatic disease including FDG/PET is not known at this time [26, 27].

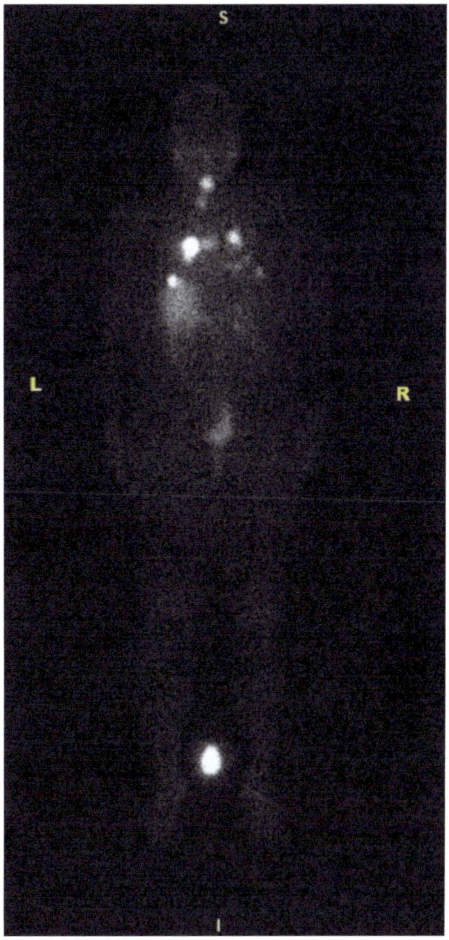

Fig. 21.2 Whole-body iodine scan (I-123) showing focal uptake of iodine-avid disease over the lower neck and lungs

Indications for Radioactive Iodine in Differentiated Thyroid Cancer

The use of RAI in the treatment of differentiated thyroid cancer is reserved for clinical situations in which its benefits outweigh the potential risks and burden associated with treatment. RAI use should be considered in the following clinical situations: (i) remnant ablation after thyroidectomy, (ii) as adjuvant therapy for micrometastases, (iii) local recurrent disease not amenable to surgery, and (iv) treatment of metastatic disease [4]. The first two indications are covered elsewhere in this book (see Chap. 23). In this chapter, we will focus on the treatment of recurrent and metastatic disease.

Rationale for Therapy

Recurrent disease after initial surgical treatment of DTC can occur, locally in the anterior neck or cervical lymph nodes or in distant sites, most commonly lungs and bones, although rarely other less frequent sites such as kidney, liver, and brain can be affected [4, 8]. Most recurrences occur in the lymph nodes during the first few years of follow-up, suggesting that lymph node involvement could represent persistent (rather than recurrent) disease, followed by subsequent enlargement [4, 8, 28]. The difference between true local recurrence and lymph node metastases is important from a surgical perspective, since local recurrence is defined as newly formed tumor within the soft tissue, in comparison with well-defined disease found in lymph nodes [28].

The treatment options for recurrent disease include observation, RAI, reoperation, and radiation therapy [4, 28]. Percutaneous ethanol ablation has also been used successfully in selected centers with experience in this procedure, for treatment of limited locoregional recurrences involving nodules in the thyroid bed or lymph nodes in the central or lateral neck [29, 30]. The use of RAI is usually reserved for cases in which treatment is needed but surgery is not advisable/feasible [4, 31].

There seems to be an association between recurrent local disease and patient outcomes such as mortality. A large study of almost 6000 patients found rates of recurrence during follow-up of 7 % for local lymph nodes, 2 % for lung, and 0.6 % for bone metastases, in addition, 1 % of the patients died from causes related to DTC [32]. The strongest predictors for death related to thyroid carcinoma were age older than 55 years, extra nodal tumor extension, and large nodal metastases. The authors suggested that recurrent lesions in older patients with evidence of extra nodal extension can represent life-threatening disease and should be aggressively managed [32]. Another study that evaluated 201 patients with DTC also found an association between the presence of locoregional recurrence and distant metastases with increased mortality on univariate analysis, but these finding remained statistically significant only for distant metastases on multivariate analyses [33].

In a study of approximately 1000 patients with DTC, 42 were found to have lung metastases during follow-up using iodine WBS and were treated with RAI with stabilization or resolution of tumor noted in 7 and 10 patients, respectively. The mean cumulative I^{131} activity was 410 ± 240 mCI [34]. Another study evaluated 101 patients with lung metastases from thyroid cancer, noting that the 5- and 10-year survival rate was higher in those with positive iodine uptake compared with those without uptake [35]. Another study that evaluated 444 patients with metastatic disease from DTC, including 223 with lung metastases, 114 with bone disease, and 82 with both bone and lung disease, found 10-year survival of 92 % in those patients who responded to therapy compared to 19 % without treatment response. Patients in this cohort were treated with 100 mCi of I^{131} after thyroid hormone withdrawal every 3–9 months for 2 years and then yearly until response (defined as negative scan) was achieved. Negative imaging studies were achieved in 43 % of the patients, most commonly in younger patients, with well-differentiated tumors and limited extent of disease. The negative studies were achieved after cumulative doses of 100–600 mCi. In the case of bone metastases, only 17 % achieved remission in comparison to 74 % of those with lung disease [36].

Preparation for Radioactive Iodine Treatment

To enhance the effectiveness of RAI therapy (its uptake and retention by malignant thyroid follicular cells), two strategies are commonly utilized: (1) depleting iodine stores and (2) increasing serum TSH levels [4, 12].

Low Iodine Diet

Current treatment guidelines recommend restriction on dietary iodine before RAI with the goal of achieving depletion of the body iodine stores and increasing RAI uptake by thyroid cells [4]. This recommendation is supported by a systematic review and meta-analysis that found that a low iodine diet decreases urinary levels of iodine, increases RAI uptake, and can possibly increase the efficacy of treatment. The most common approach is to limit dietary iodine to $\leq$50 mcg/day for 1–2 weeks [37]. During that period, avoidance of iodized salt (non-iodized salt may be used instead) and other foods rich in iodine, such as kelp, seaweed, and shellfish, is recommended. A study that evaluated 125 patients who followed a restrictive iodine diet found that 15 days were sufficient to achieve iodine depletion when measured both by a 24-hours and by a spot urinary iodine measurement [38].

However, there is conflicting data from other centers where dietary iodine restriction has not been associated with significant clinical benefits [39].

Increasing TSH

An arbitrary level of TSH stimulation of more than 30 IU/L is generally used as the cutoff above which adequate I^{131} uptake by the thyroid cells is expected to result in increased effectiveness of RAI therapy. Two main approaches are currently used to achieve thyroid stimulation: (1) thyroid hormone withdrawal (THW) and (2) recombinant human TSH stimulation (rhTSH) [3, 4, 40].

Many methods on how to perform THW have been described. These include (a) discontinuation of levothyroxine therapy 3 weeks before RAI treatment and (b) reducing the levothyroxine dose for 3 weeks followed by its discontinuation and replacement with T3 therapy (shorter half-life) for 2–4 weeks, which is then discontinued 2 weeks before RAI treatment. There does not appear to be a major difference in terms of symptoms of hypothyroidism or time to TSH elevation to necessarily prefer one method over the other. The main disadvantage of these withdrawal methods is the expected symptoms of hypothyroidism [3, 41–43].

Alternatively, rhTSH is often used to stimulate the iodine uptake to achieve ablation. However, although rhTSH has been approved for diagnostic purposes and for thyroid remnant ablation (see Chap. 23), it has not been approved by the US Food and Drug Administration for treatment of metastatic disease [12]. When RAI is used for remnant ablation, levothyroxine is continued and rhTSH is injected daily for 2–3 days before therapy. The main advantage of this approach is the avoidance of symptoms of hypothyroidism; the main disadvantage is its high cost. In addition, long-term studies regarding safety and efficacy outcomes in patients with metastatic disease are scarce [3]. However, some experience has accumulated from small studies in which this approach was used on a compassionate basis in patients unable to tolerate THW or mount an appropriate TSH response after withdrawal or in whom THW was contraindicated for medical reasons, showing that the use of rhTSH appeared to be safe and resulted in clinical improvement or stabilization of tumor burden in the majority of patients [44, 45]. Current ATA guidelines indicate there is insufficient evidence to recommend this therapy in all patients with distant metastatic disease, but allow for consideration of the use of rhTSH for treatment of metastases in selected patients in which iatrogenic hypothyroidism might be considered risky (e.g., patients with multiple comorbidities) and those with pituitary disease in whom TSH cannot be raised [4, 44, 45].

There are no randomized controlled trials evaluating the effect of rhTSH vs THW on safety and efficacy outcomes of the treatment of metastatic or recurrent disease. A review of observational studies found that patients prepared with rhTSH had positive post-therapy scans in 75 % of the cases and achieved complete or partial disease remission in 65 % of the cases [46]. In addition, observational studies comparing these preparation strategies are available, suggesting similar outcomes between these modalities. For example, an observational study that evaluated 84 patients with well DTC and RAI-avid lesions mostly in the regional neck (64 with rhTSH and 20 with THW) found no statistically significant difference between the rates of successful therapy in patients with RAI-avid metastatic disease prepared with one approach or the other [47]. In the study by Klubo-Gwiezdzinska et al., 56 patients with RAI-avid distant metastases treated with one of these approaches were followed for 72 months, and after adjusting for confounders, no difference in rates of clinical response or progression-free survival was found [48]. Another study of patients with metastatic thyroid cancer found no difference at 5.5 years of follow-up in terms of overall survival between patients prepared with rhTSH stimulation, THW, or THW followed by rhTSH stimulation [49].

The use of one approach over the other will then depend on the patient's characteristics (age, comorbidities, and potential complications in case of hypothyroidism) and other system variables (e.g., costs).

RAI Dosing

The selection of the dose to use in cases of local or metastatic disease in patients with DTC can be determined using an empiric approach, measuring the upper bound limit of blood and body dosimetry, or by quantitative tumor dosimetry [4, 12]. There are no randomized controlled trials evaluating efficacy and safety outcomes between these various approaches or comparing different radiation doses. Using the empiric approach, doses of 100–150 mCi are used for local disease (with higher doses used in cases of extrathyroidal invasion). In the case of pulmonary metastases, doses of 150–200 mCi are used (lower doses in patients with very high uptake, due to risk of lung injury). These doses can be repeated every 6–12 months as long as there is evidence of RAI avidity [4, 12].

Alternatively, dosimetry can be used to select the treatment dose based on calculations that maximize the dose delivered to the tumor lesions, while limiting whole-body retention to 80 mCi at 48 h, or by calculating the maximum tolerated activity to the bone marrow (estimated at 200 cGy) [4, 12]. The dosimetry approach is currently practiced in only a limited number of institutions, despite evidence suggesting possible benefits. For example, in a study of 535 patients in which the majority had normal renal function, an empiric dose of 200 mCI would exceed the maximum tolerated activity in 8–15 % of patients < 70 years and in 22–38 % of patients 70 years or older [50]. Another analysis of 127 dosimetry studies found that using empiric doses between 100 and 300 mCi, the proportion of patients that would exceed the maximum tolerated activity ranged from 1 to 22 %, while 78–98 % could have received a higher dose, suggesting that dosimetry would be helpful in clinical practice [51].

Value of RAI Therapy in Patients with Non-RAI-Avid Structural Disease

Empiric RAI therapy of patients with elevated Tg and known or suspected structural disease, but negative iodine WBS, is controversial. There have been no randomized controlled trials assessing the benefit of this treatment in such patients. A systematic review of 13 observational studies assessing the efficacy of RAI treatment in patients with elevated serum Tg levels but negative iodine WBS found that Tg levels decreased after therapy in 62 % of the cases and positive post-therapy scans were seen in 56 % of the patients, suggesting a possible benefit [52]. However, 44 % of the patients included in five studies had reduction of Tg levels without treatment during follow-up. In two of these studies, no patient showed a decreased or normalized Tg during follow-up. Rigorous comparison between patients treated with one approach and the other is required to provide more reliable conclusions regarding the benefits of RAI in these patients [52]. One study compared 42 patients with positive serum Tg and negative diagnostic scan with 28 patients with similar characteristics but who were not treated. In the treated group, 70 % of patients had a positive post-therapy scan. Normalization of the serum Tg or resolution of the initial iodine uptake during follow-up was seen in 56 % of the cases showing lung uptake at the first post-therapy scan, and in 60 % of the cases showing cervical node metastases at the first post-therapy scan. In the untreated group, 70 % of patients had Tg levels that became undetectable during follow-up [53]. Current treatment recommendations suggest observation in patients without structurally evident disease and low Tg levels (Tg < 10 ng/dL with thyroid hormone withdrawal or < 5 ng/mL with rhTSH). Empiric therapy with RAI should be reserved for those with significantly elevated Tg (or rapidly rising levels) without a structural target amenable to directed therapy (surgery, alcohol ablation, external radiation, etc.) [4].

Post-therapy Scan

The utility of performing a post-therapy scan in patients who received therapy with RAI is also controversial; however, current ATA guidelines recommend obtaining a post-therapy scan [4]. A study of 143 I^{131} scans in 93 patients with DTC performed 5–12 days after RAI therapy found discordance between the scans in 22 % of the cases, with detection of new areas of uptake in 9 % of the cases (lung and cervical lymph node uptake). In addition, 12 % of the cases show increased areas of uptake in locations already diagnosed by the pretreatment scan. The authors concluded that in the majority of the cases, the new areas of uptake do not change clinical management; however, the post-therapy scan can help confirm the uptake of the iodine treatment and identify more clearly cervical lymph node disease [54]. Another study evaluated the concordance between pre- and post-therapy scans in 177 pairs and found concordance in up to 94 %. In 11 pairs of scans (6 %), the new focus of disease was found in the thyroid (6 pairs), cervical lymph nodes (3), lung (1), and bone (1). The new findings would have changed the clinical management in only 2 pairs (1 %) of scans (new lung and bone disease)[55].

Complications and Side Effects of RAI Therapy

The decision to utilize RAI for the treatment of DTC should be based on an evaluation of the benefits associated with treatment as well as risks. RAI therapy is associated with both acute and chronic side effects [56, 57].

The administration of RAI is generally well tolerated. Nausea and vomiting may occur in the acute setting in 50–70 % of the patients. These symptoms usually occur within a few hours of RAI administration and resolve by 1–2 days [57].

Another important side effect is sialadenitis that can lead to xerostomia, in up to 30 % of adults. This is thought to be due to the ability of the salivary glands to concentrate significant amount of iodine from the plasma [56]. Symptoms suggestive of salivary gland dysfunction are reported in approximately 60 % of patients treated with RAI, with most cases occurring within the first 6 months; the overall incidence of these symptoms increases as the RAI dose increases [56, 58].

A systematic review of two large observational studies found an increased relative risk for secondary malignancies and leukemia in patients treated with RAI compared to those that were not; the risk for other specific cancers was not elevated [59].

Other described side effects of therapy include bone marrow suppression, hyponatremia, hypospermia, and nasolacrimal duct obstruction [56, 57]. Radiation pulmonary fibrosis has been described in patients with high lung uptake who are treated with high doses of RAI [23].

Conclusions

RAI is an effective treatment option for patients with DTC who are found to have recurrent or metastatic disease during follow-up. Patients who will undergo treatment with RAI should be placed on a low iodine diet (to deplete iodine stores) and have elevated TSH levels at the time of treatment (achieved with rhTSH or THW). The dose of RAI to be given can be based on empiric regimen strategies or estimated with the use of dosimetry. Patients should be counseled about the potential acute and chronic side effects and treatment burden of RAI.

References

1. Davies L, Welch HG. Current thyroid cancer trends in the United States. JAMA Otolaryngol Head Neck Surg. 2014;140(4):317–22. doi:10.1001/jamaoto.2014.1.
2. Pellegriti G, Frasca F, Regalbuto C, Squatrito S, Vigneri R. Worldwide increasing incidence of thyroid cancer: update on epidemiology and risk factors. J Cancer Epidemiol. 2013;2013:965212. doi:10.1155/2013/965212.
3. Lepoutre-Lussey C, Deandreis D, Leboulleux S, Schlumberger M. Postoperative radioactive iodine administration for differentiated thyroid cancer patients. Curr Opin Endocrinol Diabetes Obes. 2014;21(5):363–71. doi:10.1097/MED.0000000000000100.
4. Haugen BR, Alexander EK, Bible KC, Doherty GM, Mandel SJ, Nikiforov YE, Pacini F, Randolph GW, Sawka AM, Schlumberger M, Schuff KG, Sherman SI, Sosa JA, Steward DL, Tuttle RM, Wartofsky L. 2015 American Thyroid Association Management Guidelines for Adult Patients with Thyroid Nodules and Differentiated Thyroid Cancer: the American Thyroid Association Guidelines Task Force on Thyroid Nodules and Differentiated Thyroid Cancer. Thyroid. 2016;26(1):1–133. doi:10.1089/thy.2015.0020.
5. Carvalho DP, Ferreira AC. The importance of sodium/iodide symporter (NIS) for thyroid cancer management. Arq Bras Endocrinol Metabol. 2007;51(5):672–82.
6. Haymart MR, Banerjee M, Stewart AK, Koenig RJ, Birkmeyer JD, Griggs JJ. Use of radioactive iodine for thyroid cancer. JAMA. 2011;306(7):721–8. doi:10.1001/jama.2011.1139.
7. Cooper DS, Doherty GM, Haugen BR, Kloos RT, Lee SL, Mandel SJ, Mazzaferri EL, McIver B, Pacini F, Schlumberger M, Sherman SI, Steward DL, Tuttle RM. Revised American Thyroid

Association management guidelines for patients with thyroid nodules and differentiated thyroid cancer. Thyroid. 2009;19(11):1167–214. doi:10.1089/thy.2009.0110.
8. Mazzaferri EL, Kloos RT. Clinical review 128: current approaches to primary therapy for papillary and follicular thyroid cancer. J Clin Endocrinol Metab. 2001;86(4):1447–63. doi:10.1210/jcem.86.4.7407.
9. Scheffel RS, Zanella AB, Antunes D, Dora JM, Maia AL. Low recurrence rates in a cohort of differentiated thyroid carcinoma patients: a referral center experience. Thyroid. 2015;25(8):883–9. doi:10.1089/thy.2015.0077.
10. Suh YJ, Kwon H, Kim SJ, Choi JY, Lee KE, Park YJ, Park do J, Youn YK. Factors affecting the locoregional recurrence of conventional papillary thyroid carcinoma after surgery: a retrospective analysis of 3381 patients. Ann Surg Oncol. 2015;22(11):3543–9. doi:10.1245/s10434-015-4448-9.
11. Giovanella L, Clark PM, Chiovato L, Duntas L, Elisei R, Feldt-Rasmussen U, Leenhardt L, Luster M, Schalin-Jantti C, Schott M, Seregni E, Rimmele H, Smit J, Verburg FA. DIAGNOSIS OF ENDOCRINE DISEASE Thyroglobulin measurement using highly sensitive assays in patients with differentiated thyroid cancer: a clinical position paper. Eur J Endocrinol. 2014;171(2):R33–46. doi:10.1530/Eje-14-0148.
12. Jonklaas J. Role of radioactive iodine for adjuvant therapy and treatment of metastases. J Natl Compr Canc Netw. 2007;5(6):631–40.
13. Schlumberger M, Baudin E. Serum thyroglobulin determination in the follow-up of patients with differentiated thyroid carcinoma. Eur J Endocrinol. 1998;138(3):249–52.
14. Giovanella L, Ceriani L, Suriano S, Ghelfo A, Maffioli M. Thyroglobulin measurement before rhTSH-aided 131I ablation in detecting metastases from differentiated thyroid carcinoma. Clin Endocrinol (Oxf). 2008;69(4):659–63. doi:10.1111/j.1365-2265.2008.03244.x.
15. Toubeau M, Touzery C, Arveux P, Chaplain G, Vaillant G, Berriolo A, Riedinger JM, Boichot C, Cochet A, Brunotte F. Predictive value for disease progression of serum thyroglobulin levels measured in the postoperative period and after (131)I ablation therapy in patients with differentiated thyroid cancer. J Nucl Med. 2004;45(6):988–94.
16. Aygun N. Imaging of recurrent thyroid cancer. Otolaryngol Clin North Am. 2008;41(6):1095–106. doi:10.1016/j.otc.2008.05.003. viii.
17. Westbury C, Vini L, Fisher C, Harmer C. Recurrent differentiated thyroid cancer without elevation of serum thyroglobulin. Thyroid. 2000;10(2):171–6.
18. do Rosario PWS, Borges MAR, Fagundes TA, Franco ACHM, Purisch S. Is stimulation of thyroglobulin (Tg) useful in low-risk patients with thyroid carcinoma and undetectable Tg on thyroxin and negative neck ultrasound? Clin Endocrinol (Oxf). 2005;62(2):121–5. doi:10.1111/j.1365-2265.2005.00212.x.
19. Persoon AC, Jager PL, Sluiter WJ, Plukker JT, Wolffenbuttel BH, Links TP. A sensitive Tg assay or rhTSH stimulated Tg: what's the best in the long-term follow-up of patients with differentiated thyroid carcinoma? PLoS One. 2007;2(8):e816. doi:10.1371/journal.pone.0000816.
20. Rosario PW, Furtado Mde S, Mineiro Filho AF, Lacerda RX, Calsolari MR. Value of diagnostic radioiodine whole-body scanning after initial therapy in patients with differentiated thyroid cancer at intermediate and high risk for recurrence. Thyroid. 2012;22(11):1165–9. doi:10.1089/thy.2012.0026.
21. de Meer SG, Vriens MR, Zelissen PM, Borel Rinkes IH, de Keizer B. The role of routine diagnostic radioiodine whole-body scintigraphy in patients with high-risk differentiated thyroid cancer. J Nucl Med. 2011;52(1):56–9. doi:10.2967/jnumed.110.080697.
22. Hoang JK, Sosa JA, Nguyen XV, Galvin PL, Oldan JD. Imaging thyroid disease: updates, imaging approach, and management pearls. Radiol Clin North Am. 2015;53(1):145–61. doi:10.1016/j.rcl.2014.09.002.
23. Al-Qahtani KH, Al Asiri M, Tunio MA, Aljohani NJ, Bayoumi Y, Munir I, AlAyoubi A. Nasolacrimal duct obstruction following radioactive iodine 131 therapy in differentiated thyroid cancers: review of 19 cases. Clin Ophthalmol. 2014;8:2479–84. doi:10.2147/OPTH.S71708.

24. Kucuk ON, Gultekin SS, Aras G, Ibis E. Radioiodine whole-body scans, thyroglobulin levels, 99mTc-MIBI scans and computed tomography: results in patients with lung metastases from differentiated thyroid cancer. Nucl Med Commun. 2006;27(3):261–6.
25. Piekarski JD, Schlumberger M, Leclere J, Couanet D, Masselot J, Parmentier C. Chest computed tomography (CT) in patients with micronodular lung metastases of differentiated thyroid carcinoma. Int J Radiat Oncol Biol Phys. 1985;11(5):1023–7.
26. Lal G, Fairchild T, Howe JR, Weigel RJ, Sugg SL, Menda Y. PET-CT scans in recurrent or persistent differentiated thyroid cancer: is there added utility beyond conventional imaging? Surgery. 2010;148(6):1082–9. doi:10.1016/j.surg.2010.09.015; discussion 1089–1090.
27. Leboulleux S, Schroeder PR, Schlumberger M, Ladenson PW. The role of PET in follow-up of patients treated for differentiated epithelial thyroid cancers. Nat Clin Pract Endocrinol Metab. 2007;3(2):112–21. doi:10.1038/ncpendmet0402.
28. Grant CS. Recurrence of papillary thyroid cancer after optimized surgery. Gland Surg. 2015;4(1):52–62. doi:10.3978/j.issn.2227-684X.2014.12.06.
29. Lewis BD, Hay ID, Charboneau JW, McIver B, Reading CC, Goellner JR. Percutaneous ethanol injection for treatment of cervical lymph node metastases in patients with papillary thyroid carcinoma. AJR Am J Roentgenol. 2002;178(3):699–704. doi:10.2214/ajr.178.3.1780699.
30. Lim CY, Yun JS, Lee J, Nam KH, Chung WY, Park CS. Percutaneous ethanol injection therapy for locally recurrent papillary thyroid carcinoma. Thyroid. 2007;17(4):347–50. doi:10.1089/thy.2006.0251.
31. Magarey MJ, Freeman JL. Recurrent well-differentiated thyroid carcinoma. Oral Oncol. 2013;49(7):689–94. doi:10.1016/j.oraloncology.2013.03.434.
32. Ito Y, Kudo T, Kobayashi K, Miya A, Ichihara K, Miyauchi A. Prognostic factors for recurrence of papillary thyroid carcinoma in the lymph nodes, lung, and bone: analysis of 5,768 patients with average 10-year follow-up. World J Surg. 2012;36(6):1274–8. doi:10.1007/s00268-012-1423-5.
33. Patron V, Hitier M, Bedfert C, Le Clech G, Jegoux F. Occult lymph node metastases increase locoregional recurrence in differentiated thyroid carcinoma. Ann Otol Rhinol Laryngol. 2012;121(5):283–90.
34. Ilgan S, Karacalioglu AO, Pabuscu Y, Atac GK, Arslan N, Ozturk E, Gunalp B, Ozguven MA. Iodine-131 treatment and high-resolution CT: results in patients with lung metastases from differentiated thyroid carcinoma. Eur J Nucl Med Mol Imaging. 2004;31(6):825–30. doi:10.1007/s00259-004-1460-x.
35. Samaan NA, Schultz PN, Haynie TP, Ordonez NG. Pulmonary metastasis of differentiated thyroid carcinoma: treatment results in 101 patients. J Clin Endocrinol Metab. 1985;60(2):376–80. doi:10.1210/jcem-60-2-376.
36. Durante C, Haddy N, Baudin E, Leboulleux S, Hartl D, Travagli JP, Caillou B, Ricard M, Lumbroso JD, De Vathaire F, Schlumberger M. Long-term outcome of 444 patients with distant metastases from papillary and follicular thyroid carcinoma: benefits and limits of radioiodine therapy. J Clin Endocrinol Metab. 2006;91(8):2892–9. doi:10.1210/jc.2005-2838.
37. Sawka AM, Ibrahim-Zada I, Galacgac P, Tsang RW, Brierley JD, Ezzat S, Goldstein DP. Dietary iodine restriction in preparation for radioactive iodine treatment or scanning in well-differentiated thyroid cancer: a systematic review. Thyroid. 2010;20(10):1129–38. doi:10.1089/thy.2010.0055.
38. Padovani RP, Maciel RM, Kasamatsu TS, Freitas BC, Marone MM, Camacho CP, Biscolla RP. Assessment of the effect of two distinct restricted iodine diet durations on urinary iodine levels (collected over 24 h or as a single-spot urinary sample) and Na(+)/I(−) symporter expression. Eur Thyroid J. 2015;4(2):99–105. doi:10.1159/000433426.
39. Jury HPT, Castagna MG, Fioravanti C, Cipri C, Brianzoni E, Pacini F. Lack of association between urinary iodine excretion and successful thyroid ablation in thyroid cancer patients. J Clin Endocr Metab. 2010;95(1):230–7. doi:10.1210/jc.2009-1624.

40. Schlumberger M, Lacroix L, Russo D, Filetti S, Bidart JM. Defects in iodide metabolism in thyroid cancer and implications for the follow-up and treatment of patients. Nat Clin Pract Endocrinol Metab. 2007;3(3):260–9. doi:10.1038/ncpendmet0449.
41. Leboeuf R, Perron P, Carpentier AC, Verreault J, Langlois MF. L-T3 preparation for whole-body scintigraphy: a randomized-controlled trial. Clin Endocrinol (Oxf). 2007;67(6):839–44. doi:10.1111/j.1365-2265.2007.02972.x.
42. Lim DJ, Kim WB, Kim BH, Kim TY, Jo YS, Kang HC, Park YJ, Yi KH, Shong M, Kim IJ, Park do J, Kim SW, Chung JH, Lee J, Koong SS, Shong YK. Differences in physicians' and patients' perception of acute hypothyroid symptoms induced by thyroid hormone withdrawal in thyroid cancer patients: a multicenter survey in Korea. Eur Thyroid J. 2015;4(1):48–54. doi:10.1159/000371512.
43. Marturano I, Russo M, Spadaro A, Latina A, Malandrino P, Regalbuto C. Comparison of conventional L-thyroxine withdrawal and moderate hypothyroidism in preparation for whole-body 131-I scan and thyroglobulin testing. J Endocrinol Invest. 2015;38(9):1017–22. doi:10.1007/s40618-015-0318-3.
44. Luster M, Lassmann M, Haenscheid H, Michalowski U, Incerti C, Reiners C. Use of recombinant human thyrotropin before radioiodine therapy in patients with advanced differentiated thyroid carcinoma. J Clin Endocr Metab. 2000;85(10):3640–5. doi:10.1210/jc.85.10.3640.
45. Robbins RJ, Driedger A, Magner J. Recombinant human thyrotropin-assisted radioiodine therapy for patients with metastatic thyroid cancer who could not elevate endogenous thyrotropin or be withdrawn from thyroxine. Thyroid. 2006;16(11):1121–30. doi:10.1089/thy.2006.16.1121.
46. Luster M, Lippi F, Jarzab B, Perros P, Lassmann M, Reiners C, Pacini F. rhTSH-aided radioiodine ablation and treatment of differentiated thyroid carcinoma: a comprehensive review. Endocr Relat Cancer. 2005;12(1):49–64. doi:10.1677/erc.1.00830.
47. Tuttle RM, Lopez N, Leboeuf R, Minkowitz SM, Grewal R, Brokhin M, Omry G, Larson S. Radioactive iodine administered for thyroid remnant ablation following recombinant human thyroid stimulating hormone preparation also has an important adjuvant therapy function. Thyroid. 2010;20(3):257–63. doi:10.1089/thy.2009.0401.
48. Klubo-Gwiezdzinska J, Burman KD, Van Nostrand D, Mete M, Jonklaas J, Wartofsky L. Radioiodine treatment of metastatic thyroid cancer: relative efficacy and side effect profile of preparation by thyroid hormone withdrawal versus recombinant human thyrotropin. Thyroid. 2012;22(3):310–7. doi:10.1089/thy.2011.0235.
49. Tala H, Robbins R, Fagin JA, Larson SM, Tuttle RM. Five-year survival is similar in thyroid cancer patients with distant metastases prepared for radioactive iodine therapy with either thyroid hormone withdrawal or recombinant human TSH. J Clin Endocrinol Metab. 2011;96(7):2105–11. doi:10.1210/jc.2011-0305.
50. Tuttle RM, Leboeuf R, Robbins RJ, Qualey R, Pentlow K, Larson SM, Chan CY. Empiric radioactive iodine dosing regimens frequently exceed maximum tolerated activity levels in elderly patients with thyroid cancer. J Nucl Med. 2006;47(10):1587–91.
51. Kulkarni K, Van Nostrand D, Atkins F, Aiken M, Burman K, Wartofsky L. The relative frequency in which empiric dosages of radioiodine would potentially overtreat or undertreat patients who have metastatic well-differentiated thyroid cancer. Thyroid. 2006;16(10):1019–23. doi:10.1089/thy.2006.16.1019.
52. Chao M. Management of differentiated thyroid cancer with rising thyroglobulin and negative diagnostic radioiodine whole body scan. Clin Oncol (R Coll Radiol). 2010;22(6):438–47. doi:10.1016/j.clon.2010.05.005.
53. Pacini F, Agate L, Elisei R, Capezzone M, Ceccarelli C, Lippi F, Molinaro E, Pinchera A. Outcome of differentiated thyroid cancer with detectable serum Tg and negative diagnostic (131)I whole body scan: comparison of patients treated with high (131)I activities versus untreated patients. J Clin Endocrinol Metab. 2001;86(9):4092–7. doi:10.1210/jcem.86.9.7831.

54. Sherman SI, Tielens ET, Sostre S, Wharam Jr MD, Ladenson PW. Clinical utility of posttreatment radioiodine scans in the management of patients with thyroid carcinoma. J Clin Endocrinol Metab. 1994;78(3):629–34. doi:10.1210/jcem.78.3.8126134.
55. Alzahrani AS, Bakheet S, Al Mandil M, Al-Hajjaj A, Almahfouz A, Al Haj A. 123I isotope as a diagnostic agent in the follow-up of patients with differentiated thyroid cancer: comparison with post 131I therapy whole body scanning. J Clin Endocrinol Metab. 2001;86(11):5294–300. doi:10.1210/jcem.86.11.8030.
56. Fard-Esfahani A, Emami-Ardekani A, Fallahi B, Fard-Esfahani P, Beiki D, Hassanzadeh-Rad A, Eftekhari M. Adverse effects of radioactive iodine-131 treatment for differentiated thyroid carcinoma. Nucl Med Commun. 2014;35(8):808–17. doi:10.1097/MNM.0000000000000132.
57. Van Nostrand D, Neutze J, Atkins F. Side effects of "rational dose" iodine-131 therapy for metastatic well-differentiated thyroid carcinoma. J Nucl Med. 1986;27(10):1519–27.
58. Kim J-h, Yoo WS, Park YJ, Park DJ, Yun TJ, Choi SH, Sohn C-H, Lee KE, Sung M-W, Youn Y-K, Kim KH, Cho BY. Efficacy and safety of radiofrequency ablation for treatment of locally recurrent thyroid cancers smaller than 2 cm. Radiology 2015;276(3):909–18. doi:http://dx.doi.org/10.1148/radiol.15140079.
59. Sawka AM, Thabane L, Parlea L, Ibrahim-Zada I, Tsang RW, Brierley JD, Straus S, Ezzat S, Goldstein DP. Second primary malignancy risk after radioactive iodine treatment for thyroid cancer: a systematic review and meta-analysis. Thyroid. 2009;19(5):451–7. doi:10.1089/thy.2008.0392.

Chapter 22
Surveillance of Treated Thyroid Cancer Patients and Thyroid Hormone Replacement and Suppression

Jennifer M. Perkins

Epidemiology

Differentiated thyroid cancer is increasing in incidence. The Surveillance, Epidemiology, and End Results (SEER) program database estimates that there will be 62,450 new cases of thyroid cancer in 2015, representing 3.8 % of all new cancers, and there will be 1950 deaths resulting from thyroid cancer. The incidence has been rising at about 5 % per year [1]. Thyroid cancer affects women more than men resulting in 47,230 of the 62,450 estimated cases to be in women. Deaths estimated in 2015 will occur in 1080 women and 870 men [2]. The yearly incidence has nearly tripled from 4.9 per 100,000 in 1979 to 14.3 per 100,000 in 2009 [3]. Nearly two out of three thyroid cancers will be detected in patients under 55 [3]. Overall, the 5-year survival for differentiated thyroid cancer is 97.9 % [1]. Many investigators feel the rise in incidence is due to detection earlier of small thyroid cancers with radiologic intensity; however, some studies have shown a rise in larger tumors being diagnosed as well [4]. Several authors including Vigneri et al. feel that thyroid cancer incidence is increasing due to two processes: (1) increased detection and (2) increased incidence due to thyroid-specific carcinogens that are not fully recognized nor studied; this latter point is the focus of ongoing investigations [5]. Almost the entire increase in incidence can be attributed to papillary thyroid cancers. Additionally, 25 % of the new thyroid cancers diagnosed in 1988–1989 were <1 cm compared to 39 % in 2008–2009 [3].

Approximately 88 % of all differentiated thyroid cancers (DTC) are papillary thyroid cancer (PTC) (and its various subtypes), while 8 % are follicular thyroid cancer [6]. DTC can occur at any age, but has a median age of diagnosis of 49 years,

---

J.M. Perkins, MD, MBA
Division of Endocrinology, Duke University Health System, Durham, NC 27710, USA
e-mail: Jen.perkins@duke.edu

S.A. Roman et al. (eds.), *Management of Thyroid Nodules and Differentiated Thyroid Cancer*, DOI 10.1007/978-3-319-43618-0_22

with approximately 39 % of new cases diagnosed prior to the age of 45 years. Women are about three times more likely to develop DTC [1]. By the year 2019, one study predicts that papillary thyroid cancer will be the third most common cancer in women at a healthcare cost of $19–21 billion in the United States alone, representing a major growing healthcare concern [7].

Prognosis

Overall prognosis for DTC is quite good. The goals of initial therapy (specifically surgery) are to (1) remove the primary tumor and any disease that has extended beyond the thyroid capsule including nodal metastases that are clinically significant; (2) minimize the risk of disease recurrence; (3) facilitate radioactive iodine ablation, adjuvant, or therapeutic, when appropriate; (4) permit accurate staging and risk stratification of the disease and prognostication; (5) permit accurate long-term surveillance for disease recurrence; and (6) minimize treatment-related morbidity [8].

In patients who have PTC tumors >1 cm with no extrathyroidal extension or vascular invasion, their risk of death is nearly 0 % and risk of recurrence on average is 2 % [9]. Patients with clinical N1 disease will have an overall risk of recurrence of 13–42 %, whereas those with pathological N1 disease will have a 7–14 % risk of recurrence [10]. Those with larger metastases and extra-nodal extension are at the highest risk for recurrence [10]. In terms of survival, stage I and II patients have a near 96–99.7 % relative 5-year survival rate vs. 91 % for stage III and 50 % for stage IV [11, 12].

Surveillance of DTC

Although most patients with DTC have a favorable long-term survival, up to 30 % of patients may experience a recurrence overall, but this is very dependent on initial staging and clinical findings [13]. Clinically evident disease recurrence has been reported up to 30 or 40 years after initial therapy, but large retrospective studies consistently show that the vast majority of recurrences are detected within 10–15 years after initial therapy [14].

Short-term and long-term surveillance strategies continue to evolve based on ongoing scientific investigations. Typically, current surveillance regimens for most patients with DTC include serial thyroglobulin measurements coupled with cervical ultrasound at a minimum to identify residual or recurrent disease, which commonly occurs within the thyroidectomy bed or lateral cervical lymph node chains [15]. In order to recommend how best to provide surveillance for a patient with treated thyroid cancer in the postoperative setting, it is important to use all of the available clinical data to individually risk-stratify patients [12]. This would include the original pathology report; pre- or postoperative neck imaging, which is typically in the form of an ultrasound; and postoperative serum thyroglobulin levels. A careful analysis of these data points can provide initial estimates for risk of recurrence, risk of having persistent disease, disease-specific mortality, and TSH suppression goals; it can guide providers in choosing the best imaging modalities for surveillance [16]. Tailoring a risk-stratified approach to individual patient care could lead to a more cost-effective approach, and possibly higher quality of life by reducing the burden of adverse treatment effects, and the stress and costs of ongoing surveillance. Providers are encouraged to stage patients postoperatively to provide prognostic information that is of value when considering disease surveillance and therapeutic strategies. In addition, this allows tracking of patients for communication among other healthcare professionals, tracking by various cancer registries and for research purposes [8].

The first-line therapy in nearly all patients is surgery, followed by radioactive iodine in some intermediate- and high-risk patients. The ATA has developed risk categories to help guide clinicians in initial treatment and subsequent surveillance as defined below.

ATA low-risk patients include papillary thyroid cancer with all of the following:

- No local or distant metastases.
- All macroscopic tumor has been resected.
- No invasion into locoregional tissues.
- Tumor does not have aggressive histology including tall cell, insular, columnar cell, Hurthle cell, or follicular cell thyroid carcinoma (FTC).
- No vascular invasion.
- No I131 uptake outside the thyroid bed if an I123 or I131 scan is done.
- Clinical N0 or ≤5 pathological N1 micrometastases (<0.2 cm in largest dimension).
- Intrathyroidal, encapsulated follicular variant of PTC.
- Intrathyroidal, well-differentiated FTC with capsular invasion and no or minimal (<4 foci), vascular invasion.
- Intrathyroidal, papillary microcarcinoma (<1 cm), unifocal, or multifocal, including V600E BRAF mutated if known.

ATA intermediate-risk patients include:

- Microscopic invasion into the perithyroidal soft tissues (minimal extrathyroidal extension [ETE])
- Cervical lymph node metastases or I131 uptake outside the thyroid bed on post-treatment scan done after thyroid remnant ablation
- Tumor with aggressive histology or vascular invasion (e.g., tall cell, insular, columnar, Hurthle cell, hobnail, or FTC)
- Papillary thyroid cancer with vascular invasion

- Clinical N1 or >5 pathological N1 with all involved LNs <3 cm in largest dimension
- Intrathyroidal, PTC with primary tumor 1–4 cm, and V600E BRAF mutated if known
- Multifocal papillary microcarcinoma with extrathyroidal extension and BRAF 600E mutated (if known)

ATA high-risk patients include:

- Macroscopic tumor invasion into the perithyroidal soft tissues (gross ETE)
- Gross residual tumor
- Distant metastases
- Postoperative serum thyroglobulin suggestive of distant metastases
- Pathologic N1 with any metastatic LN $\geq$ 3 in largest dimension
- FTC with extensive vascular invasion (>4 foci)

[Adapted from the new American Thyroid Association guidelines, reference [8]]

Although most DTCs have a very favorable long-term prognosis, the disease can recur many years after initial diagnosis leading the provider to decide on a long-term plan for how best to provide surveillance for these treated thyroid cancer patients. No evidence of disease (NED) is defined as stimulated thyroglobulin <1 ng/ml with no other radiological or clinical evidence of disease. Studies looking at estimates of patients in each risk category who subsequently were characterized as no evidence of disease (NED) after total thyroidectomy and RAI remnant ablation found that 78–91 % of low-risk patients were NED; intermediate-risk patients, 52–64 % NED; and high risk, 31–32 % NED [8, 17–20]. Over a follow-up period of 5–10 years, structural disease recurrence was found in less than 1–2 % of ATA low-risk patients and 8 % of intermediate-risk patients who underwent thyroid surgery without RAI ablation as initial therapy [21–23].

It is also important to consider the clinical significance of "persistent disease." In ATA low-risk patients, 70–80 % of persistent disease is manifest by abnormal serum thyroglobulin levels (suppressed or stimulated thyroglobulin >1 ng/ml) without identifiable structural disease, whereas in intermediate-risk patients, this ranges from 29 to 51 % and in high-risk patients 19–21 % [17, 20]. When counseling patients on risk of recurrence and tailoring surveillance strategies, the original pathology provides critical data. For example, patients with unifocal intrathyroidal papillary microcarcinomas experience structural disease recurrence of 1–2 % [24, 25] which increases to 5–6 % in 2–4 cm intrathyroidal PTCs [26] and 8–10 % in intrathyroidal PTCs >4 cm [26]. Intermediate-risk patients with locoregional lymph node involvement can have a risk of structural disease recurrence of 4 % in patients with fewer than five metastatic lymph nodes, 5 % if all lymph nodes involved are <0.2 cm, 19 % if more than five lymph nodes are involved, 21 % if >10 lymph nodes, 22 % if macroscopic lymph nodes are clinically evident (CN1 disease), and 27–32 % if any metastatic nodes are greater than 3 cm [10, 27].

Ultimately, all imaging (including structural and functional), biochemical, and cytopathological data should be used for a dynamic, ongoing redefinition of clinical status to assess the individual response to therapy at each follow-up visit over time. This re-evaluation should direct intensity of surveillance and follow-up.

Surveillance of Treated Thyroid Cancer in the First Year Post Initial Therapy

The intensity of surveillance should depend on the original risk stratification of the patient. We now have a better understanding that risk stratification is ongoing at each visit, and dynamic. As patients move through the first year and beyond following initial therapy, providers need to undertake dynamic risk stratification based on available data and use this to re-evaluate their management plans. Our newest guidelines recommend putting patients into categories of "excellent response, biochemical incomplete, structural incomplete, and indeterminate".

Excellent response implies negative imaging, and either undetectable suppressed thyroglobulin or TSH-stimulated thyroglobulin <1 ng/ml. Patients who achieve an excellent response will have a 1–4 % risk of recurrence and a <1 % disease-specific death risk [8]. If patients are able to achieve this, they typically can undergo a decrease in intensity and frequency of follow-up and the degree of TSH suppression [8].

Patients who experience a biochemical incomplete response are characterized by negative imaging and a suppressed thyroglobulin >1 ng/ml, or a stimulated thyroglobulin >10 ng/ml, or a rising thyroglobulin antibody level. At least 30 % of these patients will spontaneously evolve to NED, 20 % will achieve NED after additional therapy, 20 % develop structural disease, and <1 % will experience disease-specific death [8]. Patients in this category who have stable or declining serum thyroglobulin levels should undergo continued observation with ongoing TSH suppression in most patients. Rising thyroglobulin or thyroglobulin antibody values should prompt additional investigations and potentially additional therapies [8].

Patients who fall into the category of structurally incomplete response will exhibit structural or functional evidence of disease with any thyroglobulin level +/− thyroglobulin antibodies. Patients in this category will continue to have persistent disease, despite additional therapy, 50–85 % of the time. The disease-specific death rate may be as high as 11 % with locoregional metastases, and 50 % with structural distant metastases. Patients with structural incomplete response may undergo additional treatments, or ongoing observation depending on multiple clinicopathologic factors including size, locations, rate of growth, RAI avidity, PET avidity, and specific pathology of the structural disease [8].

Indeterminate response includes patients with nonspecific findings on imaging studies or faint uptake in thyroid bed on RAI scanning; detectable non-stimulated thyroglobulin, but less than 1 ng/ml; detectable stimulated thyroglobulin but less than 10 ng/ml; or stable or declining thyroglobulin antibodies in the absence of structural of functional disease. Of these patients, 15–20 % will have structural disease identified during follow-up. In the remainder, the nonspecific changes are either stable or resolve. Less than 1 % will experience disease-specific death. Patients in this category should undergo continued observation with appropriate serial imaging of the nonspecific lesions and serum thyroglobulin monitoring. Nonspecific findings that become suspicious over time should be evaluated further with additional imaging or undergo therapy [8].

Thyroglobulin and cervical neck ultrasound are cornerstones of surveillance. Measurement of serum thyroglobulin is an important modality to monitor patients for persistent or recurrent disease. Following initial therapy, patients at low risk of recurrence and death can be followed with a suppressed thyroglobulin every 6–9 months in the first 2 years with no need to obtain a stimulated thyroglobulin value if there are no other suspicious clinical concerns [16]. These patients should undergo at least one follow-up neck ultrasound [16] keeping in mind that surveillance ultrasounds in this low-risk population are more likely to have false positives and lead to more procedures, including follow-up ultrasounds, FNA, and more patient anxiety.

Long-Term Surveillance of Treated Thyroid Cancer Patients

Long-term surveillance strategies also need to be individualized based on original risk of recurrence and mortality of the thyroid cancer patient. Determining accurate surveillance for possible recurrence in patients presumed disease-free is the major goal of long-term follow-up. Highly specific tests allow recognition of patients unlikely to experience disease recurrence so that less aggressive, more cost-effective, and safe management strategies can be deployed. Patients with higher risks of recurrence should be monitored more aggressively since early detection of recurrent disease is thought to offer the best opportunity for most effective care.

Most recurrences of DTC occur within the first 5–8 years after initial treatment; however, recurrences may occur even decades later, particularly in patients with PTC [28]. Long-term follow-up is guided by the evaluation of how the patient responded to therapy in the first 1–2 years of original diagnosis [12]. At each subsequent visit, patients should be classified as having one of the following clinical outcomes to direct long-term surveillance [12, 17]:

- Excellent response: no clinical or biochemical or structural evidence of disease
- Biochemical incomplete response: abnormal thyroglobulin levels in the absence of localized disease
- Structural incomplete response: persistent or newly identified locoregional or distant metastases
- Indeterminate response: nonspecific biochemical or structural findings that cannot be classified as either benign or malignant confidently

When defining an excellent response or a biochemical incomplete response, the extent of the initial therapy is key. In patients who have undergone total thyroidectomy and RAI remnant ablation, an excellent response is defined as a stimulated thyroglobulin value of <1 ng/ml or a highly sensitive non-stimulated thyroglobulin of <0.2 ng/ml with negative imaging and commonly a normal postoperative neck ultrasound. In patients who underwent total thyroidectomy without subsequent RAI therapy, a non-stimulated thyroglobulin value of <1 ng/ml is considered an excellent response. In patients treated with less than total thyroidectomy, non-stimulated thyroglobulin values less than 20 ng/ml are considered an excellent response. This equals about 50 % of the thyroglobulin expected from a normal thyroid. Any thyroglobulin value above these ranges is considered biochemical incomplete response in the absence of confirmed structural disease.

Patients classified as having an excellent response to therapy should have a decrease in the intensity of their surveillance and frequency of follow-up. They should have their TSH goal raised to 0.5–2 mU/L and be seen for physical exam and non-stimulated thyroglobulin levels yearly with surveillance neck ultrasound at 3–5-year intervals. Patients originally classified at ATA intermediate or high risk who then achieve an excellent response to therapy may benefit from closer follow-up and more intense suppression for a few more years.

Patients who demonstrate a biochemical incomplete response to therapy defined as an abnormal thyroglobulin in the absence of structurally identifiable disease should continue to be monitored every 6 months with ongoing TSH suppression and yearly neck ultrasound for several more years. Patients with stable or declining thyroglobulin values should continue routine surveillance and TSH suppression, while those with rising thyroglobulin should prompt additional imaging modalities and evaluation.

Patients deemed to have a structural incomplete response to therapy could require additional imaging or therapy depending on several clinical factors including location, rate of growth, FDG or RAI avidity, and pathology.

Patients with an indeterminate response to therapy defined as a nonspecific, biochemical, or structural imaging should continue on mild TSH suppression (0.1–0.5 mU/L) with 6-month follow-up visits for 2–3 years with yearly neck ultrasound. After that time, most patients can be reclassified [12, 17]. In summary, in terms of clinical decision making and algorithms for those who underwent partial thyroidectomy and are ATA low risk, follow-up should consist of possibly serum thyroglobulin levels and ultrasound; radioactive iodine scanning is not indicated. The TSH goal is 0.5–2 mU/L in most cases [8]. If there is an excellent response to therapy, non-stimulated thyroglobulin levels can be followed every 12–24 months with periodic neck ultrasounds [8].

In patients who received total thyroidectomy and are ATA low risk, we recommend routine use of postoperative serum thyroglobulin, and postoperative ultrasound can be used, with consideration of radioactive iodine scanning. Radioactive iodine treatment is typically not given, but if it is, low-dose ablation such as 30 mCi can be used for initial therapy [8]. Initial TSH goal is 0.1–0.5 mU/L if thyroglobulin is >0.2 and 0.5–1 mU/L if thyroglobulin <0.2. Response to therapy is evaluated by serum thyroglobulin and ultrasound, and if excellent response is detected, TSH is allowed to be 0.5–2 mU/L [8]. Once an excellent biochemical response is demonstrated, unstimulated thyroglobulin can be measured at 12–24 month intervals with periodic neck ultrasounds [8].

In ATA intermediate-risk patients who have undergone total thyroidectomy +/− prophylactic central neck and/or lateral neck dissections, routine use of postoperative serum thyroglobulin is recommended, and postoperative RAI scanning and ultrasound are to be considered [8]. For RAI remnant ablation, lower doses such as 30 mCI is generally favored over higher doses, and for adjuvant therapy, doses up to 150 mCI are administered in the absence of distant metastases [8]. The initial TSH goal is 0.1–0.5 mU/L. The response to therapy is evaluated by thyroglobulin measurement, ultrasound, and consideration of whole-body scanning. If there is an excellent response to therapy, the TSH goal can be allowed to come up to 0.5–2 mU/L and the patient be followed by periodic non-stimulated thyroglobulin and neck ultrasound imaging [8].

In ATA high-risk patients who have undergone total thyroidectomy+/− prophylactic central neck and/or lateral neck dissections, routine use of postoperative thyroglobulin is recommended, and postoperative RAI scanning and ultrasound are to be considered [8]. RAI should be considered, and adjuvant therapies up to 150 mCi are administered in the absence of distant metastatic disease. For known structural disease, 100–200 mCi or dosimetry is generally used [8]. Initial TSH goal is <0.1 mu/L. Initial response to therapy is assessed via thyroglobulin measurement and neck ultrasound, and consideration should be given to CT/MRI and/or FDG/PET scanning as well as whole-body scanning [8]. If there is an excellent response to therapy, the TSH goal should then become 0.1–0.5 mU/L for at least 5 years with yearly follow-up of thyroglobulin for 5 years and consideration of ultrasound +/−CT/MRI. If there is a biochemical or structural incomplete response, the TSH goal should be <0.1 indefinitely in the absence of contraindications [8].

Long-term survivorship care is becoming more recognized as an important area that requires future research. The American Cancer Society estimates that over 63,000 thyroid cancers were diagnosed in 2014, but there were only 1900 deaths [29]. There are over 50,000 thyroid cancer survivors alone in the United States [30]. Despite this, there remains a small amount of peer-reviewed literature on survivorship care.

Thyroglobulin in Patients With and Without RAI Treatment

Thyroid cells are assumed to the be the only source of thyroglobulin in the human body, and hence circulating thyroglobulin levels serve as a biochemical marker of persistent or recurrent disease in DTC follow-up [31]. Thyroglobulin is a large glycoprotein that in normal thyroid tissue is found in the follicular colloid where it serves as a substrate for thyroid hormone synthesis. Since it is only produced by normal or well-differentiated malignant thyrocytes, it serves as a suitable tumor marker [32]. Thyroglobulin assays became available in the 1980s and have greatly improved in sensitivity and precision [33], and have become a cornerstone in surveillance of patients post initial treatment. Since thyroglobulin has a half-life of 65 h, the levels typically nadir 4–6 weeks post-surgery [33].

The Presence of Thyroglobulin Antibodies and Challenges with Interpreting Thyroglobulin Levels

Most thyroglobulin assays are immunometric, but unfortunately are prone to interference from autoantibodies to thyroglobulin, which can occur in approximately 25 % of thyroid cancer patients and 10 % of the general population, particularly in patients with Hashimoto's thyroiditis [34, 35].

The presence of thyroglobulin antibodies may cause a falsely low serum thyroglobulin measurement [36]. Given this, it is recommended to measure concomitant serum thyroglobulin antibodies when measuring serum thyroglobulin. No method reliably eliminates thyroglobulin antibody interference, but radioimmunoassays (RIA) for thyroglobulin may be less prone to antibody interference [37–39]. RIA assays, however, are often not as sensitive (lower limit of detection) compared to immunometric assays. Recurrent or progressive disease should be suspected in patients with rising positive antithyroglobulin antibodies, while falling levels may indicate successful therapy [40, 41]. In most patients who have undergone total thyroidectomy and RAI remnant ablation, thyroglobulin antibodies tend to disappear over a median of 3 years in patients without recurrent or persistent disease [42–44]. Several studies have shown an increased risk of recurrence or persistent disease associated with either a new appearance of antithyroglobulin antibodies or a rising titer, and thus should prompt further investigation [40, 42, 45, 46].

Imaging Modalities Used in Surveillance of DTC

Ultrasound

Ultrasound is widely used in patients with both thyroid nodules and thyroid cancer from initial detection, diagnosis, preoperative planning, and finally to postoperative surveillance. Cervical ultrasound is well suited for surveillance since most recurrences of differentiated thyroid cancer and metastases occur within the thyroid bed and in the cervical lymph node chains; it is low cost and noninvasive without radiation exposure [15]. Once a patient has had either total thyroidectomy or partial thyroidectomy, ultrasonography can be used to monitor the thyroid bed for recurrence or for evaluating for suspicious nodules in the remaining thyroid [47].

Ultrasonography can also evaluate for abnormal appearing lymph nodes in the central compartment (in a postsurgical neck) and in the lateral compartments [47].

Differentiated thyroid carcinoma, especially PTC, has been found to involve cervical lymph node metastases in 20–50 % of patients in several studies [48–50], and may be present even in the stetting of a primary tumor that is small and intrathyroidal [51, 52]. However, the clinical significance of small volume, occult lymph node metastases is still unclear.

Abnormal lymph nodes on ultrasound examination may include calcifications, cystic changes, rounded shape, hyperechogenicity, absence of a fatty hilum, abnormal vascularity, and an increased short-axis diameter [53]. Nodal microcalcifications and cystic changes are highly indicative of malignancy, and several studies have shown these two characteristics together to have reported specificities near 100 % [54]. No single sonographic feature, however, is adequately sensitive to identify malignant cervical lymph nodes with thyroid cancer.

Normal thyroid remnant tissue appears as vascular lobules of tissue with the same echogenicity of surrounding tissue. Once patients have undergone radioablation, thyroid remnants may appear as hypoechoic, heterogeneous nodules, without internal vascularity [55]. On the other hand, thyroid bed malignant recurrences typically appear as well-defined hypoechoic oval nodules. Sometimes vascularity and microcalcifications can be seen [56]. Since these features are not specific, many entities need to be considered in the differential diagnosis for recurrence, including remnant thyroid, fibrosis, suture granulomas, reactive lymph nodes, and fat necrosis [56].

If an abnormal lymph node or soft tissue is appreciated on ultrasound, confirmation of malignancy with FNA for cytology and/or measurement of thyroglobulin in the needle washout is recommended, particularly if surgical intervention will be recommended [57].

Nuclear Medicine Imaging: I123 vs. I131

Nuclear medicine imaging was once the mainstay imaging modality in the surveillance of thyroid cancer but has largely been replaced by cervical ultrasound as the primary imaging modality. Some studies have reported that whole-body scintigraphy (WBS) has a sensitivity for detection of local recurrence of 20 % vs. cervical ultrasound at 70 % [58]. Routine use of diagnostic WBS for surveillance is not recommended for low-risk patients who did not show uptake outside of the thyroidectomy bed on their initial posttreatment WBS. We still employ diagnostic WBS in patients with intermediate or high risk of recurrence. Additionally, patients with elevated or rising thyroglobulin levels with negative cervical ultrasound should also undergo WBS to assess for recurrence of radioiodine-avid disease [15].

Some thyroid cancers become radioiodine refractory. By definition this includes (1) disease that does not take up iodine at known sites of metastatic disease, (2) continued growth of disease despite RAI therapy and confirmed uptake, (3) distant disease that grows over a 1-year period after RAI, and (4) total cumulative dose of RAI of >600 mCi [59]. It is estimated that 5–15 % of patients will develop RAI refractory disease [60]. The 5-year disease-specific survival rate in DTC that is deemed non-RAI avid is 66 % [61], and the 10-year survival rate is only 10 %. Studies have shown that the overall median survival for patients with RAI refractory disease and distant metastases is 2.5–3.5 years [62].

Cross-Sectional Imaging: CT and MRI

The utilization for computed tomography (CT) and magnetic resonance imaging (MRI) is much less common for surveillance given the advantages and efficacy of ultrasound, particularly in surveillance of treated, lower-risk DTC, as ultrasonography is the preferred method coupled with thyroglobulin determination. One could employ CT in patients with positive serum thyroglobulin levels and negative cervical ultrasound, although, in some circumstances, PET-CT may be more useful. Many use CT of the chest for surveillance of pulmonary metastases in higher-risk patients or those with known previous metastases, as this is a frequent location for metastases in PTC [15]. CT can detect both macro- and micronodular lung disease, in addition to military disease, the latter of which can be missed on WBS or PET imaging due to limited resolution [63].

MRI is not generally used for routine surveillance, but can be utilized to further define anatomy and presence of invasion for aggressive recurrences. In these cases, it can aid in surgical planning. Some studies have shown MRI to be comparable to ultrasonography for detection of recurrence, but US is less invasive, less costly, and easier to perform [64]. Lastly, MRI can be valuable for localizing retroesophageal/retrotracheal tumors and mediastinal disease [15]. The sensitivity of MRI for the detection of cervical metastases in some studies has been shown to be around 30–40 % [65]. MRI can be affected by respiratory artifacts and may be more difficult to interpret than CT scanning, especially in low-volume nodal disease [66].

Positron Emission Tomography with FDG (PET Scan)

PET scanning is generally not useful in patients with no evidence of recurrence or who maintain radioiodine avidity. It is however useful in patients who have a recurrence that is no longer radioiodine avid. When tumors dedifferentiate, there is a decrease in sodium-iodide symporter expression and an increase in glucose transporter-1 expression, the transporter by which FDG is taken up by cells. In this circumstance, PET scan becomes a valuable imaging modality [67]. It is recommended to obtain a PET scan in patients with a negative whole-body I123 or I131 scan and a stimulated thyroglobulin >5–20 ng/ml [8].

TSH Suppression

Goals and Rationale

After total thyroidectomy, thyroxine therapy is required for all patients to maintain TSH levels, whether or not radioactive iodine is given. Partial thyroidectomies may not require thyroxine therapy. Levothyroxine also can limit potential TSH stimulation of tumor growth by keeping the serum TSH suppressed. The American Thyroid Association guidelines for the treatment of thyroid cancer recommend that low-risk disease patients maintain a serum TSH level between 0.1 and 0.5 mU/L until the patient demonstrates an excellent response to therapy, which usually occurs in the first 6–12 months. At that point, the TSH can be kept between 0.5 and 2.0 mU/L. This latter level is also recommended in patients who have undergone lobectomy only for their low-risk disease. For ATA intermediate-risk disease, the serum TSH level should be 0.1–0.5 mU/L [8]. Obviously, the patient's comorbidities, such as active heart disease or bone loss, may dictate that lower doses be utilized. Per the guidelines published in 2015, those patients who have demonstrated an excellent biochemical response can have their serum TSH level kept at 0.5–2.0 mU/l, while for those with an indeterminate response, it may be more appropriate to aim for a TSH level of 0.1–0.5 mU/L, and unless they have age >60 years, osteoporosis, or atrial fibrillation, then their goal is best kept at 0.5–2.0 mU/L [8]. For those patients with no known risks and a biochemical incomplete response or known structural disease, their serum TSH goal should be <0.1 mu/L [8]. Those with active atrial fibrillation tend to be the highest-risk patients for worsening of cardiac disease from serum TSH over-suppression, and unless they have structural disease, their goal should be kept at 0.5–2.0 mU/L. If structural disease is present, even with atrial fibrillation, patients' serum TSH level should be kept at 0.1–0.5 mU/L [8]. Once patients remain disease-free for 5–10 years, the TSH can be allowed to come into the normal range [12]. Practice guidelines recommend combining patient comorbidity with tumor prognostic indicator (excellent response, indeterminate, biochemically incomplete, and structurally incomplete) to determine the best-suited TSH suppression goal [8].

The data supporting TSH suppression to below the normal range impacting thyroid cancer morbidity and mortality is controversial. There is a lack of general consensus as to what degree of suppression is needed across stages to best reduce recurrence and thyroid cancer-related death. It is thought that most well-differentiated thyroid carcinomas express TSH receptors on their cell membrane and respond to TSH stimulation by increasing the expression of several thyroid-specific proteins, such as thyroglobulin, and thus increasing rates of cell/tumor growth [68]. Goitrogens, iodine deficiency, and partial thyroidectomy may promote the development of thyroid cancer, but these tumors can be prevented by the oral administration of levothyroxine or by hypophysectomy, both of which reduce or suppress the secretion of TSH [69]. DTC tissues have functional TSH receptors, and thyroid cancer cells in primary culture respond to TSH stimulation by activating the cyclic-AMP cascade that promotes cell growth [70]. TSH receptors and other thyroid-specific proteins are not well expressed in poorly differentiated thyroid cancers [71]. The first study published describing the regression of PTC in two patients treated with thyroid extracts was published by Dunhill in 1937 [72]. Many years later, Mazzaferri and Jiang published a retrospective analysis of 30 years of follow-up data showing that patients treated with thyroxine therapy had 25 % fewer recurrences and 50 % fewer cancer deaths than those who did not receive hormonal therapy and who had serum TSH levels within the hypothyroid range [73]. Based on these findings and others, suppressing TSH became a cornerstone to therapy in patients with DTC. Although earlier studies found that TSH suppression below physiological levels have reduced thyroid cancer recurrence and disease-specific mortality, this has remained controversial and not well studied by large randomized controlled trials. There are risks to long-term suppression including iatrogenic thyrotoxicosis, bone loss, arrhythmia, angina, and others. Sugitani and Fujimoto evaluated 441 patients with a proven diagnosis of PTC who were randomized to receive serum TSH suppression to <0.01 μU/ml or to not receive any TSH suppression. They excluded patients with tumors less than 1 cm or patients too high risk to undergo suppression (already with known heart disease or bone loss). At 5 years of median follow-up, disease-free survival and recurrence did not differ among these two groups [74]. Carhill et al. performed a multi-institutional disease registry evaluating 4941 patients with DTC. Of these, 88 % had PTC, 8 % had follicular thyroid cancer (FTC), and 4 % had Hurthle cell carcinoma (HCC). Median follow-up was 6 years, but ranged from 0 to 25 years. TSH suppression was graded as serum TSH level undetectable, TSH subnormal but detectable, TSH normal range, and TSH above normal range. In all stages, moderate TSH suppression (subnormal but detectable) was shown to have improved overall and disease-specific survival. Even in the presence of distant metastases, TSH suppression to undetectable levels was not found to improve overall survival above modest TSH suppression. This suggests there may be no benefit across any stage to suppress TSH to an undetectable level [75]. Wang et al. studied 771 patients with ATA low- or intermediate-risk DTC to see if a median TSH <0.4 μU/ml vs. a median TSH >0.4 μU/ml improved recurrence over a median follow-up of 6.5 years. Osteoporosis incidence was evaluated in women only. They found that suppression of serum TSH level <0.4 μU/ml did not change recurrence rates in low- to intermediate-risk patients with DTC but did increase osteoporosis incidence in women [76]. Studies have shown that doses of levothyroxine that reduce circulation TSH to <0.4 mIU/L induce maximum suppression of serum thyroglobulin [77], suggesting that increasing the degree of TSH suppression beyond this point may not further decrease tumor function [78]. Others have found that serum thyroglobulin continues to decline when TSH is further suppressed to levels that are undetectable <0.01 mIU/L [79]. These findings have added to the controversy of optimal TSH suppression levels in patients with thyroid cancer.

Morbidity Associated with TSH Suppression

For decades, all patients with thyroid cancer were put on thyroid hormone suppression to suppress serum TSH to undetectable levels. We now have a better understanding that with suppression comes the price of morbidity, including bone loss, arrhythmias, particularly atrial fibrillation, and symptoms of hyperthyroidism. We also have a better understanding of long-term mortality and the often favorable prognosis in most patients with DTC. Given this, it is critical to weigh the risks and benefits of thyroid hormone suppression at each follow-up visit.

Bone Loss

Bone loss is a concern in patients with overt and subclinical hyperthyroidism, particularly in elderly patients. Since patients with DTC often undergo TSH suppression as part of their therapy, it is important to consider the effects on bone metabolism and clinically significant bone loss. In postmenopausal women, several studies have reported a negative effect of long-term serum TSH suppression on the bone mineral density (BMD) of patients with DTC [80, 81], while other studies have not confirmed such a negative effect [82, 83]. BMD analysis is important because it is correlated with the risk of fracture in postmenopausal women [84]. Wang et al. retrospectively examined a total of 771 patients (569 women) with ATA low or intermediate DTC with a mean age of 48 +/− 14 years who underwent thyroidectomy between the years 2000–2006. They were followed for a median of 6.5 years. They were divided into two groups, a median serum TSH level of >0.4 mIU/L or <0.4 mIU/L. Primary outcomes were structural recurrence of thyroid cancer, postoperative development of atrial fibrillation, and osteoporosis (the latter in women only). A total of 5.6 % of patients recurred (43/771) and 3.9 % (29/739) developed osteoporosis. The rates of recurrences were similar among the two groups, but patients suppressed to a TSH of <0.4 mIU/L were at a higher risk for osteoporosis (HR 2.1, $p = 0.05$) compared to those patients with a TSH of >0.4 mIU/L [81]. Gomes de Melo et al. performed a cross-sectional study that assessed BMD and risk factors for decreased BMD in 109 postmenopausal women under TSH suppression for DTC therapy. They compared this cohort to age-matched, euthyroid women as a control. They found that low body mass index and low serum TSH levels were correlated with lower BMD, but there was no increased prevalence of osteopenia or osteoporosis compared to the age-matched, euthyroid controls [85]. Sugitani and Fujimoto performed a randomized controlled trial in female patients with PTC. They were randomized to suppressive therapy or non-suppressive therapy. The mean TSH in the suppressed group was 0.07 mU/L ($n = 144$) and 3.14 mU/L ($n = 127$) in the non-suppressed group. They measured annual lumbar spine BMD. They found that there were significant decreases in T scores within the first year postoperatively in the suppressed group in women ≥50 years old but not those <50 years of age. In the non-suppressed group, there was no significant decline in lumbar spine BMD until

5 years postoperatively [86]. One can appreciate that risk factors for lower BMD and fracture risk should be taken into account along with benefits of TSH suppression when treating patients for DTC.

Atrial Fibrillation

Hyperthyroidism has a well-known association with atrial fibrillation (AF) [87]. Even subclinical hyperthyroidism has been shown to have a greater risk of AF in patients over the age of 60 years [88]. Abonowara et al. evaluated 136 patients with a mean age of 52 years (85 % female and mean follow-up of 11 years) to evaluate the risk of developing AF. The mean serum TSH level was 0.17 mIU/L and 14 patients were found to have AF. The mean age of those patients with AF was 61.6 years vs. 51.4 years in those patients who did not develop AF. The prevalence of AF in this study was 10.3 % in DTC patients over the age of 60 years, which is >17.5 % higher than the rate of published data for the incidence of AF in the normal population of the same age group [89]. In addition to AF, other important cardiovascular risk factors can develop in young and middle-aged patients undergoing long-term TSH suppression therapy including increased heart rate, increased left ventricular mass, increased mean arterial pressure, and diastolic dysfunction [90].

Symptoms of Hyperthyroidism

TSH-suppressive therapy can also be associated with signs of hyperthyroidism including insomnia, racing heart, tremor, palpitations, diarrhea, excessive sweating, anxiety, heat intolerance, and weight loss. Several studies have shown that TSH-suppressive doses of levothyroxine can impair quality of life as measured by psychological, social, and physical items, particularly when the serum TSH is undetectable [90].

Conclusion

Thyroid cancer overall has a favorable long-term prognosis and low risk of death in most cases. Risk of recurrence can be estimated based on original pathology and clinical data at time of initial treatment. At each follow-up visit, patients should be re-evaluated and considered in either one of four categories: (1) excellent response, (2) biochemical incomplete response, (3) structural incomplete response, or (4) indeterminate response. This information should then be used to guide the clinician in long-term surveillance decisions. Ongoing risk stratification is essential to guide surveillance strategies and degree of desired TSH suppression, weighing the risks and the benefits. Lifelong suppression is no longer recommended in patients who have been shown to have an excellent response to treatment. Over surveillance and over treatment with thyroxine can lead to anxiety in the patient, unnecessary studies, and morbidity. Ongoing dynamic risk stratification at each visit can avoid negative outcomes while providing appropriate surveillance to patients with treated DTC.

References

1. SEER cancer statistics. http://seer.cancer.gov/statfacts/html/thyro.html. Accessed 9/15/2015.
2. American Cancer Society. http://www.cancer.org/cancer/thyroidcancer/detailedguide/thyroid-cancer-key-statistics. Accessed 9/15/2015.
3. Davies L, Welch HG. Current thyroid cancer trends in the United States. JAMA. 2014;140:317–22.
4. Pellegriti G, et al. Worldwide increasing incidence of thyroid cancer: update on epidemiology and risk factors. J Cancer Epidemiol. 2013;2013:965212, epub.
5. Vigneri R, Malandrino P, Vigneri P. The changing epidemiology of thyroid cancer: why is incidence increasing? Curr Opin Oncol. 2015;27(1):1–7.
6. Davies L, Welch HG. Increasing incidence of thyroid cancer in the united state, 1973–2002. JAMA. 2006;295(18):2164–7.
7. Aschebrook-Kilfoy B, et al. The clinical and economic burden of a sustained increase in thyroid cancer incidence. Cancer Epidemiol Biomarkers Prev. 2013;22:1252–9.
8. Haugen B, et al. The American thyroid association management guidelines for adult patients with thyroid nodules and differentiated thyroid cancer. Thyroid. 2015. doi:10.1089/thy.2015.0020.
9. Wada N, et al. Clinical outcomes in older or younger patients with papillary thyroid carcinoma: impact of lymphadenopathy and patient age. Eur J Surg Oncol. 2008;34:202–7.
10. Randolph GW, et al. The prognostic significance of nodal metastases from papillary thyroid carcinoma can be based on size and number of metastatic lymph nodes as well as presence of extra-nodal extension. Thyroid. 2012;22(11):1144–52.
11. American Cancer Society. http://www.cancer.org/cancer/thyroidcancer/detailedguide/thyroid-cancer-survival-rates Accessed Sept 2015.
12. Cooper DS, et al. Revised American thyroid association guidelines for patients with thyroid nodules and differentiated thyroid cancer. Thyroid. 2009;19:1167–214.
13. Tuttle RM, Leboeuf R. Follow up approaches in thyroid cancer: a risk adapted paradigm. Endocrinol Metab Clin North Am. 2008;37:419–35.
14. Burch H. Follow –up strategy in papillary thyroid cancer. In: Wartofsky L, Van Nostrand D, editors. Thyroid cancer: a comprehensive guide to clinical management. 2nd ed. Totowa: Humana Press; 2006. p. 289–92.
15. Johnson N, LeBeau S, Tublin M. Imaging surveillance of differentiated thyroid cancer. Radiol Clin North Am. 2011;49:473–87.
16. Tala H, Tuttle RM. Contemporary post surgical management of differentiated thyroid carcinoma. Clin Oncol. 2010;22:419–29.
17. Tuttle RM, et al. Estimating risk of recurrence in differentiated thyroid cancer after total thyroidectomy and radioactive iodine remnant ablation: using response to therapy variables to modify the initial risk estimates predicted by the new American Thyroid Association staging system. Thyroid. 2010;20:1341–9.
18. Vasiman F, et al. Spontaneous remission in thyroid cancer patients after biochemical incomplete response to initial therapy. Clin Endocrinol. 2012;77:132–8.
19. Castagna MG, et al. Delayed risk stratification to include the response to initial treatment (surgery and radioiodine ablation), has better outcome predictivity in differentiated thyroid cancer patients. Eur J Endocrinol. 2011;165:441–6.

20. Pitoia F, et al. Outcomes of patients with differentiated thyroid cancer risk-stratified according to the American Thyroid Association and Latin American thyroid society risk of recurrence classification systems. Thyroid. 2013;23:1401–7.
21. Vaisman F, et al. Initial therapy with either thyroid lobectomy or total thyroidectomy without radioactive iodine remnant ablation is associated with very low rates of structural disease recurrence in properly selected patients with differentiated thyroid cancer. Clin Endocrinol. 2011;75:112–9.
22. Schvartz C, et al. Impact on overall survival of radioiodine in low-risk differentiated thyroid cancer patients. J Clin Endocrinol Metab. 2012;97:1526–35.
23. Durante C, et al. Long-term surveillance of papillary thyroid cancer patients who do not undergo postoperative radioiodine remnant ablation: is there a role for serum thyroglobulin measurement? J Clin Endocrinol Metab. 2012;97:2748–53.
24. Mazzaferri EL. Management of low-risk differentiated thyroid cancer. Endocr Pract. 2007;13:498–512.
25. Roti E, et al. Thyroid papillary microcarcinoma: a descriptive and meta analysis study. Eur J Endocrinol. 2008;159:659–73.
26. Ito Y, et al. Prognosis of low-risk papillary thyroid carcinoma in patients: its relationship with the size of primary tumors. Endocr J. 2012;59:119–25.
27. Lee J, Song Y, Soh EY. Prognostic significance of the number of metastatic lymph nodes to stratify the risk of recurrence. World J Surg. 2014;38:858–62.
28. Shaha AR, Loree TR, Shah JP. Prognostic factors and risk group analysis in follicular carcinoma of the thyroid. Surgery. 1995;118:1131.
29. American Cancer Society. http://www.cancer.org/cancer/thyroidcancer/detailedguide/thyroid-cancer-key-statistics. Accessed 9/21/2015.
30. SEER Database. http://seer.cancer.gov/statfacts/html/thyro.html. Accessed 9/25/2015.
31. Giovanella L, et al. Diagnosis of endocrine disease. Thyroglobulin measurement using highly sensitive assays in patients with differentiated thyroid cancer: a clinical position paper. Eur J Endocrinol. 2014;171(2):R33–46.
32. Grebe SKG. Diagnosis and management of thyroid carcinoma: focus on serum thyroglobulin. Expert Rev Endocrinol Metab. 2009;4:25–43.
33. Giovanella L. Highly sensitive thyroglobulin measurements in differentiated thyroid carcinoma management. Clin Chem Lab Med. 2008;46:1067–73.
34. Spencer CA, et al. Detection of residual and recurrent differentiated thyroid carcinoma by serum thyroglobulin measurement. Thyroid. 1999;9:435–41.
35. Hollowell JG, et al. Serum TSH, T(4), and thyroid antibodies in the United States population (1988 to 1994): national health and nutrition examination survey (NHANES III). J Clin Endocrinol Metab. 2002;87:489–99.
36. Spencer CA. Clinical review: clinical utility of thyroglobulin antibody (TgAb) measurements for patients with differentiated thyroid cancers (DTC). J Clin Endocrinol Metab. 2011;96:3615–27.
37. Stanojevic M, et al. Comparison of the influence of thyroglobulin antibodies on serum thyroglobulin values from two different immunoassays in post surgical differentiated thyroid carcinoma patients. J Clin Lab Anal. 2009;23:341–6.
38. Stanojevic M, et al. Correlation of thyroglobulin concentrations measured by radioimmunoassay and immunoradiometric assay and the influence of thyroglobulin antibody. J Immunoassay Immunochem. 2009;30:197–207.
39. Giovanella L, Ceriani L. Comparison of thyroglobulin antibody interference in first and second-generation thyroglobulin immunoassays. Clin Chem Lab Med. 2011;49:1025–7.
40. Wg K, et al. Change of serum antithyroglobulin antibody levels is useful for prediction of clinic recurrence in thyroglobulin-negative patients with differentiated thyroid carcinoma. J Clin Endocrinol Metab. 2008;93:4683–9.
41. Spencer C, Fatemi S. Thyroglobulin antibody (TgAb) methods-strengths, pitfalls and clinical utility for monitoring TgAb-positive patients with differentiated thyroid cancer. Best Pract Res Clin Endocrinol Metab. 2013;27:701–12.

42. Chiovata L, et al. Disappearance of humoral thyroid autoimmunity after complete removal of thyroid antigens. Ann Intern Med. 2003;139:346–51.
43. Thomas D, et al. Possible reasons for different pattern disappearance of thyroglobulin and thyroid peroxidase autoantibodies in patients with differentiated thyroid carcinoma following total thyroidectomy and iodine-131 ablation. J Endocrinol Invest. 2007;30:173–80.
44. Gorges R, et al. Development and clinical impact of thyroglobulin antibodies in patients with differentiated thyroid carcinoma during the first 3 years after thyroidectomy. Eur J Endocrinol. 2005;153:49–55.
45. Seo JH, Lee SW, Ahn BC, Lee J. Recurrence detection in differentiated thyroid cancer patients with elevated serum level of antithyroglobulin antibody: special emphasis on using (18)F-FDG PET/CT. Clin Endocrinol. 2010;72:558–63.
46. Adil A, et al. Frequency and clinical importance of anti-Tg auto-antibodies (ATG). J Coll Physicians Surg Pak. 2003;13:504–6.
47. Coquia SF, et al. The role of sonography in thyroid cancer. Radiol Clin North Am. 2014;52:1283–94.
48. Grebe SK, Hay ID. Thyroid cancer nodal metastases: biologic significance and therapeutic considerations. Surg Oncol Clin N Am. 1996;5:43–63.
49. Scheumann GF, et al. Prognostic significance and surgical management of locoregional lymph node metastases in papillary thyroid cancer. World J Surg. 1994;18:559–67.
50. Ito Y, et al. An observation trial without surgical treatment in patients with papillary microcarcinoma of the thyroid. Thyroid. 2003;13:381–7.
51. Qubain SW, et al. Distribution of lymph node micrometastasis in pN0 well-differentiated thyroid carcinoma. Surgery. 2002;131:249–56.
52. Arturi F, et al. Early diagnosis by genetic analysis of differentiated thyroid cancer metastases in small lymph nodes. J Clin Endocrinol Metab. 1997;82:1638–41.
53. Rosario PW, de Faria S, Bicalho L, et al. Ultrasonographic differentiation between metastatic and benign lymph nodes in patients with papillary thyroid carcinoma. J Ultrasound Med. 2005;24(10):1385–9.
54. Kuna SK, Bracic I, Tesic V, et al. Ultrasonographic differentiation of benign from malignant neck lymph-adenopathy in thyroid cancer. J Ultrasound Med. 2006;25(12):1531–7.
55. Ko MS, Lee JH, Shong YK, et al. Normal and abnormal sonographic findings at the thyroidectomy sites in postoperative patients with thyroid malignancy. AJR Am J Roentgenol. 2010;194(6):1596–609.
56. Shin JH, Han BK, Ko EY, et al. Sonographic findings in the surgical bed after thyroidectomy: comparison of recurrent tumors and nonrecurrent lesions. J Ultrasound Med. 2007;26(10):1359–66.
57. Snozek CL, et al. Serum thyroglobulin, high-resolution ultrasound and lymph node thyroglobulin in diagnosis of thyroid carcinoma nodal metastases. J Clin Endocrinol Metab. 2007;92:4278–81.
58. Pacini F, Molinaro E, Castagna MG, et al. Recombinant human thyrotropin-stimulated serum thyroglobulin combined with neck ultrasonography has the highest sensitivity in monitoring differentiated thyroid carcinoma. J Clin Endocrinol Metab. 2003;88(8):3668–73.
59. Dadu R, Cabanillas ME. Optimizing therapy for radioactive iodine-refractory differentiated thyroid cancer: current state of the art and future directions. Minerva Endocrinol. 2012;37(4):335–56.
60. Pacini F, Castagna MG. Approach to and treatment of differentiated thyroid cancer. Med Clin North Am. 2012;96(2):369–383 and Xing M, Haugen BR, Schlumberger M. Lancet. 2013;381(9871):1058–69.
61. Nixon IJ, et al. The impact of distant metastases at presentation on prognosis in patient s with differentiated carcinoma of the thyroid gland. Thyroid. 2012;22(9):884–9.
62. Durante C, et al. Long term outcome of 444 patients with distant metastases from papillary and follicular thyroid carcinoma: benefits and limits of radioiodine therapy. J Clin Endocrinol Metab. 2006;91(8):2892–9.

63. Zoller M, Kohlfuerst S, Igerc I, et al. Combined PET/CT in the follow up of differentiated thyroid carcinoma: what is the impact of each modality. Eur J Nucl Med Mol Imaging. 2007;34(4):487–95.
64. King AD, Ahuja AT, To EW, et al. Staging papillary thyroid carcinoma of the thyroid: magnetic resonance imaging vs ultrasound of the neck. Clin Radiol. 2000;55(3):222–6.
65. Jeong HS, et al. Integrated 18F-FDG PET/CT for the initial evaluation of cervical node level of patients with papillary thyroid carcinoma: comparison with ultrasound and contrast-enhanced CT. Clin Endocrinol. 2006;65:402–7.
66. Kaplan SL, et al. The role of MR imaging in detecting nodal disease in thyroidectomy patients with rising thyroglobulin levels. AJNR Am J Neuroradiol. 2009;30:608–12.
67. Lazar V, Bidart JM, Calliou B, et al. Expression of the Na+/I− symporter gene in human thyroid tumors: a comparison study with other thyroid-specific genes. J Clin Endocrinol Metab. 1999;84(9):3228–34.
68. Ichikawa Y, Saito E, Abe Y, et al. Presence of TSH receptor in thyroid neoplasms. J Clin Endocrinol Metab. 1976;42:395–8.
69. Nadler NJ, et al. The effect of hypophysectomy on the experimental production of rat thyroid neoplasms. Cancer Res. 1970;30:1909–11.
70. Carayon P, et al. Human thyroid cancer: membrane thyrotropin binding and adenylate cylase activity. J Clin Endocrinol Metab. 1989;51:915–20.
71. Tanaka K, et al. Relationship between prognostic score and thyrotropin receptor (TSH-R) in papillary thyroid carcinoma: immunohistochemical detection of TSH-R. Br J Cancer. 1997;76:594–9.
72. Dunhill TP. Surgery of the thyroid gland (the Lettsomian Lectures). BMJ. 1937;1:460–1.
73. Mazzaferri EL, Jhiang SM. Long-term impact of initial surgical and medical therapy on papillary and follicular thyroid cancer. Am J Med. 1994;97:418–28.
74. Sugitani I, Fujimoto Y. Does postoperative thyrotropin suppression therapy truly decrease recurrence in papillary thyroid carcinoma? A randomized controlled trial. J Clin Endocrinol Metab. 2010;95(10):4576–83.
75. Carhill AA, et al. Long-term outcomes following therapy in differentiated thyroid carcinoma: NTCTCS registry analysis 1987–2012. J Clin Endocrinol Metab. 2015;100(9):3270–9.
76. Wang LY, et al. Thyrotropin suppression increases the risk of osteoporosis without decreasing recurrence in ATA low and intermediate risk patients with DTC. Thyroid. 2015;25(3):300–7.
77. Burmeister LA, et al. Levothyroxine dose requirements for thyrotropin suppression in the treatment of differentiated thyroid cancer. J Clin Endocrinol Metab. 1992;75:344–50.
78. Kamel N, et al. Degree of thyrotropin suppression in differentiated thyroid cancer without recurrence or metastases. Thyroid. 1999;9:1245–8.
79. Spencer CA, et al. Thyrotropin secretion in thyrotoxic and thyroxine-treated patients: assessment by a sensitive immunoenzymometric assay. J Clin Endorinol Metab. 1986;63:349–55.
80. Diamond T, Nery L, Hales I. A therapeutic dilemma: suppressive doses of thyroxine significantly reduce bone mineral measurements in both pre menopausal and post menopausal women with thyroid carcinoma. J Clin Endocrinol Metab. 1991;72(6):1184–8.
81. Wang LY, et al. Thyrotropin suppression increases the risk of osteoporosis without decreasing recurrence in ATA low-and intermediate risk patients with differentiated thyroid carcinoma. Thyroid. 2015;9:300–6.
82. Heijckmann AC, et al. Hip bone mineral density, bone turnover and risk of fracture in patients on long term suppressive therapy L-thyroxine therapy for differentiated thyroid carcinoma. Eur J Endocrinol. 2005;153:23–9.
83. Lee MY, et al. Bone mineral density and bone turnover markers in patients on long-term suppressive levothyroxine therapy for differentiated thyroid cancer. Ann Surg Treat Res. 2014;86(5):55–60.
84. National Osteoporosis Foundation. Clinicians guide to prevention and treatment of osteoporosis. 2008. www.nof.org.

85. Gomes de Melo T, et al. Low BMI and low TSH value as risk factors related to lower bone mineral density in post menopausal women under levothyroxine therapy for differentiated thyroid carcinoma. Thyroid Res. 2015;8:1–7.
86. Sugitani I, Fujimoto Y. Effect of postoperative thyrotropin suppressive therapy on bone mineral density in patients with papillary thyroid carcinoma: a prospective controlled study. Surgery. 2011;150(6):1250–7.
87. Camm A, Kirchhof P, Lip G, et al. European heart rhythm association: European association for cardio –thoracic surgery. Guidelines for the management of atrial fibrillation: the task force for the management of atrial fibrillation of the European society of cardiology. Europace. 2010;12:1360–420.
88. Sawin C, Geller A, Wolf P, et al. Low serum thyrotropin concentrations as a risk factor for atrial fibrillation in older persons. N Engl J Med. 1994;10(31):1249–52.
89. Abonowara A, et al. Prevalence of atrial fibrillation in patients taking TSH suppression therapy for management of thyroid cancer. Clin Invest Med. 2012;35(3):E152–6.
90. Biondi B, Cooper DS. Benefits of thyrotropin suppression versus the risks of adverse effects in differentiated thyroid cancer. Thyroid. 2010;20(2):135–46.

Chapter 23
Integrative Approaches to Patients Undergoing Thyroid Surgery

Beatriz Olson

Rationale for Use of Integrative Approaches to Patients Who Have Undergone Thyroidectomy

Wellness of patients is a complex issue, however, most broadly, it is defined as the state or condition of being in good physical and mental health. A substantial number of patients lack wellness after thyroidectomy and thyroid cancer diagnosis, despite appropriate therapies. Lack of wellness is manifested by nonspecific symptoms of fatigue, loss of physical or mental vigor, pain and/or loss of range of motion, weight gain, mental "fog," cognitive deficiency, and mood changes such as anxiety or depression. Our current therapies and/or our involvement with these groups of patients may not be sufficient to make them 'whole'. Recent data on patients with hypothyroidism, especially surgically induced, have confirmed that

1. Quality of life or perceived sense of wellness is negatively affected in these patients [1].
2. Cancer-related worry is high despite the indolent nature and low mortality generally associated with the disease [2].
3. Fatigue is a persistent problem [3]; adequacy or intensity of thyroid replacement may play a role [4–8].
4. Patient support needs are not being met by our current approaches [9].
5. Thyroid patients view psychosocial aspects of the illness as very relevant to their daily lives/ongoing treatment, whereas clinicians place relevance and focus on clinical signs related to disease [10].

Dedication: To my patients and my mentors

B. Olson, MD, FACP
Endocrinology, Yale University School of Medicine, Middlebury, CT, USA
e-mail: Beatrizmd@snet.net

S.A. Roman et al. (eds.), *Management of Thyroid Nodules and Differentiated Thyroid Cancer*, DOI 10.1007/978-3-319-43618-0_23

These patients who lack of wellness have no abnormal physical findings and usually have thyroid-stimulating hormone (TSH) levels in the "normal" range, yet they often seek nonstandard treatments and non-allopathic health providers, and use supplements to try to help themselves. Past studies have suggested that 50–75 % of patients were using supplements, complementary and alternative medical (CAM) therapies, and many did not share this information with their doctors [11, 12]. For definition purposes, complementary therapies are used in conjunction with established therapies, whereas alternative therapies replace standard therapies to address health conditions.

Integrative medicine combines conventional evidence-based medicine with complementary healing practices to address lack of wellness in these types of patients. The Center for Complementary and Integrative Health at the National Institutes of Health supports evidence-based research on integrative medicine and notes that integrative approaches are particularly useful for patients who lack wellness, those with illness without diagnosis, patients with cancer, and patients with chronic illnesses for whom Western medicine has no good options. Many of these categories fit patients undergoing thyroid surgery for whom physical illness, illness-related fears and concerns, and other psychosocial sequelae are intertwined. This body-mind interaction matters to patients, and may affect ultimate sense of wellness after treatment. Therefore, these patients are prime candidates for receiving integrative holistic care and for participation in research on the effectiveness of combination of allopathic and CAM therapies.

The focus of a holistic and integrative approach is to address mind-body issues around the illness that affects the whole person in order to help them achieve wellness. Patient concerns and beliefs are acknowledged even when they cannot be fully understood, fully medically explained, or fully fixed. This enhances mutual trust in the patient-physician relationship and accepts the inexactness of medicine. This allows for flexibility for, negotiation of, and consent to the types of therapies used, some of which may be complementary or alternative, subject for evidence-based research, and may be best monitored by physicians who have expertise. Patients are empowered to access their own healing capacities (activating their innate healing response or placebo effects) and beliefs (hope) as part of the healing process. Nutrition, lifestyle adjustments, mindfulness, and stress-reducing mind-body-centering techniques are used to enhance health, counteract unwanted effects of therapy, alleviate anxiety and depression, and allow acceptance for one's reality. Herbal medicines are neither discussed nor recommended by this author for the management of hypothyroidism or thyroid cancer treatment.

Mitigating Risks in the Preoperative Period: Dealing with Supplements and Vitamin D Status

Herbal and homeopathic medicines, vitamins, supplements, cooking spices, and teas are widely used by patients. Often patients do not think it is important and/or are afraid to share with doctors that they are actively taking supplements or using alternative therapies [13, 14]. Preoperatively it is important to know if patients are taking supplements that may not have been listed as part of their medications. Just as prescription medicines, herbal and non-herbal supplements such as fish oils, vitamin E, or spices can interfere with various aspects of platelet aggregation or the coagulation pathway, anesthesia, and perioperative care [15, 16]. A cross-sectional survey of 100 consecutive patients with nodular disease preparing for thyroid surgery noted that 51 % of participants were actively using oral supplements and 31 % used supplements that would affect hemostasis [17, 18]. The safest approach to mitigate risk of perioperative bleeding complications that minimizes withdrawal symptoms for the patients is to wean off over a week and stop supplements preoperatively 2–3 weeks ahead of time for surgery and to hold on retaking the supplements until 2 weeks after surgery [19, 20].

To prepare for the risk of prolonged hypocalcemia postoperatively, it is useful to address the preoperative vitamin D status [21]. Vitamin D deficiency is common in North American patients. [22]. Many patients undergoing thyroidectomy and/or parathyroidectomy for primary hyperparathyroidism present with coexistent secondary hyperparathyroidism due to chronic vitamin D deficiency and increased metabolism of 25 (OH) vitamin D to 1,25(OH)$_2$ vitamin D [23]. These patients cannot absorb dietary calcium and have underlying metabolic bone disease as a result of chronic parathyroid hormone (PTH)-mediated bone resorption to maintain calcium homeostasis. Such patients are at risk of prolonged duration of hypocalcemia postoperatively. Patients with obesity, history of bariatric surgery, or malabsorption and African Americans are at greatest risk [22]. While the active form of vitamin D such as calcitriol (1,25(OH)$_2$, 1,25 dihydroxycholecalciferol) plus oral calcium is the replacement of choice in acute hypoparathyroidism in hospital and long-term PTH deficiency states, it makes sense to normalize serum vitamin D to levels of 30–40 ng/ml, where maximum dietary calcium absorption can be expected [24]. A retrospective analysis examining outcome after 264 total or completion thyroidectomies in patients whose preoperative vitamin D status was known showed that preoperative vitamin D deficiency was independently associated with the need for postoperative 1,25-dihydroxyvitamin D3 [25]. Patients with lasting residual hypoparathyroidism may not feel well after surgery despite adequate replacement of calcium; this could be due to the complication of hypoparathyroidism itself, given that PTH is currently not routinely given to treat PTH deficiency [26]. A new preparation of parathyroid hormone replacement is available in a daily injectable form (parathyroid 1–84) made by recombinant DNA technology; its use is reserved for patients that cannot be well managed with routine treatment of calcium and calcitriol. However, the preparation carries a black box warning for the rare potential risk for osteosarcoma, which limits wider use.

Perioperative Period: Stress and Anxiety Around Surgery

Some patients experience significant stress and anxiety in the perioperative period and can be helped by use of relaxation techniques and guided imagery [27]. Relaxation techniques are generally considered safe in children and adults without severe psychiatric illness or uncontrolled seizure disorders and include progressive relaxation, guided imagery, self-hypnosis, biofeedback, and deep breathing exercises. In guided imagery, people are taught to focus on pleasant images or intentions to replace negative or stressful feelings. This may be self-directed or lead by a practitioner or recording [28]. These techniques have been used in other surgical fields to effectively decrease of stress and anxiety in the peri- and postoperative period, and to shorten length of stay in hospitals. In a study in otolaryngology regarding elective surgery in children, a child-life specialist prepared 80 children pre-surgery by measuring and addressing preoperative anxiety, and 62 received no intervention. Anxiety scores were significantly lower in children who received the child-life intervention [29]. In a randomized study of 44 adults undergoing head and neck surgery, patients received 28 minutes of privacy before surgery, during which the treatment group listened to a guided imagery compact disk. The preoperative intervention group experienced significantly lower anxiety levels, less pain, and shorter length of stay than the group who had conventional surgery [30]. Similarly, a prospective randomized trial at a tertiary care center used guided imagery tapes daily for 3 days before surgery, music-only tape during induction and surgery and in the recovery room, and daily guided imagery for 6 days postoperatively. Patients randomized to guided imagery had lower anxiety preoperative, lower pain scores, opiate requirements, and shorter time to first bowel movement postoperatively, whereas perioperative complications did not differ between groups [31]. The conclusion from these and other studies is that understanding anxiety and addressing it preoperatively lower its levels, improve patient postoperative experience, and can be accomplished with low cost.

Physical and Emotional Recovery from Thyroidectomy

The postoperative period after thyroidectomy is a vulnerable time for patients. Often patients are uncomfortable; awaiting pathology; experiencing new fear-evoking symptoms, such as hypocalcemia, pain, and hoarseness; and wondering if they will see normalcy again. It is helpful to let patients know what they might experience in the days to weeks after surgery and that there are methods to help them through the process and decrease anxiety. Time of healing increases with extent of the surgery, with the fastest healing occurring from thyroid lobectomies and longest from total thyroidectomy and bilateral neck dissection. Often patients have already been discharged from the hospital when more insidious physical and emotional issues arise. Most patients experience throat pain for an extended period of time. Patients with preoperative cervical degenerative disk disease may experience neck pain and cervicogenic headaches. The patients with unilateral and bilateral neck dissections experience moderate head and neck swelling that takes a significant time to resolve. After bilateral neck dissection, patients may also experience loss of range of motion of cervical spine and more residual pain. These patients have numbness in neck area that may last months to years. There may be also voice changes that are transient or longer lasting due to recurrent laryngeal nerve injuries or they may be subtle, from injury to the external branches of the superior laryngeal nerves (more detail in Chap. 22). Despite the good prognosis that generally accompanies differentiated thyroid cancer (DTC), many patients with DTC experience anxiety, depressive symptoms, and declines in perception of health. Older patients and patients with more advanced stages are at highest risk [32, 33]. Asking open-ended questions, such as "Just wondering how you feel with all the news?", can create the opportunity for patients to express openly the stress and fears related to their cancer diagnosis. It can be helpful for them to grieve openly the fact that they are dealing with malignancy and the repercussions that this may have for them and their family. Listening for those few minutes, without trying to "fix" anything, can be incredibly healing for the patient at this time. It is often useful to mention that part of the armamentarium we use with all patients includes counseling to encompass issues from thyroid loss to thyroid cancer and worry, gentle massage after surgical healing has occurred, and physical therapy with and without craniosacral approaches by qualified therapists to improve mobility and relax tight guarding muscles and fascia to help process surgical trauma memory of the tissues. Support from family and friends, as well as joining focused support groups after cancer diagnosis, is invaluable to relieve pain, anxiety, and suffering in these patients [34].

For those requiring radioiodine ablation or adjuvant therapies, the use of recombinant TSH instead of thyroid hormone withdrawal makes a positive difference for these patients (see also section "Dealing Well with Radioactive Iodine: Addressing Mind-Body Concerns and Complementary Approaches to Patients Receiving Radioiodine Therapy" of this chapter) [35].

Understanding and Avoiding Weight Gain After Thyroidectomy

Most patients are not aware that they may gain weight after thyroidectomy. This weight gain is observed despite returning patients back to a euthyroid state or having thyroid tests in the normal range. In a retrospective analysis of 120 preoperatively euthyroid thyroidectomized patients, treated with levothyroxine monotherapy and maintained within the normal range (TSH 0.5–4.5) with mean serum TSH of 1.4–1.7 mIU/L, an average of 80 % of patients gained weight after thyroidectomy. Weight increased by 3.1 kg and BMI of 1.1 kg/m^2, and postmenopausal women had the greatest weight gain with mean of 4.4 kg. Patients with TSH suppressive therapy for thyroid cancer had less weight gain [36, 37]. Significant weight gains also occur after treatment for hyperthyroidism, regardless of the method used. Lönn et al. showed weight gains of 2.7 kg at 3 months and 8.7 kg at 12 months after treatment of thyrotoxicosis with either medicine or thyroidectomy [38]. In this study metabolic rate analysis showed a decline of basal metabolic rate from 2087 Cal/24 h at diagnosis to 1601 Cal/24 h at 12 months, and energy intake dropped from 3244 to

2436 Cal/24 h. Similarly, a retrospective analysis documented rapid weight increases in the first 3 months after treatment of thyrotoxicosis with an average weight gain of 6.5 kg after thyroidectomy, 5.4 kg after antithyroid medicine carbimazole, and 7.4 kg after radioiodine therapy [39]. It is not clear if it is the lower basal metabolic rate or continued increased caloric intake or both that result in such weight gain [40, 41]. Lastly, similar observations have been noted after thyroidectomy for benign multinodular goiter (MNG), with a mean increase in weight of 2.2 kg despite adequate levothyroxine treatment, particularly in patients older than 45 years of age [42]. Efforts at caloric reduction lessen weight gain in thyrotoxic patients made euthyroid with antithyroid medicine [43]. Taken together, the data show that weight gain ensues after thyroidectomy and postoperative treatment of hypothyroidism and that weight gain is higher in thyrotoxic patients. This may be associated with onset of a "new" relative hypothyroid state at the tissue level compared to tissue experience in the pretreatment or pre-thyroidectomy state. Importantly, continued higher caloric intake, inactivity, and other coexisting conditions that affect negatively resting metabolic rate, such as estrogen deficiency [44–46], sleep disturbances [47], and prior obesity [48], can contribute to weight gain.

A major assumption by patients and professionals has been that weight gain could be prevented with appropriate thyroid hormone replacement. Unfortunately, this has not been the case. Giving more levothyroxine to bring the serum TSH to a lower range does not improve weight gain [49]. The few combination therapy trials with liothyronine (T3) and levothyroxine have not consistently shown beneficial effects on weight, and T3 therapy alone has not, up to now, been recommended to treat hypothyroidism or weight gain (see section "Combination Thyroid Therapy Trials Levothyroxine and Liothyronine (T3) and Alternative Therapy Trials with Levothyroxine and Desiccated Thyroid for Patients with Persistent Hypothyroid Symptoms and Lack of Wellness" of this chapter for combination therapy). There is evidence, however, for an important metabolic role of T3 in weight regulation after thyroidectomy; a recent randomized double-blind crossover trial by Celi et al. evaluated the therapeutic substitution of T3 monotherapy for levothyroxine monotherapy to define bioequivalence of these hormones in ten patients who underwent total thyroidectomy [50]. Their data showed that TSH levels between 0.5 and 1.5 mIU/L could be achieved with total daily doses of 40.3 ± 11.3 mcg (0.57 ± 0.08 mcg/kg/day) of T3 administered as three doses and that this was equivalent to 115.2 ± 38.5 mcg (1.59 ± 0.28 mcg/kg/day) of levothyroxine once daily dosage, with bioequivalence T3 levothyroxine ratio of 0.36 ± 0.06 or approximately 1/3 [50]. Patients who were on the T3 arm of the study experienced more weight loss and improvement in lipid parameters without adverse effects [51]. Studies like this support the use of more T3-based therapies and the need for development of better commercially available T3 replacement options for patients and trials with these preparations.

There are no evidence-based recommendations that can be given to patients to prevent weight gain after thyroidectomy, other than maintaining efforts at caloric restriction, which do lessen the weight gain [43]. This author uses an integrative approach to weight loss and recommends a multipronged approach to help prevent weight gain after thyroidectomy. These recommendations include:

1. Caloric restriction for weight loss [52]
2. Avoidance of processed foods and use of whole foods [53–55] (see supplement for some of commercially available diets)
3. Daily 30–60 min per day physical activity [56, 57] using motivating goal-monitoring gadgets [58]
4. Improvement of sleep environment and quality and quantity of sleep [47, 59]
5. Stress identification [60] and mindfulness-based stress reduction (MBSR) training (see supplement for description) [61, 62].

Complementary Therapies for Fatigue and Mind-Body Issues Faced by Thyroid Cancer Patients

Thyroid cancer survivors, unlike survivors of other types of cancer, deal with lifelong thyroid hormone deficiency. There may be a cumulative impact of having a cancer diagnosis and thyroid deficiency on quality of life and wellness perception of thyroid cancer survivors. Fatigue is a common complaint in close to half of all thyroid cancer survivors for whom quality of life is also negatively affected [63–65]. Some patients have lack of wellness, fatigue, and psycho-neurocognitive complaints, prior to their thyroid cancer diagnosis, and after they undergo thyroid cancer therapy, the same complaints persist, but may be then attributed to hypothyroidism and/or thyroid cancer diagnosis. For others, these complaints develop and affect quality of life after thyroidectomy and thyroid cancer treatment. Table 23.1 shows a list of differential diagnoses for lack of wellness and fatigue in the average patient with or without thyroid cancer. It is important to identify, rule out, and/or correct coexistent medical and psychiatric conditions that may be contributing to fatigue in these patients. Once these medical problems are addressed or ruled out, the therapeutic focus is to sort out which physical and psychological complaints are due to the cancer diagnosis itself and its treatment sequelae (burden of disease; age at time of diagnosis; physical, emotional, and financial impact of diagnosis and treatment to patient and family; social support; etc.) and which are attributable to hypothyroidism (type and quality of thyroid hormone replacement and management, individual absorption and metabolism of levothyroxine, degree and duration of TSH suppression).

There are no current recommendations that therapeutically address cancer-related complaints in thyroid cancer patients. Therefore we can be guided by evidence-based data from complementary therapy trials effective at improving cancer-related complaints (low quality of life, cancer-related fatigue, anxiety, and depression) in patients with non-thyroid cancers. Table 23.2 summarizes modalities discussed in this section. The Society for Integrative Oncology (http://www.integrativeonc.org/) has issued guidelines for complementary therapies in breast cancer [66]. In this population, behavioral therapies (mindfulness/meditation, relaxation, and yoga) have strong evidence (Grade A) for improvement of mood in the context of depression during cancer treatment and meditation for improvement of quality

Table 23.1 Differential diagnosis of fatigue and lack of wellness in hypothyroid patients with TSH in normal range

Anemia
Other autoimmune disorder (celiac disease, adrenal insufficiency, pernicious anemia, atrophic gastritis, primary biliary cirrhosis, multiple sclerosis)
Lyme or tick-borne disease infections
Sleep apnea
Impaired sleep (shift work, bad habits or sleep hygiene, menopause, partner with sleep issue)
Previous chronic illness and perception of being worse after thyroid or other cancer diagnosis
Multiple hormone deficiencies (patients with pituitary issues or traumatic brain injury)
Estrogen deficiency (menopause) androgen deficiency (andropause)
Inflammation (infection, diabetes, rheumatoid arthritis, inflammatory bowel disease, poor diet ± abnormal microbiome, food sensitivities, allergies, estrogen deficiency, obesity)
Work-related and/or home-related financial and/or caretaker stress
Endogenous or situational depression and/or anxiety
Chronic fatigue or myalgic encephalomyelitis of uncertain etiologies
PTSD from prior traumatic event including childhood trauma
Malignancy – synchronous or prior to current thyroid cancer diagnosis
Drug and alcohol abuse
Anxiety specific to not understanding illness/treatment or what will happen to self or family
Postoperative hypo- or eucalcemic hypoparathyroidism
T3 deficiency and/or relative hypothyroidism at various tissue levels

Table 23.2 Complementary mind-body modalities effective in cancer-related symptoms

Symptom	Modality
Anxiety	Music therapy, meditation, MBSR, yoga, CBT, exercise
Depression	MBSR, relaxation, yoga, massage, acupuncture, acupressure, music therapy
Quality of life	Meditation, acupuncture, yoga, exercise[a]
Cancer-related fatigue	Energy conservation, yoga, acupuncture, CBT + H (radiotherapy), exercise (resistance training)
Physical function	Meditation, CBT, yoga, exercise
Nausea	Acupressure, electroacupuncture

[a]Also evaluated in thyroid cancer patients. *MBSR* mindfulness-based stress reduction, *CBT+ H* cognitive behavioral therapy + hypnosis. Data from Refs. [66–75]

of life and physical functioning. Moderate evidence (Grade B) exists for music therapy, mindfulness meditation, and stress management for reduction of long-term anxiety during and after treatment; massage, acupuncture/pressure, and music therapy for reducing depression; energy conservation for fatigue; and acupressure and electroacupuncture in addition to antiemetics to help control nausea during chemotherapy [66]. Acupuncture at three points (ST36, SP6, LI4 with alternatives at GB34 and SP9) for 20 min for 6 weeks is also significantly effective for improving cancer-related fatigue, on physical and psychological measures including quality of life in a randomized control trial of 302 breast cancer patients [67].

Meta-analysis of randomized control trials of yoga and cancer patients has documented a large effect ($d=-69$ to -0.75) in reductions in distress, anxiety, and depression and moderate effect in reduction of fatigue ($d=0.49$) and improvement quality of life ($d=0.33$) and functional well-being ($d=0.31$) [68].

Fatigue and muscle weakness were significantly lower at 4 weeks and 6 months after radiotherapy in cancer patients randomized to weekly cognitive behavioral therapy (CBT) sessions and hypnosis during the radiotherapy treatment, in comparison to those that just received compassionate listening [69]. In CBT, the patients identify negative unhelpful beliefs, and the negative consequence these cause for them, and are taught behavioral strategies counteract negative thought patters and to manage fatigue. During the 5–15 min sessions of hypnosis, the suggestion was given for increased well-being and reduced fatigue. Multivitamins are ineffective in reducing cancer-related fatigue [70]. Given these data, it appears that trials of mind-body therapies that include mindfulness meditation, yoga, acupuncture/acupressure, and CBT + hypnosis (H) can be safely recommended to thyroid cancer patients without causing harm and with the expectation of improvement in well-being. In this regard CBT + H may be particularly useful in preparing patients who need to receive radioiodine therapies.

Meta-analysis of the effect of exercise trials in breast and prostate cancer survivors shows a moderate reduction of cancer-related fatigue with effect size of 0.31 (95 % CI: 0.22–0.40) [71]. These investigators noted that moderate intensity resistance training of 3–6 Mets is more effective than lower intensity or aerobic exercise, and older patients benefited more from this than younger patients. Exercise may improve biobehavioral variables that impact quality of life for patients with cancer such as improving quality of sleep, decreasing psychological stress, increasing muscle mass, and functional capacity [72]. Studies that use trans-theoretical models, where patients progressively analyze pros and cons of their own behavioral change in exercise, are more effective at maintaining behaviors [73] and at lowering cancer-related fatigue [71]. A second meta-analysis of trials evaluating the effect of exercise on quality of life and/or quality of life domains (fatigue, anxiety, emotional health) included 40 trials and 3,694 patients. The modes of the exercise intervention included strength training, resistance training, walking, cycling, yoga, Qigong, or Tai Chi. A positive effect of exercise was seen on the global quality of life, breast cancer concerns, emotional well-being, sleep disturbances, anxiety, fatigue, and pain [74]. Quality of life improvements have also been documented in 16 thyroid cancer patients on TSH-suppressive therapy (TSH = 0.2–0.02) who participated in twice weekly exercise for 3 months compared to 16 who remained sedentary [75]. Based on these data, it is sound to recommend exercise with a goal of twice weekly sessions that include resistance training for 45–60 min for thyroid cancer survivors.

Thyroid Hormone Replacement with Levothyroxine Monotherapy and Monitoring Adequacy of Replacement with Thyroid-Stimulating Hormone (TSH)

Thyroid hormone replacement is necessary for all patients undergoing total thyroidectomy, patients with lobectomies who have underlying Hashimoto's thyroiditis and positive TPO-AB, and for those rendered hypothyroid after radioactive iodine treatment for Graves' disease or thyrotoxicosis. Levothyroxine is taken orally for thyroid hormone replacement therapy and serum thyrotropin. TSH is measured to determine adequacy of therapy using a normative TSH range derived from individuals without thyroidectomies. This section delineates data on nuances of thyroid hormone replacement and its management and provides a data-based rationale for maintaining TSH $\leq$ 2.5 mIU/L, after thyroidectomy, in most healthy patients who do not have cancer.

The replacement of thyroid hormone is complex [6–8] due to the multiple biological steps required for the active form of thyroid hormone, T3, to reach target tissues, and the patient-specific factors involved in achieving tissue euthyroidism. All endocrine societies currently recommend that only levothyroxine monotherapy be given for thyroid hormone replacement [8, 76]. This is because it is possible to normalize TSH to the normal range and achieve peripheral conversion of T4 to the active hormone T3 with levothyroxine monotherapy [77, 78], and there are no definitive data to support that combination levothyroxine/T3 therapy is better [8, 79]. A functional guide to dosing of levothyroxine monotherapy is offered in this section. For an in-depth evidence-based discussion of the literature on how levothyroxine therapy is derived and described below, the reader is referred to the 2014 American Thyroid Association (ATA) guidelines for treatment of hypothyroidism [76] Generally, the dose calculation is based on weight, age, and state of health of the patient and indications for therapy. Patients who have had thyroidectomy need full replacement doses. For levothyroxine monotherapy in patients without thyroid cancer, the average replacement dose required is approximately 1.6–1.8 mcg/kg/day for most patients. Higher doses of 2.1–2.7 mcg/kg/day are recommended for patients with thyroid cancer, particularly those with moderate and high risk of recurrence who need TSH suppression as therapy with TSH goals 0.1–0.5 mIU/L and <0.1 mIU/L, respectively [80] (see also Chap. 22).

Patient-related factors influence effectiveness of levothyroxine therapy [76]. We rely on (1) patients to be compliant to taking the medicine daily, or as prescribed, on an empty stomach and in the absence of competing medicines for best absorption, (2) a healthy digestive tract without malabsorption, (3) consistency of drug preparation taken whether generic or brand, and (4) normal thyroid hormone metabolism resulting in adequate T3 conversion from levothyroxine at the tissue level (see below). Elderly patients need lower doses of thyroid hormone, but tend to absorb thyroid hormone less, so particular caution is needed in these patients. Higher doses may be needed in patients with malabsorption syndromes and women who are pregnant or on birth control pills. Different formulations of levothyroxine, such as gel or liquid preparations, may be needed for patients with sensitivity to gluten and lactose intolerances, allergy to color dyes, using proton pump inhibitors, or diagnosed with atrophic gastritis.

In euthyroid individuals, prior to thyroidectomy, 20 % of their bioavailable T3 is secreted directly from the thyroid gland; the rest, or 80 %, is derived from peripheral conversion of T4 by peripheral tissue by enzymes called deiodinases and 5′deiodination of T4 [81]. Patients without thyroid glands cannot produce the 20 % of T3 that their thyroids used to make and secrete and have to rely entirely on the deiodinases (D1 and D2) for the peripheral conversion of T4 to its active form T3. Some individuals have variations or polymorphisms on how their deiodinases convert active hormone T3 from T4, and this may affect their thyroid hormone replacement. Some polymorphisms of the iodothyronine deiodinase 1 (D1) (found in the liver, kidney, and thyroid) gene lead to more peripheral-free T3 from T4 [82], whereas polymorphism of D2 deiodinase activity, normally found in the brain, pituitary, muscular and cardiovascular tissue, and fat (D2 Thr92ala polymorphism, present in 16 % of the population), results in decreased peripheral conversion of T4 to T3 [83]. These latter patients need higher levothyroxine doses to normalize TSH after thyroidectomy [84]. They also feel better with combination levothyroxine/T3 replacement therapy (discussed in section "Combination Thyroid Therapy Trials Levothyroxine and Liothyronine (T3) and Alternative Therapy Trials with Levothyroxine and Desiccated Thyroid for Patients with Persistent Hypothyroid Symptoms and Lack of Wellness" of this chapter) [85]. In addition there are polymorphisms of genes that regulate thyroid pathways and contribute to an individual's unique thyroid set point by defining how much TSH is needed to create the perfect T4/T3 environment for the individual [86]. Currently we do not have routine ways to detect which individuals carry such polymorphism.

While each individual has its unique set point for the regulation of their thyroid axis and intraindividual variability is narrow [87] after thyroidectomy, the adequacy of thyroid hormone replacement is determined by measuring serum TSH and ascertaining that this TSH value falls within a "normative TSH range," based on population data of euthyroid people who have not had thyroidectomies. While TSH goal for low-risk thyroid cancer patients is 0.5–2.0 mIU/L, based on recurrence risk assessment (see Chap. 22), for most patients without thyroid cancer, the accepted normal TSH range is broader, 0.45–4.12 mIU/L. This range is based on National Health and Nutrition Survey III population study, which excluded those with personal or family history of thyroid disease or positive antibodies [88]. However, data from national academy of clinical biochemists in the United States suggests that 95 % of individuals without evidence of thyroid disease have TSH below 2.5 mU/L [89]. There are population-based data showing that the upper limit of normal or 97.5 percentile of TSH appears to be age, gender, and ethnicity specific [90, 91]. In fact, there is not just a TSH reference range, but rather a series of shifting curves of TSH distribution defining ranges specific to gender, racial ethnicity, age [92], and iodine exposure history [93]. Given these nuances and patient-specific set points of TSH regulation, it is possible to understand how, after thyroidectomy, even if an individual's TSH falls within the "normal range," TSH may not represent euthyroidism at the tissue level for that individual. Most relevant for the patient who has had thyroidectomy, and a major point of this chapter's section, is that in the cross-sectional assessment of 22,116 patients without thyroid disease used to define normative data for ranges and reference limits for TSH by Bocai et al. [92], 80 % of patients age 59 years or less had TSH < 2.5 mU/L and that 90 % of patients age 70 and above had TSH < 4.5 mIU/l and at all ages analyzed less than 6 % of the population had TSH > than 4.5 mIU/L [92]. This latter point is important because higher TSH values are associated with higher cardiovascular risks [94, 95] and T3 levels cannot be normalized with levothyroxine monotherapy at TSH > 4.5 mU/L [88]. Thus for individuals who have undergone thyroidectomy and do not have thyroid cancer, unless the baseline characteristics of TSH and free T4 relationship are understood prior to surgery, efforts should be made to keep TSH ≤ 2.5 mIU/L in most patients age less than 60 years and the healthy older ones raised in iodine-sufficient countries, and no higher than 4.5 mIU/L for elderly patients.

TSH range in pregnancy after thyroidectomy is similar to that of patients with thyroid disease who receive thyroid hormone therapy during pregnancy to prevent adverse effects of maternal hypothyroidism or hyperthyroidism on maternal and fetal outcomes [96]. All these patients cannot compensate for increased thyroid hormone demands in normal pregnancy [97]. It is necessary to increase thyroid hormone replacement doses by about 30 % more than nonpregnant values [98]. This can be accomplished by increasing the prepregnancy dose by adding an extra thyroid pill 2 days of the week during the first trimester and closely monitoring patients thereafter [98]. The TSH ranges recommended are 0.1–2.5 mIU/L in the first trimester, 0.2–3.0 mIU/L in the second trimester, and 0.3–3.0 mIU/L in the third trimester and a total T4 that is 1.5 times the normal range [99–101].

Combination Thyroid Therapy Trials Levothyroxine and Liothyronine (T3) and Alternative Therapy Trials with Levothyroxine and Desiccated Thyroid for Patients with Persistent Hypothyroid Symptoms and Lack of Wellness

Levothyroxine monotherapy may not be the ideal replacement after thyroidectomy for some individuals [102, 103]. Studies suggest that 12 % of hypothyroid patients do not feel well on levothyroxine alone and have symptoms that are suggestive of hypothyroidism despite having TSH in the normal range [104]. This is a particular group of patients that may benefit from combination therapy trials [77, 105]. While it has been reported that combination therapy with levothyroxine and slow release liothyronine (T3) at a dose of 6 mcg resulted in more physiologic thyroid parameters and more normal free T4/T3 molar ratios [106], to date, there are no reliable slow release preparations of liothyronine available (or FDA approved). The concern for adverse effects due liothyronine overdosage, the rapid onset and short half-life of currently available liothyronine preparations, and the high content of T3 in commercially available porcine-derived desiccated thyroid preparations have all become hurdles to the routine use of liothyronine therapy alone or in combination therapy for patients after thyroidectomy.

The literature available on combination levothyroxine + liothyronine therapy is difficult to interpret due to the heterogeneity of patient populations treated, different dosing protocols, short duration, and different endpoints which may or may not reflect hypothyroid symptoms, or the tissue response at a biological meaningful level [6, 8, 107]. One study found benefit of combined therapy after thyroidectomy [108] but others have not [109]. Even though meta-analyses of randomized controlled trials have not found benefit of combined levothyroxine/liothyronine replacement versus levothyroxine monotherapy, combined therapy is preferred by hypothyroid patients in these trials [8, 110–113].

Both the ATA and European Thyroid Association (ETA) recognize that it is reasonable to give an experimental trial of combined levothyroxine and liothyronine to patients who continue to not feel well on levothyroxine monotherapy [8, 76]. Because liothyronine is rapidly absorbed and results in a peak 4 h after ingestion, it is prudent to use the lowest amount possible per dose, and to avoid use in patients with arrhythmia, cardiovascular compromise, osteoporosis, or pregnant women. Table 23.3 offers suggestions for the use of combination therapies for patients who desire such trials with combination therapy or alternative therapy (see below) with levothyroxine and/or desiccated thyroid (like Armour or Nature-Throid). These combinations are based on bioequivalence data of the hormones [50, 51], knowledge that the molar ratio of T4 to T3 secretion in humans is 14:1 [78], and supported by the suggested calculations of physiologic ratios with T3 and T4 hormones from the ETA [8]. They suggest methods of accounting for potential individual differences in levothyroxine and liothyronine absorption and for calculating levothyroxine and liothyronine doses, in such patients, that maintain the physiologic T4/T3 molar ratio using molar ratios of 13:1–20:1. It is suggested that the liothyronine dose is split, if possible, with the largest dose given at bedtime [8] to attempt to simulate the circadian rise in T3 that naturally happens in normal patients around 3 AM following the TSH surge [114]. This calculation (see T4:T3 ratios in Table 23.3) allows for liothyronine doses much lower than doses used in randomized controlled trials. The higher T4:T3 ratios could be used in patients with moderate to higher adverse risks to thyroid hormone. Another simple approach, used by this author, to do combination trials in healthy individuals, solely based on bioequivalence data [51, 52], is to replace 35 mcg of levothyroxine monotherapy with 10 mcg of liothyronine per day, the latter split in two doses.

An advantage of levothyroxine and liothyronine combinations over desiccated thyroid preparations is the fact that each hormone can be adjusted individually and that one can avoid the undesirable high content of T3 in available fixed doses desiccated thyroid preparations, such as Armour or Nature-Throid, where the molar ratio is 4.3:1 (60 mg having 38 mcg T4 and 9 mcg T3, 15 mg 9.5 mcg T4 and 2.37 T3) [115] or that of European preparations with T4:T3 combinations of 10:1 in Prothyroid, 5:1 in Novothyral, and 4:1 in Thyreotom, and deal with the fact that the bio-availability of T4 and T3 is similar after ingestion from all the oral preparations [116].

Table 23.3 Dose approximations for alternative thyroid replacement therapy trials using combinations of levothyroxine (LT4 mcg) with liothyronine (T3 mcg) or desiccated thyroid (DT, grain) equivalent that maintain T4:T3 daily dosing ratios[a] between 14:1 and 19:1

Baseline LT4 mcg dose	LT4:T3 ratios 14:1 16:1 19:1	LT4 × tablets/week + T3 dose × tablets/week	LT4 tablets/week + DT × tablets/week
25	20:1.6 20:1.47 21:1.25		0 mcg × 7+0.25 g × 7
50	40:3.3 41:2.9 43:2.3	50 mcg × 5.5 +2.5 mcg × 7	25 mcg × 7 +0.25 g × 7
75	60:5 61.7:4.4 63.7:3.75	50 mcg × 8 +5 mcg × 7	50 mcg × 5.5 +0.50 g × 7
88	70:5.6 72:5.17 74.8:4.4	75 mcg × 5 +5 mcg × 7	50 mcg × 7 + 0.50 g × 7
100	80:6.6 82:5.88 85:5	75 mcg × 7 + 5 mcg × 7	50 mcg × 7.5 + 0.50 g × 7
112	89:7.4 92:6.5 95:5.6	88 mcg × 7 + 7.5 mcg × 7	75 mcg × 7.5 + 0.50 g × 7
125	100:8.3 103:7.35 106:6.25	100 mcg × 7 + 7.5 mcg × 7	75 mcg × 7 + 0.75 g × 7
137	109:9.1 113:8.0 116:6.85	112 mcg × 7 + 7.5 mcg × 7	88 mcg × 7 +0.75 g × 7

Individual adjustments of liothyronine or T3 are usually necessary to increase serum free T3 and lower free T4 (fT4). Giving more levothyroxine only increases fT4 dose but does not increase endogenous free T3, as the deiodinases are suppressed at higher fT4 and suppressed TSH levels. This author aims for serum free T3/free T4 ratio of about 3, which is found in healthy individuals [117].

This author likes 3-month cycles for combination and alternative therapy (see below) trials in order to bypass a potential placebo effect, which can last up to 6 weeks, and allow patients to have an honest assessment of their well-being. Some patients return to standard levothyroxine monotherapy, while others have a clear preference for combination therapies. Some patients find it a nuisance to take thyroid more than once a day, or to cut liothyronine in small doses, or pay multiple co-pays using two thyroid preparations.

An example for trial of combination levothyroxine + liothyronine therapy based on ETA recommendations, from Table 23.3, is a patient who was on 50 mcg

Table 23.3 (continued)

Baseline LT4 mcg dose	LT4:T3 ratios 14:1 16:1 19:1	LT4 × tablets/week + T3 dose × tablets/week	LT4 tablets/week + DT × tablets/week
150	120:10 123:8.8 127:7.5	125 × 7 +10 mcg × 7	88 mcg × 7 +1.0 grain
175	140:11.6 144:10.2 148:8.75	137 mcg × 7 + 10 mcg × 7	112 mcg × 7 + 1.0 grain
200	160:13.3 164:11.7 170:10	175 mcg × 7 + 10 mcg × 7	125 mcg × **7** + 1.25 grain
300	240:19.8 246:17.6 255:15	200 mcg × 9 + 15–20 mcg × 7	200 mcg × 7 + 1.5 grain

Legend: calculations use liothyronine in 5 mcg tablets and desiccated thyroid in doses 0.25–0.5 g tablets to allow the daily dose to be divided into two to three portions for separate daily dosing, given short half-life of T3. One grain desiccated thyroid is = 60 mg, the T4:T3 ratio in DT ~ 4.3:1. Content per grain of desiccated thyroid (g) of T4-T3 (mcg) and approximate T4 equivalent for each dose of desiccated thyroid is (0.25 g) 9.5–2.25 ~ 20 mcg, (0.5 g) 19–4.5 ~ 35 mcg, (0.75 g) 28.5–6.75 ~ 50 mcg, (1) 38–9 ~ 65 mcg, (1.25) 47.5–11.25 ~ 80 mcg, (1.5) 57–13.5 ~ 100 mcgs

[a]Calculations for T4:T3 ratios were adapted from Wiersinga et al. [8]; for each ratio the total baseline LT4 dose is divided by 15, 17, and 20, respectively, to attain T3 dose for each of the three ratios calculated. The T3 dose (1/15, 1/17, and 1/20 of total) is multiplied by 3 (to address 1/3: T3/T4 bioequivalence based on data from Celi et al. [51], and this value is subtracted from the initial LT4 dose to derive the new T4 dose to be used in combination with T3 dose calculated. Rounding off to most achievable dosing. Liothyronine or Cytomel is manufactured in 5, 12.5, and 25 mcg doses. The 5 and 12.5 doses could be cut in ½ or quarters to achieve 2.5 and 3.1 doses, respectively

levothyroxine daily and in a trial could take the equivalent of 40 mcg daily by taking 50 mcg tab per day for 5 days and ½ tab the 6th day, and none on the 7th day + 1/2 tablet of 5 mcg liothyronine daily at night to achieve the 14:1 ratio dosing.

In addition to trials of combination therapy with standard levothyroxine and liothyronine, patients want to try compounded thyroid preparations or desiccated "natural" thyroid. The Endocrine Society, ATA, and ETA do not recommend that thyroid combinations be compounded by pharmacies, because of potential for errors leading to iatrogenic hypo- and hyperthyroidism, and this author strongly supports this recommendation. Similarly desiccated thyroid hormone preparation is not recommended for thyroid replacement due to its high T3 content. Therefore the use of desiccated thyroid is considered nonstandard therapy or alternative therapy. For physicians, this is an ethical dilemma, as we are bound to help with evidence-based treatments and to cause no harm. Education and flexibility in negotiation is recommended so that patients, with their preferences considered, are appropriately treated while protecting them from harm. It is important to acknowledge patients' interest in self-regulation and to work toward a long-term healing partnership with the right therapy. This may discourage patients from pursuing alternative care by nonmedically trained practitioners, who may administer even more unregulated "thyroid" preparations. Physicians always have the choice of opting out of participation in these trials and refering patients to another practice. From an integrative medicine perspective, it would be safer for our patients and more rewarding for us as physicians to oversee our patients' individual trials of thyroid preparations. This can be achieved by having mutual agreements on the goals for treatment and potential risks of the therapy (which symptom(s) will be addressed by the trial and a signed consent), making sure there are no contraindications and that potential causes of lack of wellness, as noted in Table 23.1, have been addressed.

This author finds that small doses of desiccated thyroid may be used judiciously and safely, alone or in combination therapy with levothyroxine for patients who want to try it and are deemed to be reliable and healthy. Desiccated thyroid offers dried entire thyroid contents minus connective tissue, including other thyronines, T1 and T2, which may have physiologic metabolic functions [118]. 3,5-T2 is also made by peripheral tissue conversion, it is measurable in athyreotic patients, and it is not regulated as T3 and T4 are by TSH [119]. An example of such alternative trial from Table 23.3 is a patient whose initial dose is 75 mcg/day of levothyroxine monotherapy. He or she can take the equivalent of 40 mcg daily of levothyroxine by taking 50 mcg tab per day for 5 days and ½ tab the 6th day, and none on the 7th day and adding 0.5 grain desiccated Armour daily: The Armour dose should be split to 0.25 g for twice daily dosing. Most patients are not compliant with the ideal thrice daily dosing for any T3-containing preparations. It is best to avoid doses of desiccated thyroid above the 1–1.5 grain (60–90 mg) range, and to add levothyroxine as needed to achieve treatment goals, while avoiding adverse risk or use in at-risk populations. This author uses the 0.25 grain or 15 mg tablet dose of desiccated thyroid to supplement levothyroxine and 5 mcg tablets of liothyronine to supplement T3 for combination therapy trials.

Patients receiving combination therapies should aim for goal TSH recommended for their diagnosis (section "Thyroid Hormone Replacement with Levothyroxine Monotherapy and Monitoring Adequacy of Replacement with Thyroid-Stimulating Hormone (TSH)") and have free T3 and T4 levels measured 6–8 weeks after each dose change. Note that measurements of serum total or free T3 are currently discouraged and not considered or recommended as outcome measure in the treatment of hypothyroidism. Neither the levothyroxine, liothyronine, nor desiccated thyroid should be taken the morning of blood testing to avoid transient peaks in hormone levels (17 % for T4 and up to 42 % for T3) which occur after ingestion [120].

Dealing Well with Radioactive Iodine: Addressing Mind-Body Concerns and Complementary Approaches to Patients Receiving Radioiodine Therapy

The goal of this section is to address emotional issues experienced by patients when they undergo radioiodine ablations or adjuvant therapy and create awareness of potential confounders with iodine-containing supplements in patients receiving I^{131}.

Patients experience considerable stress over the process of undergoing radioactive iodine scans, ablations, and adjuvant treatments [34]. After agreeing to receive radioiodine, dietary changes need to render the patient iodine deficiency for optimization of tissue ablation. During the exposure to radioiodine, patients are concerned about contaminating their homes and their families, particularly children. Patients do not like the isolation necessary for the process and much less the potential side effects of nausea, fatigue, acute and chronic sialadenitis, xerostomia, dysgeusia, and small (1 %) but significant increased risks for future secondary malignancy, particularly leukemia [121–124]. The ATA issued guidelines to limit the public's risk of radiation exposure after a patient receives radioiodine treatment, provided useful outlines to identify patient's capability to manage the process, and help identify patients who need more guidance or are best served by hospitalization during the treatment process [125]. Education of patients using patient decision aids helps them be more confident about the decision to receive radioiodine [126]. Meeting with radiation safety staff and a nuclear physicist can further assist with safety concerns regarding exposures to family and home.

Recombinant TSH stimulation is preferable to thyroid withdrawal in most cases for multiple reasons: (1) patients feel better and are therefore more emotionally stable to manage their care during the treatment, (2) the tissue exposure and toxicity to non-thyroid tissue is lessened [127], and (3) effectiveness of the treatment is not compromised [128]. Risk is further mitigated by use of smaller doses of radioiodine doses which are equally effective for ablation and adjuvant treatments [129] and less likely to result in radiotoxicity [130].

For patients who must receive radioiodine therapy because they have moderate to high risk disease, education and anxiety reduction techniques before treatment help patients deal with their issues. As mentioned in section "Complementary Therapies for Fatigue and Mind-Body Issues Faced by Thyroid Cancer Patients" of this chapter, CBT + H trials may be helpful during this time. The process is cumbersome even for the most capable, so planning, patience, having access to social media to stay in touch emotionally during isolation, and participation in cancer support groups are useful. Preparation for the iodine deficient diet (<50 mcg/day) has been improved by the availability of downloadable cookbooks from the internet [see Supplement for section "Dealing Well with Radioactive Iodine: Addressing

Mind-Body Concerns and Complementary Approaches to Patients Receiving Radioiodine Therapy"].

Patients often want to be told exactly what they can eat, and not just what they need to avoid. A reasonable way to help patients prepare for radioiodine therapy and possibly lose weight at the same time in preparation for a post-thyroidectomy hypothyroid state is to use the "Paleo" diet but excluding fish, eggs, seaweed, kelp, and salt (see also supplement section "Understanding and Avoiding Weight Gain After Thyroidectomy"). This diet is primarily composed of whole foods consistent of meat protein, fruits, and vegetables and free of dairy, grain, and processed foods. Patients should avoid all vitamins or supplements particularly those containing iodine [see supplement section "Dealing Well with Radioactive Iodine: Addressing Mind-Body Concerns and Complementary Approaches to Patients Receiving Radioiodine Therapy" for examples]. A recent survey of thyroid cancer patients reported high kelp use in thyroid cancer patients [131]. Patients use iodine for its reported antioxidative and antineoplastic properties on other organs at doses of 3–5 mg/day, because studies suggest iodine may have a protective effect in preventing malignancies [132].

If patients have received a high iodinated contrast load, such as a contrasted CT scan, it is suggested to wait 8 weeks to achieve normal urinary iodine <164 mcg/L, prior to starting iodine depletion protocols, scans, and/or ablative or adjuvant radioiodine treatment [133]. The same advice may be used for patients who have high iodine intake from supplements. These patients may benefit from assessment of 24h urinary iodine levels to ascertain deficiency (<50 mcg/day) and reassure them that they are ready for diagnostic scans and radioiodine treatment.

Summary

The care of patients who undergo thyroidectomy is complex, and the process affects the whole patient. These patients face the lifelong task of managing hypothyroidism and have cumulative burdens if they also have a thyroid cancer diagnosis. Weight gain is common and lack of wellness due to fatigue, psychological and neurocognitive issues, and a decrease in quality of life may occur and persist long-term after thyroidectomy. We currently do not have a clear differentiation of which symptoms are directly related to the thyroid cancer diagnosis or treatment and which are related to how and how well thyroid therapy is replaced following thyroidectomy. Our current approach to thyroid hormone replacement with levothyroxine monotherapy is adequate, but not optimal. New thyroid replacement therapies are clearly needed, including better bioavailable slow release liothyronine preparations, to normalize thyroid axis parameters more physiologically, and perhaps address hypothyroid symptoms better. In addition to counseling patients about caloric restriction to prevent weight gain after thyroidectomy, it is also reasonable to have a goal of maintaining TSH ≤ 2.5 mIU/L for most healthy patients who do not have thyroid cancer. Combination thyroid replacement with T3 and T4 therapy may be tried safely in patients with persistent hypothyroid symptoms with mutual goals set and consent. In addition until we have better understanding of, and therapies for, the psychological and physical symptoms attributable to a thyroid cancer diagnosis, we can safely use complementary mind-body therapies shown to be effective in improving well-being in patients with non-thyroid cancers. Addressing mind and body issues together, before and after thyroidectomy, and integrating safe complementary treatments to standard conventional therapies broaden the options we can offer, and provide a more comprehensive and holistic approach to and for our patients.

Supplement Section for Chapter 23

Chapter 23 section "Perioperative Period: Stress and Anxiety Around Surgery"

Relaxation and guided imagery: Integrative medicine centers recommend and use several commercially available "relaxation and guided imagery instructional materials" available online (http://www.amazon.com). Dr. Olson has experience with and tends to use for her thyroid patients Peggy Huddleston's Relaxation/Healing CD plus instructional CD or Huddleston's book and CD, *Prepare for Surgery, Heal Faster with Relaxation and Quick Start CD: A Guide of Mind-Body Techniques.*

Chapter 23 section "Understanding and Avoiding Weight Gain After Thyroidectomy"

Commercially available whole food diets include the Mediterranean diet [53] or Paleo diet programs that are reasonable guides for these patients [54, 55].

Mindfulness-based stress reduction (MBSR) is the process of training the mind to pay attention without judgment to oneself or what is happening in the moment. Mindfulness practice leads to greater awareness of one's physical and mental state leading to better understanding of self, better self-regulation, and to making choices that support well-being and health. For mindfulness reading and available CDs recommended by Dr. Olson, search on the web Jon Kabat-Zinn, and mindfulness meditation CDs and reading lay press publications on the topic by Pickert K. 2014. For tertiary centers to initiate their own MBSR program, inquiry may be made through the University of Mass Center for Mindfulness.

Chapter 23 section "Dealing Well with Radioactive Iodine: Addressing Mind-Body Concerns and Complimentary Approaches to Patients Receiving Radioiodine Therapy"

Thyroid cancer survivor websites:

1. ThyCa website (http://www.thyca.org/download/document/231/Cookbook.pdf)

2. Light of Life Foundation, checkyourneck.com, see The Light of life Foundation Cook book, which also has recipes for low iodine diet.

Iodine-containing supplements examples: spirulina, seaweed, a high concentration iodine brands such as Iodoral (brand name for high iodine preparation), and kelp.

References

1. Abraham-Nordling M, Törring O, Hamberger B, Lundell G, Tallstedt L, Calissendorff J, Wallin G. Graves' disease: a long-term quality-of-life follow up of patients randomized to treatment with antithyroid drugs, radioiodine, or surgery. Thyroid. 2005;15(11):1279–86.
2. Bresner L, Banach R, Rodin G, Thabane L, Ezzat S, Swaska AM. J Clin Endocrinol Metab. 2015;100:977–85.
3. To J, Goldberg AS, Jones J, Zhang J, Lowe J, Ezzat S, Gilbert J, Zahedi A, Segal P, Swaska AM. A systematic review of randomized control trials for management of post-treatment fatigue in thyroid cancer survivors. Thyroid. 2014;25:198–210.
4. Benevicius R, Prange AJ. Mental improvement after replacement therapy with thyroxine plus triiodothyronine: relationship to cause of hypothyroidism. Int J Neuropsychopharmacol. 2000;3:167–74.
5. Eustatia-Reuten CF, Corssmit EP, Pereira AM, Frolich M, Baxx JJ, Romijn JA, Smit JW. Quality of life in long-term exogenous subclinical hyperthyroidism and the effects of restoration of euthyroidism, a randomized controlled trial. Clin Endocrinol (Oxf). 2006;64:284–91.
6. Biondi B, Wartofsky L. Treatment with thyroid hormone. Endocr Rev. 2014;35(3):433–512. doi:10.1210/er.2013-1083. Epub 2014 Jan 16. Review.
7. Andreas Schäffler, Prof. Dr. med. Hormone replacement after thyroid and parathyroid surgery. Dtsch Arztebl Int. 2010;107(47): 827–34. Published online 2010 Nov 26. doi:10.3238/arztebl.2010.0827.
8. Wiersinga WM, Duntas L, Fadeyev V, et al. 2012 ETA guidelines: the use of L-T4+L-T3 in the treatment of hypothyroidism. Eur Thyroid J. 2012;1(2):55–71. Published online 13 Jun 2012. doi:10.1159/000339444.
9. Morley S, Goldfarb M. Support needs and survivorship concerns of thyroid cancer patients. Thyroid. 2015;25:649–56.
10. Watt T, Hegedüs L, Rasmussen AK, Groenvold M, Bonnema SJ, Bjorner JB, Feld-Rasmussen U. Which domains of thyroid related quality of life are most relevant? Patients and clinicians provide complementary perspectives. Thyroid. 2007;17:647–54.
11. Eisenberg DM, Davis RB, Ettner SL, et al. Trends in alternative medicine use in the United States, 1990–1997: results of a follow-up national survey. JAMA. 1998;280:1569–75.
12. Rosen JE, Gardiner P, Saper RB, et al. Complementary and alternative medicine use among patients with thyroid cancer. Thyroid. 2013;23(10):1238–46. doi:10.1089/thy.2012.0495.
13. Sadovsky R, Collins N, Tighe AP, Brunton SA, Safeer R. Patient use of dietary supplements: a clinician's perspective. Curr Med Res Opin. 2008;24(4):1209–16.
14. Ashar BH, Rice TN, Sisson SD. Physicians' understanding of the regulation of dietary supplements. Arch Intern Med. 2007;167(9):966–9.
15. Ang-Lee MK, Moss J, Yuan C. Herbal medicines and perioperative care. JAMA. 2001;286(2):208–16. doi:10.1001/jama.286.2.208.
16. Abe A, Kaye AD, Gritsenko K, Urman RD, Kate AM. Perioperative analgesia and the effects of dietary supplements. Clin Anesthesiol. 2014;28(2):183–9.

17. Brake MK, Bartlett C, Hart RD, Trites JR, Taylor SM. Complementary and alternative medicine use in the thyroid patients of a head and neck practice. Otolaryngol Head Neck Surg. 2011;145(2):208–12. doi:10.1177/0194599811407564.
18. Saw JT, Bahari MB, Ang HH, Lim YH. Potential drug-herb interaction with antiplatelet/anticoagulant drugs. Complement Ther Clin Pract. 2006;12(4):236–41.
19. Wong WW, Gabriel A, Maxwell GP, Gupta SC. Bleeding risks of herbal, homeopathic, and dietary supplements: a hidden nightmare for plastic surgeons? Aesthet Surg J. 2012;32(3):332–46. doi:10.1177/1090820X12438913.
20. Dinehart SM, Henry L. Dietary supplements: altered coagulation and effects on bruising. Dermatol Surg. 2005;31(7 Pt 2):819–26.
21. Leinung M, Beyer T. Postoperative hypocalcemia after thyroidectomy: can it be prevented? Endocr Pract. 2015;21:452–3.
22. Holick MF. Vitamin D, deficiency. N Engl J Med. 2007;357:266–81.
23. Grey A, Lucas J, Horne A, Gamble G, Davidson JS, Reid IR. Vitamin D repletion in patients with primary hyperparathyroidism and coexistent vitamin D insufficiency. J Clin Endocrinol Metab. 2005;90:2122–6.
24. Heany RP. Health is better at serum 25(OH) D above 30 ng/ml. J Steroid Biochem Mol Biol. 2013;136:224–8.
25. Falcone TE, Stein DJ, Jumaily JS, Pearce E, Holick MF, McAneny DB, Jalisi S, Grillone GA, Stone MD, Devaiah AK, Noordzij JP. Correlating pre-operative vitamin D status with post-thyroidectomy hypocalcemia. Endocr Pract. 2015;21:348–54.
26. Arlt W, Fremerey C, Callies F, Reincke M, Schneider P, Timmermann W, Allolio B. Well being, mood, and calcium homeostasis in patients with hypoparathyroidism receiving standard treatment with calcium and vitamin D. Eur J Endocrinol. 2002;146:215–22.
27. Pritchard MJ. Managing anxiety in the elective surgical patient. Br J Nurs. 2009;18(7):416–9.
28. Relaxation techniques for health: what you need to know. https://nccih.nih.gov/sites/nccam.nih.gov/files/Get_The_Facts_Relaxation_Techniques_02-06-2015.pdf.
29. Brewer S, Gleditsch SL, Syblik D, Tietiens ME, Vacik HW. Pediatric anxiety: child life intervention in day surgery. J Pediatr Nurs. 2006;21(1):13–22.
30. Gonzales EA, Ledesma RJ, McAllister DJ, Perry SM, Dyer CA, Maye JP. Effects of guided imagery on postoperative outcomes in patients undergoing same-day surgical procedures: a randomized, single blind study. AANA J. 2010;78(3):181–8.
31. Tussek DL, Church JM, Strong SA, Grass JA, Fazio VW. Guided imagery: a significant advance in the care of patients undergoing elective colorectal surgery. Dis Colon Rectum. 1997;40(2):172–8.
32. Guisti M, Melle G, Fenocchio M, et al. Five-year longitudinal evaluation of quality of life in a cohort of patients with differentiated thyroid carcinoma. J Zhejiang Univ Sci B. 2011;12(3):163–73.
33. Almeida J, Vartanian JG, Kowalshi LP. Clinical predictors of quality of life in patients with initial differentiated thyroid cancers. Arch Otolaryngol Head Neck Surg. 2009;135(4):342–6. doi:10.1001/archoto.2009.16.
34. Olson BR's patient communications, and Olson BR, Insights of 51 patients on their thyroid cancer treatment (manuscript under review).
35. Giusti M, Sibilla F, Cappi C, Dellepiane M, Tombesi F, Ceresola E, Augeri C, Rasore E, Minuto F. A case-controlled study on the quality of life in a cohort of patients with history of differentiated thyroid carcinoma. J Endocrinol Invest. 2005;28(7):599–608.
36. Jonklaas J, Nsouli-Maktabi H. Weight changes in euthyroid patients undergoing thyroidectomy. Thyroid. 2011;21(12):1343–51.
37. Weinreb JT, Yang Y, Braunstein GD. Do patients gain weight after thyroidectomy for thyroid cancer? Thyroid. 2011;21(12):1339–42.
38. Lönn L, Stenlöf K, Ottosson M, Lindroos AK, Nyström E, Sjöström L. Body weight and body composition changes after treatment of hyperthyroidism. J Clin Endocrinol Metab. 1998;83:4269–73.

39. Pears J, Jung RT, Gunn A. Long-term weight changes in treated hyperthyroid and hypothyroid patients. Scott Med J. 1990;35(6):180–2.
40. van Veenendaal NR, Rivkees SA. Treatment of pediatric Graves' disease is associated with excessive weight gain. J Clin Endocrinol Metab. 2011;96(10):3257–63.
41. Tigas S, Idiculla J, Beckett G, Toft A. Is excessive weight gain after ablative treatment of hyperthyroidism due to inadequate thyroid hormone therapy? Thyroid. 2000;10(12):1107–11.
42. Ozdemir S, Ozis ES, Gulpinar K, Aydin TH, Suzen B, Korkmaz A. The effects of levothyroxine substitution on body composition and body mass after total thyroidectomy for benign nodular goiter. Endocr Regul. 2010;44(4):147–53.
43. Laurberg P, Knudsen N, Andersen S, et al. Thyroid function and obesity. Eur Thyroid J. 2012;1(3):159–67.
44. Lovejoy JC, Champagne CM, de Jonge L, Xie H, Smith SR. Increased visceral fat and decreased energy expenditure during the menopausal transition. Int J Obes (Lond). 2008;32(6):949–58.
45. Santen RJ, Allred DC, Ardoin SP, et al. Postmenopausal hormone therapy: an Endocrine Society scientific statement. J Clin Endocrinol Metab. 2010;95(7 Suppl 1):s1–66.
46. Davis SR, Castelo-Branco C, Chedraui P, Lumsden MA, Nappi RE, Shah D, Villaseca P; Writing Group of the International Menopause Society for World Menopause Day 2012. Understanding weight gain at menopause. Climacteric. 2012;15(5):419–29.
47. Penev PD. Update on energy homeostasis and insufficient sleep. J Clin Endocrinol Metab. 2012;97:1792–801.
48. Sumithran P, Prendergast LA, Delbridge E, Purcell K, Shulkes A, Kriketos A, Proietto J. Long-term persistence or hormonal adaptations to weight loss. N Engl J Med. 2011;365:1597–609.
49. Walsh JP, Ward LC, Burke V, Bhagat CI, Shiels L, Henley D, Gillett MJ, Gilbert R, Tanner M, Stuckey BG. Small changes in thyroxine dosage do not produce measurable changes in hypothyroid symptoms, well-being, or quality of life: results of a double-blind, randomized clinical trial. J Clin Endocrinol Metab. 2006;91(7):2624–30.
50. Celi FS, Zemskova M, Linderman JD, Babar NI, Skarulis MC, Csako G, Wesley R, Costello R, Penzak SR, Pucino F. The pharmacodynamic equivalence of levothyroxine and liothyronine: a randomized, double blind, cross-over study in thyroidectomized patients. Clin Endocrinol. 2010;72:709–15.
51. Celi FS, Zemskova M, Linderman JD, Smith S, Drinkard B, Sachdev V, Skarulis MC, Kozlosky M, Csako G, Costello R, Pucino F. Metabolic effects of liothyronine therapy in hypothyroidism: a randomized, double-blind, crossover trial of liothyronine versus levothyroxine. J Clin Endocrinol Metab. 2011;96:3466–74.
52. Miller WC, Koceja DM, Hamilton EJ. A meta-analysis of the past 25 years of weight loss research using diet, exercise or diet plus exercise intervention. Int J Obes Relat Metab Disord. 1997;21(10):941–7.
53. Castro-Quezada I, Román-Viñas B, Serra-Majem L. The mediterranean diet and nutritional adequacy: a review. Nutrients. 2014;6(1):231–48. Published online 3 Jan 2014. doi:10.3390/nu6010231. PMCID: PMC3916858.
54. Stephenson N, Cordain L. The paleo diet and cookbook. John Wiley & Sons, Hoboken, NJ, 2011.
55. Klonoff DC. The beneficial effects of a paleolithic diet on type 2 diabetes and other risk factors for cardiovascular disease. J Diabetes Sci Technol. 2009;3(6):1229–32. Published online Nov 2009. PMCID: PMC2787021.
56. Donnelly JE, Blair SN, Jakicic JM, et al. American College of Sports Medicine Position Stand. Appropriate physical activity intervention strategies for weight loss and prevention of weight regain for adults. Med Sci Sports Exerc. 2009;41(2):459–71.
57. Swift DL, Johannsen, NM, Lavie CJ, et al. The role of exercise and physical activity in weight loss and maintenance. Prog Cardiovasc Dis. 2014;56(4):441–7. Published online 11 Oct 2013. doi:10.1016/j.pcad.2013.09.012.

58. Bravata DM, Smith-Spangler C, Sundaram V, Gienger AL, Lin N, Lewis R, Stave CD, Olkin I, Sirard JR. Using pedometers to increase physical activity and improve health: a systematic review. JAMA. 2007;298(19):2296–304.
59. Xiao Q, Arem H, Moore SC, Hollenbeck AR, Matthews CE. A large prospective investigation of sleep duration, weight change, and obesity in the NIH-AARP Diet and Health Study cohort. Am J Epidemiol. 2013;178(11):1600–10.
60. Wing RR, Marcus MD, Epstein LH, Kupfer D. Mood and weight loss in a behavioral treatment program. J Consult Clin Psychol. 1983;51(1):153–5.
61. Kabat-Zinn J. Mindfulness-based interventions in context: past, present, and future. Clin Psychol Sci Pract. 2003;10(2):144–56. doi:10.1093/clipsy/bpg016.
62. Kabat-Zinn J. Full catastrophe living: using the wisdom of your body and mind to face stress, pain and illness. New York: Delacourt; 1990.
63. Swaka AM, Naeem A, Jones J, Lowe J, Segal P, Goguen J, Gilbert J, Zahedi A, Kelly C, Ezzat S. Persistent post-treatment fatigue in thyroid cancer survivors: a Scoping review. Endocrinol Metab Clin North Am. 2014;43:475–94.
64. Singer S, Lincke T, Gamper E, Baskharan K, Schreiber S, Hinz A, Schulte T. Quality of life in patients with thyroid Cancer Compared to the general population. Thyroid. 2012;22:117–24.
65. Husson O, Mols F, van de Poll-Franse L, de Vries J, Schep G, Thong MS. Variation in fatigue among 6011 (long-term) cancer survivors and a normative population: a study from the population-based PROFILES registry. Support Care Cancer. 2015;23(7):2165–74. doi:10.1007/s00520-014-2577-5. Epub 6 Jan 2015.
66. Greenlee H, Balneaves LG, Carlson LE, et al. Clinical practice guidelines on the use of integrative therapies as supportive care in patients treated for breast cancer. J Natl Cancer Inst Monogr. 2014;50:346–58.
67. Molassiotis A, Bardy J, Finnegan-John J, et al. Acupuncture for cancer-related fatigue in patients with breast cancer: a pragmatic randomized controlled trial. J Clin Oncol. 2012;30:4470–6. doi:10.1200/jco.2012.41.6222.
68. Buffart LM, VanUffelen JGZ, Riphagen II, et al. Physical and psychosocial benefits of yoga in cancer patients and survivors, a systematic review and metaanalysis of randomized controlled trials. BMC Cancer. 2012;12:559. doi:10.1186/1471-2407-12-559.
69. Montgomery GH, Kangas M, David D, Hallquist MN, Green S, Bovbjerg DH, Schnur JB. Fatigue during breast cancer radiotherapy: an initial randomized study of cognitive behavioral therapy plus hypnosis. Health Psychol. 2009;28:317–22. doi:10.1037/a0013582.
70. Finnegan-John J, Molassiotis A, Richardson A, Ream E. A systematic review of complementary and alternative medicine interventions for the management of cancer-related fatigue. Integr Cancer Ther. 2013;12:276–90.
71. Brown JC, Huedo-Medina TB, Pescatello LS, Pescatello SM, Ferrer RA, Johnson BT. Efficacy of exercise interventions in modulating cancer-related fatigue among adult cancer survivors: a meta-analysis. Cancer Epidemiol Biomarkers Prev. 2011;20:123–33. doi:10.1158/1055-9965.epi-10-0988.
72. Sadeeka Al-Majid S, Gray DP. A biobehavioral model for the study of exercise interventions in cancer-related fatigue. Biol Res Nurs. 2009;10(4):381–91.
73. Marcus BH, Simkin LR. The transtheoretical model: applications to exercise behavior. Med Sci Sports Exerc. 1994;26(11):1400–4.
74. Mishra SI, Scherer RW, Geigle PM, Berlanstein DR, Topaloglu O, Gotay CC, Snyder C. Exercise interventions on health-related quality of life for cancer survivors. Cochrane Database of Systematic Reviews 2012;(8):CD007566. doi:10.1002/14651858.CD007566.pub2.
75. Vigårio Pdos S, Chachamovits DS, Teixiera PF, Rocque Mde L, Santos ML, Vaisman M. Exercise is associated with better quality of life in patients on thyrotropin-suppressive therapy with levothyroxine for differentiated thyroid carcinoma. Arq Bras Endocrinol Metabol. 2014;58:274–81.
76. Jonklaas J, Bianco AC, Bauer AJ, Burman KD, Cappola AR, Celi FS, Cooper DS, Kim BW, Peeters RP, Rosenthal MS, Swaka AM. Guidelines for the treatment of hypothyroidism. Thyroid. 2014;24:1670–751.

77. Jonklaas J, Davidson B, Bhagat S, Soldin SJ. Triiodothyronine levels in athyreotic individuals during levothyroxine therapy. JAMA. 2008;299:769–77.
78. Pilo A, Iervasi G, Vitek F, Ferdeghini M, Cazzuola F, Bianchi R. Thyroidal and peripheral production of 3,5,3′-triiodothyronine in humans by multicompartmental analysis. Am J Physiol. 1990;258:E715–26.
79. Grozinsky-Glasberg S, Fraser A, Nahshoni E, Weizman A, Leibovici L. Thyroxine-triiodothyronine combination therapy versus thyroxine monotherapy for clinical hypothyroidism: meta-analysis of randomized controlled trials. J Clin Endocrinol Metab. 2006;91:2592–9.
80. Haugen BR, Alexander EK, Bible KC, et al. American thyroid association management guidelines for adult patients with thyroid nodules and differentiated thyroid cancer. Thyroid. 2015;26(1):1–133.
81. Bianco AC, Salvatore D, Gereben B, Berry MJ, Larsen PR. Biochemistry, cellular and molecular biology, and physiological roles of the iodothyronine selenodeiodinases. Endocr Rev. 2002;23:38–89.
82. Panicker V, Cluett C, Shields B, et al. A common variation in deiodinase 1 gene DIO1 is associated with the relative levels of free thyroxine and triiodothyronine. J Clin Endocrinol Metab. 2008;93(8):3075–81.
83. Peeters RP, van der Deure WM, Visser TJ. Genetic variation in thyroid hormone pathway genes; polymorphisms in the TSH receptor and the iodothyronine deiodinases. Eur J Endocrinol. 2006;155:655–62.
84. Torlantano M, Durante C, Torrente I, et al. Type 2 deiodinase polymorphism (threonine 92 alanine) predicts L-thyroxine dose to achieve target thyrotropin levels in thyroidectomized patients. J Clin Endocrinol Metab. 2008;93:910–3.
85. Panicker V, Saravanan P, Vaidya B, et al. Common variation in the DIO2 gene predicts baseline psychological well-being and response to combination thyroxine plus triiodothyronine therapy in hypothyroid patients. J Clin Endocrinol Metab. 2009;94(5):1623–9.
86. Dayan CM, Panicker V. Novel insights into thyroid hormones from the study of common genetic variation. Nat Rev Endocrinol. 2009;5:211–8.
87. Andersen S, Pedersen KM, Bruun NH, Laurberg P. Narrow individual variations in serum T(4) and T(3) in normal subjects: a clue to the understanding of subclinical thyroid disease. J Clin Endocrinol Metab. 2002;87:1068–72.
88. Hollowell JG, Staehling NW, Flanders WD, et al. Serum TSH, T_4, and thyroid antibodies in the United States population (1988 to 1994): National Health and Nutrition Examination Survey (NHANES III). J Clin Endocrinol Metab. 2002;87:489–99. Abstract, ISI.
89. Baloch Z, Carayon P, Conte-Devolx B, et al.; Guidelines Committee, National Academy of Clinical Biochemistry. Laboratory medicine practice guidelines. Laboratory support for the diagnosis and monitoring of thyroid disease. Thyroid. 2003;13:3–126.
90. Boucai L, Hollowell JG, Surks MI. An approach for development of age-, gender-, and ethnicity-specific thyrotropin reference limits. Thyroid. 2011;21:5–11.
91. Vadiveloo T, Donnan PT, Murphy MJ, Leese GP. Age- and Gender specific TSH reference interval in people with no obvious thyroid disease in Tayside Scotland: the thyroid epidemiology, audit and research study (TEARS). J Clin Endocrinol Metab. 2013;98:1147–53.
92. Boucai L, Surks M. Reference limits of serum TSH and free T4 are significantly influenced by race and age in an urban outpatient medical practice. Clin Endocrinol (Oxf). 2009;70:788–93. doi:10.1111/j.1365-2265.2008.03390.x.
93. Van den Ven AC, Netea-Maier RT, Smit JW, et al. Thyrotropin versus age relation as an indicator of historical iodine intakes. Thyroid. 2015;25:629–634. doi:10.1089thy.2014.0574.
94. Biondi B. Thyroid and obesity: an intriguing relationship. J Clin Endocrinol Metab. 2010;95:3614–7.
95. Cappola AR, Ladenson PW. Hypothyroidism and atherosclerosis. J Clin Endocrinol Metab. 2003;88:2438–44.
96. Okosieme O, Lazarus JH. Thyroid dysfunction in pregnancy. Rev Endocrinol. 2008;2(4):50–3.

97. Glinoer D. The regulation of thyroid function in pregnancy: pathways of endocrine adaptation from physiology to pathology. Endocr Rev. 1997;18:404–33.
98. Alexander EK, Marqusee E, Lawrence J, Jarolim P, Fischer GA, Larsen PR. Timing and magnitude of increases in levothyroxine requirements during pregnancy in women with hypothyroidism. N Engl J Med. 2004;351:241–9.
99. Abalovich M, Amino N, Barbour LA, et al. Management of thyroid dysfunction during pregnancy and postpartum: an Endocrine Society clinical practice guideline. J Clin Endocrinol Metab. 2007;92:S1–47.
100. Stagnaro-Green A, Abalovich M, Alexander E, et al. Guidelines of the American Thyroid Association for the diagnosis and management of thyroid disease during pregnancy and postpartum. Thyroid. 2011;21:1081–125.
101. De Groot L, Abalovich M, Alexander EK, et al. Management of thyroid dysfunction during pregnancy and postpartum: an Endocrine Society clinical practice guideline. J Clin Endocrinol Metab. 2012;97:2543–65.
102. Biondi B, Wartofsky L. Combination treatment with T4 and T3: toward personalized replacement therapy in hypothyroidism? J Clin Endocrinol Metab. 2012;97(7):2256–71.
103. McAninch EA, Bianco AC. The history and future treatment of hypothyroidism. Ann Intern Med. 2016;164:50–6.
104. Canaris GJ, Manowitz NR, Mayor G, Ridgway EC. The Colorado thyroid disease prevalence study. Arch Intern Med. 2000;160:526–34.
105. Fish LH, Schwartz HL, Cavanaugh J, Steffes MW, Bantle JP, Oppenheimer JH. Replacement dose, metabolism, and bioavailability of levothyroxine in the treatment of hypothyroidism. Role of triiodothyronine in pituitary feedback in humans. N Engl J Med. 1987;316:764–70.
106. Hennemann G, Docter R, Visser TJ, Postema PT, Krenning EP. Thyroxine plus low-dose, slow-release triiodothyronine replacement in hypothyroidism: proof of principle. Thyroid. 2004;14:271–5.
107. McDermott MT. Does combination therapy make sense? Endocr Pract. 2012;18:750–7.
108. Bunevicius R, Jakuboniene N, Jurkevicius R, Cernicat J, Lasas L, Prange Jr AJ. Thyroxine vs thyroxine plus triiodothyronine in treatment of hypothyroidism after thyroidectomy for Graves' disease. Endocrine. 2002;18(2):129–33.
109. Walsh JP, Shiels L, Lim EM, Bhagat CI, et al. Combined thyroxine/liothyronine treatment does not improve well-being, quality of life, or cognitive function compared to thyroxine alone: a randomized controlled trial in patients with primary hypothyroidism. J Clin Endocrinol Metab. 2003;88(10):4543–50.
110. Bunevicius R, Kazanavicius G, Zalinkevicius R, Prange Jr AJ. Effects of thyroxine as compared with thyroxine plus triiodothyronine in patients with hypothyroidism. N Engl J Med. 1999;340:424–9.
111. Appelhof BC, Fliers E, Wekking EM, et al. Combined therapy with levothyroxine and liothyronine in two ratios, compared with levothyroxine monotherapy in primary hypothyroidism: a double-blind, randomized, controlled clinical trial. J Clin Endocrinol Metab. 2005;90:2666–74.
112. Escobar-Morreale HF, Botella-Carretero JI, Gómez-Bueno M, et al. Thyroid hormone replacement therapy in primary hypothyroidism: a randomized trial comparing L-thyroxine plus liothyronine with L-thyroxine alone. Ann Intern Med. 2005;142:412–24.
113. Nygaard B, Jensen EW, Kvetny J, et al. Effect of combination therapy with thyroxine (T4) and 3,5,3′-triiodothyronine versus T4 monotherapy in patients with hypothyroidism, a double-blind, randomised cross-over study. Eur J Endocrinol. 2009;161:895–902.
114. Russell W, Harrison RF, Smith N, et al. Free triiodothyronine has a distinct circadian rhythm that is delayed but parallels thyrotropin levels. J Clin Endocrinol Metab. 2008;93(6):2300–6.
115. Rees-Jones RW, Larsen PR. Triiodothyronine and thyroxine content of desiccated thyroid tablets. Metabolism. 1977;26(11):1213–8.
116. LeBoff MS, Kaplan MM, Silva JE, Larsen PR. Bioavailability of thyroid hormones from oral replacement preparations. Metabolism. 1982;31(9):900–5.

117. Gullo D, Latina A, Frasca F, Le Moli R, Pelligriti G, Vigneri R. Levothyroxine monotherapy cannot guarantee euthyroidism I all athyreotic patients. PLoS One. 2011;6:e22552. PMID: 21829633.
118. Peitzner M, Lehmphul I, Friedrich N, et al. Translating pharmacological findings from hypothyroid rodents to euthyroid humans: is there a functional role of endogenous 3,5-T2? Thyroid. 2015;25:188–97.
119. Lehmphul I, Brabant G, Wallaschofski H, Ruchala M, Strausberger CJ, Kohrle J, Wu Z. Detection of 3,5 diiodothyronine in sera of patients with altered thyroid status using new monoclonal antibody-based chemiluminescence immunoassay. Thyroid. 2015;24:1350–9.
120. Saravanan P, Siddique H, Simmons DJ, Greenwood R, Dayan CM. Twenty-four hour hormone profiles of TSH, Free T3 and free T4 in hypothyroid patients on combined T3/T4 therapy. Exp Clin Endocrinol Diabetes. 2007;115(4):261–7.
121. Mandel SJ, Mandel L. Radioactive iodine and the salivary glands. Thyroid. 2003;13:265–71.
122. Lee S. Complications of radioactive iodine treatment of thyroid carcinoma. J Natl Compr Canc Netw. 2010;8:1277–87.
123. Sawka AM, Thabane L, Parlea L, Ibrahim-Zada I, Tsang RW, Brierley JD, Straus S, Ezzat S, Goldstein DP. Second primary malignancy risk after radioactive iodine treatment in thyroid cancer: a systematic review and meta-analysis. Thyroid. 2009;19:451–7.
124. Kim C, Bi X, Pan D, Chen Y, Carling T, Ma S, Udelsman R, Zhang Y. The risk of secondary cancers after diagnosis of thyroid cancer is elevated in thyroid microcarcinomas. Thyroid. 2013;23:575–82.
125. Sisson JC, et al. Radiation safety in treatment of patients with thyroid diseases by ^{131}I: practice recommendations of the American thyroid association. Thyroid. 2011;21(4):335–46.
126. Swaka AM, Straus S, Rodin G, et al. Thyroid cancer patient perceptions of radioactive iodine treatment choice: follow up from a decision-aid randomized trial. Cancer. 2015. doi:10.1002/cncr.29548.
127. Taieb D, Sebag F, Farman-Ara B, et al. Iodine biokinetics and radioiodine exposure after recombinant human thyrotropin-assisted remnant ablation in comparison with thyroid hormone withdrawal. J Clin Endocrinol Metab. 2010;95:3283–90.
128. Tuttle RM, Brokhin M, Omry G, et al. Recombinant human TSH-assisted radioactive iodine remnant ablation achieves short-term clinical recurrence rates similar to those of traditional thyroid hormone withdrawal. J Nucl Med. 2008;49:764–70.
129. Schlumberger M, Catargi B, Borget I, et al. Strategies of radioiodine ablation in patients with low-risk thyroid cancer. N Engl J Med. 2012;366:1663–73.
130. Cooper DS, Doherty GM, Haugen BR, Kloos RT, Lee SL, Mandel SJ, Mazzaferri EL, McIver B, Pacini F, Schlumberger M, Sherman SI, Steward DL, Tuttle RM. Revised American Thyroid Association management guidelines for patients with thyroid nodules and differentiated thyroid cancer. Thyroid. 2009;19:1167–214.
131. Rosen JE, Gardiner P, Saper RB, Pearce EN, Hammer K, Gupta-Lawrence RL, Lee SL. Kelp use in patients with thyroid cancer. Endocrine. 2014;46:123–30.
132. Aceves C, Anguiano B, Delgado G. The extrathyronine actions of iodine as antioxidant, apoptotic, and differentiation Factor in various tissues. Thyroid. 2012;23(8):938–46.
133. Lee SY, Chang DLF, He X, Pearce EN, Braverman LE, Leung AM. Urinary iodine excretion and serum thyroid function in adults after iodinated contrast administration. Thyroid. 2015;25(5):471–7. doi:10.1089/thy.2015.0024.

Part VII
Other Differentiated and Advanced Thyroid Cancer

Chapter 24
Follicular and Hürthle Cell Carcinoma

Naris Nilubol, Xavier Keutgen, and Electron Kebebew

Follicular neoplasms of the thyroid comprise a wide range of pathology, such as follicular adenoma, follicular thyroid carcinoma (FTC), and oxyphilic variant of follicular neoplasm (Hürthle cell adenoma and carcinoma). Despite the more aggressive behavior and worse prognosis of Hürthle cell carcinoma (HCC), the World Health Organization (WHO) considers it the oxyphilic variant of FTC [1], while others classify HCC in a separate subtype of thyroid neoplasms, different from FTC [2, 3].

Because the cytologic features of FTC and HCC are indistinguishable from their benign counterparts, the diagnosis of FTC or HCC is made based on the evidence of capsular and/or vascular invasion or lymph node or distant metastasis. FTC is the second most common of the histologic subtypes, accounting for 10–20 % differentiated thyroid cancer, while HCC is uncommon, accounting for 3 % of differentiated thyroid cancer. Patients with FTC usually present in the fourth to sixth decades of life. The female/male ratio is 2:1–3:1. The prevalence and incidence of FTC is higher in iodine-deficient areas, accounting for 25–40 % of all thyroid cancer cases in such areas [4, 5]. Unlike PTC, FTC is more likely to have hematogenous metastasis to distant organs than to regional lymph nodes [6]. Distant metastasis at presentation occurs in 10–15 % of patients with FTC [7, 8], but the average rate of lymph node metastasis in patients with FTC is less than 10 %, ranging from 3 to 19 % [9]. Multifocality is uncommon in FTC.

N. Nilubol, MD (✉)
Endocrine Oncology Branch, National Cancer Institute, Maryland, MD, USA
e-mail: naris.nilubol@nih.gov

X. Keutgen, MD
Department of Surgery, Rush University Medical Center, Chicago, IL, USA

E. Kebebew, MD
Endocrine Oncology Branch, National Cancer Institute, National Institute of Health, Bethesda, MD, USA

S.A. Roman et al. (eds.), *Management of Thyroid Nodules and Differentiated Thyroid Cancer*, DOI 10.1007/978-3-319-43618-0_24

The WHO has classified FTC into minimally invasive and widely invasive [1]. The key differences in natural history, diagnosis, and management are discussed below.

The initial description of Hürthle cell by Karl Hürthle in 1894 was for the canine parafollicular C cells, not those that are now known as Hürthle cells. The historic misnomer first appeared in James Ewing's description of a thyroid carcinoma, in which he referred to the large cells containing fine, granular, eosinophilic cytoplasm as hypertrophic Hürthle cells [10]. Similar to FTC, patients with HCC are predominantly female (female/male ratio is 2:1). Patients with HCC typically present in the fourth to sixth decades of life [11]. A dominant thyroid nodule is a common presentation. Due to the rarity of Hürthle cell neoplasm, the natural history and optimal management of patients with these tumors have been the subject of ongoing debates because of the variable biologic behavior reported. The rate of extrathyroidal extension varies from 5 to 39 %, lymph node metastasis from 2.7 to 56 %, and distant metastasis from 5 to 50 % [9]. Multifocality is common in HCC, ranging from 33 to 70 % [12–14].

While the majority of patients with FTC often present with an asymptomatic solitary thyroid nodule, typically larger than 2 cm [5], 20 % of patients have a dominant nodule in a multinodular goiter. An initial presentation with distant metastasis to the lungs and bones occurs infrequently [15]. Minimally invasive follicular thyroid carcinoma (MIFTC) usually presents in younger patients, with median age between 35 and 49 years, and with a presentation and indolent clinical course that are similar to those of follicular adenoma [16]. Widely invasive FTC (WIFTC) presents in the older patients, with a median age of 60 years, and has a more aggressive clinical course.

Similarly, HCC is categorized as minimally invasive or widely invasive [17]. Although minimally invasive HCC has a more favorable prognosis than its widely invasive counterpart, the natural history and optimal management remain unclear because of the rarity of the disease.

Diagnosis

Ultrasonography

In a retrospective study, Sillery et al. compared the sonographic features of FTC with those of follicular adenoma and found that FTC were more frequently hypoechoic, were larger, had fewer occurrences of sonographic halo, and had fewer cystic changes [18]. However, these features overlapped with those of follicular adenoma (Fig. 24.1). Others have found that iso- or hypoechoic appearance, predominantly solid or mixed echotexture, and the presence of microcalcifications or rim calcifications are more commonly seen in FTC than in follicular adenoma [19].

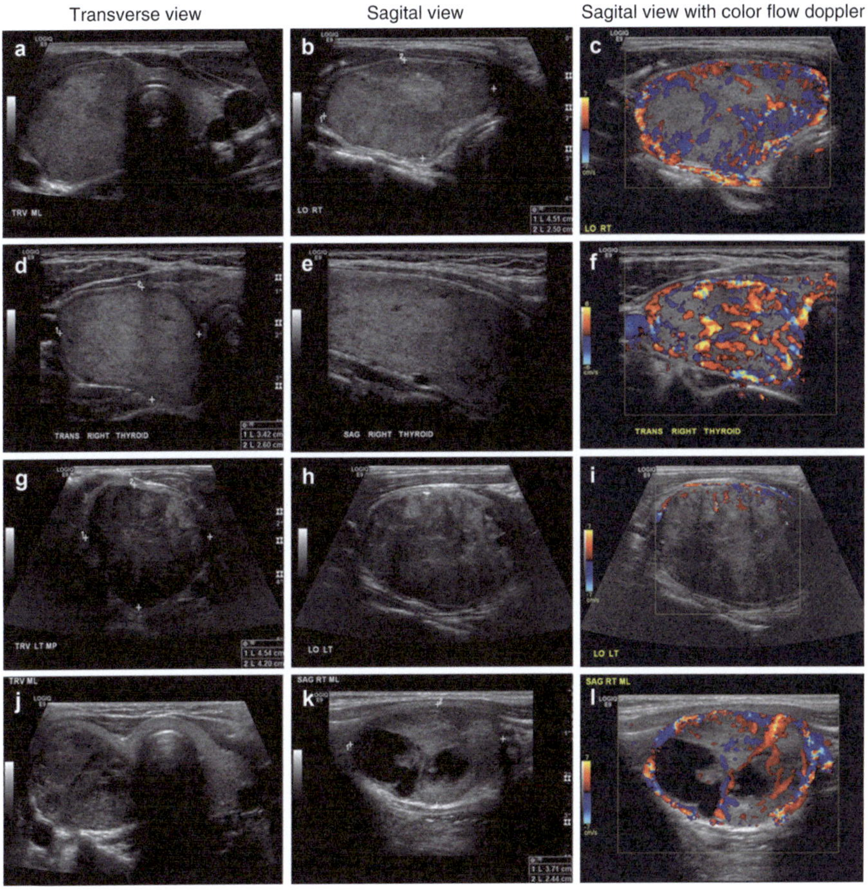

Fig. 24.1 A high-resolution ultrasonography images of (1) follicular adenoma (**a**–**c**), (2) Hürthle cell adenoma (**d**–**f**), (3) follicular thyroid carcinoma (**g**–**i**), and (4) Hürthle cell carcinoma (**j**–**l**)

However, many of these features overlap with those of follicular adenoma. An additional feature that may help distinguish follicular adenoma from FTC is the absence of blood flow in the thyroid nodule, which has 96 % negative predictive value for carcinoma [20].

Hürthle cell neoplasms have a wide range of sonographic appearances from predominantly hypoechoic to hyperechoic lesions with various degrees and patterns of vascularization. Ultrasonography cannot distinguish Hürthle cell adenoma from HCC, unless obvious local invasion or lymphadenopathy is seen. Common sonographic features of Hürthle cell neoplasms include a hypoechoic or isoechoic appearance, with heterogeneity. Cystic changes and sonographic halo signs are common. Coarse calcification occurs in 20 % of cases. Most HCC have internal and peripheral vascularity (Fig. 24.1) [21, 22].

Fine-Needle Aspiration Biopsy

Although fine-needle aspiration biopsy (FNAB) is the most commonly used diagnostic test to guide management of a patient with a thyroid nodule (s), it cannot distinguish FTC or HCC from their benign counterparts because capsular and vascular invasion cannot be assessed by FNAB. Thus, most FNAB results for follicular neoplasms fall into an indeterminate category, such as follicular lesion of undetermined significance or follicular neoplasm, and surgical excision to obtain a tissue diagnosis is indicated. The diagnostic criteria for follicular neoplasm on FNAB include the presence of abundant follicular cells in microfollicles in the absence of colloid material (Fig. 24.2a, b) (see Chap. 5).

Hürthle cells are thyroid follicular cells characterized by a large polygonal shape with an abundant eosinophilic, granular cytoplasm that is rich in mitochondria and a large nucleus with a prominent nucleolus. Hürthle cell changes are seen in various thyroid conditions, including nonneoplastic pathology such as Hashimoto's thyroiditis, Graves' disease, and nodular goiter [23].

Hürthle cell neoplasms are uncommon, accounting for 4–10 % of thyroid neoplasms [24]. Cytologic features of Hürthle cell neoplasms on FNAB include hypercellular lesions with Hürthle cell predominance >75 % and a paucity of colloid and absence of lymphocytes (Fig. 24.2c, d).

Molecular Markers

Although significant progress has been made in the molecular diagnosis of thyroid nodules in recent years, none of the available modalities can accurately differentiate FTC from follicular adenoma. A gene expression classifier (GEC) uses an expression panel of messenger RNAs to distinguish benign from malignant lesions in patients with indeterminate nodules. Afirma (Veracyte, San Francisco, CA) is a commercially available test that uses a messenger expression panel of 142 genes. The test has high sensitivity and a negative predictive value of >90 % in indeterminate nodules (atypia or follicular lesion of undetermined significance and follicular or Hürthle cell neoplasm), but the specificity is only 50 %. Thus, approximately half of benign nodules with indeterminate cytology are falsely classified as "suspicious for malignancy" [25, 26].

Because the false-negative rate (5–8 %) of the Afirma test is similar to the rate of malignancy in patients with atypia or follicular lesion of undetermined significance (5–15 %), it remains unclear whether the test will alter a surgical decision. Li et al. conducted a cost-effective analysis and suggested that GEC testing may reduce the overall cost due to 74 % fewer surgeries for benign nodules, with no greater number of untreated cancers [27].

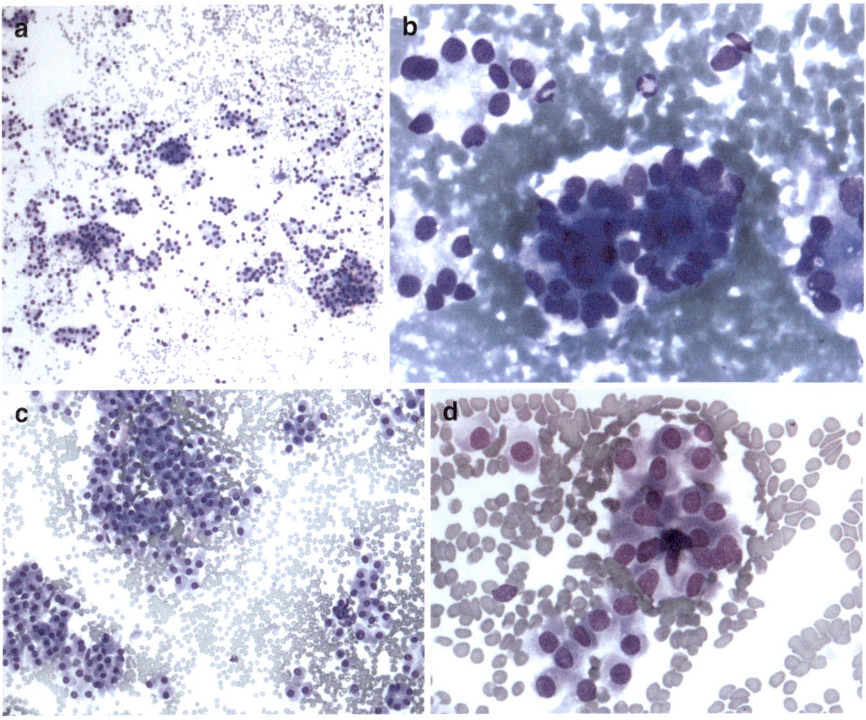

Fig. 24.2 Cytologic features of (**a**) follicular neoplasm (low power): cellular aspirate showing follicular cells in crowded clusters, pseudorosettes, tubule-like formations, and singly, in a background of red blood cells and no colloid present. Diff-Quik, 100×; (**b**) follicular neoplasm with microfollicle pseudorosettes: follicular cells with diffuse nuclear enlargement arranged in microfollicles and pseudorosettes in a background of red blood cells. Diff-Quik, 600×; (**c**) Hürthle cell neoplasm (low power): cellular aspirate showing Hurthle cells with diffuse nuclear enlargement arranged in crowded clusters, pseudorosettes, and singly, in a background of red blood cells and no colloid. Diff-Quik, 200×; (**d**) Hürthle cell neoplasm with microfollicle pseudorosettes: Hürthle cells with diffuse nuclear enlargement and abundant granular cytoplasm, arranged singly, in pseudorosettes and a microfollicle, in a background of red blood cells. Diff-Quik, 400× (Courtesy of Dr. Armando Filie, Laboratory of Pathology, National Cancer Institute, NIH)

Point mutations in *BRAF* V600E and *RAS (H-RAS, N-RAS, K-RAS)* and RET/PTC and PAX8/PPARg gene arrangements have been identified in >70 % of thyroid cancer with high positive predictive values. The performance of previous-generation tests was not accurate enough to distinguish FTC or HCC from adenoma [28–30]. A recent study by Nikiforov et al. of 143 FNABs with a cytologic diagnosis of follicular neoplasm showed promising results in a comprehensive panel (ThyroSeq v2 NGS) that tests for point mutations in 13 genes and 42 types of gene fusions that occur in thyroid cancers. The authors reported 90 % sensitivity, 93 % specificity, and 92 % overall accuracy [31].

Pathological Diagnosis

The WHO defined FTC as "a malignant epithelial tumor showing follicular cell differentiation and lacking the diagnostic nuclear features of papillary thyroid carcinoma" [1]. Two main features in diagnosing FTC are evidence of capsular and or vascular invasion and the absence of the nuclear features of PTC in a tumor arising from follicular thyroid cells [17]. The combination of using strict diagnostic criteria for recognizing capsular and/or vascular invasion in the absence of the nuclear features of PTC and the trend toward an increase diagnosis of follicular variant of PTC has resulted in the increasing number of PTC diagnoses and a decrease in the percentage of FTCs among well-differentiated thyroid carcinomas [1, 17, 32].

Follicular adenoma commonly presents as a solitary lesion in an otherwise normal thyroid gland without evidence of invasive growth. Histologic features of adenomas include a microfollicular or macrofollicular growth pattern and lack degenerative changes, such as hemorrhage, fibrosis, and cyst formation [33] (Fig. 24.3a).

Most FTCs are well-encapsulated solid tumors with a grayish tan to brown color at the cut surface [34]. MIFTCs typically have thicker and more irregular capsules than follicular adenomas, but are otherwise grossly indistinguishable. The presence of a capsule is an important feature that distinguishes MIFTC from WIFTC. WIFTCs may occur as partially encapsulated tumors with extensive penetration of the capsule or as multinodular, bulky tumors without a capsule, occasionally showing permeation of the thyroid blood vessels [34] (Fig. 24.3b–d). Multifocality in FTC is uncommon. The term MIFTC covers a wide range of pathology, from tumors with minimal capsular invasion only to those with extensive vascular invasion [16]. Vascular invasion is defined as the presence of tumor cells that are attached to the wall of capsular vessels [35]. Rosai has classified encapsulated tumors, or MIFTC, into three categories based on the presence and the extent of vascular invasion: (1) capsular invasion only, (2) limited vascular invasion (fewer than four sites), and (3) extensive vascular invasion (four or more sites) [36]. Others consider MIFTC as tumors with capsular invasion only [37, 38]. Because vascular invasion is an adverse prognostic feature that is associated with higher rates of recurrence and mortality [6, 39], it is suggested that MIFTC be categorized by the presence of vascular invasion, as MIFTC without vascular invasion has an excellent prognosis [40], as compared with MIFTC with vascular invasion [6]. In a large cohort of patients with FTC, Ito et al. demonstrated that extensive vascular invasion and tumor size >4 cm were independently associated with mortality in patients with MIFTC [41]. MIFTC with extensive vascular invasion was associated with higher recurrence and distant metastasis [42, 43].

Similar to patients with MIFTC, those with minimally invasive HCC that have four or more foci of vascular invasion or with tumor size >4 cm have a higher risk for recurrent disease [44] (Fig. 24.3e–g). Histology of Hürthle cell adenoma is shown in Fig. 24.3h.

Treatments

Surgical Management

A patient who has a cytologic diagnosis of follicular or Hürthle cell neoplasm should at least undergo a diagnostic thyroid lobectomy and isthmusectomy because the risk of malignancy is 15–30 % [45]. A total thyroidectomy should be considered in patients who are at risk for thyroid cancer, such as those who have had prior head/neck irradiation or a family history of thyroid cancer or those who have contralateral nodules, hypothyroidism, or clinical evidence of malignancy, such as signs of local invasion, suspicious sonogram findings, or lymphadenopathy.

Because the diagnosis of FTC and HCC is based on evidence of vascular or capsular invasion, intraoperative frozen section analysis of the thyroid nodule is inaccurate, as it is impractical to examine the entire capsule of the nodule and the histologic morphology of frozen tissue is inferior to that of formalin-fixed tissue because of the presence of frozen artifacts [46, 47].

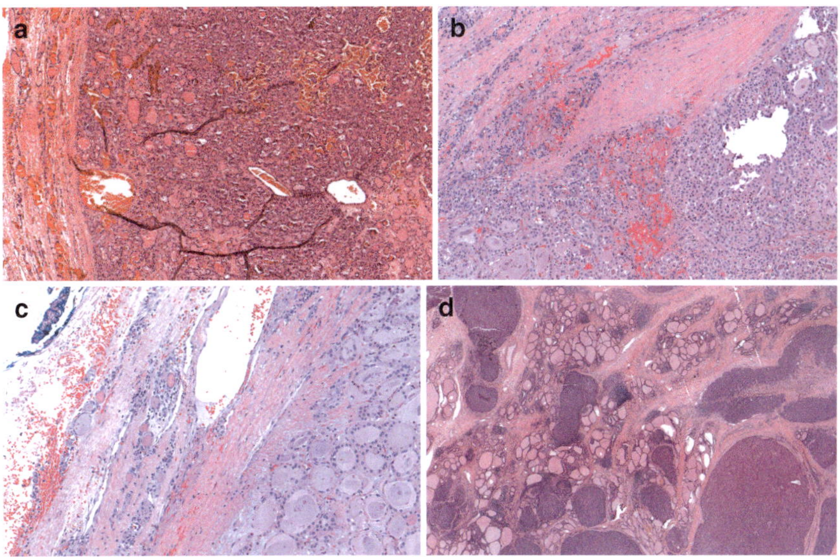

Fig. 24.3 Histologic features of (**a**) follicular adenoma: tumor with follicular cells, thick capsule, without any evidence of vascular or capsular invasion. Hematoxylin and eosin, 8×; (**b**) minimally invasive follicular thyroid carcinoma with capsular invasion. Hematoxylin and eosin, 12×; (**c**) minimally invasive follicular thyroid carcinoma with vascular invasion. Hematoxylin and eosin, 15×; (**d**) widely invasive follicular carcinoma with no complete capsule and extensive invasion. Hematoxylin and eosin, 2×; (**e**) minimally invasive Hürthle cell carcinoma with capsular invasion. Hematoxylin and eosin.10×; (**f**) minimally invasive Hürthle cell carcinoma with vascular invasion. Hematoxylin and eosin. 30×; (**g**) widely invasive Hürthle carcinoma. Hematoxylin and eosin. 0.7×; (**h**) Hürthle cell adenoma with no evidence of caspsular or vascular invasion. Hematoxylin and eosin. 8× (Courtesy of Drs. Drew Pratt and Martha Quezado, Laboratory of Pathology, National Cancer Institute, NIH)

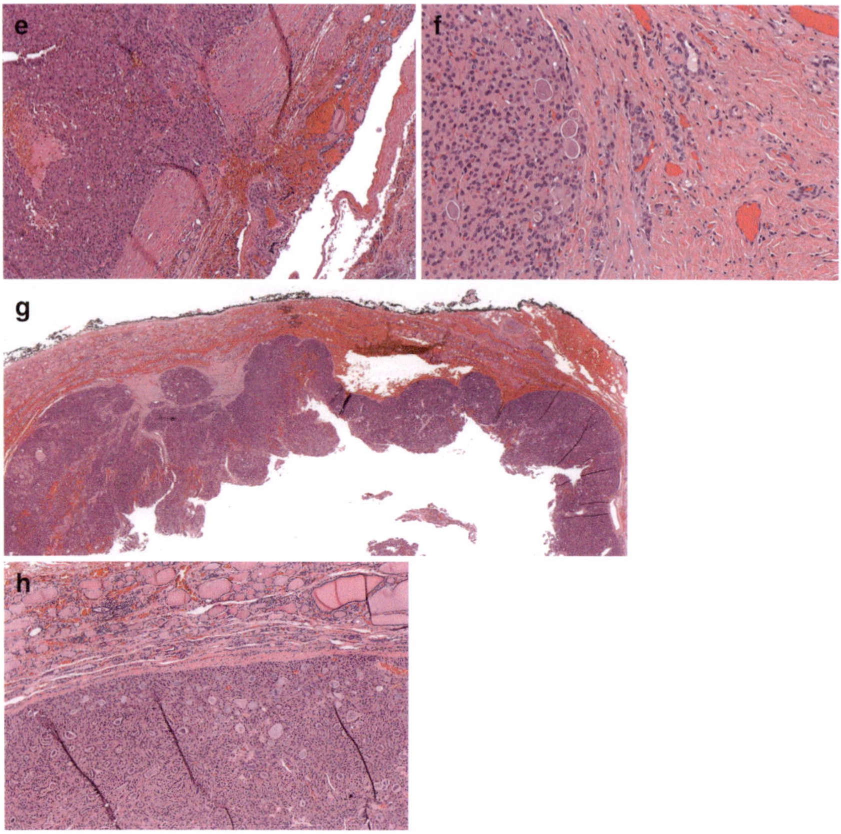

Fig. 24.3 (continued)

However, intraoperative frozen section analysis is accurate in detecting lymph node metastasis. Once lymph node metastasis is confirmed, total thyroidectomy with a compartment-oriented lymph node dissection should be performed.

Published papers on MIFTC and HCC are limited and often lack statistical power due to the rarity of the disease. The classification of FTC and HCC by the degree of invasion stratifies patients into high-risk (WIFTC) and low-risk (MIFTC) groups. The optimal surgical management of patients with MIFTC remains controversial. The 2015 American Thyroid Association guidelines recommend either a thyroid lobectomy or a total thyroidectomy for low-risk PTC or FTC between 1 and 4 cm. in size without extrathyroidal extension and without evidence of lymph node metastasis [48]. However, several centers consider a thyroid lobectomy as an adequate procedure for MIFTC with capsular invasion only, without vascular invasion, with a tumor size <4 cm, no evidence of nodal or distant metastasis, and patient age less than 45 years old. Candidates for total thyroidectomy are those who are more than 45 years old, have a tumor size >4 cm, or have a presence of vascular invasion or evidence of nodal or distant metastasis [40, 49–51]. A large series of MIFTC from Japan demonstrated that age greater than 45 years was the only independent prognostic factor for survival, while tumor size >4 cm and distant metastasis were significant adverse prognostic factors in univariate analysis. Findings suggest that younger patients with MIFTC have a good prognosis despite having large tumors or distant metastases [52]. A series from the Mayo Clinic showed 10-year cause-specific mortality and distant metastases of 28 and 19 %, respectively, in patients with MIFTC and vascular invasion, while none of the patients with capsular invasion only developed distant metastases or had mortality [40]. Thus, a completion thyroidectomy should be considered for patients with MIFTC who are more than 45 years old, have a tumor size >4 cm, and have a presence of vascular invasion or evidence of nodal or distant metastasis. Patients with WIFTC should undergo a total thyroidectomy to remove macroscopic disease, if recognized intraoperatively, or a completion thyroidectomy. Because the rate of lymph node metastasis in patients with FTC is low, a prophylactic compartmental lymphadenectomy is not recommended [16].

Optimal surgical management of a thyroid nodule with cytologic diagnosis of Hürthle cell neoplasm has been controversial but should include at least a diagnostic thyroid lobectomy. The clinical factors associated with HCC include gender (male), age (older), tumor size (>4 cm), and prior childhood head and neck irradiation [53–58]. A total thyroidectomy may be considered in patients with these clinical factors. Any suspicious lymph nodes found intraoperatively should be submitted for frozen section analysis. A compartment-oriented lymphadenectomy should be performed if lymph node metastasis is confirmed. The role of prophylactic central compartment lymph node dissection for HCC is not known. However, it should be considered in patients with risk factors or who are suspected to have widely invasive HCC (WIHCC), as lymph node metastasis is not uncommon and many HCCs do not take up radioiodine (RAI). McDonald et al. used AMES (age, metastasis, extent, and size) risk stratification to identify high-risk patients and found that the extent of the operation was the strongest risk factor for recurrence. Thus, the authors advocate more aggressive surgery for patients with one or more AMES risk factors [56].

Because patients with minimally invasive HCC (MIHCC), defined as either HCC with a minimal capsular invasion only [57] or a focus of capsular or vascular invasion [58], have an excellent prognosis, a thyroid lobectomy and isthmusectomy may be adequate. Two studies, one by Stojadinovic et al. ($n=23$) and another by Sanders and Silverman ($n=12$), found that none of the patients with MIHCC who underwent a thyroid lobectomy developed recurrence or mortality after a median follow-up of 8 and 14 years, respectively [57, 58].

Postoperative Management

Thyroid-Stimulating Hormone (TSH) Suppression Therapy

The 2015 American Thyroid Association management guidelines for differentiated thyroid cancer recommended the use of 2009 guidelines with additional clinical features to stratify patients into three categories by the risk of recurrence. The initial assessment for the risk of recurrence should be continually modified during the follow-up because the risks of recurrence or mortality can change as the result of change in clinical course or treatments:

1. Low-risk patients: (a) no local or distant metastasis; (b) all macroscopic tumor tissue is removed; (c) no tumor invasion of locoregional tissues; (d) no aggressive histology or vascular invasion; (e) no RAI uptake outside the thyroid bed on the first whole-body scan; (f) clinical N0 or ≤5 pathologic N1 micrometastasis (<0.2 cm. in greatest dimension); (g) intrathyroidal FTC with capsular invasion and no or minimal (<4) foci of vascular invasion; (h) intrathyroidal papillary microcarcinoma including *BRAF* V600E mutation.
2. Intermediate-risk patients: (a) microscopic tumor invasion into the perithyroidal soft tissues found at initial surgery; (b) ^{131}I uptake outside the thyroid bed on the RAI whole-body scan performed after thyroid remnant ablation; (c) tumor with aggressive histology or vascular invasion; (d) clinical N1 or >5 pathological N1 with all involved lymph nodes <3 cm in greatest dimension; (e) multifocal papillary microcarcinoma with extrathyroidal extension and *BRAF* V600E mutation.
3. High-risk patients: (a) macroscopic tumor invasion; (b) incomplete tumor resection; (c) distant metastases; (d) thyroglobulinemia out of proportion to what is seen on the posttreatment scan; (e) pathologic N1 with any metastatic lymph node >3 cm. in greatest dimension; (f) FTC with extensive (≥4 foci) vascular invasion.

The initial dose of levothyroxine in patients with thyroid cancer is 2 μg/kg. Patients with excellent response, defined as non-stimulated Tg < 0.2 ng/ml or TSH-stimulated Tg < 1 ng/ml with no radiographic evidence of tumor, do not require TSH suppression. TSH should be maintained at 0.5–2.0 mU/L. If non-stimulated Tg ≥ 0.2 ng/ml in low-risk patients (indeterminate or incomplete response), TSH should be maintained at 0.1–0.5 mU/L. Initial TSH goal for intermediate-risk and high-risk patients should be at 0.1–0.5 mU/L and <0.1 mU/L, respectively [48]. Thyroid function tests should be monitored every 6–8 weeks after initial administration of levothyroxine until no adjustment is needed.

Radioactive Iodine Treatment

RAI is the most effective treatment option for microscopic foci of distant metastatic differentiated thyroid carcinoma. An additional benefit of using RAI is that it facilitates the use of serum Tg as a marker for recurrent or persistent disease in the absence of thyroid tissue. RAI is not routinely recommended in low-risk patients. RAI should be considered following a total thyroidectomy or a completion thyroidectomy in patients with WIFTC or WIHCC, who are more than 45 years old and have a tumor size >4 cm. RAI is recommended as it improves disease-specific and disease-free survival in patients who have extensive vascular invasion or gross extrathyroidal invasion or evidence of distant metastasis [16, 48, 52].

Because MIFTC has an excellent prognosis, there is no evidence that the use of RAI following a total thyroidectomy improves patient outcome. A population-based study of survival among 1200 patients with MIFTC suggested that the use of RAI following total thyroidectomy did not improve patient survival [11].

In contrast to other differentiated cancers of follicular cell origin, HCCs are less RAI avid. Less than 10 % of HCC concentrate iodine in patients with known distant metastasis [12]. However, postoperative RAI ablation should still be performed to facilitate surveillance using serum Tg. The revised ATA guidelines recommend 100–200 mCi and 30–100 mCi ^{131}I for patients with known or suspected residual disease and those without, respectively, followed by post-therapy whole-body scan [59].

Follow-Up

Appropriate and accurate active surveillance for disease recurrence in patients with no evidence of disease is important. The rates of recurrent FTC or HCC vary from 7 to 53 %, depending on the length of the follow-up and the definition of recurrence [9]. As with PTC, over 80 % of FTC recurs within 10 years after initial diagnosis. Thus, long-term follow-up is necessary. The recurrence rates are the highest at the extreme age (less than 20 years old and more than 59 years old) [60]. Early recurrence, within a year after diagnosis, is associated with high mortality, as most patients who experience early recurrence developed distant metastasis [61].

In patients with FTC or HCC, initial follow-up after a total or a completion thyroidectomy should include determining whether RAI treatment is indicated based on the patient's risks of recurrence and metastasis. Both FTC and HCC usually secrete Tg, making Tg an accurate tumor marker following total thyroidectomy when patients are anti-Tg antibody negative [62]. Postoperative TSH-stimulated thyroglobulin level, either by thyroid hormone withdrawal or by administration of recombinant TSH, should be performed to assess for residual thyroid tissue or disease.

If initial post-therapy whole-body scan shows uptake in the thyroid bed only, a high-resolution ultrasonography of the neck is the initial modality that should be used to surveil patients postoperatively every 6–12 months. TSH-stimulated Tg (with or without diagnostic whole-body scan) should be performed 6–12 months after remnant ablation [59]. In the absence of anti-Tg antibodies, which can result in falsely low serum Tg, serum Tg has a high sensitivity and specificity in detecting thyroid cancer after total thyroidectomy and remnant ablation. Because serum Tg level that is measured during TSH suppression may fail to identify patients with low-volume disease, TSH-stimulated Tg provides the highest sensitivity in detecting patients with residual disease, with a negative predictive value of 95–99 % [63, 64]. However, TSH-stimulated Tg may identify patients with clinically insignificant disease. Patients with elevated serum Tg (>0.3 ng/ml for TSH-suppressed Tg level, or >2 ng/ml for TSH-stimulated Tg level) should undergo neck ultrasonography. A diagnostic RAI whole-body scan should be considered if neck ultrasonography is negative. Additional imaging studies, such as computed tomography (CT) or magnetic resonance imaging of the neck and chest or ^{18}F-fludeoxyglucose positron emission tomography/CT, are recommended for patients with elevated or rising serum Tg without evidence of disease, as found on radioactive diagnostic iodine whole-body scan and neck ultrasonography [59]. FNAB for cytology and Tg wash should be performed for any suspicious lesions.

Prognosis

Several risk stratification and staging systems have been developed for patients with differentiated thyroid cancers. These include AGES (age, tumor grade, extent, and size), AMES (age, metastasis, extent, and size), MACIS (metastasis, age, completeness of resection, invasion, and size), and the TNM staging system by the American Joint Committee on Cancer. These systems demonstrate important prognostic factors that influence patient survival. Overall, the 5- and 10-year survival rates of patients with FTC are 82–92 % and 67–90 %, respectively [9]. Patients with MIFTC typically have an excellent prognosis, one that is comparable to benign adenoma. A population-based study of 1200 patients showed that distant metastases were rare in patients with MIFTC, and the overall survival rate of these patients was comparable to that of the general population in the United States [65]. Compared with MIFTC, WIFTC is associated with worse prognosis, with a 10-year disease-specific mortality of 15–25 % [40, 41, 66].

It is controversial whether the prognosis is worse for HCC than for FTC. A study from the National Cancer Data Base revealed a lower 10-year survival rate in patients with HCC (75 %) than those with FTC (85 %) or PTC (93 %) [67]. Other studies reported worse outcomes, with 5- and 10-year survival rates of 45–95 % and 45–80 %, respectively [9], and that more than half of the patients with HCC died during long-term follow-up [12, 58]. However, a population-based study showed that patients with HCC had a comparable overall survival of those with demographically and clinically matched FTC. Older age at diagnosis, men, and larger tumor size were associated with shorter overall survival in patients with HCC [68].

References

1. DeLellis RA, Lloyd RV, Heitz PU. World Health Organization classification of tumours. In: Pathology and genetics of tumours of endocrine organs. Lyon: IARC Press; 2004.
2. Franssila KO, Ackerman LV, Brown CL, Hedinger CE. Follicular carcinoma. Semin Diagn Pathol. 1985;2(2):101–22.
3. Kushchayeva Y, Duh QY, Kebebew E, D'Avanzo A, Clark OH. Comparison of clinical characteristics at diagnosis and during follow-up in 118 patients with Hurthle cell or follicular thyroid cancer. Am J Surg. 2008;195(4):457–62.
4. Correa P, Chen VW. Endocrine gland cancer. Cancer. 1995;75(1 Suppl):338–52.
5. Baloch ZW, LiVolsi VA. Our approach to follicular-patterned lesions of the thyroid. J Clin Pathol. 2007;60(3):244–50.

6. Kim HJ, Sung JY, Oh YL, Kim JH, Son YI, Min YK, et al. Association of vascular invasion with increased mortality in patients with minimally invasive follicular thyroid carcinoma but not widely invasive follicular thyroid carcinoma. Head Neck. 2014;36(12):1695–700.
7. Shaha AR, Shah JP, Loree TR. Patterns of nodal and distant metastasis based on histologic varieties in differentiated carcinoma of the thyroid. Am J Surg. 1996;172(6):692–4.
8. Lo CY, Chan WF, Lam KY, Wan KY. Follicular thyroid carcinoma: the role of histology and staging systems in predicting survival. Ann Surg. 2005;242(5):708–15.
9. Phitayakorn R, McHenry CR. Follicular and Hurthle cell carcinoma of the thyroid gland. Surg Oncol Clin N Am. 2006;15(3):603–23, ix–x.
10. Ewing J. Neoplastic disease: a treatise on tumors. 3rd ed. Philadelphia: W. B. Saunders Company; 1928.
11. Goffredo P, Roman SA, Sosa JA. Hurthle cell carcinoma: a population-level analysis of 3311 patients. Cancer. 2013;119(3):504–11.
12. Lopez-Penabad L, Chiu AC, Hoff AO, Schultz P, Gaztambide S, Ordonez NG, et al. Prognostic factors in patients with Hurthle cell neoplasms of the thyroid. Cancer. 2003;97(5):1186–94.
13. Arganini M, Behar R, Wu TC, Straus 2nd F, McCormick M, DeGroot LJ, et al. Hurthle cell tumors: a twenty-five-year experience. Surgery. 1986;100(6):1108–15.
14. Gundry SR, Burney RE, Thompson NW, Lloyd R. Total thyroidectomy for Hurthle cell neoplasm of the thyroid. Arch Surg. 1983;118(5):529–32.
15. Panda SK, Patro B, Samantaroy MR, Mishra J, Mohapatra KC, Meher RK. Unusual presentation of follicular carcinoma thyroid with special emphasis on their management. Int J Surg Case Rep. 2014;5(7):408–11.
16. Dionigi G, Kraimps JL, Schmid KW, Hermann M, Sheu-Grabellus SY, De Wailly P, et al. Minimally invasive follicular thyroid cancer (MIFTC) – a consensus report of the European Society of Endocrine Surgeons (ESES). Langenbecks Arch Surg. 2014;399(2):165–84.
17. Rosai J, Carcargiu ML, DeLellis RA. Tumors of the thyroid gland, 3rd series. In: Rosai J, Sobin L, editors. Atlas of tumor pathology. Washington, DC: Armed Forces Institute of Pathology; 1992.
18. Sillery JC, Reading CC, Charboneau JW, Henrichsen TL, Hay ID, Mandrekar JN. Thyroid follicular carcinoma: sonographic features of 50 cases. AJR Am J Roentgenol. 2010;194(1):44–54.
19. Seo HS, Lee DH, Park SH, Min HS, Na DG. Thyroid follicular neoplasms: can sonography distinguish between adenomas and carcinomas? J Clin Ultrasound JCU. 2009;37(9):493–500.
20. Iared W, Shigueoka DC, Cristofoli JC, Andriolo R, Atallah AN, Ajzen SA, et al. Use of color Doppler ultrasonography for the prediction of malignancy in follicular thyroid neoplasms: systematic review and meta-analysis. J Ultrasound Med Off J Am Inst Ultrasound Med. 2010;29(3):419–25.
21. Lee SK, Rho BH, Woo SK. Hurthle cell neoplasm: correlation of gray-scale and power Doppler sonographic findings with gross pathology. J Clin Ultrasound JCU. 2010;38(4):169–76.
22. Maizlin ZV, Wiseman SM, Vora P, Kirby JM, Mason AC, Filipenko D, et al. Hurthle cell neoplasms of the thyroid: sonographic appearance and histologic characteristics. J Ultrasound Med Off J Am Inst Ultrasound Med. 2008;27(5):751–7; quiz 9.
23. LiVolsi VA. Surgical pathology of the thyroid. Philadelphia: Saunders; 1990.
24. McLeod MK, Thompson NW. Hurthle cell neoplasms of the thyroid. Otolaryngol Clin North Am. 1990;23(3):441–52.
25. Alexander EK, Kennedy GC, Baloch ZW, Cibas ES, Chudova D, Diggans J, et al. Preoperative diagnosis of Benign thyroid nodules with indeterminate cytology. N Engl J Med. 2012;367:705–15.
26. Mathur A, Olson MT, Zeiger MA. Follicular lesions of the thyroid. Surg Clin North Am. 2014;94(3):499–513.
27. Li H, Robinson KA, Anton B, Saldanha IJ, Ladenson PW. Cost-effectiveness of a novel molecular test for cytologically indeterminate thyroid nodules. J Clin Endocrinol Metab. 2011;96(11):E1719–26.

28. Nikiforov YE, Steward DL, Robinson-Smith TM, Haugen BR, Klopper JP, Zhu Z, et al. Molecular testing for mutations in improving the fine-needle aspiration diagnosis of thyroid nodules. J Clin Endocrinol Metab. 2009;94(6):2092–8.
29. Yip L, Kebebew E, Milas M, Carty SE, Fahey 3rd TJ, Parangi S, et al. Summary statement: utility of molecular marker testing in thyroid cancer. Surgery. 2010;148(6):1313–5.
30. Ohori NP, Nikiforova MN, Schoedel KE, LeBeau SO, Hodak SP, Seethala RR, et al. Contribution of molecular testing to thyroid fine-needle aspiration cytology of "follicular lesion of undetermined significance/atypia of undetermined significance". Cancer Cytopathol. 2010;118(1):17–23.
31. Nikiforov YE, Carty SE, Chiosea SI, Coyne C, Duvvuri U, Ferris RL, et al. Highly accurate diagnosis of cancer in thyroid nodules with follicular neoplasm/suspicious for a follicular neoplasm cytology by ThyroSeq v2 next-generation sequencing assay. Cancer. 2014;120(23):3627–34.
32. Alevizaki M, Papageorgiou G, Rentziou G, Saltiki K, Marafelia P, Loukari E, et al. Increasing prevalence of papillary thyroid carcinoma in recent years in Greece: the majority are incidental. Thyroid. 2009;19(7):749–54.
33. Baloch ZW, Fleisher S, LiVolsi VA, Gupta PK. Diagnosis of "follicular neoplasm": a gray zone in thyroid fine-needle aspiration cytology. Diagn Cytopathol. 2002;26(1):41–4.
34. Sobrinho-Simoes M, Eloy C, Magalhaes J, Lobo C, Amaro T. Follicular thyroid carcinoma. Mod Pathol. 2011;24 Suppl 2:S10–8.
35. LiVolsi VA, Baloch ZW. Follicular-patterned tumors of the thyroid: the battle of benign vs. malignant vs. so-called uncertain. Endocr Pathol. 2011;22(4):184–9.
36. Rosai J. Handling of thyroid follicular patterned lesions. Endocr Pathol. 2005;16(4):279–83.
37. Ghossein R. Update to the College of American Pathologists reporting on thyroid carcinomas. Head Neck Pathol. 2009;3(1):86–93.
38. Saade N, Sadler C, Goldfarb M. Impact of regional lymph node dissection on disease specific survival in adrenal cortical carcinoma. Horm Metab Res. 2015;47:820–5.
39. Lang W, Choritz H, Hundeshagen H. Risk factors in follicular thyroid carcinomas. A retrospective follow-up study covering a 14-year period with emphasis on morphological findings. Am J Surg Pathol. 1986;10(4):246–55.
40. van Heerden JA, Hay ID, Goellner JR, Salomao D, Ebersold JR, Bergstralh EJ, et al. Follicular thyroid carcinoma with capsular invasion alone: a nonthreatening malignancy. Surgery. 1992;112(6):1130–6; discussion 6–8.
41. Ito Y, Hirokawa M, Masuoka H, Yabuta T, Kihara M, Higashiyama T, et al. Prognostic factors of minimally invasive follicular thyroid carcinoma: extensive vascular invasion significantly affects patient prognosis. Endocr J. 2013;60(5):637–42.
42. Lang BH, Lo CY, Chan WF, Lam KY, Wan KY. Staging systems for follicular thyroid carcinoma: application to 171 consecutive patients treated in a tertiary referral centre. Endocr Relat Cancer. 2007;14(1):29–42.
43. Goldstein NS, Czako P, Neill JS. Metastatic minimally invasive (encapsulated) follicular and Hurthle cell thyroid carcinoma: a study of 34 patients. Mod Pathol. 2000;13(2):123–30.
44. Ghossein RA, Hiltzik DH, Carlson DL, Patel S, Shaha A, Shah JP, et al. Prognostic factors of recurrence in encapsulated Hurthle cell carcinoma of the thyroid gland: a clinicopathologic study of 50 cases. Cancer. 2006;106(8):1669–76.
45. Cibas ES, Ali SZ, Conference NCITFSotS. The bethesda system for reporting thyroid cytopathology. Am J Clin Pathol. 2009;132(5):658–65.
46. Chen H, Nicol TL, Udelsman R. Follicular lesions of the thyroid. Does frozen section evaluation alter operative management? Ann Surg. 1995;222(1):101–6.
47. LiVolsi VA, Baloch ZW. Use and abuse of frozen section in the diagnosis of follicular thyroid lesions. Endocr Pathol. 2005;16(4):285–93.
48. Haugen BR, Alexander EK, Bible KC, Doherty GM, Mandel SJ, Nikiforov YE, et al. 2015 American Thyroid Association management guidelines for adult patients with thyroid nodules and differentiated thyroid cancer: the American Thyroid Association guidelines task force on thyroid nodules and differentiated thyroid cancer. Thyroid. 2016;26(1):1–133.

49. Huang CC, Hsueh C, Liu FH, Chao TC, Lin JD. Diagnostic and therapeutic strategies for minimally and widely invasive follicular thyroid carcinomas. Surg Oncol. 2011;20(1):1–6.
50. Collini P, Sampietro G, Pilotti S. Extensive vascular invasion is a marker of risk of relapse in encapsulated non-Hurthle cell follicular carcinoma of the thyroid gland: a clinicopathological study of 18 consecutive cases from a single institution with a 11-year median follow-up. Histopathology. 2004;44(1):35–9.
51. Gemsenjager E, Heitz PU, Martina B. Selective treatment of differentiated thyroid carcinoma. World J Surg. 1997;21(5):546–51; discussion 51–2.
52. Sugino K, Kameyama K, Ito K, Nagahama M, Kitagawa W, Shibuya H, et al. Outcomes and prognostic factors of 251 patients with minimally invasive follicular thyroid carcinoma. Thyroid. 2012;22(8):798–804.
53. Chen H, Nicol TL, Zeiger MA, Dooley WC, Ladenson PW, Cooper DS, et al. Hurthle cell neoplasms of the thyroid: are there factors predictive of malignancy? Ann Surg. 1998;227(4):542–6.
54. Zhang YW, Greenblatt DY, Repplinger D, Bargren A, Adler JT, Sippel RS, et al. Older age and larger tumor size predict malignancy in hurthle cell neoplasms of the thyroid. Ann Surg Oncol. 2008;15(10):2842–6.
55. Thompson NW, Dunn EL, Batsakis JG, Nishiyama RH. Hurthle cell lesions of the thyroid gland. Surg Gynecol Obstet. 1974;139(4):555–60.
56. McDonald MP, Sanders LE, Silverman ML, Chan HS, Buyske J. Hurthle cell carcinoma of the thyroid gland: prognostic factors and results of surgical treatment. Surgery. 1996;120(6):1000–4; discussion 4–5.
57. Sanders LE, Silverman M. Follicular and Hurthle cell carcinoma: predicting outcome and directing therapy. Surgery. 1998;124(6):967–74.
58. Stojadinovic A, Ghossein RA, Hoos A, Urist MJ, Spiro RH, Shah JP, et al. Hurthle cell carcinoma: a critical histopathologic appraisal. J Clin Oncol. 2001;19(10):2616–25.
59. Cooper DS, Doherty GM, Haugen BR, Kloos RT, Lee SL, Mandel SJ, et al. Revised American Thyroid Association management guidelines for patients with thyroid nodules and differentiated thyroid cancer. Thyroid. 2009;19(11):1167–214.
60. Mazzaferri EL, Jhiang SM. Long-term impact of initial surgical and medical therapy on papillary and follicular thyroid cancer. Am J Med. 1994;97(5):418–28.
61. Lin JD, Hsueh C, Chao TC. Early recurrence of papillary and follicular thyroid carcinoma predicts a worse outcome. Thyroid. 2009;19(10):1053–9.
62. Besic N, Hocevar M, Zgajnar J, Petric R, Pilko G. Aggressiveness of therapy and prognosis of patients with Hurthle cell papillary thyroid carcinoma. Thyroid. 2006;16(1):67–72.
63. Gonzalez C, Aulinas A, Colom C, Tundidor D, Mendoza L, Corcoy R, et al. Thyroglobulin as early prognostic marker to predict remission at 18–24 months in differentiated thyroid carcinoma. Clin Endocrinol (Oxf). 2014;80(2):301–6.
64. Kloos RT, Mazzaferri EL. A single recombinant human thyrotropin-stimulated serum thyroglobulin measurement predicts differentiated thyroid carcinoma metastases three to five years later. J Clin Endocrinol Metab. 2005;90(9):5047–57.
65. Goffredo P, Cheung K, Roman SA, Sosa JA. Can minimally invasive follicular thyroid cancer be approached as a benign lesion?: a population-level analysis of survival among 1,200 patients. Ann Surg Oncol. 2013;20(3):767–72.
66. Ito Y, Hirokawa M, Masuoka H, Yabuta T, Fukushima M, Kihara M, et al. Distant metastasis at diagnosis and large tumor size are significant prognostic factors of widely invasive follicular thyroid carcinoma. Endocr J. 2013;60(6):829–33.
67. Hundahl SA, Fleming ID, Fremgen AM, Menck HR. A National Cancer Data Base report on 53,856 cases of thyroid carcinoma treated in the U.S., 1985–1995 [see comments]. Cancer. 1998;83(12):2638–48.
68. Bhattacharyya N. Survival and prognosis in Hurthle cell carcinoma of the thyroid gland. Arch Otolaryngol Head Neck Surg. 2003;129(2):207–10.

Chapter 25
Locally Advanced Differentiated Thyroid Cancer

Ming Yann Lim, Mark Zafereo, and Elizabeth Grubbs

Definition of Locally Advanced Thyroid Cancer

Well-differentiated thyroid carcinoma (WDTC) comprises the majority (>90 %) of thyroid cancers [1], with 10–15 % presenting as locally advanced [2, 3]. Locally advanced thyroid cancers are those that extend beyond the thyroid capsule to invade surrounding structures, including muscles, recurrent laryngeal nerve(s), trachea, larynx, esophagus, and major blood vessels in the neck and chest. McCaffrey et al. described 262 patients with locally advanced papillary thyroid carcinoma (PTC) treated over a 60-year period at the Mayo Clinic; sites of invasion included the muscle (53 %), trachea (37 %), recurrent laryngeal nerve (47 %), esophagus (21 %), larynx (12 %), and other sites (30 %) [4]. Su et al. recently published a contemporary review of 69 patients with WDTC invading the upper aerodigestive tract, reporting complete tumor excision with negative margins in 62 % of patients. The authors showed 85 % locoregional control, with 23 % of patients developing distant metastases, and 5-year overall survival of 71 % [5].

M.Y. Lim
Department of Otolaryngology, Tan Tock Seng Hospital, Singapore, Singapore
e-mail: mingyannl@yahoo.com

M. Zafereo
Departments of Head and Neck, University of Texas MD Anderson Cancer Center, Houston, TX, USA
e-mail: MZafereo@mdanderson.org

E. Grubbs (✉)
Departments of Surgical Oncology, University of Texas MD Anderson Cancer Center, 1400 Pressler Street, Unit 1461, Houston, TX 77030, USA
e-mail: eggrubbs@mdanderson.org

S.A. Roman et al. (eds.), *Management of Thyroid Nodules and Differentiated Thyroid Cancer*, DOI 10.1007/978-3-319-43618-0_25

Ortiz et al. performed a retrospective study of 200 patients undergoing surgery for papillary thyroid cancer, of whom 47 (23.5 %) presented with extrathyroidal spread. The study demonstrated that the presence of extrathyroidal spread is more common in older patients and is associated mostly with tumors greater than 4 cm, nonencapsulated, with lymph node metastasis and aggressive histological subtypes or variants (diffuse sclerosis, tall-cell, solid, and poorly differentiated) [6].

General Principles of Management

Management of locally advanced WDTC is complex and controversial. Debate exists in the literature surrounding whether radical resection of involved viscera [7–11] leads to a more favorable outcome than simpler shaving procedures [12, 13] with potential for residual microscopic disease. Kowalski et al. found no significant difference in survival between patients who underwent radical surgery versus those who underwent a "shave resection" followed by radioactive iodine (RAI) [14], with resection utilized mainly for invasion into muscle or recurrent laryngeal nerve and shaving reserved for disease involving tracheal, laryngeal, or esophageal involvement.

Although management of specific invaded local structures bears scrutiny, a resounding principle remains that all gross disease should be resected [14–16], as extirpation of gross disease has been shown to improve overall and disease-free survival [14]. Preservation of speech and swallowing function, while an extremely important second principle, is not alone a justification for incomplete surgery, especially since gross residual disease will ultimately compromise function as it continues to invade involved structures. However, the morbidity of a radical resection must be weighed against its potential benefit in each individual patient, taking into account overall disease status, age, comorbidities, and other factors.

In addition to the principles above, management of locally advanced WDTC also requires thoughtful consideration of the complex interplay of the surgeon, patient, and disease factors. It is imperative that a patient with locally advanced WDTC undergo assessment by an experienced surgeon prior to consideration of initial surgery, or postoperative adjuvant therapy. If the planned surgery could potentially involve a laryngotracheal or esophageal resection, a less experienced surgeon should consider referral to a tertiary care center [3].

Patient factors play an important role in the decision-making process. For an elderly patient with significant comorbidities or an individual with aggressive distant metastatic disease, the clinical scenario may not favor a complex local resection. Additionally, a child or adolescent is more likely to have less biologically aggressive disease and also to demonstrate response of microscopic disease to RAI, also suggesting a less morbid local approach [17, 18].

Disease factors also influence management. For example, a shave procedure is not suitable for a thyroid cancer that has invaded through the trachea to involve tracheal mucosa. Bilateral internal jugular vein involvement would necessitate reconstruction of at least one of the sacrificed veins. Preoperative functioning status is also important. For example, if the thyroid cancer is adherent to the recurrent laryngeal nerve, the preoperative functioning status of the nerve should be taken into consideration in determining the extent of efforts made to preserve the structural integrity of the nerve.

The use of adjuvant therapy in the form of external beam radiation and systemic and targeted therapy also requires a careful consideration of patient and disease factors with surgeon input in the decision.

The purpose of this chapter is to provide a thorough consideration of each of these factors, allowing the clinician to make educated decisions about a complex disease process.

Preoperative Evaluation

History

Patients with locally advanced WDTC may be asymptomatic. The nature of symptoms, if present, depends on the extent and location of invasion. Symptoms indicating airway invasion include hoarseness, hemoptysis, and dyspnea, though extraluminal invasion of the larynx is often not associated with any symptoms. Patients with invasion into the esophagus may complain of dysphagia. Individuals with invasion and occlusion of the jugular vein may report facial flushing and swelling or a potential globus sensation secondary to vascular engorgement [19]. Superior vena cava syndrome may occur if involvement of the thoracic inlet and mediastinal venous structures occurs. Acute symptoms that present abruptly with a rapidly growing neck mass should lead to consideration of a pathology that includes a poorly differentiated or anaplastic component.

Examination

General inspection should include observation of body habitus and ability to extend the neck. Transcervical access to the mediastinum and tracheal mobilization (in the event of a tracheal resection) can be challenging with obese patients; those with short, stocky necks; and individuals who cannot extend well for other reasons such as previous cervical fusion. Surgeons should be prepared for potential upper sternotomy dependent upon these factors and location of disease in the superior mediastinum. Presence of facial edema and distended neck vessels should be assessed.

The thyroid mass should be carefully examined to determine fixation to surrounding structures including the larynx, trachea, and overlying strap muscles. The vocal cords should be assessed for subtle weakness (or paralysis) of the vocal cords. Intraluminal laryngeal invasion may be seen on laryngoscopy as tumor growing along the mucosal surfaces of the true or false vocal folds or ventricles. There may be ecchymosis or gross invasion into the pyriform sinus.

It is imperative that the relevant history and examination findings, particularly with regard to recurrent laryngeal nerve status, are adequately documented prior to undertaking further treatment.

Preoperative Workup

In the preoperative workup, all patients with locally advanced WDTC should have a comprehensive thyroid/neck ultrasound and CT neck with contrast (and often CT chest), with consideration for PET if there is concern for a component of aggressive histopathology (poorly differentiated, anaplastic). Addition of contrast with CT is invaluable in properly delineating disease extent and should not be compromised in anticipation of potential postoperative RAI. RAI can usually be given 6 weeks after contrast administration without significant impact on treatment. MRI with gadolinium can also be considered as an alternative to CT with contrast imaging, especially in the setting of a severe contrast allergy, or if vascular involvement is suspected.

Bronchoscopy or esophagoscopy may be performed, either prior to or at the time of surgery, for patients with radiographically equivocal tracheal or esophageal disease. Sometimes, despite the preoperative workup, local invasion into surrounding structures can only be assessed and identified intraoperatively, and the surgeon must be prepared for these eventualities.

Laboratory workup should include thyroid function tests and, for those who have previously undergone thyroid surgery, calcium and parathyroid hormone levels. 25-Hydroxy vitamin D levels should be evaluated and repleted prior to surgery.

Involvement of Extrathyroidal Muscles (Straps, Inferior Constrictor, Cricothyroid)

The strap muscles (sternothyroid, sternohyoid) are the structures most commonly involved in locally advanced thyroid cancer because of the numerous fascial bands and blood vessels that connect the muscles to the underlying thyroid gland. Patients with strap muscle invasion as the only locally invaded structure do not have a worse prognosis [13]. Surgical management requires resection of the involved muscles. Although the strap muscles are accessory muscles for swallowing and respiration, there is generally no significant morbidity from resection of these muscles, and there should be a low threshold for sacrificing the sternothyroid muscles with recurrent/advanced disease.

Similarly, involvement of nearby cricothyroid muscle and inferior constrictor muscle requires resection of these structures to obtain negative margins. The cricothyroid muscle plays a role in vocal pitch and resection of this may lead to altered vocal pitch, especially when singing. The inferior constrictor plays a role in deglutition, and resecting this may cause some dysphagia, though this is generally temporary.

Larynx

Locally advanced WDTC can invade the larynx by one of several routes. Anteriorly, the carcinoma can invade through the cricothyroid membrane. The carcinoma can also invade laterally via the thyroid cartilage into the adjacent paraglottic space or can extend superoposteriorly into the pyriform fossa. Similarly, direct invasion through the cricoid cartilage can occur.

It is important to distinguish, both on preoperative imaging and intraoperative findings, between partial thickness invasion of the laryngeal skeleton and intraluminal invasion. Intraluminal invasion, though rare in WDTC, generally necessitates a total laryngectomy, while a partial laryngectomy with excision of involved cartilage is generally sufficient for partial invasion of the thyroid cartilage only.

Involvement of Thyroid Cartilage

For partial thickness involvement, shaving of the involved cartilage is appropriate to remove all gross disease and to preserve the larynx. Shaving is indicated if there is cartilage invasion with no intraluminal involvement. Partial removal of the external thyroid cartilage will result in thinning of this structure with no adverse sequelae. If disease involves the cricothyroid joint, shave excision of this joint is required, with or without sacrifice of the recurrent laryngeal nerve to remove all gross disease. Microscopic disease may be addressed by RAI or external beam radiotherapy (EBRT), if appropriate.

Full-thickness involvement of the thyroid cartilage with intraluminal involvement will require open partial or total laryngectomy [17]. Shave excision is not sufficient for cases with intraluminal involvement. Hemilaryngectomy and supraglottic or supracricoid laryngectomy can be performed as appropriate, dictated by disease extent in order to preserve organ function.

Involvement of Cricoid Cartilage

Cricoid cartilage resection and reconstruction should be managed based upon the degree of cartilage involvement. Partial thickness involvement of the cricoid cartilage may be suitably addressed by shaving the involved cartilage. If there is full-thickness involvement, up to 30 % of the total cricoid circumference can be resected as a wedge and reconstructed with a local muscle flap [20]. If up to half the cricoid cartilage is resected, a rib graft can be used to reconstruct the defect, keeping the costal perichondrium intact and positioning this intraluminally to allow for remucosalization [21]. More extensive resection of the cricoid cartilage requires either a cricotracheal resection, where a small portion of the cricoid cartilage is preserved posteriorly for the arytenoid support, or a total laryngectomy.

Involvement of the Trachea

Invasion of the trachea can occur via direct extension through the tracheal ring cartilages or through the intercartilaginous space into the tracheal lumen [9]. The management of tracheal invasion is similar to the larynx; the abiding principle is removal of all gross disease.

Shin and colleagues described five stages of trachea invasion by papillary thyroid carcinoma. In Stage 0, the papillary carcinoma is limited within the substance of the thyroid gland. Stage I comprises of cases of carcinoma with extracapsular spread of the thyroid gland and abutting of the external tracheal perichondrium without eroding the cartilage or invading between the cartilaginous plates. Stage II comprises of cases that either invade between the rings of the cartilage or destroy the cartilage. In Stage III, the carcinoma extends through the cartilage or between the cartilaginous plates into the lamina propria of the tracheal mucosa, but does not elevate or invade the epithelium. Stage IV consists of carcinoma that is extending through the entire thickness of the trachea and expanding the tracheal mucosa. This would be visible through a bronchoscope as a nodule or an ulcerated mass [22].

Several studies have shown that limited superficial invasion can be treated successfully by shaving of the involved trachea and that those with deep invasion should be treated by resection of the invaded trachea [4, 23]. Unlike the larynx, segmental resection of the trachea can usually be achieved without compromising organ function, since small tracheal segmental resections can be primarily anastomosed.

In contrast to the laryngeal cartilage, it is more difficult to obtain disease clearance with a shave of the trachea. The trachea wall is much thinner, and if disease infiltrates the thick fibrous adhesions between tracheal cartilage rings, it is difficult to clear without breaching the tracheal lumen. Additionally, rarely tumor can involve the tracheal lumen even in the absence of direct invasion via mechanism of lymphatic spread [22, 24].

The difficulty in clearing disease with a shave procedure was demonstrated in a study of 432 thyroid carcinoma patients, 16 with tracheal cartilage invasion. Cartilage shaving was the primary treatment in all patients, removing gross disease. Subsequent radioactive iodine or external beam radiotherapy was administered to control any potential microscopic disease. The patients were followed over a mean of 71 months. Only 4 of the 16 patients remained disease-free: the disease was not controlled in the other 12, and seven of this latter group eventually died of their disease. This led the authors to suggest that a more extensive resection procedure than cartilage shaving should be considered, even in patients with superficial tracheal invasion [11].

A tracheal shave excision is best reserved for a short segment of the trachea invaded with superficial cartilage invasion. Appropriate local control can be achieved by shaving if the tumor does not extend beyond the perichondrium [25]. However, intraluminal tracheal involvement or significant cartilage invasion mandates a circumferential sleeve resection.

Care must be taken during the tracheal resection to avoid injury to the recurrent laryngeal nerves. Circumferential resection may, depending on the number of rings resected, require further mobilization of the proximal larynx and distal trachea to allow tension-free closure (Fig. 25.1a, b). This may require the employment of a suprahyoid release (with additional 5 cm of lengthening) as well as inferior dissection of the anterior tracheal wall caudally toward the carina. In general, up to five tracheal rings can be resected with primary anastomosis, though up to eight have been described [26].

When segmental tracheal resection is performed with end-to-end anastomosis, consideration should be given to raising a pectoralis major flap, especially if there is anticipation for postoperative radiotherapy. The addition of the pectoralis major flap in this situation may reduce complications such as fistula. Oftentimes in these cases, the strap muscles are resected, and the soft tissue coverage over the trachea prevents the skin/subcutaneous tissue from adhering to the trachea with the radiation. The pectoralis major flap also permits great vessel coverage and eliminates dead space.

In certain situations, other techniques may be appropriate. Limited involvement of the anterior wall of the trachea may be addressed by resection of a tracheal window. The resultant defect may be restored by the insertion of a temporary tracheostomy, or for slightly larger defects, a myofascial flap may be rotated in to fill the defect.

If segmental resection results in more than eight tracheal rings being removed, the involved anterior trachea can be resected as a long window and the anterior defect reconstructed with a free flap, although it remains extremely challenging to reconstruct the rigidity of the trachea with free tissue transfer. In some instances, the defect may be a composite anterior tracheal defect in combination with a cricoid and thyroid cartilage defect. A free radial forearm flap can be stitched to a PolyMax mesh (Synthes, Paoli, PA) and Hemashield vascular graft (Boston Scientific, Natick, MA) for rigid support and employed as a rigid, single construct to repair the defect [27]. Circumferential tracheal defects repaired with a free flap supported by prosthetic materials have also been described [28]. Reconstruction may involve the use of a temporary tracheostomy to ensure airway patency in the initial postoperative period.

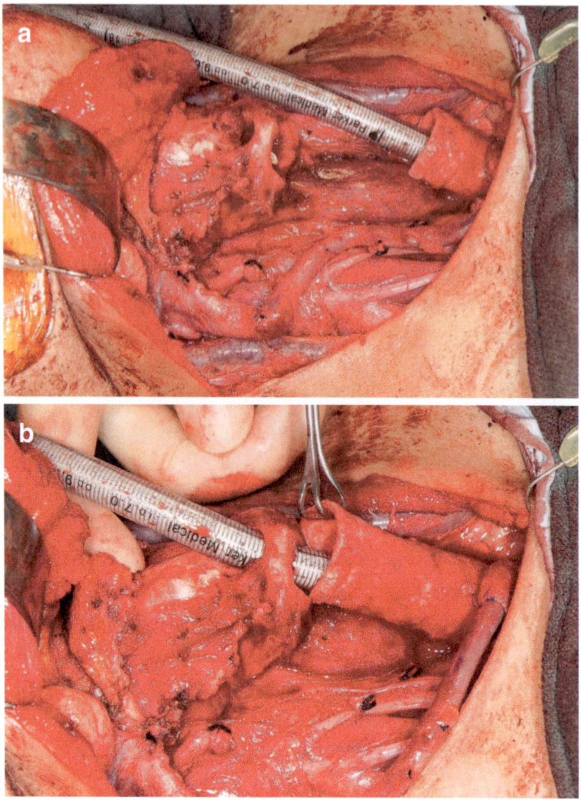

Fig. 25.1 (**a**) Five ring tracheal resection for Stage IV tracheal invasion in which well differentiated thyroid cancer extended through the entire thickness of the trachea wall. (**b**) Mobilization of the larynx and trachea to allow-tension free closure

Pharynx and Esophagus

Isolated pharyngeal involvement is unusual without concomitant laryngeal and esophageal involvement. If isolated pharyngeal involvement occurs, the involved pharynx can be resected via a lateral pharyngotomy. More often however the larynx is also involved and partial laryngectomy with pharyngectomy is performed [15].

Esophageal involvement occurs either as a result of direct posterior extrathyroidal spread or, less commonly, from extranodal spread from central lymph node involvement [29]. When pharyngeal or esophageal involvement occurs, most commonly the muscularis is involved but the mucosa and submucosa are usually spared [15, 30]. If esophageal invasion is limited to the esophageal muscularis, the mucosa and submucosa can be preserved by finding the plane of dissection between the muscularis and submucosa, allowing complete resection and preserving the integrity of the esophageal lumen (Fig. 25.2).

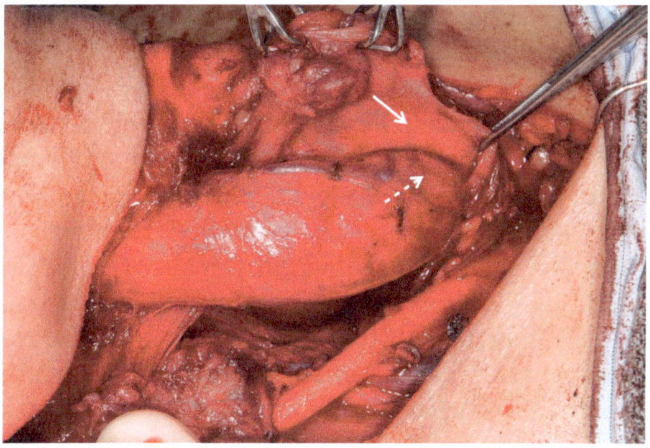

Fig. 25.2 Tumor involving esophageal muscularis, with dissection of the esophageal muscularis (*solid arrow*) off the esophageal submucosa (*dashed arrow*) in order to preserve the integrity of the esophageal lumen

If there is full-thickness intraluminal involvement of the esophagus but the area involved is small, full-thickness resection can be performed with tension-free closure in a layered fashion, and consideration may be given to rotating pectoralis muscle to cover the closure. For larger or circumferential defects of the cervical esophagus, reconstruction with a tubed pedicled or free flap is necessary. Free flap options include tubed radial free forearm, anterolateral thigh, or jejunal free flap. If the resection involves the thoracic esophagus, a gastric pull-up will be necessary.

Recurrent Laryngeal Nerve

The recurrent laryngeal nerve can be involved as a result of direct tumor extension from the thyroid or from paratracheal nodal involvement. The recurrent laryngeal nerve is involved relatively frequently in locally advanced thyroid cancer. A study performed at the Mayo Clinic of 262 patients with locally advanced papillary thyroid cancer showed that 123 (46 %) of these patients were found at surgery to have invasion of the recurrent laryngeal nerve with or without invasion of other structures. However, isolated recurrent laryngeal nerve involvement is rare with only 16 of these patients having recurrent laryngeal nerve involvement without invading other local structures [31].

The guiding principle of recurrent laryngeal nerve management is based upon several studies which demonstrate that leaving microscopic disease on the recurrent laryngeal nerve does not lead to decreased survival or increased recurrence, in comparison with resection of the nerve [31, 32].

Nishida et al. performed a retrospective study of 50 patients with differentiated thyroid cancer and intraoperative evidence of recurrent laryngeal nerve invasion.

The 50 patients were divided into two groups: 27 patients had the recurrent laryngeal nerve resected with the tumor, and 23 patients had the recurrent laryngeal nerve preserved by dissection of tumor off the nerve. The two groups had similar demographic backgrounds and similar local, regional, and distant involvement. No patients received prophylactic use of radioiodine. The study found that the incidence of postoperative recurrence was not different between the two groups. Rates of local, regional, and distant metastatic recurrences were similar between the groups. Postoperative overall survival of the preserved group was similar to that of the resected group. Mean postoperative survival periods of the resected and preserved groups were 8.55 ± 1.17 and 10.23 ± 1.04 years, respectively [32].

In the retrospective study by Falk et al., 24 patients with papillary carcinoma infiltrating the recurrent laryngeal nerve were analyzed. Five of the subjects had vocal cord paralysis, and 19 had normal vocal cord function. All five patients with paralysis received complete excision of the tumor and involved nerve. Of the 19 patients with normal cord function, 12 received complete and 7 received incomplete excision. Patients with complete excision had resection of all visible tumor and this necessitated excision of the involved recurrent laryngeal nerve. When the two groups of complete versus incomplete excision were compared, no significant difference was found in survival. The authors concluded that because complete excision of papillary carcinoma with resection of the recurrent laryngeal nerve did not improve survival over incomplete microscopic excision, incomplete excision of papillary carcinoma infiltrating a functioning recurrent laryngeal nerve should be performed to preserve the nerve. Postoperative RAI and thyroid-stimulating hormone suppression should be added as adjunct treatment in these situations [31].

Our treatment algorithm for approaching a recurrent laryngeal nerve infiltrated with tumor is often dependent upon the nerve's baseline function. Therefore, we strongly recommend preoperative evaluation of nerve function by means of either direct or indirect laryngoscopy when concern exists for a locally advanced thyroid cancer. If the nerve is infiltrated or encased with tumor and is functioning preoperatively, every attempt should be made to dissect disease off the nerve, leaving at most microscopic disease behind in order to preserve the function of the nerve. Adjuvant therapy in the form of RAI, T4 suppression, and potentially ERBT should be considered postoperatively and such treatment discussed by the surgeon with the multidisciplinary team. Being most intimately involved with the completeness of resection, the surgeon must play a key role in these decisions.

If the recurrent laryngeal nerve is infiltrated or encased by tumor, and vocal cord paresis or paralysis is present preoperatively (Fig. 25.3), in most cases the nerve should be fully resected in order to completely resect the disease. However, great care should be taken to preserve uninvolved posterior branches and preserve as much unaffected nerve as possible. It is also important to evaluate the status of the contralateral nerve prior to recurrent laryngeal nerve sacrifice, as bilateral involvement requires the surgeon to carefully assess degree of involvement on both sides before deciding on which (if any) unilateral nerve may be potentially sacrificed.

In the unusual circumstance that the contralateral vocal cord is paretic/paralyzed despite the absence of tumor, disease should be shaved off the involved recurrent

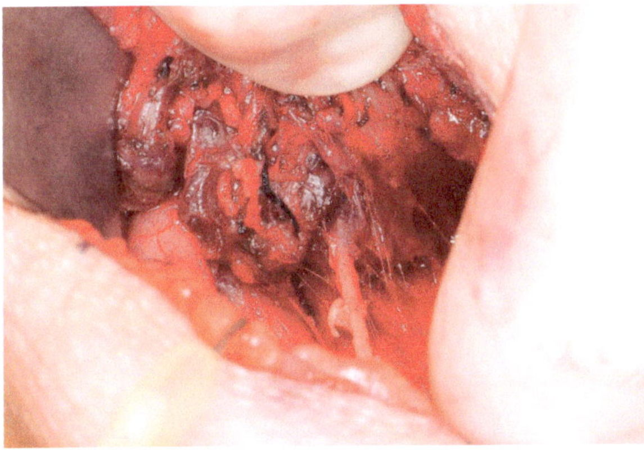

Fig. 25.3 Recurrent laryngeal nerve encased and invaded with well differentiated thyroid carcinoma

laryngeal nerve in attempts to preserve nerve function. Surgeons should counsel patients about the possibility of the need for a tracheostomy in such cases as shaving tumor off the nerve may result in temporary paresis or permanent paralysis. Because the functional status of the nerve plays such an important role in intraoperative decision-making regarding its handling, preoperative evaluation of the vocal cords when advanced disease is suspected is imperative before embarking on surgery. This information also allows a frank and informative preoperative conversation with the patient about the potential for temporary or permanent airway management.

Reconstruction of Recurrent Laryngeal Nerve

Laryngeal reinnervation after sacrifice of a recurrent laryngeal nerve can allow restoration of muscle tone and achievement of good voice quality. Reconstruction of a recurrent laryngeal nerve can be performed primarily or by means of a nerve graft. If the length of remaining recurrent laryngeal nerve allows direct anastomosis without tension, the nerve can be primarily opposed using three to four stitches of 8–0 or 9–0 nylon or Prolene under an operating microscope or Loupe magnification. If the defect does not allow primary anastomosis without tension, a free nerve graft can be used as a segmental interposition graft. These can be taken from the transverse cervical, supraclavicular, or ansa cervicalis nerves. In situations where the proximal end of the recurrent laryngeal nerve is not available for anastomosis post resection, the proximal end of the ansa cervicalis can also be employed to directly anastomose to the distal end of the recurrent laryngeal nerve (Fig. 25.4a, b) [33].

Several studies have shown good long-term results of both immediate and delayed direct recurrent laryngeal nerve reconstruction. Reinnervation can restore muscle tone, improve glottal closure, confer an improved mucosal wave, and reduce air leak, allowing a better voice outcome to be achieved. Sanuki et al.

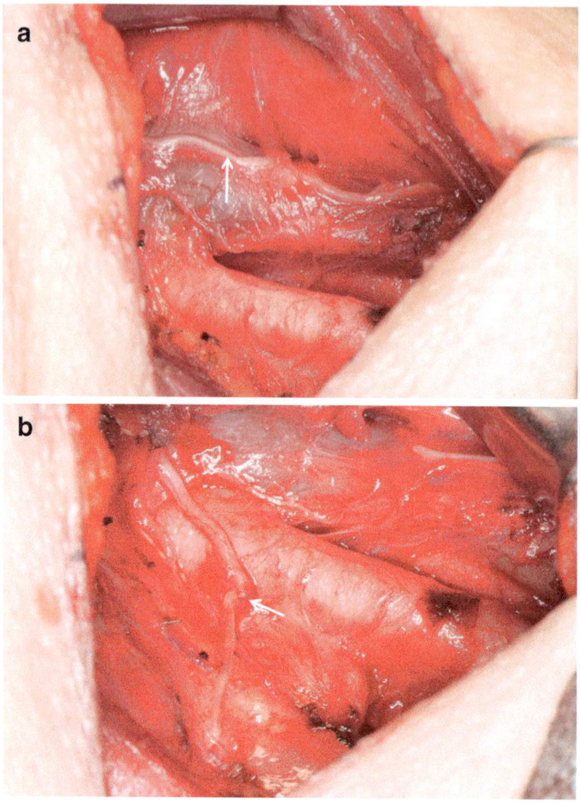

Fig. 25.4 (**a**) Ansa cervicalis nerve (*arrow*) in the lateral neck overlying internal jugular vein. (**b**) Ansa cervicalis nerve to recurrent laryngeal nerve anastomosis (*arrow* marks the anastomosis)

examined 12 patients with thyroid carcinoma who had preoperative unilateral vocal fold paralysis ($n=6$) or who had a unilateral recurrent laryngeal nerve that required sacrifice intraoperatively due to tumor involvement ($n=6$). Immediate reconstruction of recurrent laryngeal nerve was performed in all 12 patients by means of direct anastomosis ($n=1$), free nerve grafting ($n=9$), or ansa cervicalis ($n=2$) grafting to recurrent laryngeal nerve. The patients were assessed with the follow-up period ranging from 7 to 103 months (average of 34.6 months). The patients were assessed in the postoperative period in three domains: videostroboscopy findings, aerodynamic findings, and perceptual findings. Scrutinizing patients with known preoperative vocal fold paralysis enabled direct comparison of pre- and postoperative findings in the three domains. For videostroboscopy, although no visible vocal fold movement was detected during the follow-up period, the postoperative mucosal wave and glottal closure score were significantly greater than the preoperative score. Aerodynamic analysis showed that the postoperative recordings of maximum phonation time in this group had significant improvement, and the postoperative mean airflow leak rate had significant reduction. The mean perceptual voice evaluation scores for grade, breathiness, and roughness also showed significant improvement in the postoperative period [33].

Immediate reconstruction of the recurrent laryngeal nerve during thyroid cancer extirpation was described in the study by Yumoto et al. in which 22 patients with advanced thyroid cancer underwent resection of the primary lesion and involved recurrent laryngeal nerve. Recurrent laryngeal nerve paralysis was seen in 12 patients preoperatively and involvement of the RLN was noted intraoperatively in 10. Immediate reconstruction of the RLN was performed in eight patients using the great auricular nerve and by direct anastomosis of the RLN in one; nine patients had no reconstruction. The majority of patients who underwent immediate reconstruction showed minimal or no glottal gap during phonation, whereas those in the nonreconstructed group exhibited a large gap along the entire length of the fold. Phonatory function of harmonics-to-noise ratio, maximum phonation time, and mean airflow rate were also significantly better in the reconstructed group [34].

Wang et al. studied 237 patients with unilateral vocal cord paralysis secondary to thyroid surgery who underwent ansa cervicalis main branch-to-RLN anastomosis. Reconstruction was performed in delayed fashion, with at least 6 months between initial paralysis and reconstruction date. Videostroboscopy, vocal function assessment, and electromyography were performed preoperatively and postoperatively. The mean follow-up period was 5.2 years (ranging from 2 to 12 years). Analysis of videostroboscopic findings indicated that the glottic closure, vocal fold edge, vocal fold position, phase symmetry, and regularity were significantly improved in the postoperative period. The postoperative parameters of vocal function assessment (acoustic analysis, perceptual evaluation, and maximum phonation time) were also significantly improved. Postoperative laryngeal electromyography confirmed successful reinnervation of laryngeal muscle. The authors concluded that delayed laryngeal reinnervation with the ansa cervicalis was effective in restoring laryngeal phonatory function to normal or a nearly normal voice quality in unilateral vocal cord palsy secondary to thyroid surgery [35].

Involvement of Vessels

Invasion of vascular structures in papillary thyroid carcinoma has been shown to have prognostic significance. Both intrathyroidal and extrathyroidal vascular invasion are associated with a higher incidence of distant metastases at diagnosis [36]. Fortunately, well-differentiated thyroid cancer is rarely associated with substantial extrathyroidal vascular invasion or encasement [37].

Venous Involvement

The internal jugular vein is the most common extrathyroidal major vascular structure affected by tumor invasion or occlusion, with or without tumor thrombus. It is most frequently involved by large metastatic lateral neck lymph nodes and less likely to be directly invaded from the thyroid primary [38]. Due to impairment of venous drainage, patients with internal jugular vein involvement may present preoperatively with edema, dilated neck veins, fascial flushing, dyspnea, or dysphagia, though they may be asymptomatic. Further involvement of the superior vena cava with thrombus propagation may manifest with Pemberton's sign, a triad marked by the presence of facial congestion, cyanosis, and respiratory distress on arm elevation.

CT scanning with intravenous contrast may demonstrate venous involvement with evidence of enlarged veins, tumor invasion, compression, or filling defects [37]. It is important for the clinician not only to appreciate tumor invasion into the internal jugular vein on imaging preoperatively but also to determine if the level of invasion allows sacrifice of the vein to clear disease through a purely transcervical approach. Low-lying level 4 nodal disease with internal jugular vein involvement and extension into the brachiocephalic vein necessitates planning for intrathoracic access. The clavicle or upper ribs may have to be divided or sternotomy performed to safely allow adequate exposure of the vessel and clearance of gross disease.

If only a small patch of vein is involved, the area involved can be excised and the vein repaired either primarily or with a patch using either autologous vein or synthetic material. If however a significant portion of the vessel is involved, the vein should be sacrificed in order to clear disease. In unilateral internal jugular vein involvement, resection of the vessel can be performed with minimal morbidity. However, if both veins are involved, then at least one vein should be reconstructed. Typically, the resections of the veins can be staged, with initial resection and reconstruction of the vein with greater involvement. Staging allows collaterals to form after reconstruction of the first vein so that even if thrombosis develops within the reconstructed vein, sufficient time (usually 6 weeks) is given for collaterals to form before resection of the second vein. Reconstruction can be performed with autologous vein graft or ringed expanded polytetrafluoroethylene graft, though autologous vein graft is preferred as this has a lower risk of thrombosis [39]. Superior vena cava involvement will require cardiothoracic involvement, and successful resection of these tumors through a median sternotomy or right thoracotomy can be performed [40, 41].

Arterial Involvement

Carotid artery involvement is much less common than internal jugular vein involvement and its presence is usually asymptomatic. Carotid artery involvement should be suspected clinically when there is a mass in the area of the carotid artery that is fixed to the bony thoracic inlet. Involvement of the carotid artery is usually picked up on initial imaging (CT with contrast). However, if there is evidence of carotid artery involvement on the initial scan, evaluation may be performed with either CT angiogram or MR angiogram for further delineation. If carotid resection is planned, then MRA or conventional angiography may be employed to determine if shunting is necessary based upon the pattern of collateral intracranial blood flow and the integrity of the circle of Willis [3]. A balloon occlusion test will also be useful in determining if an artery can be sacrificed without shunting.

Depending on the degree of carotid invasion and degree of cross arterial supply, surgical resection can include shave resection, patch excision with autologous vein patch, en bloc excision with ligation, or en bloc resection and reconstruction [37] (Fig. 25.5a, b). Arterial reconstruction is usually performed using polytetrafluoroethylene or vein grafts. It may require a branched "Y" graft if the carotid-subclavian-brachiocephalic junction is involved [42]. Expert colleagues in vascular surgery should be involved in cases that required reconstruction.

Adjuvant Therapy

Role of Radioactive Iodine (RAI)

The current American Thyroid Association (ATA) guidelines recommend the use of RAI in all patients with known distant metastases or gross extrathyroidal extension of the tumor regardless of tumor size. It is also recommended that RAI be considered for selected patients with adverse features such as advancing age, aggressive histologies, or increasing number of large lymph nodes [43]. In patients with invasive WDTC in whom remaining microscopic disease is known or highly suspected after adequate surgical resection, such as with preservation of structures by the utilization of shaving, RAI is an excellent adjuvant treatment. However, RAI is less likely to be effective in achieving complete tumor response in cases in which there is gross residual disease after surgery [3].

Patients with high-risk features who have a known history of poor response to RAI or have a lower chance of responding to RAI, such as those with unfavorable histology, older age, recurrent disease, high FDG uptake, and/or low RAI uptake in known residual disease may be considered for EBRT in specific circumstances (please see section on EBRT below).

Systemic therapy, mainly in the form of kinase inhibitors, has been shown to improve progression-free survival in certain clinical contexts in patients with radioiodine-refractory well-differentiated thyroid cancer. Three randomized placebo-controlled trials with kinase inhibitors have been performed [44–46], two of which specifically addressed advanced local disease in their included cohorts [44, 45]. In a phase 3 trial with sorafenib which included both well and poorly differentiated thyroid cancer, progression-free survival was improved in

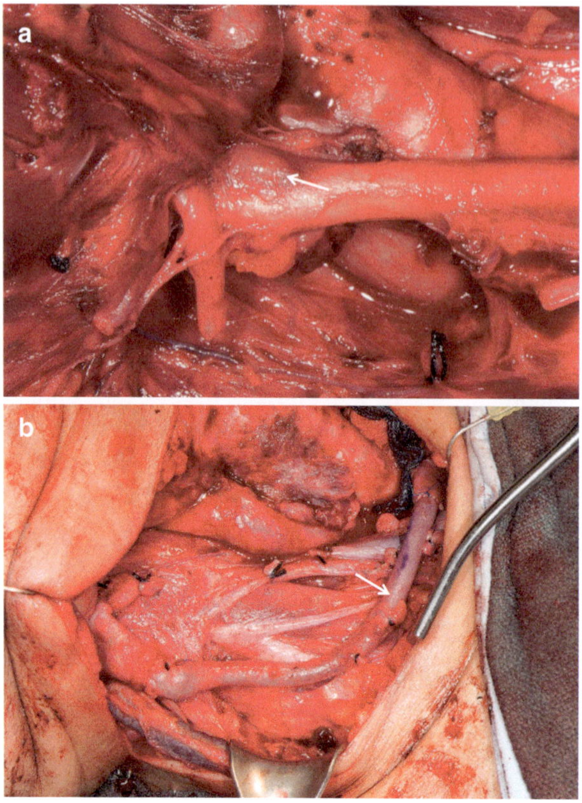

Fig. 25.5 (**a**) Metastatic thyroid cancer encasing carotid artery and involving the wall of the artery (*arrow*). (**b**) En bloc resection and reconstruction of carotid artery with saphenous vein graft (*arrow*)

the drug arm (10.8 months vs. 5.8 months, HR 0.59, 95 % CI 0.45–0.76). However, while 67 of the 417 participants (16 %) were reported to have metastatic lesions sites within the head and neck, only 15 (4 %) had locally advanced disease alone, making interpretation of treatment effect on this variable prohibitive [44]. Similarly in the phase 2 vandetanib trial, in which 61 % of patients had well-differentiated thyroid cancer, only 3 of the 145 participants (2 %) had advanced local disease alone, making conclusions about drug effect in the advanced local setting impossible to generate [45]. Though data specifically related to locally advanced disease is not available, the initial success of these kinase inhibitors in advanced disease makes them important treatment modalities to consider. However, the use of these agents should be performed by clinicians who are well versed in their advantages and adverse effects and always after careful consideration of the more standard therapy of RAI and TSH suppression has been performed.

Role of External Beam Radiation Therapy (EBRT)

The use of EBRT in well-differentiated thyroid carcinoma has often been debated. A complexity of factors influences the clinician's decision to use this modality (see Chap. 26 also). Prior to making a decision about the use of EBRT, it is imperative that the patient has a thorough assessment by an experienced surgeon, as adequate surgery is the most important treatment in curing a patient with well-differentiated thyroid carcinoma. Patients who have had inadequate surgery, with gross residual disease, need an appropriate definitive surgery prior to any consideration for EBRT.

The decision to employ EBRT is not to be taken lightly, especially in younger patients. In patients less than 45 years old, EBRT is usually not recommended after complete resection, as these patients have lower risk of locoregional recurrence, and RAI and/or further surgery are likely to achieve long-term control. A greater risk exists in younger patients regarding late toxicities and second malignancies. EBRT to the thyroid bed/central compartment generally closes the door to further surgery for a patient, short of a total laryngectomy as it makes further surgery much more technically difficult. Hence it is important, especially for younger patients, to be extremely judicious and cautious with the use of radiation in this situation. We would recommend, in general, to avoid radiation and allow the potential for further future surgery whenever possible. Because of the complexity of decision-making surrounding EBRT in well-differentiated thyroid carcinoma, a multidisciplinary discussion should always be undertaken in deciding upon the optimal treatment for the individual patient.

Rather than listing absolute indications for EBRT, given the complexity of the decision, we have included common presenting profiles of patients and whether EBRT would be considered in these scenarios:

1. *Patients with gross residual locoregional disease following initial surgery and deemed inappropriate for further surgery or patients felt to have primary unresectable locoregional disease.* Patients who have been evaluated for further resectability by a thyroid surgeon experienced in laryngotracheal resection and reconstruction and have been deemed not to be a candidate suitable for initial or further surgery. EBRT may be considered.
2. *Patients with extensive laryngotracheal and/or esophageal disease who have had appropriate surgery.* In general, EBRT should not be routinely used as adjuvant therapy after complete resection of gross disease. However, EBRT should be considered in patients with extensive laryngotracheal and/or esophageal disease that has been resected and reconstructed, requiring laryngectomy, tracheal resection, and/or esophageal resection, such that the experienced surgical team understands that the patient will not be a candidate for further surgery in the future. EBRT may be considered in such a scenario regardless of margin status, due to the extensive nature of the disease with high risk of recurrence and lack of further surgical options, as assessed by an experienced surgeon. Table 25.1 illustrates factors that should be considered in making a decision in such a scenario.

Table 25.1 Factors to consider when deciding upon administration of external beam radiation therapy in well-differentiated thyroid cancer

Factors favoring observation	Factors favoring radiation
Age ≤45	Age >45
Well differentiated	Poorly differentiated
Non-visceral involvement	High-risk visceral involvement
First presentation	Recurrent disease
No or few surgeries performed in the past by an experienced surgeon	Multiple surgeries in past and experienced surgeon feels surgical options exhausted
RAI naïve	Previous administration of RAI reaching maximum dose or disease unresponsive to RAI
Low FDG uptake and/or high RAI uptake in known residual disease	High FDG uptake and/or low RAI uptake in known residual disease
Presence of distant disease	Absence of distant disease

3. *Patients who have had surgical resection with concern/proof for microscopic residual disease postoperatively for which RAI may be adequate.* There is higher likelihood of microscopic residual disease in cases where tumor is shaved off the RLN, trachea, or larynx, which may occur in the setting of gross extrathyroidal extension or revision surgery for persistent or recurrent disease. Individually, microscopic positive margins are not an indication for EBRT. Postoperative RAI versus close observation is indicated and further surgery can be undertaken by an experienced surgeon if disease recurs in the future. EBRT is not generally indicated in this clinical scenario.
4. *Patients who have had surgical resection with concern/proof for microscopic residual disease in which further surgery short of laryngectomy will not be possible.* In this scenario surgical options have been exhausted by an experienced surgeon, and a period of observation is indicated before committing the patient to laryngectomy. EBRT may be considered in such a case, to potentially avoid or prolong time to laryngectomy. Table 25.1 illustrates factors which may be considered in such a scenario
5. *Patients with isolated distant metastases amenable to radiation therapy.* In disease that has metastasized, EBRT may be considered as local treatment of isolated distant metastases. Localized and/or unresectable metastases in the spine, bone, or brain may be treated with EBRT, particularly if the disease has been shown to be radioiodine-refractory.

Gross residual disease that is not amenable to further surgery (clinical scenario #1 above) can be controlled or even cured with the use of radiotherapy. Several studies have been performed looking at the effectiveness of EBRT in the treatment of macroscopic residual disease after surgery. Chow et al. performed a study in which after primary thyroid surgery (including biopsy only), 217 patients were classified as having gross locoregional residual disease. Among these 217 patients, 23 % had RAI alone, 7.4 % had EBRT, 52.1 % had both RAI and EBRT and 17.5 % had no radiation therapy. While there is clearly selection bias in such a study, the authors found that those groups that received EBRT had a 10-year locoregional failure-free survival improvement from 24 to 63.4 %, while the 10-year cause-specific survival was improved from 49.7 to 74.1 % [47]. In the study by Tsang et al., 33 patients with macroscopic residual disease who were treated with EBRT +/− RAI had a 5-year cause-specific survival of 65 % and a 5-year local relapse-free rate of 62 % [48]. Sheline et al. reported 8 of 15 patients with tumor control over a 2- to 15-year period [49]. The response of macroscopic disease to radiotherapy is variable, with some patients having no effect while others may have complete response. The study by O'Connell et al. reported 49 patients with gross residual disease (both follicular and papillary) treated with EBRT; complete regression was obtained in 37.5 %, partial regression in 25 %, and no regression in 37.5 % [50].

A small minority of patients with WDTC have extensive visceral disease and laryngotracheal disease that has been completely resected and reconstructed, requiring laryngectomy, tracheal resection, or esophageal resection, such that the experienced surgical team feels that further surgery in the future would not be feasible (clinical scenario #2 above). Although there are no studies that specifically examine ERBT in this scenario, it is generally agreed that select patients with pT4 PTC with visceral invasion have better failure-free survival, locoregional recurrence rates, and disease-specific survival with the addition of EBRT [47]. Although we do not recommend EBRT routinely based on pT4 PTC status alone, this adjuvant treatment modality should be considered in patients with invasive visceral disease in which further surgical options as assessed by an experienced thyroid surgeon are limited. On the contrary, microscopic positive margins are not a reason for EBRT in patients with well-differentiated thyroid cancer in the absence of aggressive poorly differentiated histopathology. EBRT should be generally reserved for older patients with aggressive histopathology and/or extensive laryngotracheal or esophageal invasion, resection, and reconstruction.

Prognostic Significance of Extrathyroidal Spread

Extrathyroidal spread has been shown to impact disease-free interval following surgery. Ortiz found that the 1-year, 5-year, and 10-year disease-free interval rates in patients with papillary thyroid carcinoma without extrathyroidal spread were 95 %, 87 %, and 82 %, respectively, whereas the disease-free interval rates in the group of patients with extrathyroidal spread were 66 %, 46 %, and 31 %, respectively [6]. Extrathyroidal spread in this study was defined as invasion by the primary tumor of the thyroid capsule and infiltration of the fat and tissue adjacent to the thyroid gland (prethyroid muscles, trachea, larynx, blood vessels, or recurrent larynx nerve). However, the degree of extrathyroidal spread may be important. In a study by Ito et al., extrathyroidal extension was classified into no extension, minimal extension (extension to sternothyroid muscle or perithyroid soft tissues), and massive extension (extension to subcutaneous soft tissue, larynx, trachea, esophagus, or recurrent laryngeal nerve). Patients with massive extension showed a significantly worse relapse-free survival rate than those with no or minimal extension ($P<0.0001$).

There was, however, no difference in the relapse-free survival rate between patients with no extension and those with minimal extension [51].

The site of invasion is also important in determining prognosis. In the study by McCaffrey of 262 patients with papillary thyroid carcinoma, the factors that had significant influence on survival were invasion of the trachea and the esophagus. Muscle invasion, laryngeal invasion, and recurrent laryngeal nerve invasion had no significant independent influence on survival [12]. It is likely that this significance of invasion relates to the relative ease at which disease can be grossly cleared by the operating surgeon.

Various studies have shown that 36–80 % [26, 52, 53] of patients who succumb to papillary thyroid carcinoma die with active local disease. This observation underscores the importance of thoughtful multidisciplinary planning and treatment of locally advanced well-differentiated thyroid carcinoma.

References

1. Sherman SI. Thyroid carcinoma. Lancet (London, England). 2003;361(9356):501–11.
2. Shaha AR. Thyroidectomy for locally advanced cancer. In: Duh W-Y, editor. Atlas of endocrine surgical techniques. 1st ed. Philadelphia: Saunders; 2010. p. 25–46. Townsend and Evers.
3. Shindo ML, Caruana SM, Kandil E, McCaffrey JC, Orloff LA, Porterfield JR, et al. Management of invasive well-differentiated thyroid cancer: an American Head and Neck Society consensus statement. AHNS consensus statement. Head Neck. 2014;36(10):1379–90.
4. McCaffrey JC. Aerodigestive tract invasion by well-differentiated thyroid carcinoma: diagnosis, management, prognosis, and biology. Laryngoscope. 2006;116(1):1–11.
5. Su SY, Milas ZL, Bhatt N, Roberts D, Clayman GL. Well-differentiated thyroid cancer with aerodigestive tract invasion: long-term control and functional outcomes. Head Neck. 2016;38(1):72–8. doi:10.1002/hed.23851. Epub 2015 Apr 6.6.
6. Ortiz S, Rodriguez JM, Soria T, Perez-Flores D, Pinero A, Moreno J, et al. Extrathyroid spread in papillary carcinoma of the thyroid: clinicopathological and prognostic study. Otolaryngol Head Neck Surg Off J Am Acad Otolaryngol Head Neck Surg. 2001;124(3):261–5.
7. Andersen PE, Kinsella J, Loree TR, Shaha AR, Shah JP. Differentiated carcinoma of the thyroid with extrathyroidal extension. Am J Surg. 1995;170(5):467–70.
8. Fujimoto Y, Obara T, Ito Y, Kodama T, Yashiro T, Yamashita T, et al. Aggressive surgical approach for locally invasive papillary carcinoma of the thyroid in patients over forty-five years of age. Surgery. 1986;100(6):1098–107.
9. Grillo HC, Zannini P. Resectional management of airway invasion by thyroid carcinoma. Ann Thorac Surg. 1986;42(3):287–98.
10. Melliere DJ, Ben Yahia NE, Becquemin JP, Lange F, Boulahdour H. Thyroid carcinoma with tracheal or esophageal involvement: limited or maximal surgery? Surgery. 1993;113(2):166–72.
11. Park CS, Suh KW, Min JS. Cartilage-shaving procedure for the control of tracheal cartilage invasion by thyroid carcinoma. Head Neck. 1993;15(4):289–91.
12. McCaffrey TV, Bergstralh EJ, Hay ID. Locally invasive papillary thyroid carcinoma: 1940–1990. Head Neck. 1994;16(2):165–72.
13. Czaja JM, McCaffrey TV. The surgical management of laryngotracheal invasion by well-differentiated papillary thyroid carcinoma. Arch Otolaryngol Head Neck Surg. 1997;123(5):484–90.

14. Kowalski LP, Filho JG. Results of the treatment of locally invasive thyroid carcinoma. Head Neck. 2002;24(4):340–4.
15. Shaha AR. Implications of prognostic factors and risk groups in the management of differentiated thyroid cancer. Laryngoscope. 2004;114(3):393–402.
16. Breaux Jr GP, Guillamondegui OM. Treatment of locally invasive carcinoma of the thyroid: how radical? Am J Surg. 1980;140(4):514–7.
17. Ballantyne AJ. Resections of the upper aerodigestive tract for locally invasive thyroid cancer. Am J Surg. 1994;168(6):636–9.
18. Frankenthaler RA, Sellin RV, Cangir A, Goepfert H. Lymph node metastasis from papillary-follicular thyroid carcinoma in young patients. Am J Surg. 1990;160(4):341–3.
19. Wada N, Masudo K, Hirakawa S, et al. Superior vena cava (SVC) reconstruction using autologous tissue in two cases of differentiated thyroid carcinoma presenting with SVC syndrome. World J Surg Oncol. 2009;7:75.
20. Michael E. Kupferman, Randal S. Weber. Surgical management of locally advanced thyroid cancer. In: RE Pollack, editor. Advanced therapy in surgical oncology. 2008 BC Decker INC. Ontario: PMPH-USA; 2008. p. 353–60.
21. Friedman M. Surgical management of thyroid carcinoma with laryngotracheal invasion. Otolaryngol Clin North Am. 1990;23(3):495–507.
22. Shin DH, Mark EJ, Suen HC, Grillo HC. Pathologic staging of papillary carcinoma of the thyroid with airway invasion based on the anatomic manner of extension to the trachea: a clinicopathologic study based on 22 patients who underwent thyroidectomy and airway resection. Hum Pathol. 1993;24(8):866–70.
23. Nishida T, Nakao K, Hamaji M. Differentiated thyroid carcinoma with airway invasion: indication for tracheal resection based on the extent of cancer invasion. J Thorac Cardiovasc Surg. 1997;114(1):84–92.
24. Ozaki O, Sugino K, Mimura T, Ito K. Surgery for patients with thyroid carcinoma invading the trachea: circumferential sleeve resection followed by end-to-end anastomosis. Surgery. 1995;117(3):268–71.
25. Tsukahara K, Sugitani I, Kawabata K. Surgical management of tracheal shaving for papillary thyroid carcinoma with tracheal invasion. Acta Otolaryngol. 2009;129:1498–502.
26. Patel KN, Shaha AR. Locally advanced thyroid cancer. Curr Opin Otolaryngol Head Neck Surg. 2005;13(2):112–6.
27. Yu P, Clayman GL, Walsh GL. Human tracheal reconstruction with a composite radial forearm free flap and prosthesis. Ann Thorac Surg. 2006;81(2):714–6.
28. Yu P, Clayman GL, Walsh GL. Long-term outcomes of microsurgical reconstruction for large tracheal defects. Cancer. 2011;117(4):802–8.
29. Machens A, Hinze R, Lautenschlager C, Thomusch O, Dralle H. Thyroid carcinoma invading the cervicovisceral axis: routes of invasion and clinical implications. Surgery. 2001;129(1):23–8.
30. Gillenwater AM, Goepfert H. Surgical management of laryngotracheal and esophageal involvement by locally advanced thyroid cancer. Semin Surg Oncol. 1999;16(1):19–29.
31. Falk SA, McCaffrey TV. Management of the recurrent laryngeal nerve in suspected and proven thyroid cancer. Otolaryngol Head Neck Surg Off J Am Acad Otolaryngol Head Neck Surg. 1995;113(1):42–8.
32. Nishida T, Nakao K, Hamaji M, Kamiike W, Kurozumi K, Matsuda H. Preservation of recurrent laryngeal nerve invaded by differentiated thyroid cancer. Ann Surg. 1997;226(1):85–91.
33. Sanuki T, Yumoto E, Minoda R, Kodama N. The role of immediate recurrent laryngeal nerve reconstruction for thyroid cancer surgery. J Oncol. 2010;2010:846235.
34. Yumoto E, Sanuki T, Kumai Y. Immediate recurrent laryngeal nerve reconstruction and vocal outcome. Laryngoscope. 2006;116(9):1657–61.
35. Wang W, Chen D, Chen S, Li D, Li M, Xia S, et al. Laryngeal reinnervation using ansa cervicalis for thyroid surgery-related unilateral vocal fold paralysis: a long-term outcome analysis of 237 cases. PLoS One. 2011;6(4):e19128.

36. Gardner RE, Tuttle RM, Burman KD, Haddady S, Truman C, Sparling YH, et al. Prognostic importance of vascular invasion in papillary thyroid carcinoma. Arch Otolaryngol Head Neck Surg. 2000;126(3):309–12.
37. Kebebew E, Clark OH. Locally advanced differentiated thyroid cancer. Surg Oncol. 2003;12(2):91–9.
38. Lee YS, Chung WY, Chang HS, Park CS. Treatment of locally advanced thyroid cancer invading the great vessels using a Y-shaped graft bypass. Interact Cardiovasc Thorac Surg. 2010;10(6):1039–41.
39. Wada N, Masudo K, Hirakawa S, Woo T, Arai H, Suganuma N, et al. Superior vena cava (SVC) reconstruction using autologous tissue in two cases of differentiated thyroid carcinoma presenting with SVC syndrome. World J Surg Oncol. 2009;7:75.
40. Thompson NW, Brown J, Orringer M, Sisson J, Nishiyama R. Follicular carcinoma of the thyroid with massive angioinvasion: extension of tumor thrombus to the heart. Surgery. 1978;83(4):451–7.
41. Lalak NJ, Campbell PR. Infiltrating papillary carcinoma of the thyroid with macroscopic extension into the internal jugular vein. Otolaryngol Head Neck Surg Off J Am Acad Otolaryngol Head Neck Surg. 1997;117(6):S228–30.
42. Lee YS, Chung WY, Chang HS, Park CS. Treatment of locally advanced thyroid cancer invading the great vessels using a Y-shaped graft bypass. Interact Cardiovasc Thorac Surg. 2010;10:1039–41.
43. Haugen BR, Alexander EK, Bible KC, Doherty GM, Mandel SJ, Nikiforov YE, Pacini F, Randolph GW, Sawka AM, Schlumberger M, Schuff KG, Sherman SI, Sosa JA, Steward DL, Tuttle RM, Wartofsky L. 2015 American Thyroid Association Management Guidelines for adult patients with thyroid nodules and differentiated thyroid cancer: the American Thyroid Association guidelines task force on thyroid nodules and differentiated thyroid cancer. Thyroid. 2016;26(1):1–133. doi:10.1089/thy.2015.0020.
44. Brose MS, Nutting CM, Jarzab B, Elisei R, Siena S, Bastholt L, de la Fouchardiere C, Pacini F, Paschke R, Shong YK, Sherman SI, Smit JW, Chung J, Kappeler C, Pena C, Molnar I, Schlumberger MJ. Sorafenib in radioactive iodine-refractory, locally advanced or metastatic differentiated thyroid cancer: a randomised, double-blind, phase 3 trial. Lancet. 2014;384:319–28.
45. Leboulleux S, Bastholt L, Krause T, de la Fouchardiere C, Tennvall J, Awada A, Gomez JM, Bonichon F, Leenhardt L, Soufflet C, Licour M, Schlumberger MJ. Vandetanib in locally advanced or metastatic differentiated thyroid cancer: a randomised, double-blind, phase 2 trial. Lancet Oncol. 2012;13:897–905.
46. Schlumberger M, Tahara M, Wirth LJ, Robinson B, Brose MS, Elisei R, Habra MA, Newbold K, Shah MH, Hoff AO, Gianoukakis AG, Kiyota N, Taylor MH, Kim SB, Krzyzanowska MK, Dutcus CE, de las Heras B, Zhu J, Sherman SI. Lenvatinib versus placebo in radioiodine-refractory thyroid cancer. N Engl J Med. 2015;372:621–30.
47. Chow SM, Yau S, Kwan CK, Poon PC, Law SC. Local and regional control in patients with papillary thyroid carcinoma: specific indications of external radiotherapy and radioactive iodine according to T and N categories in AJCC 6th edition. Endocr Relat Cancer. 2006;13(4):1159–72.
48. Tsang RW, Brierley JD, Simpson WJ, Panzarella T, Gospodarowicz MK, Sutcliffe SB. The effects of surgery, radioiodine, and external radiation therapy on the clinical outcome of patients with differentiated thyroid carcinoma. Cancer. 1998;82(2):375–88.
49. Sheline GE, Galante M, Lindsay S. Radiation therapy in the control of persistent thyroid cancer. Am J Roentgenol Radium Ther Nucl Med. 1966;97(4):923–30.
50. O'Connell ME, A'Hern RP, Harmer CL. Results of external beam radiotherapy in differentiated thyroid carcinoma: a retrospective study from the Royal Marsden Hospital. Eur J Cancer (Oxford, England: 1990). 1994;30A(6):733–9.

51. Ito Y, Tomoda C, Uruno T, Takamura Y, Miya A, Kobayashi K, Matsuzuka F, Kuma K, Miyauchi A. Prognostic significance of extrathyroid extension of papillary thyroid carcinoma: massive but not minimal extension affects the relapse-free survival. World J Surg. 2006;30(5):780–6.
52. McConahey WM, Hay I, Woolner LB, van Heerden JA, Taylor WF. Papillary thyroid cancer treated at the Mayo Clinic, 1946 through 1970: initial manifestations, pathologic findings, therapy and outcome. Mayo Clinic Proc. In: Edge SE, Byrd D, Compton CC, et al., editors. AJJ cancer staging manual. 7th ed. New York: Springer; 2009.
53. Tovi F, Goldstein J. Locally aggressive differentiated thyroid carcinoma. J Surg Oncol. 1985;29(2):99–104.

Chapter 26
External Beam Radiation for Locally Advanced and Metastatic Differentiated Thyroid Cancer

James D. Brierley, Meredith E. Giuliani, and Richard W. Tsang

Introduction

The mainstay in the management of differentiated thyroid cancer is surgery and in intermediate-/high-risk patients postoperative administration of radioactive iodine (RAI). Systemic radiation in the form of RAI is beneficial not only in reducing the risk of recurrence in the neck but also in diagnosing and treating local and distant disease. A significant amount of work has been done in recent years in trying to classify risk with respect to which patients can benefit from RAI. In contrast, external beam radiation therapy (EBRT) is a focused treatment, and as such, is only expected to be of benefit when the risk of recurrence is chiefly local. Given the effectiveness of surgery and RAI in intermediate- and some high-risk patients, the number of patients expected to benefit from EBRT is small; all studies examining the role of EBRT have been retrospective, with one exception described below. Given the lack of consensus in identifying patients who may benefit from RAI, it is not surprising that there is little consensus for whom EBRT should be routinely recommended.

To review the role of EBRT in differentiated thyroid cancer, it is useful to consider the three scenarios in which EBRT may be used:

1. Treatment of unresectable cancer in the neck. This may be after the surgical procedure is unable to remove all gross disease, or when no surgery was attempted initially, either because of the known extent of local disease or because the patient was not considered fit for surgery.

J.D. Brierley, MBBS, MRCP, FRCR, FRCPC (✉) • M.E. Giuliani, MBBS, MEd, FRCPC • R.W. Tsang, MD, FRCPC
Department of Radiation Oncology, University of Toronto, Princess Margaret Cancer Centre, 610 University Ave, Toronto, ON M5G2M9, Canada
e-mail: James.Brierley@rmp.uhn.on.ca

S.A. Roman et al. (eds.), *Management of Thyroid Nodules and Differentiated Thyroid Cancer*, DOI 10.1007/978-3-319-43618-0_26

2. Adjuvant therapy after surgery (and RAI) in patients who have had all gross tumor resected in the neck but who are considered to be at significant risk of local recurrence. This is usually in the setting of a large primary tumor with significant extrathyroidal extension into the soft tissue and important structures of the neck, such as the recurrent laryngeal nerve, trachea, larynx, and esophagus.
3. Treatment of metastatic disease. As noted earlier EBRT has a limited value in treating systemic disease, however:
(a) If the metastases are symptomatic, EBRT can help control the symptoms.
(b) In certain situations when the number of known metastases is small (oligometastatic disease), EBRT may achieve long-term control of these metastases.

This review will consider these scenarios separately.

Treatment of Unresectable Cancer in the Neck

The TNM defines T4b disease as advanced disease invading the prevertebral fascia, encasing the carotid artery and/or mediastinal vessels [1]; however, less advanced disease may also be unresectable or, if resectable, will leave gross residual disease because complete extirpation requires extensive surgery, such as pharyngolaryngectomy, to achieve negative margins. The role for EBRT in these cases has been suggested by many studies over the last 50 years [2]. In a study from Hong Kong in 124 patients with gross residual disease after surgery, the 69 patients who had EBRT had a local relapse-free survival of 64 %, but it was only 29 % in the 55 patients who did not have EBRT [3]. Like all retrospective studies on the effectiveness of EBRT, this study has the problems of selection bias. However, it shows that EBRT is effective in patients with gross residual disease in improving local control. It also demonstrated that even at 10 years after surgery, not all patients with local gross residual disease progress and have uncontrolled cancer in the neck, or die from metastatic disease. However, we cannot predict who are the patients who will have very slowly growing disease and may not require EBRT. Patients with FDG-PET scan negative distant metastatic disease have excellent prognosis because such metastases with low metabolic activity are slow growing and tend to be stable for many years [4]. However, there are no prospective data to confirm that patients with gross residual disease who are FDG-PET negative can be safely observed.

In another study from our own institution, albeit with a smaller sample size, the use of EBRT for gross residual neck disease resulted in a 10-year local relapse-free rate of 90 % [5]. However, the corresponding cause-specific survival (CSS) was only 48 % suggesting that even if local control is achieved, there is a significant risk of distant metastases developing and patients dying of metastatic disease. This is not surprising given that patients with unresectable cancer tend to be older and have less well-differentiated disease that is iodine resistant. Data on EBRT from the MD Anderson Cancer Center and from the Christie Hospital in patients with gross residual or unresectable thyroid cancer showed local control rates of 60 % and 69 %, respectively, although these studies were small with only 15 and 19 patients, in each study [6, 7]. The American Thyroid Association 2009 guidelines recommended EBRT for those patients with gross residual tumor in whom further surgery or RAI would likely be ineffective [8]. The 2015 guidelines do not address the situation of unresected tumor, but comment that for tumors that invade the upper aerodigestive tract, surgery combined with additional therapy such as ^{131}I and/or EBRT is generally advised [9]. Similarly, the British Thyroid Association recommends EBRT for residual or recurrent tumor that fails to concentrate RAI, i.e., locoregional disease where further surgery or RAI is ineffective or impractical [10].

In summary EBRT can control unresectable or gross residual disease in the neck preventing the potentially devastating effects of uncontrolled thyroid cancer in the neck, such as voice impairment or loss, airway obstruction, dysphagia, and esophageal obstruction. This is also true for cancer that has recurred in the neck after initial therapy but the disease extent is such that it is unresectable. EBRT does not replace high-quality surgery.

Adjuvant Therapy

The American Thyroid Association recommended that the adjuvant use of EBRT should be considered in patients over age 45 years with grossly visible extrathyroidal extension at the time of surgery and a high likelihood of postoperative microscopic residual disease [8]. The 2015 guidelines state that there is no role for routine adjuvant EBRT, but note that it can be used selectively in patients with residual disease after surgery and in patients after repeated surgeries for recurrent nodal involvement especially if the risks of further surgery outweigh the risk from EBRT [9]. The British Thyroid Association recommends adjuvant EBRT for patients with a high risk of recurrence or progression, specifically those with gross evidence of local tumor invasion at surgery and those with significant macroscopic residual disease [10]. However, the only randomized controlled trial on the use of adjuvant EBRT was negative and did not show a benefit. Unfortunately the entry criterion for the study was any patient with pathological T4 differentiated thyroid cancer. Therefore, many patients could potentially be entered who did not meet either of these two recommendations in that they may have had no evidence of clinical extrathyroidal extension or risk of microscopic or macroscopic residual disease after surgery. In addition, recruitment was poor and only 45 of a planned 311 patients consented, so the study was converted to an open cohort study, and ultimately only 26 patients received EBRT. The local failure rate in the observation group without EBRT was only 3 % confirming that this was indeed a group of patients with a low local recurrence risk [11].

Retrospective single-institution studies appear to show a benefit to EBRT in selected patients with high risk of local recurrence (Table 26.1). In a study from our institution patients over 60 years of age with extrathyroidal extension and no gross residual disease after surgery had improved 10-year cause-specific survival (81.0 %

Table 26.1 10-year recurrence free rates in patients with high risk of local recurrence. All series are retrospective and use of RAI not standardized

First author and publication date	Recurrence-free rate after surgery ± RAI and EBRT (%)	Recurrence-free rate after surgery ± RAI(%)
Tubiana (1985) [12]	86	79
Farahati (1996) [13]	90	50
Tsang (1998) [14]	93	78
Chow (2002) [15]	88	84
Kim (2003) [16][a]	95	63
Phlips (2004) [17]	97	79
Brierley (2005) [18][b]	86	66
Keum (2006) [19][c]	89	38
Azrif (2008) [6][a]	81	Not reported
Schwartz (2009) [7][d]	79	Not reported

[a]At 5 years
[b]For patients over 60 with ETE. Note some patient overlap with report from Tsang (1998)
[c]All patient had tracheal invasion
[d]At 4 years

vs. 64.6%) and also improved local relapse-free rates (86.4% vs. 65.7%). Patients under 60 years had improved local control only (10-year LRFR 95.9% with EBRT vs. 85.4% with no EBRT, $p=0.03$) [18]. This study confirmed the results of an earlier study from Germany [13]. In that series of 137 patients, all who had extrathyroid extension, surgery, and RAI, 85 received radiotherapy EBRT to the thyroid bed and cervical and upper mediastinal lymph nodes. The patients in the EBRT group had fewer local and regional recurrences ($P=0.004$). More recent institutional reports have not compared outcomes with and without EBRT because in those institutions EBRT has become standard in patients at high risk of recurrence. A group from the Christie Hospital in the UK reported that in patients with macroscopic residue or inoperable disease treated with EBRT, the local regional control rate was 89% [6]. A group from the MD Anderson Cancer Center in the USA reported that for patients with microscopic residual disease, the four-year regional control rate was 86% and four-year cause-specific survival, 82% [7]. A recent review from France that included 13 papers concluded that there was a role for EBRT in patient at high risk of recurrence. They developed a scoring system to define patients who would benefit from EBRT. Any patient who scores 6 or more points would be recommended EBRT. Being over 60 years of age, extrathyroidal extension and microscopic residual disease, all score two points each [20].

Although lacking proof from randomized controlled studies, EBRT appears to benefit patients at high risk of local recurrence. Risk is usually defined by older age, extrathyroidal extension, and microscopic residual disease. It is our current institutional policy to recommend EBRT in older patients (usually over 50 years of age) with gross extrathyroidal extension noted at the time of surgery that invades posteriorly into the trachea-esophageal groove. Invariably, there is a risk of microscopic disease after surgery in this region, unless an extirpative operation such as a laryngectomy was performed. We believe such disease is unlikely to be controlled by radioactive iodine alone. It is important to involve the surgeon in the discussion to ensure that the extrathyroidal extension was significant and that salvage surgery would be difficult if not impossible without extensive radical surgery, and that recurrence would have a significant impact on speech, swallowing, and quality of life. Patients with gross extrathyroidal extension that invades anteriorly into the strap muscles can usually be resected with clear margins and do not require EBRT. There may also be a role for EBRT in patients who have repeated surgery for recurrent cervical nodal involvement and in whom further surgery may result in unacceptable risks or complications.

Radiation Therapy

If patients are to have RAI and adjuvant EBRT, our preference is usually to give ^{131}I and then perform postoperative CT scans after the post-RAI therapy scan and reassess the extent of disease after surgery, as seen on post-RAI scan and CT scan. A PET scan if available may provide additional information. Although in theory EBRT could reduce the effectiveness of RAI, there is no good evidence to support this, and therefore if there is concern about the extent of local disease that may cause an oncological emergency without control of that disease, such as gross residual disease after spinal cord decompression, then we will give EBRT before RAI.

A preoperative CT scan with intravenous contrast is a great aid in planning any postoperative radiation therapy. In our institution, surgeons routinely perform CT scans with intravenous contrast in any patients with a large mass, fixation, pain, or hoarseness that suggest a possible T4 tumor. Past concerns that iodinated contrast may interfere with the effectiveness of RAI have been allayed with modern water-soluble contrast media (see Chap. 6). A 1 or 2 months delay only is now required for the urinary iodine levels to fall after a contrast enhanced CT [21]. An alternative to CT with contrast is a cervical MRI; however, the ability to identify laryngeal cartilage or lymph node involvement may be inferior.

It is our practice to include in the volume to be irradiated the surgical thyroidectomy bed and levels III, IV, and VI and part of level V. The volumes extend from the hyoid bone superiorly to the aortic arch inferiorly. Sixty Gray in 30 fractions is usually prescribed to the thyroid bed and areas of surgical dissection if there is concern for microscopic residual disease, and a lower dose of 54 Gy in 30 fractions to undissected areas at risk of microscopic disease. In patients with gross residual disease, unresectable or unresected disease, a higher dose of 66 Gy in 33 fractions to 70 Gy in 35 fractions is given to the gross disease, with 56 Gy in 33 or 35 fractions to the areas at risk of microscopic disease (Fig. 26.1). For patients with unresected gross disease and poor performance status unable to tolerate 66 Gy, occasionally we will give 50 Gy in 20 fractions over 4 weeks. For palliation in patients with local symptoms and disseminated disease and limited performance status radiation such as 20 Gy in 5 fractions or 30 Gy in 10 fractions may be prescribed.

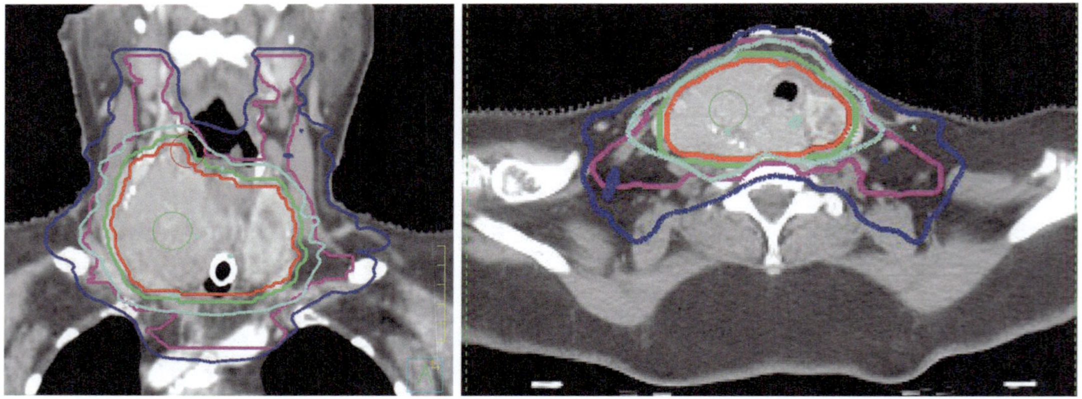

Fig. 26.1 A 76-year-old woman presents with a short history of shortness of breath but a long-standing history of a thyroid mass. Biopsy shows differentiated thyroid cancer. CT scan is reported as extensive thyroid mass with tracheal involvement and involvement of the carotid. The tumor is considered unresectable. She is referred for EBRT. A tracheostomy is performed and she is prescribed 70 Gy in 35 fractions over 7 weeks. Sagittal and axial view of radiation treatment plan. The *red line* is the gross target volume (GTV). The *lime green line* is the 70 Gy isodose line (all the tissue with that volume described by the 70 Gy isodose line received a minimum of 70 Gy). The *dark blue line* is the 56 Gy isodose line

Volume and Toxicity

There is controversy on the appropriate volume to treat with EBRT. Our philosophy has been to give EBRT to control disease in the thyroid bed and tracheoesophageal groove. Consequently our volumes are smaller than in other institutions that treat the entire cervical nodal basin (levels II to V and some include the retropharyngeal lymph nodes). Although this volume may result in fewer nodal recurrences (which hopefully can be salvaged with further surgery), the radiation-induced acute and late toxicity will be greater. Minimizing toxicity from EBRT is critically important, especially in patients who are already at risk from xerostomia because of RAI. Both acute and late effects following EBRT are dependent on the volumes radiated as well as the dose to normal structures. Structures of particular concern include the parotid glands, radiation to which potentiates the risk of xerostomia. Other volumes of concern include the pharyngeal constrictors which may result in dysphagia and, in rare circumstance, feeding tube dependence, and the mandible which is associated with a risk of osteoradionecrosis, although this is rare. Second malignancy can occur after any radiation treatment but is exceedingly rare and has not to our knowledge been reported following EBRT for thyroid cancer but should always be a consideration especially in treating young patients. Not surprisingly in a study on quality of life in patients treated for thyroid cancer, those who had EBRT and RAI fared less well than those who had RAI only after surgery [22]. Intensity-modulated radiation therapy (IMRT, Table 26.2) which is now the standard for treating head and neck cancers in many centers, has been reported to be associated with less late morbidity than older techniques [7].

In general however well-planned EBRT results in acceptable levels of acute toxicity. Serious complications are rare and EBRT does not preclude future surgical intervention by surgeons with experience in operating in previously irradiated tissues. Acute toxicity that occurs toward the end of a course of radiation therapy includes moderate skin erythema, and rarely moist desquamation and mucositis of the esophagus, trachea, and larynx. Larger radiation volumes to treat nodal areas extending to the salivary glands result in changes in taste, sensation, and xerostomia. Late toxicity is uncommon, and may comprise skin telangiectasias, skin pigmentation, soft tissue fibrosis, and mild lymphedema, usually appearing just below the chin. Esophageal stenosis in our experience can usually be treated by dilatation. We have not seen G-tube dependency or tracheal stenosis in our patients, although it has been reported by others [7]. Two large series on the use of EBRT reported no radiation therapy oncology group grade IV toxic effects [13, 14).

Treatment of Metastatic Disease

The role of EBRT as part of the armamentarium to control the symptoms of metastatic disease is well established. In patients with distant metastases from thyroid cancer, 42 % have bone involvement, the third highest incidence after breast and

Table 26.2 Glossary of terms used in radiation therapy

Intensity-modulated radiotherapy (IMRT). The intensity of the radiation and the shape of the radiation fields are varied (modulated) so that the radiation is conformed (or tailored) to the target to be treated. The toxicity to normal structures is reduced and therefore a higher radiation dose can potentially to be given to the cancer
Radiosurgery and stereotactic body radiotherapy. This is highly conformed precision radiation. A *single* large fraction of radiation is given
Stereotactic radiosurgery (SRS). SRS usually refers to radiosurgery (a single large fraction of radiation) to the brain (Gamma Knife © is an example of SRS)
Stereotactic body radiosurgery (SBRS). SBRS usually refers to radiosurgery that is administered to parts of the body other than the brain (CyberKnife © and X-Knife © are examples)
Stereotactic body radiotherapy (SBRT). SBRT usually refers to highly conformal radiotherapy given in 3–6 fractions rather than a single fraction

prostate cancer; therefore, EBRT is a valuable tool to help control pain from bone metastases [23]. Single fractions such as 8 Gy or multiple fractions (20 Gy in 5 fractions or 30 Gy in 10 fractions) of radiotherapy are commonly used. However, not all bone metastases are widespread, and because RAI is less effective in controlling bone metastases even if they concentrate RAI (in comparison to lung metastases), an aggressive surgical approach for patients with isolated bone metastases is warranted. This depends on the site of the metastases and the performance status of the patient, as an aggressive surgical approach is not always clinically wise or even possible. We recommend EBRT after RAI to unresectable bone metastases or multiple bone metastases. For solitary metastases, we usually give 50 Gy in 25 fractions or 40 Gy in 15 fractions. Some specific anatomic sites, when involved with small volume of disease, can be considered for hypofractionated high-dose stereotactic body radiotherapy (SBRT, see Table 26.2). All patients with painful bone metastases should be referred for EBRT to aid pain control. Palliative radiation is also valuable to control brain metastases, hemoptysis from lung metastases, and distal lung collapse secondary to bronchial obstruction from mediastinal or hilar lymphadenopathy.

Stereotactic radiotherapy allows for higher doses of radiotherapy to be given safely over a short time period with the aim of long-term control. There are different names and types of stereotactic radiotherapy, but essentially they are similar in that they allow for higher dose per fraction of radiation, usually given with few fractions (most commonly 1–6), with very high precision. They differ in their modes of delivery (see Table 26.2). Figures 26.2, 26.3, and 26.4 give example of stereotactic radiotherapy given for isolated bone metastases, lung metastases, and brain metastases in different patients. There is no high-level evidence that stereotactic radiotherapy is superior to other forms of ablative therapy such as radiofrequency ablation in thyroid cancer; however, its use is less restricted by

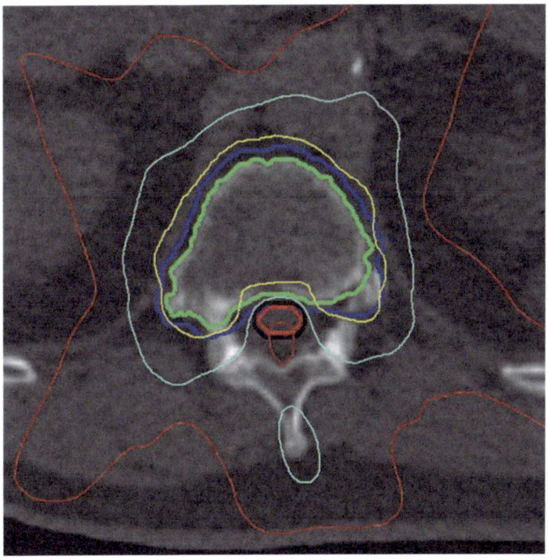

Fig. 26.2 A 61-year-old man has a thyroidectomy for a 5 cm papillary carcinoma with angioinvasion. Post-RAI scan shows uptake in the thyroid bed and in the T12 vertebrae. There is no evidence of any other metastases. He is given stereotactic RT to the vertebral body 24 Gy in 2 fractions. The green line is the clinical target volume (CTV). The *blue line* is the planning target volume (PTV). The *red line* is the spinal cord. The *yellow line* is the 24 Gy isodose line (all the tissue with that volume described by the 24 Gy isodose line received a minimum of 24 Gy). The *light blue line* is the 17 Gy isodose line. The *maroon line* is the 10 Gy isodose line. Note the spinal cord is outside the 17 Gy isodose line and therefore receives less than 17 Gy

consideration of size and certain adjacent structures such as major vessels. The choice of stereotactic radiotherapy or other ablative forms of treatment is often dependent on local availability and expertise. SBRT should be considered in the context of limited or oligometastatic disease where RAI is not felt to be of benefit because of failure to uptake RAI or progression despite RAI avidity. The benefit of local disease control should be balanced against the risk of toxicity from SBRT, and the natural history of metastatic differentiated thyroid cancer being one usually of widespread dissemination. We advocate for a multidisciplinary approach with case review with surgeons, as surgical metastasectomy may also be an option.

For small number of brain metastases, generally less than 5, stereotactic radiation is an alternative to whole brain radiotherapy. SBRT may be an important advantage in patients with differentiated thyroid cancer and brain metastases who may have a more prolonged survival than many other patients with metastases from other sites and therefore spare the long-term side effects of whole brain radiotherapy.

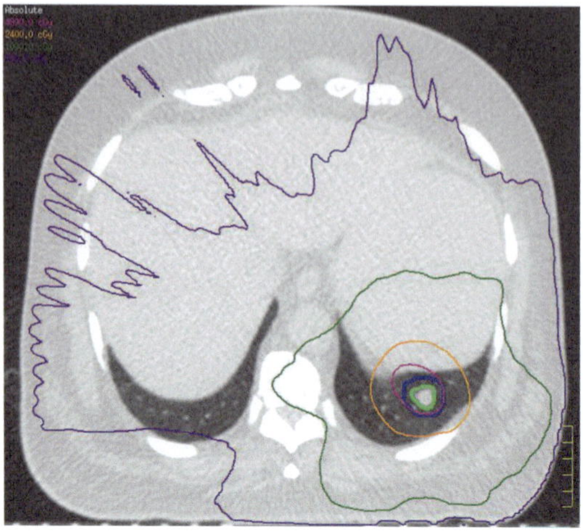

Fig. 26.3 A 73-year-old man with a previous history of thyroid cancer has an episode of cough and chest pain. A CT scan shows two small lung nodules. His suppressed TG is undetectable. A biopsy confirms differentiated thyroid cancer. He receives 5550 MBq of RAI. Post-RAI therapy scan is negative. Two years later a repeat CT scan is unchanged. There are no new lesions. He agrees to stereotactic radiotherapy to the two lung lesions to 48 Gy in 4 fractions. The *green line* is the gross target volume (CTV). The *blue line* is the planning target volume (PTV). The *purple line* is the 48 Gy isodose line (all the tissue with that volume described by the 48 Gy isodose line received a minimum of 48 Gy). The *orange line* is the 24 Gy isodose line. The green line is the 10 Gy isodose line. The *dark purple line* is the 5 Gy isodose line

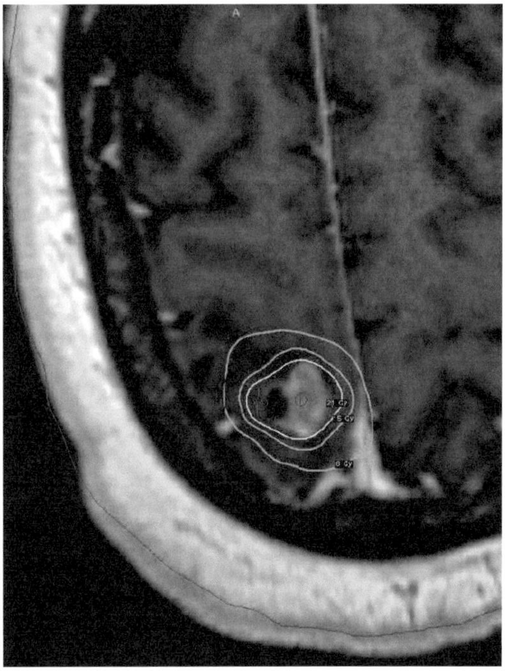

Fig. 26.4 A 51-year-old man presents with a large thyroid mass with extrathyroidal extension. Surgery is performed and the mass is dissected off the carotid sheath. He receives RAI and EBRT. Six years later he has focal motor seizures affecting his left leg. MRI reveals two lesions in his right parietal lobe and left occipital lobe. He is treated with whole brain radiation with radiosurgery boost from Gamma-Knife ©. Four years later he remains free from disease. The *red line* is the gross target volume (CTV). The blue line is the planning target volume (PTV). The *yellow line* is the 21 Gy isodose line (all the tissue with that volume described by the 21 Gy isodose line received a minimum of 21 Gy). The *inner green line* is the 15 Gy isodose line. The *outer green line* is the 8 Gy isodose line

Conclusion

The evidence for the role of EBRT in controlling unresectable differentiated thyroid cancer in the neck has been reviewed; we believe there is sufficient evidence to also confirm its role in reducing the risk of local regional recurrence, but only in carefully selected high-risk patients. The most appropriate radiation volumes and doses are reviewed but. There is a clearly defined role for EBRT in the palliation of symptoms from metastatic disease, and patients with oligometastatic disease can be irradiated but it is yet to be determined if this results in a significant change in the natural history of metastatic differentiated thyroid cancer.

References

1. Edge SB, Byrd DR, Compton CC, Fritz AG, Greene FL, Trotti A. AJCC staging cancer manual. 7th ed. New York: Springer; 2010.
2. Brierley JD, Tsang RW. External-beam radiation therapy in the treatment of differentiated thyroid cancer. Semin Surg Oncol. 1999;16(1):42–9. Epub 1999/01/16.
3. Chow S-M, Law SCK, Mendenhall WM, Au S-K, Chan PTM, Leung T-W, et al. Papillary thyroid carcinoma: prognostic factors and the role of radioiodine and external radiotherapy. Int J Radiat Oncol Biol Phys. 2002;52(3):784–95.
4. Robbins RJ, Wan Q, Grewal RK, Reibke R, Gonen M, Strauss HW, et al. Real-time prognosis for metastatic thyroid carcinoma based on 2-[18F]fluoro-2-deoxy-D-glucose-positron emission tomography scanning. J Clin Endocrinol Metab. 2006;91(2):498–505.
5. Sia MA, Tsang RW, Panzarella T, Brierley JD. Differentiated thyroid cancer with extrathyroidal extension: prognosis and the role of external beam radiotherapy. J Thyroid Res. 2010;2010:183461. Epub 2010/11/05.
6. Azrif M, Slevin NJ, Sykes AJ, Swindell R, Yap BK. Patterns of relapse following radiotherapy for differentiated thyroid cancer: implication for target volume delineation. Radiother Oncol. 2008;89(1):105–13.
7. Schwartz DL, Lobo MJ, Ang KK, Morrison WH, Rosenthal DI, Ahamad A, et al. Postoperative external beam radiotherapy for differentiated thyroid cancer: outcomes and morbidity with conformal treatment. Int J Radiat Oncol Biol Phys. 2009;74(4):1083–91. Epub 2008/12/20.
8. Cooper DS, Doherty GM, Haugen BR, Kloos RT, Lee SL, Mandel SJ, et al. Revised American Thyroid Association management guidelines for patients with thyroid nodules and differentiated thyroid cancer. Thyroid. 2009;19(11):1167–214. Epub 2009/10/29.
9. Haugen BR, Alexander EK, Bible KC, Doherty GM, Mandel SJ, Nikiforov YE, et al. 2015 American Thyroid Association Management Guidelines for adult patients with thyroid nodules and differentiated thyroid cancer: the American Thyroid Association Guidelines task force on thyroid nodules and differentiated thyroid cancer. Thyroid. 2016;26(1):1–133. Epub 2015/10/16.
10. Perros P, Boelaert K, Colley S, Evans C, Evans RM, Gerrard Ba G, et al. Guidelines for the management of thyroid cancer. Clin Endocrinol (Oxf). 2014;81 Suppl 1:1–122. Epub 2014/07/06.
11. Biermann M, Pixberg M, Riemann B, Schuck A, Heinecke A, Schmid KW, et al. Clinical outcomes of adjuvant external-beam radiotherapy for differentiated thyroid cancer - results after 874 patient-years of follow-up in the MSDS-trial. Nuklearmedizin. 2009;48(3):89–98; quiz N15. Epub 2009/03/27.
12. Tubiana M, Haddad E, Schlumberger M, Hill C, Rougier P, Sarrazin D. External radiotherapy in thyroid cancers. Cancer. 1985;55(9 Suppl):2062–71.

13. Farahati J, Reiners C, Stuschke M, Muller SP, Stuben G, Sauerwein W, et al. Differentiated thyroid cancer. Impact of adjuvant external radiotherapy in patients with perithyroidal tumor infiltration (stage pT4). Cancer. 1996;77(1):172–80.
14. Tsang RW, Brierley JD, Simpson WJ, Panzarella T, Gospodarowicz MK, Sutcliffe SB. The effects of surgery, radioiodine and external radiation therapy on the clinical outcome of patients with differentiated thyroid cancer. Cancer. 1998;82:375–88.
15. Chow SM, Yau S, Lee SH, Leung WM, Law SC. Pregnancy outcome after diagnosis of differentiated thyroid carcinoma: no deleterious effect after radioactive iodine treatment. Int J Radiat Oncol Biol Phys. 2004;59(4):992–1000.
16. Kim TH, Yang DS, Jung KY, Kim CY, Choi MS. Value of external irradiation for locally advanced papillary thyroid cancer. Int J Radiat Oncol Biol Phys. 2003;55(4):1006–12.
17. Phlips P, Hanzen C, Andry G, Van Houtte P, Fruuling J. Postoperative irradiation for thyroid cancer. Eur J Surg Oncol. 1993;19(5):399–404.
18. Brierley J, Tsang R, Panzarella T, Bana N. Prognostic factors and the effect of treatment with radioactive iodine and external beam radiation on patients with differentiated thyroid cancer seen at a single institution over 40 years. Clin Endocrinol (Oxf). 2005;63(4):418–27.
19. Keum KC, Suh YG, Koom WS, Cho JH, Shim SJ, Lee CG, et al. The role of postoperative external-beam radiotherapy in the management of patients with papillary thyroid cancer invading the trachea. Int J Radiat Oncol Biol Phys. 2006;65(2):474–80.
20. Sun XS, Sun SR, Guevara N, Marcy PY, Peyrottes I, Lassalle S, et al. Indications of external beam radiation therapy in non-anaplastic thyroid cancer and impact of innovative radiation techniques. Crit Rev Oncol Hematol. 2013;86(1):52–68. Epub 2012/10/24.
21. Padovani RP, Kasamatsu TS, Nakabashi CC, Camacho CP, Andreoni DM, Malouf EZ, et al. One month is sufficient for urinary iodine to return to its baseline value after the use of water-soluble iodinated contrast agents in post-thyroidectomy patients requiring radioiodine therapy. Thyroid. 2012;22(9):926–30. Epub 2012/07/26.
22. Gal TJ, Streeter M, Burris J, Kudrimoti M, Ain KB, Valentino J. Quality of life impact of external beam radiotherapy for advanced thyroid carcinoma. Thyroid. 2013;23(1):64–9. Epub 2012/09/14.
23. Coleman RE. Clinical features of metastatic bone disease and risk of skeletal morbidity. Clin Cancer Res. 2006;12(20 Pt 2):6243s–9. Epub 2006/10/26.

Chapter 27
Systemic Therapy for Advanced Metastatic Thyroid Cancer

Dwight Owen and Manisha H. Shah

Introduction

Differentiated thyroid cancer (DTC) is the most common type of thyroid cancer and includes papillary, follicular, and Hürthle cell histologies [1]. The prognosis for most patients diagnosed with thyroid cancer is excellent, with a 5-year survival rate of 97.9 % with standard treatments including surgery, thyroid-stimulating hormone (TSH) suppression, and radioactive iodine (RAI) [2, 3]. However, for the 10–15 % of patients who develop disease that is resistant to RAI treatment, there have historically been limited treatment options, and median overall survival drops to 2.5–3.5 years [4]. With 62,450 patients estimated to have been diagnosed with thyroid cancer in 2015, the number of patients requiring treatment for advanced disease is expected to continue to increase [3]. Until very recently, the only Food and Drug Administration (FDA)-approved therapy for patients with metastatic, RAI-refractory disease was cytotoxic chemotherapy with doxorubicin. However, this therapy has been associated with low response rates and significant toxicities [5]. Based on a better understanding of the pathogenetics of DTC, including the relevance of BRAF mutations as well as the role of angiogenesis in tumor growth, sorafenib, a multikinase inhibitor (MKI), became the first new agent approved by the FDA in 2013 for treatment of metastatic, RAI-refractory thyroid cancer in over a quarter century. This has led to further investigations with other targeted MKIs, including lenvatinib which joined sorafenib as an FDA-approved agent for advanced DTC in early 2015 (Table 27.1). The American Thyroid Association now recommends consideration of kinase inhibitor therapy for patients with metastatic, progressive RAI-refractory DTC, either with and FDA-approved medication or in the context of a clinical trial [6]. However, an improvement

D. Owen, MD • M.H. Shah, MD (✉)
The Ohio State University Comprehensive Cancer Center, Arthur G. James Cancer Hospital and Richard J. Solove Research Institute,
A438 Starling-Loving Hall, 320 West 10th Avenue, Columbus, OH 43210, USA
e-mail: manisha.shah@osumc.edu

S.A. Roman et al. (eds.), *Management of Thyroid Nodules and Differentiated Thyroid Cancer*, DOI 10.1007/978-3-319-43618-0_27

Table 27.1 Multikinase inhibitors approved for treatment of metastatic radio-iodine refractory differentiated thyroid cancer

	Sorafenib	Lenvatinib
Year approved by Food and Drug Administration	November 2013	February 2015
Trial enrollment period	2009–2011	2011–2012
Pivotal phase III placebo-controlled Trial	DECISION[22]	SELECT[23]
Total of number of patients	417	392
Overall response rate (Partial response + complete response) (%)	12.2 (12.2 + 0)	64.8 (63.2 + 1.5)
Median progression-free survival for patients on active drug (months)	10.8	18.3
Median progression-free survival for patients on placebo (months)	5.8	3.6
Hazard ratio (*p*-value)	0.59 ($p<0.0001$)	0.21 ($p<0.001$)
Median overall survival (months)	Not reported	Not reported
Patients needing dose interruption (%)	82.4 %	66.2 %
Patients needing dose reduction (%)	64.3 %	67.8 %
Patients needing drug withdrawal (%)	18.8 %	14.2 %
Patients on active drug with BRAF mutations (%)	27 %	10 %[a]

[a]BRAF status was known in 123/261 patients on active drug and 59/131 patients on placebo

in overall survival has yet to be demonstrated with these new therapies, and the majority of patients end up discontinuing treatment either due to treatment failure or intolerable toxicities. Having learned the limitations of such MKIs with angiogenic targets, RAS-BRAF-MEK signaling pathway inhibitors are currently being evaluated in clinical trials. A separate treatment modality that is being pursued is the "redifferentiation" of thyroid cancer cells, allowing for the ability to uptake iodine and therefore rendering the tumors susceptible to therapeutic radioiodine. With multiple targeted therapeutic options pending approval, further research is needed to determine the optimal sequence of therapies. Importantly, given the non-curative intent of treatment and the lack of survival advantage, clinicians need further data to help determine the timing of initiating treatment in patients who may not be symptomatic.

In this chapter, we focus on targeted therapies with MKIs that have been developed in the last decade followed by ongoing research with such therapies and close with providing historic data on cytotoxic chemotherapy.

Multikinase Inhibitors Targeting the VEGFR Pathway

Randomized Phase II–III Clinical Trials in DTC

Lenvatinib

Lenvatinib (Lenvima) was approved by the FDA for the treatment of patients with progressive, RAI-refractory DTC in February 2015 and by the European Medicines Agency (EMA) in May 2015. Lenvatinib is an oral, multikinase inhibitor of VEGFR-1,

VEGFR-2, and VEGFR-3, FGFRs 1–4, PDGFR, RET, and KIT [7]. Based on data indicating that activation of the VEGFR signaling network may be associated with the aggressiveness of thyroid carcinoma [8], as well as based on safety and high response rates noted in a single-arm phase II trial of lenvatinib in DTC [9], lenvatinib was studied in a multicenter, international, phase III, randomized, double-blind, placebo-controlled trial (SELECT trial) of 392 patients with progressive, RAI-refractory DTC [10]. Patients were randomized in 2:1 fashion to lenvatinib 24 mg/day in 28-day cycles or a placebo. For the trial, inclusion criteria included iodine-131-refractory disease and radiologic progression per RECIST within 13 months of trial enrollment. Patients who had received at most one prior tyrosine kinase inhibitor (TKI) therapy were allowed on study. The primary endpoint was progression-free survival (PFS). Median PFS was 18.3 months with lenvatinib vs 3.6 months with placebo regardless of BRAF or RAS mutation status (HR 0.21, $p<0.0001$). Lenvatinib-treated patients had significantly higher response rates (65 %) compared to 1.5 % in the placebo arm, including four complete responses (CRs) ($p<0.0001$). The improvement in PFS compared to placebo extended to those patients previously treated with TKI therapy. Median PFS was 18.7 months among patients with no prior TKI therapy compared to 15.1 months among those who had received one prior TKI. Among patients with bone disease at study enrollment, a decrease in progression of existing bone disease was observed in those treated with lenvatinib (24 %) vs placebo (59 %). However, no difference in overall survival was observed, which was attributed to crossover of patients from placebo arm to treatment arm at disease progression. Treatment-related adverse events (AEs) of all grades occurred in 97 % of patients treated with lenvatinib vs 59 % of patients on placebo, and the incidence of grade 3 or higher was 76 % in treatment group. Adverse events included HTN most commonly (70 %) followed by fatigue, asthenia, and diarrhea (all roughly 60 %). Other serious adverse events included arterial and venous thrombotic events, renal failure, hepatic failure, QTc prolongation, posterior reversible encephalopathy syndrome (PRES), and GI fistula. More fatal adverse events occurred during treatment in the lenvatinib group (7.7 %) vs placebo group (4.6 %), and treatment-related deaths occurred in 2.3 %. Discontinuation of treatment occurred in 14 % of treatment arm, with dose interruption in 82 % of patients and dose reduction in 68 % of patients. The median PFS of 18.3 months is significantly longer than that observed in any other randomized trial in this patient population and the PFS in placebo group was significantly shorter than typically observed, possibly because of the specific inclusion of high-risk patients (due to eligibility requirement of evidence of disease progression within 13 months prior to enrollment). Limitations of study included lack of an overall survival benefit (potentially confounded by crossover to lenvatinib in the placebo arm) as well as a lack of data on quality of life of those patients treated with lenvatinib.

Sorafenib

Sorafenib (Nexavar) was the first MKI to be approved by the FDA for metastatic RAI-refractory DTC in November 2013 and by the EMA in April 2014. Sorafenib is a multikinase inhibitor with activity against VEGFR-2–3, PDGFR-β, FLT3, KIT,

Raf-1, BRAF, and RET kinases [11]. The approval was based on the results of the DECISION trial [12], which added further weight to the data from a number of open-label, single-arm phase II clinical trials of sorafenib that demonstrated combined response rates of 21 % and median progression-free survival rates of well over 1 year in a recent meta-analysis [13]. The DECISION trial was a multicenter, international, randomized, double-blinded phase III trial in RAI-refractory DTC patients comparing sorafenib 400 mg twice a day with placebo [12]. Like the SELECT trial [10], the patient population in this study was felt to be especially high risk because of the inclusion criteria of disease progression by RECIST within the 14 months prior to study enrollment. Baseline characteristics of tumor histologies included 57 % papillary, 25 % follicular, and 10 % poorly differentiated. The primary endpoint was progression-free survival. The median PFS was 10.8 months vs 5.8 months for sorafenib compared to placebo (HR 0.59, $p<0.0001$). Consistent with prior studies, no complete responses (CRs) were seen. No statistically significant difference in overall survival rates was observed (HR 0.80, $p=0.14$), which may have been expected due to the high rates of crossover (71 % of patients on placebo crossed to sorafenib at progression). By far the most common adverse events experienced in the sorafenib arm were hand-foot skin reaction (HFSR) (76 %), diarrhea (68 %), alopecia (67 %), and rash (50 %). Hypertension occurred in 40 %. Serious adverse events occurred in 37 % of patient receiving sorafenib (compared to 26 % of patients receiving placebo). In the sorafenib group, secondary malignancies occurred in nine patients, including seven squamous cell carcinomas of the skin and one diagnosis of leukemia. Dose interruptions occurred in 66 % and dose reductions occurred in 64 % of patients receiving sorafenib, while drug discontinuation due to AE occurred in 19 % of patients on sorafenib compared to 4 % receiving placebo. One death in each arm was attributed to study drug. This is consistent with prior studies of sorafenib. In the aforementioned meta-analysis, 72 % of patients were unable to tolerate the initial planned dosage of sorafenib 400 mg twice daily, with 56 % requiring dose reductions due to toxicity. Subset analysis of the DECISION trial seemed to suggest that patients with tumors harboring BRAF mutations had longer PFS than patients with wild-type tumors (median PFS in the sorafenib arm with BRAF mutation 20.5 months vs 8.9 months in BRAF wild-type tumors) [12]. However, BRAF mutation status was not associated with overall prognosis.

Vandetanib

Compared to medullary thyroid carcinoma (MTC), where germline mutations in the RET proto-oncogene occur in nearly all patients with hereditary MTC and 50 % of patients with sporadic MTC, no mutations in RET are observed in DTC, and RET/PTC rearrangements occur in approximately 20 % of tumors of DTC patients [14]. The MKI vandetanib (Caprelsa) targets RET, VEGFR, and EGFR signaling and was shown to significantly prolong PFS compared to placebo in a phase III trial in MTC patients [15]. Results of this phase III trial were the basis for FDA approval of vandetanib in patients with progressive MTC in April 2011. Based on this study, and the work showing disease activity of other tyrosine kinase inhibitors targeting angiogenesis in metastatic DTC, a randomized, double-blinded, placebo-controlled, multicenter phase II study was undertaken in Europe comparing vandetanib to placebo in locally advanced (surgically unresectable) or metastatic DTC [16]. Inclusion criteria included measurable disease by RECIST 1.0, but RAI-refractory disease and progressive disease were not required at study entry. Treatment consisted of vandetanib 300 mg orally daily or placebo. Blinded treatment continued until disease progression or 12 months of stable disease, at which point patients could cross over. The primary endpoint was progression-free survival as determined by RECIST. Vandetanib demonstrated statistically significant improvement in median PFS compared to placebo (11.1 vs 5.9 months, respectively, HR 0.63 two-sided $p=0.017$). There was a trend toward improved PFS in patients with papillary subtype (16.2 vs 5.9 months) that was not statistically significant. Notably, there was no statistical improvement in ORR or OS. The most common AEs of any grade in vandetanib arm were diarrhea (74 %), hypertension (34 %), and acneiform rash (27 %). Grade 3 or higher AEs in the treatment arm were 53 % compared with 19 % in the placebo arm, with the most common attributed to vandetanib being QTC prolongation (24 %) and diarrhea (10 %). Adverse events leading to discontinuation of treatment occurred in 33 % of vandetanib patients and 6 % of placebo patients. Grade 3 or more photosensitivity occurred in 4 % of treatment patients, less than in prior studies, which was attributed to better education about this specific side effect. Based on this, a randomized, double-blind, placebo-controlled, multicenter phase III study has been undertaken (NCT01876784).

Single-Arm Phase II Clinical Trials in DTC

Multiple MKI drugs targeting the VEGFR pathway have been tested in prospective phase II clinical trials in DTC including sorafenib, lenvatinib, and vandetanib as discussed above, but also axitinib, motesanib, pazopanib, and sunitinib in a first-line TKI setting, while cabozantinib has been tested as second- or third-line TKI therapy. Given that sorafenib and lenvatinib were already tested in phase III trials (as listed above), we will not discuss details of phase II trials of these drugs [9, 17–19]. Additionally, while motesanib showed modest activity in DTC, [20] this trial is not discussed here as further drug development was terminated.

Axitinib

Axitinib (Inlyta) is a second-generation selective VEGFR inhibitor that was studied in a multicenter, open-label, phase II trial of 52 patients with metastatic or advanced, RAI-refractory thyroid cancer [21]. Axitinib is approved by FDA for advanced renal cell carcinoma but not for thyroid cancer. Like pazopanib, axitinib does not have significant RET activity. Due to slow accrual, this trial was eventually opened up to other types of thyroid cancer (MTC and anaplastic thyroid cancer), as well as to patients without disease progression within 6 months of study entry and patients without RAI-refractory disease. The starting dose of axitinib was 5 mg orally twice daily, which could be increased incrementally if no adverse events were observed to 7.5 mg twice daily and then to 10 mg twice daily, the target therapeutic dose. The primary endpoint was ORR by RECIST. Unique among other trials, this study included a patient-reported outcome (PRO) as a secondary endpoint. This tool evaluated patients at baseline and on treatment not only for a number of symptoms (i.e., pain, fatigue, distress) but also how those symptoms impacted on their overall quality of life (QOL). The baseline clinical characteristics included 87 % of patients with DTC (54 % papillary and 33 % follicular). A partial response (PR) rate of 33 % in patients with DTC histology was observed, with median PFS of 15.2 months (95 % CI 14.5–21.2) and median OS of 24.3 months (95 % CI 13.8–33.0). All patients experienced at least one AE of any grade, with 79 % experiencing at least one grade 3 event or worse AE, which included diarrhea, hypertension, dyspnea, and lymphopenia. Evaluation of PRO demonstrated that in general, even these toxicities were not associated with deterioration of quality of day-to-day life.

Pazopanib

Pazopanib (Votrient) is a small oral kinase inhibitor of VEGF, PDGF, and c-KIT [22]. Unlike some of the other MKIs already mentioned, pazopanib does not inhibit RET, RET/PTC, or BRAF. Therefore, antitumor activity of pazopanib is hypothesized to be primarily via antiangiogenesis. Pazopanib is approved by FDA for soft tissue sarcoma and renal cell carcinoma but not for thyroid cancer. In an NCI-sponsored, multicenter, open-label phase II trial of 37 patients with RAI-refractory DTC and evidence of progressive disease defined by RECIST within 6 months of trial entry, pazopanib was given at a starting dose of 800 mg daily in continuous 4-week cycles [23]. The primary endpoint was tumor response rate, with a secondary endpoint of decrease in thyroglobulin levels. Although there were no reported complete responses, pazopanib did show disease activity with 49 % of patients achieving PR (73 % of follicular patients, 45 % of Hürthle cell patients, and 33 % of papillary patients). Dose reductions were required in 43 % of patients due to toxicities, and common all-grade AEs reported were hypertension (51 %), diarrhea (73 %), nausea (51 %), fatigue (78 %), and skin/hair hypopigmentation (80 %), which appeared to be reversible upon cessation of pazopanib. There were two patient deaths on trial (one due to myocardial infarction and the other due to bowel obstruction complicating cholecystectomy for cholecystitis) and two serious bleeding events (one grade 4 intracranial bleed and one grade 3 gastrointestinal bleed). The study was not powered to detect this, but pazopanib seemed to have better a response rate in patients with follicular compared to papillary histologies.

Sunitinib

Sunitinib (Sutent) is a MKI with activity against VEGFR-1 and VEGFR-2, PDGFR, c-KIT, FLT3, and RET that has been approved by the FDA for advanced renal cell carcinoma and gastrointestinal stromal tumors [24]. In a phase II study of 35 patients with metastatic, radioiodine-refractory DTC and MTC, sunitinib 37.5 mg orally daily was given on a continuous schedule [25]. This lower dose given continuously, as opposed to intermittent dosing of 50 mg, was evaluated in hopes of avoiding some of the toxicities associated with the intermittent dosing. The study mandated PET-avid lesions for enrollment, in order to accrue patients with aggressive disease [26]. Primary endpoint of this study was overall response rate by RECIST. An interesting exploratory study was whether 1 week of therapy would have significant change on a repeat PET-CT, and whether this would be predictive of response, as has been reported during sunitinib treatment of GIST [27]. Baseline histologic characteristics included 51 % papillary, 11 % follicular, and 14 % Hürthle cell, along with 23 % other subtypes including MTC. Sunitinib was observed to have a partial response of 28 % in DTC patients compared to 50 % in MTC patients. Dose reduction was required in 60 % of patients, and common grade 3 or worse AEs were diarrhea (17 %), neutropenia (34 %), hand-foot syndrome (17 %), and gastrointestinal bleeding (6 %). One treatment-related death occurred secondary to gastrointestinal bleeding. Patients who responded to sunitinib seemed to have a decrease in the SUV of the most PET-avid lesion after one week of treatment, whereas those patients who did not benefit from sunitinib during the trial did not have a decrease in PET avidity. This poses the attractive possibility of using early PET imaging to determine which patients will benefit most from sunitinib therapy.

Cabozantinib as a Second- or Third-Line TKI Therapy

Cabozantinib (Cometriq) is a potent, orally bioavailable receptor multikinase inhibitor of VEGFR-2, MET, and RET and less potently FLT3, KIT, and TEK [28] and is currently approved by the FDA for treatment of metastatic medullary thyroid cancer, where RET is known to play a key role. Cabozantinib was recently evaluated in a multicenter NCI- and International Thyroid Oncology Group (ITOG)-sponsored phase II trial in 25 patients with RAI-refractory DTC who had progressed on prior one or two lines of VEGFR-targeted therapy. Cabozantinib demonstrated activity in this pretreated population with observed partial response rate of 36 %, stable disease rate of 52 %, and progressive disease rate of 4 % [29]. Further study with this agent in DTC is currently underway in additional phase II trials, including in the up-front setting (NCT02041260).

Kinase Inhibitors Targeting the BRAF-MEK Signaling Pathway

"Redifferentiation" Strategy: Selumetinib (MEK Inhibitor) and Dabrafenib (BRAF Inhibitor) to Induce Reuptake of Iodine

Given the disparate 10-year survival rates of patients with radioiodine-sensitive metastatic DTC compared with RAI-refractory disease (60 % vs 10 %) [4], as well as the high potential complete response rates (up to 45 %) seen in metastatic thyroid achieved with radioiodine treatment [30], strategies aimed at regaining radioiodine avidity have been the subject of great interest. Compared with the MKIs targeting the VEGFR pathway described above with low CR rates and relatively prolonged ongoing treatment durations, this strategy aims to offer a shorter treatment duration, potentially allowing for further radioactive iodine treatments with this highly efficacious therapy, delaying the need for the toxicities associated with prolonged systemic treatment. Up until recently, studies aimed at "redifferentiation" of metastatic DTC have demonstrated minimal clinical benefit using lithium [31] and retinoids [32]. The preclinical finding that activation of mitogen-activated protein kinases (MAPK) interferes with tumor cells' ability to synthesize the sodium-iodine symporter [33], and the finding that BRAF and MEK inhibition can lead to recovery of radioiodine uptake in a mouse model of BRAF V600E thyroid cancer [34], generated the hypothesis that inhibition of MAPK kinase may cause tumors to regain their radioiodine sensitivity. This was further supported by clinical observation of decreased thyroid-specific gene expression among BRAF-mutated tumors [35]. This hypothesis was tested by Ho et al. in a single-center phase II study of selumetinib, a MEK 1 and MEK 2 inhibitor, in 24 patients with radioiodine-refractory DTC [35]. Iodine uptake was assessed pre- and posttreatment by means of an iodine-124 PET-CT, which allows for precise measurement of iodine uptake in individual lesions. Those patients who showed a clinically significant increase in uptake after treatment went on to receive therapeutic radioiodine therapy. The primary endpoint was the percent of patients with an increase in iodine uptake in index lesions, with a secondary endpoint being the effect of treatment on measurement of thyroglobulin levels. The study included 24 patients, 20 of which could be evaluated after four did not meet inclusion criteria. Baseline clinical characteristics included a variety of histological subtypes (25 % classical papillary, 40 % tall-variant papillary, and 35 % poorly differentiated carcinoma) and tumor mutational status (45 % BRAF V600E, 25 % NRAS, 15 % RET/PTC, and 15 % wild type). After 4 weeks of treatment with selumetinib 75 mg orally twice daily, 12 out of 20 (60 %) patients had iodine uptake that was new, increased, or both on posttreatment imaging. A total of eight (40 %) patients had significant enough uptake to safely tolerate therapeutic radioiodine, including all patients with NRAS-mutant tumors and one out of nine patients with

BRAF-mutant tumors. Of the eight patients subsequently treated with therapeutic radioiodine, all were observed to have reduction in tumor size. After 6 months of follow-up, five patients achieved partial response, and three achieved stable disease as best response, corresponding with a mean decrease in thyrotropin-suppressed serum thyroglobulin levels of 89 % at 2 months and 80 % at 6 months. Despite being a small study limited in scope, treatment with selumetinib appears to be an attractive option especially because the effect was observed after such a short duration of treatment. Furthermore, no grade 3 or 4 toxicities were reported. Grade 1 and 2 toxicities included fatigue (80 %), maculopapular rash (70 %), and transaminitis (70 %). One patient did go on to develop myelodysplastic syndrome which subsequently progressed to acute leukemia. The increased efficacy in NRAS-mutant tumors observed in this study has also led to interest in other cancers.

A more recent investigation of the strategy of redifferentiation involved ten patients with RAI-refractory BRAF V600E-mutant papillary thyroid cancer [36]. The authors of this study noted the higher rates of selumetinib-induced increase in radioiodine uptake in NRAS-mutant tumors (all five patients) compared with BRAF-mutant tumors (four of nine patients) in the trial by Ho et al. and hypothesized that direct inhibition of BRAF may be more effective than downstream MEK inhibition in these patients. The primary endpoint of the study was the percentage of patients with dabrafenib-induced radioiodine uptake. Unlike the selumetinib study, radioiodine resistance was defined solely as the absence of uptake on a whole-body scan within 14 months of study entry. This trial also utilized standard iodine-131 whole-body scanning as opposed to the more investigational I-124 PET-CT used in the selumetinib trial by Ho et al. Patients in this study were treated with dabrafenib 150 mg orally twice daily for 25 days before recombinant thyrotropin-stimulated iodine-131 whole-body scan. If new sites of radioiodine uptake were observed, patients continued dabrafenib for an additional 17 days and were then treated with therapeutic radioiodine. A total of ten patients were enrolled, and six of ten (60 %) patients developed new uptake while on therapy and were subsequently treated with 5.5GBq iodine-131. Of these patients, two patients had partial responses and four patients had stable disease at 3 months. Six months after therapeutic radioiodine, five of the six treated patients had reduction in the size of target lesions. All patients completed the full course of dabrafenib without dose modification. The most common AEs were new skin lesions or changes (80 %), fatigue (50 %), electrolyte abnormalities (50 %), and palmar-plantar erythrodysesthesia (40 %). There was one new squamous cell carcinoma of the skin, with all of the other AEs being grade 1 or 2. Results of this pilot study generated the hypothesis that BRAF inhibition may lead to redifferentiation of BRAF-mutant PTCs, allowing for additional doses of therapeutic radioiodine, and a larger prospective trial is in development. One interesting area of future research is combined TGF-β inhibition and BRAF/MEK inhibition, given preclinical data suggesting a role for TGF-β in promoting resistance to radioiodine in PTC cell lines [37].

Direct Antitumor Activity

Vemurafenib

Given that sorafenib is a relatively weak inhibitor of BRAF, efforts were undertaken to more potently inhibit BRAF. Vemurafenib (Zelboraf) is a potent small-molecule kinase inhibitor of BRAF V600E shown in preclinical studies to have activity against thyroid cancer cell lines harboring the V600E mutation, where it seems to exert antiproliferation and anti-migratory effects via downstream ERK 1 and 2 [38]. Three patients with metastatic PTC harboring BRAF V600E mutations were treated within a larger phase I study of vemurafenib [39]. One confirmed PR was observed and the other two patients had stable disease as best initial response. All three patients developed cutaneous keratinocytic eruptions including squamous cell carcinoma of the skin in two patients and verruca in the other. Two patients experienced rapid progression of disease including dedifferentiation to squamous cell histology in one and anaplastic transformation in another, highlighting the potential risks of BRAF pathway inhibition. Further evidence of antitumor activity of BRAF inhibitors was provided by a retrospective review of 17 patients with BRAF-mutated DTC treated with vemurafenib which demonstrated a partial response rate of 47 % and stable disease of 53 % [40].

This study was followed by a multicenter, open-label phase II trial of vemurafenib in patients with RAI-refractory PTC positive for BRAF V600E mutation [41]. The trial included 51 patients in two cohorts: those who had no prior systemic therapy with TKI and those who were previously treated (most commonly with sorafenib). In the treatment-naïve population, best overall response rate was 35 % compared to 26 % in the pretreated population. The median PFS in the previously untreated cohort was 15.6 (95 % CI, 11.2-NR) months compared to 6.8 months (95 % CI, 5.38-NR) in the pretreated cohort. Common AEs included rash, fatigue, weight loss, and increased bilirubin. Based on these data, further investigation with this agent is underway, including its use in the neoadjuvant setting (NCT01709292) as well as studying its ability to enhance radioiodine uptake in a pilot study (NCT02145143).

Dabrafenib

Dabrafenib is a RAF kinase inhibitor which most potently inhibits the BRAF V600E mutant kinase compared to other RAF kinases including wild-type BRAF [42]. In a subset analysis of a larger phase I trial, dabrafenib was also shown to have disease activity in 14 patients with BRAF-mutated thyroid carcinomas [43]. In this trial, dabrafenib therapy was associated with partial responses in four patients (29 %) and stable disease in six patients (43 %). Median PFS was 11.3 months. Grade 3 or worse AEs were fatigue, febrile neutropenia, cutaneous squamous cell carcinoma, and abnormal liver function tests. With these results in mind, it is possible that the patients in the above sensitization study had improved outcomes due to the antitumor activity of dabrafenib as opposed to re-sensitization to radioiodine therapy. Finally, the finding that secondary resistance to BRAF inhibitors may be mediated through RAF isoform switching, and that this resistance can be overcome by downstream MEK inhibition [44], has led to study of combination therapy of dabrafenib with MEK inhibition, including an ongoing multicenter phase II trial of dabrafenib with or without trametinib (NCT01723202).

Kinase Inhibitor Targeting mTOR Pathway Single Agent and in Combination

Everolimus

The PI3K-Akt-mTOR pathway has been shown to play an active role in the pathogenesis of thyroid cancer through a variety of mechanisms, including point mutations in PI3K, overexpression of PI3K, activation by RAS, as well as activation by RET/PTC and PPARγ/Pax8 rearrangements [45]. Although point mutations in PI3K are significantly less common in DTC than in anaplastic thyroid cancer [46], gene amplification is present in roughly a quarter of follicular thyroid cancers [47]. Mammalian target of rapamycin (mTOR) is downstream from Akt and regulates cell proliferation and apoptosis as well as cell metabolism and autophagy [48]. Everolimus (Afinitor) is a dual mTORC1 and mTORC2 inhibitor that has shown limited efficacy in an open-label, single-arm phase II trial of 40 patients, including patients with DTC, MTC, and ATC [49]. Confirmed objective response rates of only 5 % were reported, with treatment-related AEs including mucositis (84 %), anorexia (44 %), and transaminase elevation (26 %).

Everolimus and Sorafenib as Combination Therapy

Everolimus in combination with sorafenib was tested in a phase II trial (NCT01141309), with updated results announced at the American Society of Clinical Oncology (ASCO) 2015 meeting [50]. The trial included 28 patients with DTC and 10 patients with MTC. In patients with DTC treated with combination therapy, response rates were impressive: 61 % PR, 36 % SD, and 4 % PD. Grade 4 event reports included hepatic enzyme increase, hyperglycemia, and hypertriglyceridemia. A separate phase II trial also presented at ASCO 2015 evaluating the addition of everolimus to sorafenib at the time of disease progression on sorafenib alone reported low PR rates but a stable disease rate of 55 % [51]. Based on this data, a randomized phase II trial of sorafenib with or without everolimus is currently underway (NCT02143726).

Cytotoxic Chemotherapy for Advanced DTC

In general DTC has been viewed as relatively refractory to standard cytotoxic chemotherapy, since these tumors are typically slow growing and cytotoxic agents exert greater activity against rapidly dividing cells. Chemotherapy is noted to have minimal efficacy for metastatic DTC in National Comprehensive Cancer Network (NCCN) guidelines [2]. Currently the only FDA-approved cytotoxic agent for metastatic thyroid cancer is doxorubicin. Doxorubicin was one of the earliest agents to show promising activity in metastatic differentiated thyroid cancer, when a trial in 1974 including 19 patients with DTC demonstrated partial responses (defined as >50 % reduction in tumor area) in seven (37 %) patients [52]. However, the benefits of therapy were countered by hematologic toxicity and the development of serious cardiomyopathy. A comprehensive review over 20 years later included ten trials of single-agent doxorubicin in patients with metastatic DTC, with response rates ranging from 0 to 100 %, averaging 38.5 % [53]. These trials were limited by a small number of patients involved (range 2–19) and a uniform lack of placebo-controlled cohorts. A more recent study examining single-agent doxorubicin in 22 patients with DTC showed a more modest partial response (PR) rate of 5 % and stable disease (SD) rate of 42 % [5]. Adverse events included hair loss (42 %), nausea (23 %), respiratory infection (13 %), neutropenia (10 %), and pneumonia (7 %). With newer understanding of anthracycline-induced cardiomyopathy and dosing limits, no patients developed treatment-related cardiomyopathy. The data supported the dose of the 60 mg/m^2 every 3 weeks.

In an effort to build on the efficacy of single-agent doxorubicin, trials have attempted to combine it with a variety of other agents, including cisplatin [54, 55], vincristine and bleomycin [56], and interferon-α [57]. These trials showed modest activity at the cost of burdensome toxicities (over three-quarters of patients in the last study experienced grade 3 or 4 neutropenia, and all patients eventually had progressive disease). Other attempts to build a doxorubicin-based combination have been fraught with low accrual numbers [58].

Combination therapies based on regimens not containing doxorubicin have also been studied. The combination of gemcitabine and paclitaxel was evaluated in nine patients with DTC and MTC but showed no partial responses and one (11 %) stable disease [59]. Adverse events included hair loss (100 %), respiratory infections (22 %), peripheral neuropathy (11 %), and neutropenia (11 %). In a phase I trial of the antifolate pemetrexed in combination with paclitaxel, three (20 %) partial responses were observed among 15 DTC patients (out of a larger cohort of 95 patients) [60]. Cytopenias were frequent, with roughly half of all patients (51.7 %) experiencing grade 4 lymphopenia. The combination of gemcitabine and oxaliplatin was evaluated in 14 patients with refractory DTC and was associated with an ORR of 57 %, including 7 % CR, 50 % PR, and 28 % SD [61]. There were no grade 4 toxicities, and the most common grade 3 toxicities were asthenia, neuropathy, neutropenia, and diarrhea.

Conclusion

Great progress in the understanding of the pathogenesis of DTC has led to the approval of two new targeted therapies since 2013, with many more in development. These advances have changed the standard of care for the treatment of metastatic DTC and were only possible because of a better understanding of the RAS/RAF/MAPK and PI3K/Akt pathways, an appreciation for efficacy of antiangiogenic therapies, and the role of "redifferentiation" of thyroid tumors to allow for treatment with radioactive iodine. Building upon this foundation, there has been an explosion of novel therapeutic treatments in patients with RAI-refractory DTC that are now being evaluated in prospective trials (Table 27.2). Researchers across the globe have collaborated in forming an International Thyroid Oncology Group (ITOG) that is

Table 27.2 Selected ongoing clinical trials in differentiated thyroid cancer

Trial Identification	Phase	Title	Setting
NCT01843062	III	A Randomized, Double Blind Study to Compare the Complete Remission Rate Following a 5-Week Course of Selumetinib or Placebo and Single Dose Adjuvant Radioactive Iodine Therapy in Patients With Differentiated Thyroid Cancer	First line for local disease; randomized, double-blind, multicenter
NCT02041260	II	A Phase II Trial of Cabozantinib for the Treatment of RAI-Refractory DTC in the First-line Setting	First line; non-randomized, open-label
NCT02390934	II	Single Arm Phase II Trial Evaluating the Efficacy of Radium 223 in Radioactive Iodine Refractory Bone Metastases From Differentiated Thyroid Cancer	Metastatic, RAI-refractory; single arm, non-randomized, open-label
NCT01788982	II	Nintedanib (BIBF1120) in Thyroid Cancer	Locally advanced or metastatic disease; randomized, double-blind, multicenter
NCT01830504	II	A Multicenter Phase II Pilot Open Label Study to Evaluate the Efficacy and Safety of BKM120 in the Treatment of Patients With Advanced or Metastatic Differentiated Thyroid Cancers	Locally advanced or metastatic; single-arm, nonrandomized, open-label. Class I PI3K inhibitor
NCT01813136	II	A Randomized, Multicenter, Open-label, Phase II Study of the Optimal Scheme of Administration of Pazopanib in Thyroid Carcinoma	RAI-refractory; multicenter, open-label

(continued)

Table 27.2 (continued)

Trial Identification	Phase	Title	Setting
NCT02152995	II	A Phase 2 Study of Trametinib in Combination With RAI for RAS Mutant or RAS/RAF Wild-Type, RAI-Refractory Recurrent and/or Metastatic Thyroid Cancers	RAI-refractory, metastatic; single-arm, open label
NCT02393690	II	Randomized Double-Blind Phase II Study of RAI in Combination With Placebo or Selumetinib for the Treatment of RAI-Avid Recurrent/Metastatic Thyroid Cancers	RAI-refractory; randomized, double-blind, multicenter
NCT02472080	II	Open Labeled Phase II Study Evaluating Efficacy and Safety of Chemotherapy With Gemcitabine – Oxaliplatin Combination for Advanced Refractory Thyroid Cancer Patients	Locally advanced, metastatic, RAI-refractory; single-arm, open label
NCT01270321	II	A 3-Arm Randomized Phase II Trial Evaluating Single Agent and Combined Efficacy of Pasireotide and Everolimus in Adult Patients With Radioiodine-Refractory Differentiated and Medullary Thyroid Cancer	RAI-refractory; randomized, multicenter, open label
NCT01723202	II	A Randomized Phase 2 Study of Single Agent Dabrafenib (BRAFi) vs. Combination Regimen Dabrafenib (BRAFi) and Trametinib (MEKi) in Patients With BRAF Mutated Thyroid Carcinoma	RAI-refractory, BRAF V600 mutation positive; Randomized, open-label
NCT02456701	I	Enhancing RAI Incorporation Into BRAF Mutant, RAI Refractory Thyroid Cancers With the Combination of BRAF Inhibitor Vemurafenib and Anti-ErbB3 Antibody KTN3379: A Pilot Study With a Phase 1 Run-in	RAI-refractory, BRAF V600 mutation positive; single-arm, open-label
NCT02145143	Pilot	Enhancing RAI Incorporation Into BRAF Mutant, RAI-Refractory Thyroid Cancers With the BRAF Inhibitor Vemurafenib: A Pilot Study	RAI-refractory, BRAF V600 mutation positive; single-arm, open-label

Abbreviations: DTC differentiated thyroid cancer, *FTC* follicular thyroid cancer, *HTC* hurthle cell thyroid cancer, *mo* months, *mt* mutant, *MTC* medullary thyroid cancer, *RAI* radioiodine, *pts* patients focusing on rapid discovery to improve therapies by leading many multicenter clinical trials in thyroid cancers.

With extraordinary advances, there remain several challenges. There has yet to be a reported improvement in overall survival in a phase III randomized trial with any of these agents. Further, with multiple MKIs to choose from and more on the way, data is lacking on the precise sequence of treatments that will yield the greatest benefit to patients. As has been pointed out elsewhere [62], patients with thyroid cancer tend to be on MKI therapy longer than patients with other solid tumors such as renal cell carcinoma or hepatocellular carcinoma and therefore have a longer exposure to MKI-related toxicity. Given the lack of a survival advantage to date, it is imperative that quality of life data be included in future prospective trials, to ensure that the therapies being offered to patients are not negatively impacting their lives in a meaningful way. Further research is needed to determine the optimal doses and dosing schedules for MKIs in DTC, to optimize antineoplastic activity and minimize toxicities. Finally, the decision of when to start treatment and when to switch treatments is quite complex in thyroid cancer, considering that many patients may not be symptomatic from their disease. Therefore, treatment of their disease may not necessarily improve their symptoms and may only add toxicities related to therapy. Better predictive and prognostic biomarkers would be helpful to decide on what treatments would be most effective for individual patients.

Finally, advances in understanding pathogenesis and treatment of DTC in the last decade have fueled the field, and vital collaborations across the government agencies, industry, and academic centers are ongoing to conduct research with a goal to improve lives of patients with thyroid cancer.

References

1. Sherman SI. Thyroid carcinoma. Lancet. 2003;361(9356):501–11.
2. Tuttle RM, Haddad RI, Ball DW, Byrd D, Dickson P, Duh QY, et al. Thyroid carcinoma, version 2.2014. J Natl Compr Canc Netw. 2014;12(12):1671–80; quiz 80.
3. Siegel RL, Miller KD, Jemal A. Cancer statistics, 2015. CA Cancer J Clin. 2015;65(1):5–29.
4. Durante C, Haddy N, Baudin E, Leboulleux S, Hartl D, Travagli JP, et al. Long-term outcome of 444 patients with distant metastases from papillary and follicular thyroid carcinoma: benefits and limits of radioiodine therapy. J Clin Endocrinol Metab. 2006;91(8):2892–9.
5. Matuszczyk A, Petersenn S, Bockisch A, Gorges R, Sheu SY, Veit P, et al. Chemotherapy with doxorubicin in progressive medullary and thyroid carcinoma of the follicular epithelium. Horm Metab Res. 2008;40(3):210–3.
6. Haugen BRM, Alexander EK, Bible KC, Doherty G, Mandel SJ, Nikiforov YE, et al. American Thyroid Association management guidelines for adult patients with thyroid nodules and differentiated thyroid cancer. Thyroid. 2015;26(1):1–133.
7. Matsui J, Yamamoto Y, Funahashi Y, Tsuruoka A, Watanabe T, Wakabayashi T, et al. E7080, a novel inhibitor that targets multiple kinases, has potent antitumor activities against stem cell

factor producing human small cell lung cancer H146, based on angiogenesis inhibition. Int J Cancer. 2008;122(3):664–71.
8. Salajegheh A, Smith RA, Kasem K, Gopalan V, Nassiri MR, William R, et al. Single nucleotide polymorphisms and mRNA expression of VEGF-A in papillary thyroid carcinoma: potential markers for aggressive phenotypes. Eur J Surg Oncol J Eur Soc Surg Oncol Br Assoc Surg Oncol. 2011;37(1):93–9.
9. Cabanillas ME, Schlumberger M, Jarzab B, Martins RG, Pacini F, Robinson B, et al. A phase 2 trial of lenvatinib (E7080) in advanced, progressive, radioiodine-refractory, differentiated thyroid cancer: A clinical outcomes and biomarker assessment. Cancer. 2015;121(16):2749–56.
10. Schlumberger M, Tahara M, Wirth LJ, Robinson B, Brose MS, Elisei R, et al. Lenvatinib versus placebo in radioiodine-refractory thyroid cancer. N Engl J Med. 2015;372(7):621–30.
11. Wilhelm SM, Carter C, Tang L, Wilkie D, McNabola A, Rong H, et al. BAY 43–9006 exhibits broad spectrum oral antitumor activity and targets the RAF/MEK/ERK pathway and receptor tyrosine kinases involved in tumor progression and angiogenesis. Cancer Res. 2004;64(19):7099–109.
12. Brose MS, Nutting CM, Jarzab B, Elisei R, Siena S, Bastholt L, et al. Sorafenib in radioactive iodine-refractory, locally advanced or metastatic differentiated thyroid cancer: a randomised, double-blind, phase 3 trial. Lancet. 2014;384(9940):319–28.
13. Thomas L, Lai SY, Dong W, Feng L, Dadu R, Regone RM, et al. Sorafenib in metastatic thyroid cancer: a systematic review. Oncologist. 2014;19(3):251–8.
14. Nikiforov YE. RET/PTC rearrangement in thyroid tumors. Endocr Pathol. 2002;13(1):3–16.
15. Wells Jr SA, Robinson BG, Gagel RF, Dralle H, Fagin JA, Santoro M, et al. Vandetanib in patients with locally advanced or metastatic medullary thyroid cancer: a randomized, double-blind phase III trial. J Clin Oncol. 2012;30(2):134–41.
16. Leboulleux S, Bastholt L, Krause T, de la Fouchardiere C, Tennvall J, Awada A, et al. Vandetanib in locally advanced or metastatic differentiated thyroid cancer: a randomised, double-blind, phase 2 trial. Lancet Oncol. 2012;13(9):897–905.
17. Gupta-Abramson V, Troxel AB, Nellore A, Puttaswamy K, Redlinger M, Ransone K, et al. Phase II trial of sorafenib in advanced thyroid cancer. J Clin Oncol. 2008;26(29):4714–9.
18. Haraldsdottir S, Shah MH. New era for treatment in differentiated thyroid cancer. Lancet. 2014;384(9940):286–8.
19. Krajewska J, Handkiewicz-Junak D, Jarzab B. Sorafenib for the treatment of thyroid cancer: an updated review. Expert Opin Pharmacother. 2015;16(4):573–83.
20. Sherman SI, Wirth LJ, Droz J-P, Hofmann M, Bastholt L, Martins RG, et al. Motesanib diphosphate in progressive differentiated thyroid cancer. N Engl J Med. 2008;359(1):31–42.
21. Locati LD, Licitra L, Agate L, Ou SH, Boucher A, Jarzab B, et al. Treatment of advanced thyroid cancer with axitinib: phase 2 study with pharmacokinetic/pharmacodynamic and quality-of-life assessments. Cancer. 2014;120(17):2694–703.
22. Kumar R, Knick VB, Rudolph SK, Johnson JH, Crosby RM, Crouthamel MC, et al. Pharmacokinetic-pharmacodynamic correlation from mouse to human with pazopanib, a multikinase angiogenesis inhibitor with potent antitumor and antiangiogenic activity. Mol Cancer Ther. 2007;6(7):2012–21.
23. Bible KC, Suman VJ, Molina JR, Smallridge RC, Maples WJ, Menefee ME, et al. Efficacy of pazopanib in progressive, radioiodine-refractory, metastatic differentiated thyroid cancers: results of a phase 2 consortium study. Lancet Oncol. 2010;11(10):962–72.
24. Chow LQ, Eckhardt SG. Sunitinib: from rational design to clinical efficacy. J Clin Oncol. 2007;25(7):884–96.
25. Carr LL, Mankoff DA, Goulart BH, Eaton KD, Capell PT, Kell EM, et al. Phase II study of daily sunitinib in FDG-PET-positive, iodine-refractory differentiated thyroid cancer and metastatic medullary carcinoma of the thyroid with functional imaging correlation. Clin Cancer Res. 2010;16(21):5260–8.
26. Robbins RJ, Wan Q, Grewal RK, Reibke R, Gonen M, Strauss HW, et al. Real-time prognosis for metastatic thyroid carcinoma based on 2-[18F]fluoro-2-deoxy-D-glucose-positron emission tomography scanning. J Clin Endocrinol Metab. 2006;91(2):498–505.

27. Prior JO, Montemurro M, Orcurto MV, Michielin O, Luthi F, Benhattar J, et al. Early prediction of response to sunitinib after imatinib failure by 18F-fluorodeoxyglucose positron emission tomography in patients with gastrointestinal stromal tumor. J Clin Oncol. 2009;27(3):439–45.
28. Yakes FM, Chen J, Tan J, Yamaguchi K, Shi Y, Yu P, et al. Cabozantinib (XL184), a novel MET and VEGFR2 inhibitor, simultaneously suppresses metastasis, angiogenesis, and tumor growth. Mol Cancer Ther. 2011;10(12):2298–308.
29. Shah MHDJ, Menefee ME, et al. Cabozantinib in patients with radioiodine-refractory differentiated thyroid cancer who progressed on prior VEGFR-targeted therapy: results of NCI- and ITOG-sponsored multicenter phase II clinical trial. Presented at 15th International Thyroid Congress, Lake Buena Vista; 2015.
30. Schlumberger M, Challeton C, De Vathaire F, Travagli JP, Gardet P, Lumbroso JD, et al. Radioactive iodine treatment and external radiotherapy for lung and bone metastases from thyroid carcinoma. J Nucl Med Off Publ Soc Nucl Med. 1996;37(4):598–605.
31. Liu YY, van der Pluijm G, Karperien M, Stokkel MP, Pereira AM, Morreau J, et al. Lithium as adjuvant to radioiodine therapy in differentiated thyroid carcinoma: clinical and in vitro studies. Clin Endocrinol (Oxf). 2006;64(6):617–24.
32. Handkiewicz-Junak D, Roskosz J, Hasse-Lazar K, Szpak-Ulczok S, Puch Z, Kukulska A, et al. 13-cis-retinoic acid re-differentiation therapy and recombinant human thyrotropin-aided radioiodine treatment of non-Functional metastatic thyroid cancer: a single-center, 53-patient phase 2 study. Thyroid Res. 2009;2(1):8.
33. Knauf JA, Kuroda H, Basu S, Fagin JA. RET/PTC-induced dedifferentiation of thyroid cells is mediated through Y1062 signaling through SHC-RAS-MAP kinase. Oncogene. 2003;22(28):4406–12.
34. Wheler J, Yelensky R, Falchook G, Kim KB, Hwu P, Tsimberidou AM, et al. Next generation sequencing of exceptional responders with BRAF-mutant melanoma: implications for sensitivity and resistance. BMC Cancer. 2015;15:61.
35. Durante C, Puxeddu E, Ferretti E, Morisi R, Moretti S, Bruno R, et al. BRAF mutations in papillary thyroid carcinomas inhibit genes involved in iodine metabolism. J Clin Endocrinol Metab. 2007;92(7):2840–3.
36. Rothenberg SM, McFadden DG, Palmer EL, Daniels GH, Wirth LJ. Redifferentiation of iodine-refractory BRAF V600E-mutant metastatic papillary thyroid cancer with dabrafenib. Clin Cancer Res. 2015;21(5):1028–35.
37. Cabanillas ME, Patel A, Danysh BP, Dadu R, Kopetz S, Falchook G. BRAF inhibitors: experience in thyroid cancer and general review of toxicity. Horm Cancer. 2015;6(1):21–36.
38. Nucera C, Nehs MA, Nagarkatti SS, Sadow PM, Mekel M, Fischer AH, et al. Targeting BRAFV600E with PLX4720 displays potent antimigratory and anti-invasive activity in preclinical models of human thyroid cancer. Oncologist. 2011;16(3):296–309.
39. Kim KB, Cabanillas ME, Lazar AJ, Williams MD, Sanders DL, Ilagan JL, et al. Clinical responses to vemurafenib in patients with metastatic papillary thyroid cancer harboring BRAF(V600E) mutation. Thyroid. 2013;23(10):1277–83.
40. Dadu R, Shah K, Busaidy NL, Waguespack SG, Habra MA, Ying AK, et al. Efficacy and tolerability of vemurafenib in patients with BRAFV600E -positive papillary thyroid cancer: M.D. Anderson Cancer Center Off Label Experience. J Clin Endocrinol Metab. 2015;100(1):E77–81.
41. Brose MSCM, Cohen EEW, et al. An open-label, multi-center phase 2 study of the BRAF inhibitor vemurafenib in patients with metastatic or unresectable papillary thryoid cancer (PTC) positive for the BRAF V600E mutation. Eur J Cancer. 2013;49(3):S7–19.
42. Gibney GT, Zager JS. Clinical development of dabrafenib in BRAF mutant melanoma and other malignancies. Expert Opin Drug Metab Toxicol. 2013;9(7):893–9.
43. Falchook GS, Millward M, Hong D, Naing A, Piha-Paul S, Waguespack SG, et al. BRAF inhibitor dabrafenib in patients with metastatic BRAF-mutant thyroid cancer. Thyroid. 2015;25(1):71–7.
44. Villanueva J, Vultur A, Lee JT, Somasundaram R, Fukunaga-Kalabis M, Cipolla AK, et al. Acquired resistance to BRAF inhibitors mediated by a RAF kinase switch in melanoma can be overcome by cotargeting MEK and IGF-1R/PI3K. Cancer Cell. 2010;18(6):683–95.

45. Petrulea MS, Plantinga TS, Smit JW, Georgescu CE, Netea-Maier RT. PI3K/Akt/mTOR: a promising therapeutic target for non-medullary thyroid carcinoma. Cancer Treat Rev. 2015;41(8):707–13.
46. Wang Y, Hou P, Yu H, Wang W, Ji M, Zhao S, et al. High prevalence and mutual exclusivity of genetic alterations in the phosphatidylinositol-3-kinase/akt pathway in thyroid tumors. J Clin Endocrinol Metab. 2007;92(6):2387–90.
47. Wu G, Mambo E, Guo Z, Hu S, Huang X, Gollin SM, et al. Uncommon mutation, but common amplifications, of the PIK3CA gene in thyroid tumors. J Clin Endocrinol Metab. 2005;90(8):4688–93.
48. Wullschleger S, Loewith R, Hall MN. TOR signaling in growth and metabolism. Cell. 2006;124(3):471–84.
49. Lim SM, Chang H, Yoon MJ, Hong YK, Kim H, Chung WY, et al. A multicenter, phase II trial of everolimus in locally advanced or metastatic thyroid cancer of all histologic subtypes. Ann Oncol. 2013;24(12):3089–94.
50. Sherman EJHA, Fury MG et al. Combination of everolimus and sorafenib in the treatment of thyroid cancer: update on phase II study. J Clin Oncol. 2015;33(Suppl): (abstr 6069).
51. Brose MSTA, Yarchoan M, et al. A phase II study of everolimus (E) and sorafenib (S) in patients (PTS) with metastatic differentiated thyroid cancer who have progressed on sorafenib alone. J Clin Oncol. 2015;33(Suppl): (abstr 6072).
52. Gottlieb JA, Hill Jr CS. Chemotherapy of thyroid cancer with adriamycin. Experience with 30 patients. N Engl J Med. 1974;290(4):193–7.
53. Haugen BR. Management of the patient with progressive radioiodine non-responsive disease. Semin Surg Oncol. 1999;16(1):34–41.
54. Shimaoka K, Schoenfeld DA, DeWys WD, Creech RH, DeConti R. A randomized trial of doxorubicin versus doxorubicin plus cisplatin in patients with advanced thyroid carcinoma. Cancer. 1985;56(9):2155–60.
55. Williams SD, Birch R, Einhorn LH. Phase II evaluation of doxorubicin plus cisplatin in advanced thyroid cancer: a Southeastern Cancer Study Group Trial. Cancer Treat Rep. 1986;70(3):405–7.
56. Hoskin PJ, Harmer C. Chemotherapy for thyroid cancer. Radiother Oncol. 1987;10(3):187–94.
57. Argiris A, Agarwala SS, Karamouzis MV, Burmeister LA, Carty SE. A phase II trial of doxorubicin and interferon alpha 2b in advanced, non-medullary thyroid cancer. Invest New Drugs. 2008;26(2):183–8.
58. Sherman SI. Cytotoxic chemotherapy for differentiated thyroid carcinoma. Clin Oncol (R Coll Radiol). 2010;22(6):464–8.
59. Matuszczyk A, Petersenn S, Voigt W, Kegel T, Dralle H, Schmoll HJ, et al. Chemotherapy with paclitaxel and gemcitabine in progressive medullary and thyroid carcinoma of the follicular epithelium. Horm Metab Res. 2010;42(1):61–4.
60. Hanauske AR, Dumez H, Piccart M, Yilmaz E, Graefe T, Gil T, et al. Pemetrexed combined with paclitaxel: a dose-finding study evaluating three schedules in solid tumors. Invest New Drugs. 2009;27(4):356–65.
61. Spano JP, Vano Y, Vignot S, De La Motte Rouge T, Hassani L, Mouawad R, et al. GEMOX regimen in the treatment of metastatic differentiated refractory thyroid carcinoma. Med Oncol. 2012;29(3):1421–8.
62. Cohen AB, Brose MS. Second-line treatment for advanced thyroid cancer: an indication in need of randomized clinical trials. J Clin Endocrinol Metab. 2014;99(6):1995–7.

Index

S.A. Roman et al. (eds.), *Management of Thyroid Nodules and Differentiated Thyroid Cancer*, DOI 10.1007/978-3-319-43618-0